Voices of
Integrative Medicine
Conversations and Encounters

Voices of
Integrative Medicine
Conversations and Encounters

BONNIE J. HORRIGAN

InnoVision Communications
Encinitas, California

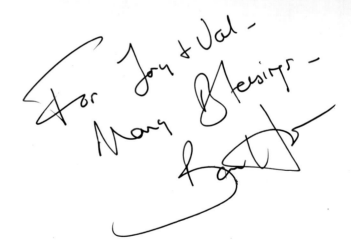

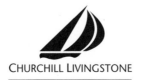

CHURCHILL LIVINGSTONE

An Imprint of Elsevier Science

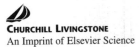
CHURCHILL LIVINGSTONE
An Imprint of Elsevier Science

11830 Westline Industrial Drive
St. Louis, Missouri 63146

NOTICE

Complementary and alternative medicine is an ever-changing field. Standard safety precautions must be followed, but as new research and clinical experience broaden our knowledge, changes in treatment and drug therapy may become necessary or appropriate. Readers are advised to check the most current product information provided by the manufacturer of each drug to be administered to verify the recommended dose, the method and duration of administration, and contraindications. It is the responsibility of the licensed prescriber, relying on experience and knowledge of the patient, to determine dosages and the best treatment for each individual patient. Neither the publisher nor the author assumes any liability for any injury and/or damage to persons or property arising from this publication.

International Standard Book Number 0-443-07278-7

Acquisitions Editor: Linda Duncan
Executive Editor: Inta Ozols
Developmental Editor: Melissa Kuster Deutsch
Publishing Services Manager: Linda McKinley
Project Manager: Ellen Forest Kunkelmann
Designer: Julia Dummitt
Cover Design: MW Design

Printed in the United States of America

Last digit is the print number: 9   8   7   6   5   4   3   2   1

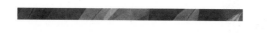

This book is dedicated to Larry Dossey, MD, whom I have had the great pleasure of working with for the past 10 years. When science creates darkness and refuses to see, Larry is a star in the night.

Many thanks to Mike Muscat and Bryna Block, both of whom worked with me on the interviews at the journal offices—it is because of them that everything is spelled correctly. Thanks also to Inta Ozols and Melissa Kuster Deutsch at Elsevier Science for sharing the vision, and thanks to my husband David, who stands besides me in the quest for truth and grace.

FOREWORD

Voices of Integrative Medicine could turn out to be one of the most significant books you will ever read. It might even save your life.

But before reading further, pause for a moment and ask yourself: If you were sick, what would it take for you to get well?

If you pay attention to conventional wisdom, you might conclude that your recovery is a matter of taking the right medication or undergoing the appropriate surgical procedure. If you have a *really* serious problem, you may decide you need a bone marrow transplant, irradiation, chemotherapy, or some other dramatic intervention. But wait...

Throughout human history, healers of every culture have recognized an essential factor in getting well that we have largely overlooked in our modern, high-tech approaches. The missing element is the compassion and caring that take place between a healer and a patient. Nothing fancy here, merely a genuine coming together between two individuals.

Too simple to make a difference? If you think so, consider what happens when your physician tries to arrive at a diagnosis of your problem. *Diagnosis* comes from words meaning "a knowing that exists through or between two people." To know what's wrong, your doctor has to engage you, enter you, in some sense *become* you. If she doesn't, she is likely to remain in the dark and you are likely to remain ill.

We often dismiss compassion, caring, and love as hopelessly old-fashioned. But that's because we have been too dazzled by all the heady talk these days about stem cells, gene chips, and DNA manipulation to focus on what healing actually involves.

To get a picture of what getting well is about, consider an event in the life of Sir William Osler (1849-1919). Osler was the most influential physician of his time and is considered the father of Western scientific medicine. After revolutionizing how medicine was taught and practiced in the United States and Canada, at the peak of his fame in 1905, he was lured to England where he became the Regius professor of medicine at Oxford. One day he went to graduation ceremonies at Oxford wearing his regal academic robes. On the way he stopped by the home of his friend and colleague, Ernest Mallam. One of Mallam's young sons was sick with whooping cough and was dying. He would not eat or respond to the ministrations of his parents, physician, or nurse. Osler greatly loved children and had a special way with them. He adored playing with them, and children would invariably admit him into their world. When Osler appeared in his majestic ceremonial robes, the little boy was captivated. Never before had he seen such a thing!

After a brief examination, Osler sat down. He selected a peach from a bowl of fruit on a bedside table, slowly peeled, cut and sugared it, and fed it bit by bit to the enthralled lad. Although Osler felt recovery unlikely, he returned for the next 40 days, each time dressed in his great robes, and personally fed the young child nourishment. Within a few days the tide had turned, and the little boy's recovery was assured.[1]

Osler knew the young boy's illness was a killer. He had no antibiotics or heroic measures at his disposal in those days. But Osler was a healer. He was able to empathize with the boy, to enter his experience, to *become* him and therefore know what would enchant and inspire him to cling to life. Osler saved a life because he cared, and because he possessed the skill to make his caring count.

[1]Golden RL: William Osler at 150. An overview of a life, JAMA Dec 15; 282(23):2252-8, 1999.

As you read about the nature of healing in *Voices of Integrative Medicine*, you will discover that this book contains a paradox. In many respects the "new" medicine is not new at all but is exceedingly ancient because it is concerned with factors long known to promote healing—the role of consciousness, the innate capacity of the body for self-repair, the power of compassion and love. But these issues are new to us because we let them slip away and are in the process of reclaiming them. The voices in these pages are not merely resurrecting earlier traditions, however; they are building on them and crafting a form of medicine that works better and feels better than that now in place.

What will the new medicine look like? It will be an integration of science and psyche, head and heart, body and soul. It will honor an individual's spirit and the beliefs and meanings that are important in his or her personal life.

In their book *Remarkable Recovery*,[2] authors Caryle Hirshberg and Marc Ian Barasch investigated nearly four dozen patients who recovered from cancers that should have been fatal. They asked them their personal opinions about why they recovered, which, oddly enough, are never reported when cases of this sort are published in scholarly medical journals. They found that the leading factor to which patients attributed their cure was prayer (68% of cases). Other factors were meditation (64%), exercise (64%), guided imagery (59%), walking (52%), music/singing (50%), and stress reduction (50%). When they inquired what psychospiritual factors the patients felt were important in their recovery, the ones most often mentioned were belief in a positive outcome (75%), a fighting spirit (71%), acceptance of disease (71%), and seeing disease as a challenge (71%). Seventy-five percent reported artistic pursuits at which they were somewhat proficient, and 68% described experiencing feelings they could not rationally explain but which seemed important. In other words, even in the midst of life-threatening illness, these patients were able to find *hope* and *meaning*, which took a variety of forms. Yet there was no specific formula for recovery that applied to everyone. People's meanings were highly individual and often different. For example, almost equal numbers of patients responded with calm acceptance of their disease as with a fighting spirit. If there was a common thread, it was hope—the rekindling of which healers such as Osler have always excelled. When hope and individual meanings are combined with the blessings of modern medicine, the result is a significant advance beyond high-tech medicine alone, which too often disempowers patients by ignoring these factors.

The new medicine is not pollyannish, however. It recognizes the harsh reality of disease and the fact that we shall all die. But for reasons you will read about, the new medicine also honors the concept that consciousness is not limited to the physical body but extends beyond it—that consciousness is infinite or nonlocal in space and time, therefore eternal and immortal. This is the most significant way in which the new medicine differs from conventional approaches, and why it is *always* possible for sick and dying individuals to find hope and meaning.

Hand on to your hat. The ideas that follow will challenge many of the assumptions you make about the nature of health and illness, and your own nature as well. But there are no preachy exhortations in these pages, just gentle invitations to consider new views. Almost all these visionaries are highly trained professionals who work within science and who honor its traditions. They are not asking you to reject modern medicine but to expand it.

It has been my honor to work with Bonnie J. Horrigan at *Alternative Therapies in Health and Medicine* since the journal's inception in 1995. In the field of complementary and alternative medicine, this journal has set a high standard of excellence and has become a beacon for those

---

[2]Hirshberg C, Barasch MI: *Remarkable Recovery*, New York, NY, 1995, Riverhead, 332-333.

navigating the difficult waters of change. Bonnie's vision is responsible for the journal's birth, growth, and maturation. I know of no one in medical publishing with her level of integrity. She interviewed all the visionaries who follow. Bonnie has a great gift for making an interview feel comfortable, and her presence permeates every paragraph in this book.

It's no secret that people are currently unhappy with our healthcare system. They often ask impatiently, "Will medicine ever change?" The question is not *whether* but *when*, for medicine has always changed; it remains one of the most dynamic institutions in our society.

When will medicine change? The answer is *now*, as you are about to see.

Larry Dossey, MD
Executive Editor,
Alternative Therapies in Health and Medicine

CONTENTS

Part 8: **Conversations About Medical Education**

Part 9: **Conversations About Healing With Hands**

Part 10: **Conversations About Indigenous Medicine**

Part 11: **Conversations About Cross-Cultural Medicine**

Part 12: **Conversations About Medicine as a Spiritual Path**

Voices of
Integrative Medicine
Conversations and Encounters

BONNIE J. HORRIGAN

Publisher, Alternative Therapies in Health and Medicine

Thanks to many people, the way our culture views health and the fundamental way we think about the world and our relationship to it is changing. The mechanistic, existential view in which you and I do not really matter is being replaced by the age-old idea that we are a vital part of life's equation and that true health involves our bodies, our minds, *and* our spirits. And as we reintegrate this knowledge into our psyche, we are beginning to understand *and experience* that the universe is not inanimate. The circle has come full swing. The ancient religions told us that our individual consciousness had an affect on the reality we experienced and now modern medical science is telling us the same. The ancient peoples knew that plants were medicine, and today we are once again recognizing the true value of nature's bounty. The concept of a "good death," known to many of our ancestors, is re-emerging as something that you and I might actually attain.

This book, *Voices of Integrative Medicine,* offers a rich collection of perspectives about the new medical paradigm that is emerging. Forty-five of our nation's brightest minds speak within these pages. The conversations are about the diverse systems of medicine that numerous societies have created throughout time and across cultures. But they are also about the deep, fundamental essence of the universe and what it means to be a human being living out one's personal destiny in a collective world.

In 1995, I was privileged to be part of a team of people who launched what was, at the time, a radical new medical journal titled *Alternative Therapies in Health and Medicine.* Our purpose was to explore the effectiveness of alternative, complementary, and cross-cultural medicines by publishing the current research in these areas, which was something other medical journals were disinclined to do at that point. We wanted to assist in the integration of *proven* alternative practices with those of conventional medicine so that physicians, nurses, and other healthcare providers would know that choices—ones perhaps more humane, less invasive, and with less side effects—did exist. And we wanted healthcare providers to recover the sacred nature of their profession.

As publisher of the journal, part of my job was to interview the leading authorities from such fields as Chinese medicine, shamanism, osteopathy, homeopathy, herbology, Ayurveda, Native American medicine, and the touch therapies. Because most of the journal was devoted to research and clinical studies, the purpose of the interviews was to expose readers to the ancient wisdom, colorful cultural traditions, thoughtful philosophies and cosmologies, and personal experiences and intuitions on which many of the alternatives were based.

I was thrilled to have such a responsibility because I suspected that interviewing people such as Dean Ornish, Andrew Weil, Rachel Naomi Remen, and Larry Dossey would be an incredibly interesting and educational experience. Eight years later, I can confirm this to be true. During the course of our conversations, the people I interviewed imparted an immense amount of knowledge about health and healing, about themselves as people and practitioners, and about the ways in which the world is ordered. Half of the time, I was on firm intellectual ground—I knew of what they were speaking—but during the other half, they led me down new paths of thought into realities I'd never visited before. Those moments are some of my fondest memories.

Read individually, the interviews contain a vast amount of information. For instance, I learned that there is an ancient text on Chinese medicine that outlines the three levels of healing needed for true health to be obtained. In the first level, the physician addresses the person's physical complaints. The second level directs the physician to understand the person's nature. And the third level is about assisting the person in fulfilling his or her destiny. I learned that many women between the ages of 25 and 50 have nutrient deficiencies of vitamin B_6, folate, B_{12}, magnesium, and zinc, any and all of which could cause a hormonal imbalance leading to depression. I learned that a tribe in the Amazon shared their dreams each morning as a way of decision-making about the tribe's future. I learned about the ancient Tibetan practice of meditating in front of a copper wall to enhance lucidity. I learned that research has shown the body system most sensitive to therapeutic touch is the autonomic nervous system. And I learned that Japanese women have one seventh the incidence of breast cancer that American women do, and that Asian men have one thirtieth the incidence of fatal prostate cancer compared with American men—two alarming facts that many believe have to do with our diet and environment.

So there is much knowledge in this book. But when the interviews are read as a *collection*, something emerges that is beyond data, beyond measure. The ancient shamanic traditions of soul retrieval, to the indigenous botanical medicines of the rainforests, to the Tibetan rituals for the care of the dying, to the use of hands to heal, to the recent clinical studies on prayer, to the detoxification rituals of Ayurveda, and to the latest scientific research on brain chemistry and how that relates to consciousness and love—rarely are these different views presented in one place and at one time. When they are, however, what becomes evident are the "Principles of Pot."

Now, I do not mean marijuana, so allow me to elucidate. Even though most medical systems are quite different in appearance and practice, if one asks of a tradition why people get sick or well, one often gets, essentially, a similar answer. These types of core principles can be likened to the reason a pot is a pot. The pot may change color, size, or shape; the method by which the pot is made or the materials from which it is fashioned may vary; its purpose may differ in that it could be a flower pot or a cooking pot or a piece of art; it may be made to hold water or dirt or grease or a plant—all these things may change. But the "Principles of Pot"—the essence of what a pot is and why it is able to hold something—remain the same.

In talking with the leaders in this field, I discovered that some of the principles at work in mind-body medicine from the 1980s and 1990s are similar to principles at work in shamanic healing ceremonies practiced 2500 years ago. It became clear that one of the great healing aspects of homeopathy is also one of the greatest healing aspects of therapeutic touch. Both Chinese and Ayurvedic medicine evolved philosophies based on a five-fold nature of the universe, and both place strong emphasis on individual treatment, a practice that has been once again blessed by modern biological research. So before passing you on to the people in this book, I would like to talk about a few of the "Principles of Pot" I believe are most important.

First, most, if not all, of the people I interviewed possessed a great reverence for life. Often, in the middle of an interview I would be awestruck by the compassion or the unconditional love I was sensing in the other person. For instance, I will never forget my afternoon with Rachel Naomi Remen, MD, whom I suspect may be a saint. She had just returned from speaking to a large crowd and was tired—she has a chronic, debilitating illness—but she willingly honored her commitment to be interviewed. As we sat together in a hotel room in Los Angeles, she spoke of being a physician and how awful it was to work in the era of managed care, in which doctors have to do what they are told instead of what they believe is right. Because of this situation, in her workshops for physicians, she asks them to tell each other stories about the things they have seen as doctors that do not make sense, things such as miracle cures and other anomalies. "As they tell these stories, their sense of awe grows," she said. "Awe evokes the wish to serve. And we serve life not because it is broken, but because it is holy."

This reverence for life spills over into the relationship between patient and provider. On another noteworthy day, this one in Santa Fe, New Mexico, David Reilly, FRCP, MRCGP, FFHom, a homeopathic physician from Scotland, explained that compassion may be every bit as important in healing a patient as the particular medicine or modality being used. "Sometimes therapies are the least of the issue," he said. "It's the question of intention and integrity, the quality of the meeting, the trust, the relationship, the shared walk together of the person and the caregiver—that's where the magic really happens. That's where things move and people experience radical changes in how they're coping or not coping, and in the quality of their life. That's where transformation occurs."

I do not experience this love and compassion when I go see the physician in my HMO or to the pediatrician who cares for my son. No one in any medical office has ever looked at me with awe in his or her eyes or in any way addressed me as something holy. But these feelings and emotions were present in the people I interviewed. Whether it is the doctor in Mill Valley who helps patients heal through the use of imagery, or the nurse-healer who lives in the mountains of Montana and has taught thousands to heal with their hands, or the ethnobotanist who is looking for healing plants in the Amazon—these scientists and practitioners have a deep and profound respect for life and for other people. And in my personal book of beliefs, this is one of the real reasons alternative medicine works so well on so many people.

Another underlying principle woven through the interviews has to do with our individuality. Over and over, I heard people telling me that who we are and the manner in which we live is intimately connected to our *experience* of health or illness. We are not disconnected from ourselves, constantly getting sick or being made well in random fashion, they say. We are not just biological machines. Our minds and souls, and the way we think and live and love, matter. In short, the patient *is* relevant to the process of healing.

One evening in Hilton Head, South Carolina, Larry LeShan, PhD, talked to me at length about his experience with cancer patients. He found that traditional psychotherapy—which takes the approach of finding out what is wrong with someone and fixing that—offered little hope or relief to his patients. Yet when he began to work with these same patients on the basis of what was *right* with them, what made them happy and gave them a zest for life, he achieved a 50% remission rate. In short, he got better results when he took the uniqueness of the individual—not the sameness—into account.

Dr. LeShan explained the underlying philosophy as this: "The heart of the western spiritual tradition is that at birth you are given a seed of an unknown and unique flower. That's your soul. Your job is to garden it to the fullest so that it blossoms most fully, and is worthy of the one who calls it back."

What he was telling me was similar to the ancient Chinese text on medicine and the three levels of healing that Harriett Beinfield, LAc, and Efrem Korngold, LAc, OMD, spoke about in their interview. Health is not simply about the biological and chemical activity within our bodies; it is also about who we are and our personal destiny.

Harriet and Efrem live in San Francisco. When you walk down their street, you pass ordinary house after ordinary house. Then you come to a house protected by a wonderful, wooden fence. As you pass through the gate, you enter an exquisite, fragrant garden, and it is as if you have passed into a completely different reality. That, in itself, told me something about this couple. While we were sitting at a wooden table in her kitchen having tea, Harriett explained, "If you understand life as a material phenomenon, then you look at humans as physical, biological, chemical entities and you define medicine as an attempt to correct pathologies within those physical, biological, chemical domains. But if you define the purpose of life as being able to experience happiness and to overcome ignorance through the development of the mind—and you see the mind as developing in a long-term sense, perhaps not even confined to one biological life span—then the goal of medicine is to help someone fulfill that purpose."

I found this viewpoint fascinating. My regular doctor barely knows my name, much less what I do for a living or what my goals and dreams may be. But if "I" am to be made well, then all of me, not just my body, must be included in the treatment because all of me, not just my body, is included in the experience of illness. Harriett put it this way, "Disease doesn't come from nowhere. It emerges from a lived life."

Now, this is not to say that when we are sick it is our fault. Not at all. But it is to say that when we are sick, we may have the resources and capacities to help make ourselves well.

This leads naturally to the conversation about consciousness and the underlying "Principle of Pot" that consciousness can affect matter.

What is giving life, and scientific respect, to this ancient idea found in most spiritual traditions are the recent round of research studies showing that acts of intentionality, such as prayer and biofeedback, can affect health outcomes in a positive way, and that healers can have an effect on people without being physically present. As people ask *why* this happens, they find themselves face-to-face with consciousness.

"Consciousness precedes matter," neuroscientist Candace Pert, PhD, told me one warm spring day as we walked along a creek bed in Potomac, Maryland. We were discussing her work regarding the biochemical mechanism for emotions. She had just explained how the brain releases neuropeptides throughout the body and how our cells have receptors that receive the information these neuropeptides carry. "But emotions are not in the head," she said. "The truth is so weird I've only recently come to believe it. And the truth comes out of Eastern thought in which molecules are secondary. The emotional energy comes first and then peptides are released all over. It's not like a peptide creates the feeling. The feeling creates the peptide."

Dr. Pert discussed how our own consciousness affects our own body, but Marilyn Schlitz, PhD, director of research at the Institute of Noetic Sciences, discussed people's ability to affect *each other* across a distance. "Healers across cultures and throughout time have demonstrated that healing can occur at a distance," Schlitz said. "We have conducted 13 experiments now. In these experiments, instead of trying to regulate one's own physiology, a healer from a distance tries to regulate the physiology of another. And overall, we found highly significant evidence for non local healing."

Dolores Kreiger, RN, PhD, one of the founders of Therapeutic Touch (TT), agrees. One day as we sat in her cabin in the mountains of Montana, she told me about the changes that happen to a person who practices TT. She said, "Over time comes the realization that not only don't you stop at your skin, but that your neighbor doesn't stop at his or her skin. Once that happens, you begin to understand more clearly that relationships are something very different from what we think they are. You now look at all animate beings, whether people or trees, as completely different experiences from what your culture taught you to expect. You know that your human energies are constantly and dynamically interacting with the vital energy fields of others in a manner not thought of in Biology 101."

Aside from bring a prolific author and internationally renowned speaker, Larry Dossey, MD, is the executive editor of our journal; so I have had the pleasure of many conversations with him, both on and off the record. In a recent conversation at his home in Santa Fe, New Mexico, he told me, "Imagine, as we speak, that part of your mind is not present in your body or brain or even in this moment. Imagine that this aspect of your consciousness spreads everywhere, extending billions of miles into space, from the beginning of time to the limitless future, linking us with the minds of one another and with everyone who has ever lived or will live. This is the infinite piece of your consciousness." This is the part of our minds that can be used in healing, he told me. "Its expressions include sharing thoughts and feelings at a distance, gaining information and wisdom through dreams and visions, knowing the future, radical breakthroughs in creativity and discovery, and more."

The next core principle I want to discuss in this introduction is simple: We (human beings) are not *alone* in this universe.

This is not a popular belief in conventional medicine or the other sciences, but it is common among alternative practitioners. The choice of words differs, but many of the people I have talked with spoke of a divine being or helping spirits or the fact that other life forms such as trees and mountains might be conscious, or that even the planet itself might be conscious, and that these conscious entities, if contacted, could be helpful to humans. We often talked about a higher intelligence and an "Other." The importance is not in the rightness or wrongness of the individual philosophy involved. The importance is that through the recognition that we are not alone, we access an opportunity for help and for healing. Or, to put it in other terms, the failure to recognize that we are not alone may be what is killing us.

On one warm fall day in Vermont in 1996, James Jealous, DO, explained to me that the natural laws are not manmade. We were eating lunch in a small, rural café and his statement was so simple that I had to put my sandwich down and laugh. Of course not, I replied. The human race didn't create things like gravity. *Everyone* knows that. But then I realized the profound implications of his statement—If not us, who? And so I was finally able to hear what he had to say and to recognize the forces about which he was talking.

In his osteopathic practice, Dr. Jealous works with the "Breath of Life." He says this force is at work in everyone. He told me, "When a patient comes into the office, we always begin by waiting and perceiving the purity and sensing the Health at work. We are listening with our hands for a story unfolding into the consciousness of each of us. Some people start crying after they do it for the first time because they realize they were handmade, on purpose, by an artist who loves his work. They feel completely embraced by life and they get the magic."

"The Health in us," he told me quietly and with reverence, "is always trying to heal us." And therefore, Dr. Jealous is never alone.

Jeanne Achterberg, PhD, with whom I have worked for many years, talks about this force greater than ourselves through the story of Shin, a Japanese musician who developed cancer. After being sent home to die, "Shin awoke the next morning and went again to a rooftop on the 18th floor of his apartment building. When the sun rose he felt the rays enter and send energy into his body. He saw the sun as God, and he saw auras around his family and he thought everyone was God. He started to cry, he was so happy to be alive. He realized that he had to love his cancer—it was a part of him, it was not an enemy. He wanted to love the whole of himself."

Dr. Achterberg asks, "What healed Shin—the image of God or God? I think both. It's difficult for me to be specific because I think God is in everything. God is in a white blood cell. God is in an image. What I believe is that we are all part of this source."

Other traditions hold a similar perspective, although the language is different. One stormy afternoon in Mill Valley, California, I spoke with anthropologist Michael Harner, PhD. It was so stormy, in fact, that the winds had blown the electric lines down and we were using the fading daylight and two candles to finish our conversation. Proving my ignorance, I asked him about shamanism and self-healing. And he said, "To an outsider it might look like a person was healing him- or herself. But the concept of self-healing excludes the spirits. From the shamanic point of view, nobody has lived into adult life without spiritual help... So the big news shamanism offers is not that the head is connected to the rest of the body, but that we are not dependent solely on ourselves for healing—there are spirits to help us."

Dr. Harner is not alone, and after that interview, neither was I.

But you cannot talk about life without also talking of about death, which leads to the last core principle. Death is *not* a failure.

When I was talking with Tracy Gaudet, MD, about physician education, she told me, "If you (the physician) are supposed to know everything and your job is to cure disease, then death is a failure." But, of course, this is an impossible stance. At some point, everyone dies. So at the Fellowship, they try to instill a different relationship with death, one that makes a distinction between curing and healing and that promotes the concept of the "good" death. "Healing can happen in death as well as life," she said.

In 1997, I had the pleasure of interviewing Joan Halifax. We met in Santa Fe, New Mexico, at Upaya, the Buddhist center where she practices and teaches. Dr. Halifax talked to me about her own mother's death and what a transforming experience it was for her. "We've marginalized dying people," she explained. "We've pushed death out of sight and characterized it in a negative way. I'm hoping through my own experience and the experience of many colleagues who currently work with dying people as a contemplative practice, that we can foster a new vision of death in the 21st century that will transform the context of dying." What is the new vision? "Fundamentally," Joan said, "death is a release from suffering and perhaps even the moment of awakening of great liberation."

Therese Schroeder-Sheker, works with music to assist dying people to make the transition. In a very intense interview, filled with words, harp music, and chanting, she told me that in death, "There is the element of the sacred, which fills us; we observe and participate within it... Sometimes dying persons come out of a coma and are without any indication of psychosis; they have one foot in each world, they're on the threshold, and begin clearly, quietly, simply relating to the presence of a being whom no one else can see or experience in the same way. I've seen their eyes shine and fill with a directed gaze. It's clear that they are in deep converse—their lips are moving silently, their hands are reaching out for or toward that which is unknowable in my cluttered heart, in my distracted everyday self. But the room is filled with such a palpable burning stillness and reverence, a quietude, an indescribable depth, witnessed by all present, clinicians and loved ones, that I cannot avoid or deny, and any desire to measure this picture would actually defy the experience. Aren't we talking about grace?"

These words do not describe a "failure."

In closing, I would like to address one final thread that wove its way through the interviews because it changed my concept of how scientific discoveries are made and how advances in medicine actually emerge. It also validated my long-time sense that our personal realities, our inner worlds that we may or may not share with others, are powerful conduits of life that should be nurtured.

Ten years ago, I had this silly idea that most scientific discoveries happen through trial and error research in the lab, that somehow the brain of a scientist was like a huge computer making millions of computations every minute and that it was only through this incredible use of logic that advances were made. It never occurred to me that a scientist's *humanity*—his or her feelings or vulnerabilities—might be involved in why they mix chemical A with chemical

B. But I came to realize that many scientific discoveries are nascent through dreams or visions or intuition. And almost all of the people I interviewed were led to conduct research or write or teach or work with patients in a new way because of a *personal experience*, not because of a lab report.

In my conversation with Dr. Pert, she talked about the experience that led to her discovery of Peptide T. She said, "The magic occurred on Maui. That's where Peptide T was actually mentally invented—hiking up Haleakala with Michael Ruff amidst lots of rainbows." Dr. Pert later proved her vision true in the lab—but the vision came first.

Jeff Levin, PhD, an epidemiologist, started down the path that led to his research on the relationship between religion and health and most recently, love and health, because of a mystical experience he had while in graduate school. Alan Davis, MD, who uses soul retrieval as part of his rehabilitation practice in Salt Lake City, was led to the study of shamanism through his own personal quest for wholeness. Mitchell Krucoff, MD, a cardiologist at Duke University, had a profound experience while visiting a hospital in India that eventually led him to design a research project testing the effect of prayer on heart disease. The list goes on, as you will shortly discover.

The real importance of this point is that meeting these people and listening to their stories about how their *personal experiences* or *visions* shaped their lives and led them to great discoveries or great doings, was extremely life affirming. And I cannot think of a better mind-set in which to journey toward wholeness and health—that it is in the listening to the soul and the following of the heart and the acceptance of help from people and god, or however you wish to name the mystery, that destiny is revealed and the dream, your dream, comes true.

NOTE: All of the interviews were conducted between the years of 1995 and 2001 and first published in the medical journal, Alternative Therapies in Health and Medicine. *In the journal, the interviews appear in a question-and-answer format. But for the purposes of this book, we have re-edited the conversations as monologues. We have, where needed, updated biographies to reflect current circumstances, and in some cases, changes, deletions, and additions were made to the interviews to reflect important changes in data in the field or in the person's perceptions and opinions. Four of the interviews are unique to this book and did not appear in the journal—David Cumes, MD; Alan Davis, MD; Wayne Jonas, MD; and Steven Weiss, DO.*

Part One

Conversations About Mind-Body-Spirit

"If the stories in the mind change, thoughts change, emotions change, and the body changes—it's as simple as that."

—JEANNE ACHTERBERG

CHAPTER 1

LARRY LESHAN, PhD

Mobilizing the Life Force

The human body comes equipped with natural healing abilities. In most cases, if one cuts a finger, the wound will heal itself; the flesh will regenerate and the finger will return to its normal state of wholeness. Once set, broken bones typically mend without intervention, and white blood cells automatically rush to the site of infection. Research psychologist Larry LeShan, PhD, has spent much of his career in search of ways to enhance these inherent healing abilities. He is perhaps best known for his therapeutic work with terminally ill cancer patients, but he has also written more than 80 professional articles and 15 books, including *Cancer as a Turning Point, Einstein's Space and Van Gogh's Sky* (with Henry Margenau), *How to Meditate,* and *The Psychology of War.* Born in 1920, LeShan earned his BS from the College of William and Mary, his MS from the University of Nebraska, and his PhD from the University of Chicago.

I interviewed Larry LeShan in December, 1994, at a conference sponsored by the National Institute for the Clinical Application of Behavioral Medicine on the Psychology of Health, Immunity, and Disease, at which LeShan was a featured speaker. The conference was held in Hilton Head, North Carolina. We agreed to meet in the lobby of his hotel. Since I had never met Dr. LeShan, I asked him how I would recognize him. "I'll be the one with a rose between my teeth," he said. And he was. And that's when I knew I was in for an interesting conversation.

Around 1950, in this country and Europe, about 40 people, completely independently and not knowing of each other's existence, started asking the same questions: Is there anything cancer patients can do to mobilize their own self-healing ability? Is there a relation between psychological factors and cancer?

And yes, there's clearly a relationship. How large it is—nobody knows. It may be as small as 5%, but think of what a difference 5% can make in a close election. Over the years, we researchers have come to much the same conclusion. What patients can do is set an example for the immune system by treating themselves as if they are really worth caring for, as if they are special, as if their life is worth fighting for.

I started out using a standard psychotherapy approach with patients in the late 1950s. I spent the first six years conducting interviews and doing projective tests. I wasn't a bad psychotherapist, and I probably did more good than harm. My patients were glad to see me, and my work seemed to make life in the hospital easier for them. But the patients all died at the same rate as if I had done nothing. Then I shifted the basis of the psychotherapy.

Now, all psychotherapy is built on a medical model, which means that when I go to my physician, he or she asks three questions. First, why is this character in my office? What are the symptoms? What's wrong with him? Second, how did he get that way? What's the hidden cause—the cyst, the lesion, the vitamin deficiency? And third, what can we do about it? But therapy based on these questions does not have any effect on the life span. It makes life easier while you're sick or dying, but it doesn't lengthen the life span. And there's no reason it should. Therapy was built to deal with problems of perception, memory, feelings—psychological factors—not to mobilize physiological healing abilities.

But when you change the basis of therapy to a quite different approach, the picture changes. You have two different basic questions. The first new question is "what's right with this person?" What's this particular person's special way of being, relating, and creating, so that when he's living this way, he has a zest for life? So that when he is tired, it's the good tired, not the dragged-down tired? The second new question is "given the reality of the situation, how can he move his life in that direction?" Then you build a therapy based on these answers.

Using the same population in which nearly 100% of my cancer patients died with the old approach, with this new approach, about 50% go into long-term remission and often begin to respond much better to medical treatment. And people I've trained and supervised are getting the same results. It's not just a one-person phenomenon.

So this is now my approach to healing—you help the person live a life of enthusiasm.

Why Does It Work?

There's nothing sacred about this approach. It's not as if I invented it; I was taught it by my patients. But it often requires a lot of support. It's hard to change your life. We've all been brought up with the basic determinants of what our behavior should be, what's the right thing to do, what does a good person do, what am I supposed to do? We're adding a fourth factor: What do I enjoy doing? What turns me on?

As far as what's happening inside the body when people start moving in this direction and finding the life they want, my feeling is that we're at a very primitive state of knowledge. We really know nothing of the relationship of mind and body except correlations. If I take alcohol into my body, my mind gets drunk. If somebody refers to my mother in certain terms and I come from a certain cultural group, my blood distribution changes. But these are just correlations. We have no idea what's between them. There's a bridge of cobwebs a mile long between our concepts of the mind and of the body.

You could do studies that would show that this kind of approach increases the activity of what we loosely call the immune system. But we use the term "immune system" to make us feel as if we know more than we do. In the beginning of my career, we didn't have the term "immune system." For self-healing abilities we had the term, "pituitary adrenocortical axis." It made us feel very learned. But it's the same thing. If I cut myself when I'm shaving, I heal. If I bruise my heel, my foot gets better. These are self-healing abilities, and they can operate at higher or lower levels.

We're operating on the theory that everybody gets cancer hundreds, maybe thousands of times a day. Individual cells, as they multiply and divide, lose their inner and outer coherence. They become cancer cells. But the body has a mechanism—we don't know for sure, but T-cells may be part of it, and killer cells may be part of it—that reaches out and goes "schloop" and takes care of the cancer cells. The strength of this mechanism is apparently set genetically, but it can be weakened by radiation, by certain pollutants, and by aging. The important question is "can we strengthen it?" This is what this work has been all about, finding a way to strengthen it.

Can You Refuse an Unwanted Favor?

George Solomon, probably our best psychosomatics man today, studied many AIDS patients. What he found was that the only thing that could predict long-term survival was this one question: "Can you refuse an unwanted favor?" The question itself doesn't mean too much. It's asking, "What is your attitude toward protecting yourself?"

Let me show you what I mean. Let's suppose you come to me and say, "Larry, I just came in from California because I know you're very sick and I love you. I've got some tickets for the Grateful Dead concert. You can't get these tickets for love or money. I've spent a fortune, and I'm taking you tonight."

Now, I hate rock music. It's the last thing I want to hear. But it's such a lovely thing you did. The question is: "Can I refuse this favor? Can I be protective enough toward myself to decline?" If you can, your chances of long-term survival are better.

Now, before you ask why everyone isn't using this, remember that the medical profession has two responsibilities. One is to give people the best treatment available. The second is to drag their heels, literally, so that all kinds of kooks who come down the road with beautiful, charismatic statements and wonderful statistics don't sweep the patients away. An awful lot of people make marvelous claims for all kinds of things. In my time alone, I've seen about four cures for schizophrenia. Lactic acid was one cure; nicotinic acid was another. Before that, they thought it was caused by poison under the teeth so they took out all the teeth of schizophrenics. Before that, it was poison at the base of the colon, so at one point thousands of schizophrenics had the last 6 inches of their colons removed. And wonderful results were reported for all these cures.

So you have to be careful. But I think this should be a part of all cancer treatment and that it someday will be. The change is taking place.

Who Should Practice?

If we want to get better results, then one of the first things we should be studying is who we allow to practice psychotherapy. If you look at who is practicing out there, it's very discouraging. For example, we do not insist that you cannot be a therapist until you've had a great deal of personal therapy yourself, until you're grown up and can earn a living in something else so you're not running to this to get away from the world. You shouldn't practice until you can bring something more than just what is in the psychology and psychiatry books to it, until you know more than what is in these books about what it means to be human. This can come from the serious study of art, history, philosophy, music, or the like, but you need at least one other field of knowledge. And last, you shouldn't practice until you yourself have touched something of life. So the first thing we need to do is clean up who we let practice.

I can't answer for the other professions, but psychotherapy is not "fixing" somebody. It doesn't make much difference who my auto mechanic is if he's just going to change the carburetor in my Chevrolet. That's fixing something. But you don't fix people. What you're trying to do with human beings is to help them grow, to "garden" them to a greater thriving in their own way, to help them on their path.

How do you do this? The first thing a therapist does is model. The therapist pays attention to the patient and thereby teaches the patient to pay attention to himself. He has respect for the patient and thereby teaches the patient to respect himself. What you're really trying to teach is an attitude, but attitudes can't be taught. They have to be caught. This is why you get the same level of results whether you're a Freudian and talk about the Oedipal complex, or a

Jungian and talk about archetypes, or a humanist and talk about getting in touch with your inner child. Therapists operate on different theories, but the thing they have in common is that they all model.

The question is "why are the results so low?" There are two reasons. One is the second level of modeling. This is the example the therapist gives about caring for his or her own life. I will not refer patients to a therapist who doesn't take as much time and energy caring for her own growth and becoming as she does for that of her most loved and most difficult patient. She should be as much involved in her own growth as she is for the patients. For example, therapists who in any 5-year period aren't having a better time and more fun in life than they had in previous 5-year periods should be barred from the profession.

The second aspect of why results are so low lies in how we design the therapy for each patient. Most therapists were raised on the idea that they had the right way to do therapy. They knew exactly how to do it. Their mentor taught them, and if they'd only do it well enough, they could cure everybody. Unfortunately, most patients don't fit their specifications. If we really want to get results, we must look at the patient and ask "what does this particular person need, different from anybody else? What special therapeutic environment, what metaphor for growth will help this person thrive?" That's probably the main thing we need in terms of research—how to treat each patient differently and how to design what this patient needs in order to thrive.

This is a part of Western spiritual development concepts. St. Theresa of Liseaux, in her book on being a spiritual director, wrote, "the hardest job for the spiritual director, harder than making the sun rise at night, is to give up his own special path, his own special likes and dislikes, and lead the patient along the particular way that will lead him to God." Dom Baker, the Benedictine mystic, said that the spiritual director is an usher who ushers people along their own special path, not the usher's path. It's different with each person. And Rabbi Nachman said, "God calls one person with a song, one with a shout, one with a whisper."

So to me, there's no one "right" way. What's right for one person is wrong for another. There's no one right diet for cancer, for example. I've seen people do beautifully on the macrobiotic diet and I've seen people damn near die of it—not of the disease, but of the diet. Mindfulness, the empty mind, is fine for some people. But meditation is wrong and right for different people and at different times. The important question is: "Given myself, the individual, unique person I am, what's the best way for me to move further on my path, so that my life is increasingly filled with zest, joy, and fun?" That is the name of the game.

One of the great spiritual documents of the West is the *Cloud of Unknowing*, a medieval manuscript. It says over and over again, the path should be "listy," which is the opposite of "listless." It means active, eager, involved. It's not a quiet, passive thing. You're trying in your own way to get more out of life. The heart of the Western spiritual tradition is that at birth you're given a seed of an unknown and unique flower. That's your soul. Your job is to garden it to the fullest so that it blossoms most fully and becomes worthy of the one who calls it back.

There are two separate streams of psychotherapy. One is the medical stream, in which the person comes in with a symptom. Your job is to heal that symptom and possibly the cause behind it. Then the person is fine, and that's the end of it. The spiritual director, which is the other stream that therapy comes from, is not concerned with that. He or she is concerned with the whole. You don't go to the spiritual director like you go to a dentist or a barber. I go to a dentist to take care of my teeth, a barber to take care of my hair. I go to a spiritual director to take care of my whole being, to help me move toward thriving, not just surviving.

Conventional medicine has been very legitimately designed to help people solve problems. If I have a hot swelling in my belly and it's tender and painful at McBurney's point, I don't want a doctor who is concerned with my lifestyle or soul or diet or anything else. I'm going to have a ruptured appendix, and I want the doctor to surgically remove it. Now, hopefully, when we move further, we will see this as a valid, crucial beginning and move then to states of more health and zest and so forth.

The World of the One

In *The Medium, Mystic, and the Physicist,* which was published in the 1970s, I drew parallels between the worldview of modern physics and the great mystics of all major religions. While I still think these parallels are true, I've come to realize it's more complicated than it looks because you have so many divisions and small groups within the mystics and the physicists. Also, at that time I didn't really understand the difference between Eastern and Western mysticism, which I now see as quite profound. But basically both say that the question of the basic nature of reality is a meaningless and fruitless question.

Around 1900, science gave up the search for reality. Up to 1900 the search was "What are the laws of reality?" In 1900 it shifted to "What is the most fruitful way we can construe reality? How can we organize it; how can we put it together?" And we found out that at different times we do it differently. For example, if you're talking about the very, very small, you have the laws of quantum mechanics. When we're talking about the very, very small, there's no such thing as cause and effect, only statistical causation. We say that things can go from one place to another without crossing the space in between or that an electron can go through two holes in the same plate at the same time without splitting.

Next you have the construction of reality within the see/touch realm, which is essentially the common sense Newtonian reality. And then when you get to the very big and very fast, you have a completely different reality, a reality where the faster you go, the larger you get, and the slower your clock runs.

Reality is construed differently in different realms of experience. That's what the physicist says. The mystic says different states of consciousness see a different reality and that they're all equally valid.

The great insight of the 17th century was that the whole world worked on the same principles. The great insight of the 20th century was that it doesn't. The world doesn't work on mechanical principles in the very small and the very large, and it doesn't work on mechanical principles in human consciousness, either.

Both the mystics and physicists say that there are different ways to construe reality. One of them, they both agree, is the "world of the One." Every serious mystical school, from the early Greeks to the present, has agreed that there are at least two basic ways of being in reality: the way of the Many, and the way of the One. We're all well trained in the world of the Many. You have to be, or you'd never grow up alive. We're highly organized in the world of the Many, but we're unorganized in the world of the One. The job for adults in every mystical school is to increase our perception of the world of the One so that when I see you, a unique, one-of-a-kind individual, I also see that you and I are one and cannot be separated, that you are part of a total, seamless garment of the universe and vice versa.

Can this idea be used in healing? The trouble is, we know so little. It's very hard to keep in mind that at least 50% of what we think we know for certain is false. We just don't know which 50% it is, as the saying goes. And if you look back, the things we're most sure of today, in 100 years we'll regard at least 50% of them as foolishness. So I don't know if it can be used in healing, but I suspect that it's the best explanation of psychic healing we have today.

The explanation is that when you change the construction of reality that the patient is in, the one that's operating at the time, and you change it to one in which you and the patient are one, you're feeding a part of him that's undernourished. And it may well be that in some cases this permits his self-healing ability to operate at a higher level.

Now, even though I've taught psychic healing and done research in this, and I do it when necessary, I don't think there is such a thing as psychic healing. It doesn't work. I think there is simply a paranormal way of stimulating the person's own self-healing abilities.

In psychic healing, the healer says, "I heal you." But actually, he didn't do anything. I can send you a message where you heal yourself, but I can't heal you. If my wife is sick, I cannot send energy to her. I'd love to, but I can't. But I can change the organismic situation. I can be with her in the most profound way two human beings can be together, and this may help her to heal herself. But you can't do anything to the other person.

One of the great insights of both Eastern and Western mystical schools is that we are "amphibians." We need to live both in the world of the One and the world of the Many. But we're almost invariably undernourished in our need for being in the world of the One. We have a "vitamin deficiency" of the organism. Ramakrishna said, "A human being is like a frog. When young, it's a tadpole. It exists in one medium only. But when the tail of ignorance drops off, it needs both."[1] When we feed that undernourished part of the person, his self-healing abilities operate at a higher level. That's the best explanation we have today of psychic healing.

I don't think the best psychic healer, on his or her best day, gets more than 20% results. But, boy, those results can be spectacular. It's a very real phenomenon, and we have a lot to learn about it. Actually, we should be studying the paranormal more, because the paranormal says something profound about human beings.

First of all, we have to remember where we are in the human race. We cannot stop killing each other. We don't know how. And we're poisoning our planet. The way you treat something depends on what you consider it is. If I consider this as wood, it's firewood. If I consider it a place to put something, it's a table. If I consider it a hard bed, I can lie on it. How I treat it depends on what I consider it is. We have a view of what a human being is. Separate, alone, related, whatever. And we treat each other on that basis. And on that basis, we can't stop killing each other.

The great thing about the paranormal is that it gives us a different conception of a human being. For example, it says that under certain conditions, we cannot be separated. We've done telepathy over 7000 miles, just as well as telepathy to the next room. The two people were connected and information was flowing. They reacted as if they were one.

If we get this new conception of what a human being is, maybe we'll be able to treat ourselves in different ways. I'd like to see a tremendous amount of money put into that, because to me, it's the greatest hope of the human race.

We're a beautiful, joyous, wonderful, crazy, sick, neurotic, pathological race. We're all these things. We've got so much possibility. We've all seen such gentleness, loving, caring, self-sacrifice, heroism, dedication, pathology, selfishness, and all seven deadly sins. We've all seen all of them.

The field of alternative medicine is just one small aspect of a hope of using certain kinds of technical tools to say, "Can we learn to be with ourselves and be with others in new ways?" Alternative medicine is really one of the trails on that approach.

---

[1]Ramakrishna lived in India between 1836 and 1886. He was a Hindu mystic whom many considered as one of God's incarnations. See *The Gospel of Sri Ramakrishna*, New York, Ramakrishna-Vivekananda Center, 1942.

A lot of people are working in many ways on it. Other ways have failed. The way of religion failed. Even in the medieval period, when the church had absolute power, it couldn't control war. They tried to pass laws saying you couldn't fight on weekends. They tried to have the crossbow outlawed as inhumane, but the church couldn't make it stick. The way of philosophy has failed; the way of politics has failed; the way of education has failed. If you look at the people who led the war in Viet Nam, they were our best college professors, educators, doctors, lawyers, businessmen, and generals, the best.

Something New Is Being Born

One important thing to remember is that an age is dying and a new age is being born. When a major transition like this happens, something very curious occurs. You can only see backward. You can't see forward. For example, take the 5th century in Rome, the 13th century, and the 17th century. What do they have in common? In all of them, an age was dying. And in each of the times, they said the same things. They said: The streets aren't safe. The generations don't understand each other. There are too many books. And the institutions we have are foundering one after another. If you read the literature from these periods, you find the same thing. All they could see was what was dying. They couldn't see that something was being born. After the death of Rome came the rich medieval society. At the death of the medieval society came the Renaissance. At the death of the Renaissance came the present.

The present is the same. Something new is being born at this time. We are in a transition period. We're seeing the birth pangs and it's horrible because all we feel is that our institutions are foundering, one after another. Our school systems are foundering, our political system is foundering, and God knows, the military system is foundering. Everything is foundering.

At each time in the past, something new and rich was born. So am I optimistic? Yes. Something new is being born.

As we begin to put the new field of alternative medicine together, I think it is crucial to remember that no two patients are alike. They are as unique as their fingerprints. If you see two patients who need the same treatment, it means that you do not know very much about one or both of them. If you see three who need the same treatment, it means you have severe tunnel vision or else you are treating them for your problems and not theirs!

There is no adequate model for human beings except that of a human being. We are not a flowering plant, a white rat, or a computer. The model, metaphor, and method your school and mentor taught you is right for some of your patients but does violence to others. Each patient is new and unique. It is more important to think, "How is this patient unique?" than it is to decide on a diagnosis.

Kurt Goldstein was a psychiatrist who, for decades, was a voice crying in the wilderness for a holistic revolution in medicine. He coined the term *self-actualization* and was a major force in developing humanistic psychology. Before a patient came into his office, Goldstein would take a quiet moment and reflect to himself, "Now I must give up all my preconceptions."

I recommend this to all of us.

CHAPTER 2

JEANNE ACHTERBERG, PhD

Imagery, Ceremony, and Healing Rituals

Part of the original team that started *Alternative Therapies in Health and Medicine* in 1995, Jeanne Achterberg, PhD, is one of the pioneers of alternative medicine. She is perhaps best known for her work with imagery and healing and for her groundbreaking practice that used imagery to help burn patients.

She received her PhD in experimental psychology and physiological psychology from Texas Christian University in 1973. A faculty member for 11 years at Southwest Medical School, University of Texas Health Science Center, she is currently a professor at Saybrook Institute in San Francisco and research director for the North Hawaii Community Hospital on the Kona Coast of the big island of Hawaii.

Achterberg was named Healer of the Year in 1994 by the Nurse Healers–Professional Associates Cooperative, the J. B. Rhine Memorial Lecturer at the 1992 annual meeting of the Parapsychology Association, the Highpoint Memorial Lecturer at California State University-Fresno in 1991, and the Gardner Murphy Lecturer for the American Society for Psychical Research in 1989. She has authored more than 100 papers and eight books, including *Imagery in Healing: Shamanism and Modern Medicine, Woman as Healer,* and *Rituals for Healing* (with Barbara Dossey). Her own journey into healing, which started when she discovered she had a tumor behind her left eye, resulted in her newest book, *Lightning at the Gate*.

Because we have worked together on the journal for the past seven years, I have had many conversations with Dr. Achterberg, but this one took place on a foggy morning in the seaside village of Del Mar, California, in the summer of 1999.

Over the last 28 years, I have watched imagery, which has an ancient lineage in the art of healing, become an acceptable part of the lexicon of mind-body medicine. Part of the acceptability of this art and science is that imagery simply *is*. Nobody can deny that we all have images, and that if we imagine certain negative events with frequency and intensity, we become sick. If the stories in the mind change, thoughts change, emotions change, and the body changes—it's as simple as that. Thoughts are biochemical reactions, and biochemistry influences thoughts.

I should say at the beginning, however, that I am becoming more and more uncomfortable with the kind of language we use to describe mind and body. As science marches on—and especially when one considers the work of Candace Pert and others like her—we cannot really discriminate body from mind. It's all created from the same stuff. We need to develop a new vocabulary, but that hasn't happened yet. You might think of imagery, though, as the way what we call "mind" and what we call "body" communicate. It's a bridge; a vital aspect of consciousness and of the way we think.

And if all of this is true—and I believe it is—imagery is an integral aspect of getting sick, getting well, and staying well.

There are many different practices that people call imagery. It is basic to many psychotherapies as well as hypnosis and biofeedback. Most people who use or teach imagery are doing some form of relaxation or meditation, with the goal of reducing stress or getting quiet enough to listen to messages from bodies or lives—"consulting their inner adviser," many call it—on a regular basis. Generally, such people also imagine themselves in a pleasant situation, feeling peaceful and well. These valuable and popular techniques are supported by a respectable body of research.

I know from my work that the regular use of "specific imagery" can result in major changes in health, including fewer side effects from treatments such as chemotherapy, more rapid healing, and even improved immunology. When I teach "specific imagery," I advise people to learn some form of relaxation, do it for about 10 minutes, and then imagine (using all the senses, not just the visual) the steps to the desired outcome, including how they will feel, think, and live after the crisis is past.

The nature of imagery goes far beyond the world of a daily therapeutic practice. If you consider that the things that are most important and human are invisible—feelings, beliefs, ideas, our connections with one another and something greater—you realize that these are represented and vested in images and symbols. Once we become conscious of the images, we might be compelled to make adjustments in our work life, our social life, even our spirit life. So, as far as I'm concerned, imagery is a wedge or an entrance into the ability to translate and transform the very nature of our being.

My training programs are usually conducted during an intense 1- to 2-week seminar or quarterly for a year with a wide array of healthcare professionals. I teach what I understand to be true about imagery, medically and psychologically, in both its healing and transformative aspects. I teach imagery as a technique—something that is helpful to health if done regularly—and as something that may well pull us together as human beings. Running through my work is the symbolic aspect of life that gives purpose and meaning.

Symbols and Images

One of the ways I introduce the imaginal aspects of thought is to ask people to describe who they are symbolically. For instance, I could tell you that I am Jeanne—this, that, and the other—and show you my curriculum vitae. But what I really am is a wildflower. When I say that, you don't even have to see me or know me—you already know many characteristics about my inner life and my lifestyle. Wildflowers are tenacious, delicate, and tough. After they bloom they can go underground for weeks or years; there is still life, but of a different sort. They are also stubborn and don't transplant or grow if forced against their will. Symbols are a great means of communication about who we are to ourselves and one another.

Once we become aware of our symbolic nature, we begin to identify our own story and wholeness; the symbol becomes a source of wisdom and power, a totem, a fetish, a power object. The wildflower teaches me things about myself. It teaches me that I am part of an organic whole that does what it does when it does because of the story. This is nothing new; it is old tribal medicine.

In the beginning of my workshops, I help participants figure out what symbol best represents them. It is a way of bringing people to a more beautiful and authentic knowledge about their own life stories and reinventing themselves if they wish. People who are seriously ill often become fully identified with their disease, the treatment, and what their doctors tell them, and this often becomes their whole story. In my experience, we don't move on our way medically, psychologically, or spiritually until we move past the diagnosis or label we've been given or have given ourselves. I think this was the purpose of many of the Greek and other ancient forms of medicine that included the arts. They would have plays, music, and dance, enacting the mythologies of the culture. And with these, the individual would see, "Oh yes, this is awful. I hurt and I am afraid and I am of value, but I am part of something so much greater."

The Collective Unconscious

The collective unconscious is one of the more controversial ideas in imagery work. Some of the images we have do seem to come from somewhere outside self-experience and personal knowledge. In my own language, there is a kind of data bank composed of the great mush of all thoughts—good and bad—that humans have ever had. In certain circumstances, especially in altered states of awareness or trances, we have access to these archives created by human consciousness. It is tempting to think of this information as a transmittal from some divine source that guides and assists us in our transformation to an elevated plane of being, but I don't think that is always true. Garbage and evil thoughts are part of this collective stew. I think many of the images people have are thoughts that bleed down from this data bank. They are "fact" in some version of reality, but not necessarily the physical reality that we all currently share. This is a huge therapeutic issue in the so-called "recovered memories" of dreaded events, which may or may not have actually happened.

But there seems to be a repository of information beyond collective thought, some level of reality that probably emerged at the time of creation and was planted like seeds for the evolution of consciousness. It has a life and energy of its own, and we have access to it as well. The images have purpose and meaning. Carl Jung is generally associated with the development of the idea of the collective unconscious. He talked about archetypes—mythological creatures—whose stories act as universal guiding principles for humanity. In Jung's later works, such as *Memory, Dreams, and Reflections,* he admitted that the most difficult aspect of these images to reconcile was that they did not seem to be buried elements of the human experience or "psyche" but were autonomous with a life and landscape of their own.

Stan Grof, who has worked with thousands of people all over the world in altered states of consciousness, agrees that the images come from some realm other than peoples' thoughts. And as I listen to people describe their imagery, I am likewise convinced that it may not be their own experience or even human consciousness that is accessed, but something different.

The few people who do talk about it continue to call it the "collective unconscious" or "mythic reality" but usually refer to the idea that it predated humanity. Some of the other terms are "alternative reality" and "parallel universes."

Imagery can be in all of these. The alternative realities—or whatever you call them—come to us in images and symbols. They don't come forth as a television show; they present themselves in symbolic forms, just as dreams do. Their meanings are hidden, and we have to work at understanding how they relate to our lives.

Healing with Imagery

You might start off with a very basic protocol for 20 minutes a day. During this time, you sit down, get comfortable, and imagine what is challenging you, imagine what is right with you, and imagine yourself healed in any way that makes sense to you. That is the basic practice that works. It just works.

If you guide or engage with another in the imaginal field, it is as though you become dancers in the same dream, and the process becomes interactive. It is a very shamanistic practice, actually. Shamans are people who have an ability to enter into altered states of consciousness at will. They do many things, but in some cultures they take your dreams and redream them. Then you share dreams, and the shaman—who has been in the dream territory many times—helps you to find meaning and healing. That is what skilled imagery therapists do, though they would certainly not consider themselves to be shamans—that is a decision made by the culture and not an individual. But they interact in the same mythic reality as the person with whom they work.

Why is this intervention healing? Perhaps because there is some mutual connection with this huge cosmic thing called *consciousness*. There is a communion of two humans in this landscape, which is what healing is about anyway: connection. It is knowing that we are not separate at some ineffable level. If we walk in one another's dream space, we are connected at a place beyond psychological description. Once there is an awareness of the connection, healing—or what feels like healing in a broad sense—takes place because one is no longer outside the fabric of humanity.

I will share two stories about my work. Both involve friends, not patients or clients. The first is about a woman I will call Jane. She was a great teacher for me about symbolic healing. She is a nurse and at one point was in an administrative position that squelched her creativity and probably her soul. She went to Rancho la Puerta, which is a health spa in northern Mexico. They offer a late afternoon meditation called "The Inner Journey," which is held at the base of Mount Kuchamia, a mountain legendary for its use for vision quests. During the first part of the meditation, Jane had the spontaneous image of being captured within brick walls, which was exactly how she felt in her life. Then, as the imagery progressed, the walls started to undulate and became wavy and movable. A bird in the center flew in a spiral fashion out of the wall. She said it was a momentous healing for her because precisely at that instant she realized she was not encased in stone and did have the freedom to fly. She went home and sketched her image, dated it, and later shared it with me.

A few months later, Rancho la Puerta invited a well-known architect to design a monument in honor of the ranch and the mountain. He appointed 12 apprentices to assist him. Before beginning their work, they visited with the people who lived in the nearby town of Tecate. They slept on the land and tried to connect to the place, especially Mount Kuchamia, in any way they could. Close to the time that they needed to get the monument finished, they stayed up all night and made individual models and then a composite drawing. It was an undulating brick wall with a spiral in the center, and that is what they built.

When Jane and her husband went back to the ranch a month later, she walked into the woods and witnessed her image in brick and stone. Later, she wrote to the architect and asked where he thought the design for the monument might have come from. He said that he and the apprentices thought the vision came from the land itself. Who knows? Coincidence? I think not—it defies any statistical odds. But we do know that there is no available scientific explanation at this point. Nonetheless, it was a personal healing for Jane, maybe a healing for the land, and certainly nurturing for anyone who visits the monument and gazes out to the sacred mountain.

The other story is about Don Campbell. Don and I have been friends for about 20 years, dating back to the time when he, the Dosseys, and I had our "Dallas days" and supported each other through our own shifting paradigms. Several years ago I received an alarming call from Don. He had been diagnosed with a blood clot over an inch and a half long in his right carotid artery that had formed because of a hemorrhage in his skull. He had what he described as a spiral clot shaped like a crescent moon. His options were major surgery with no guaranteed outcome or to watch and wait, neither of which was acceptable.

We talked for more than 2 hours and, in retrospect, seemed to fall into a state of consensual trance. He was imaging sitting in a wonderful wooden chair, in a wooden room, looking out an open window near an ocean shoreline. But I, not he, was actually in that room by the ocean. I imagined being in his brain. I asked him what was going on in there. He remembers my telling him that the imagery he was describing was harmful and must be stopped or he would have a stroke. I cannot recall ever being so blunt and directive with anyone, but I must have sensed serious consequences. I have amnesia for most of the details of the conversation, which is not uncommon with such events.

Don shifted thoughts and I heard a different sound. We both heard it. Over the phone, we worked until he found gentle visual and auditory images that he and I felt were more healing. Don's book, *The Mozart Effect*, gives details of his remarkable experience, and I recommend it highly. He is now remarkably well, for reasons that are unknown with any certainty, but I would say it was at least partially due to his imagery and certainly due to his will and creativity.

If I were to describe these events in scientific terms, I would have to acknowledge that the structure and function of a brain is not completely unknown to me. My graduate training was in physiology, and that knowledge has served me well. I really think it is important to have some kind of background in science if you are going to do the energy work in a medical setting. You don't just pick up imagery skills in a weekend workshop, and if I could stress one issue it would be that. You should approach this work from a background well grounded in the modern understanding of mind, body, and their interactions.

I heard a funny story last week. There was a woman who believed she could know what was going on in peoples' bodies but didn't know what it meant or how to describe it. She said that one person she worked with had this horrible black substance all through his belly and she worried and worried about it. Later she found that it was probably food. People have always been able to do work with images and healing whether or not they had modern ideas about science and physiology. This is crisis healing and is practiced cross-culturally. I do think, however, that people in our culture who want to work in this area should be grounded in some profession.

The second explanation is that I had known Don for some time; we trusted one another; and there were not the normal barriers you have when you don't know people very well. He was also receptive and our intentions were quite clear. I have seen too much scientific evidence that consciousness is not contained in the body. We are enmeshed consciously—not totally enmeshed, or we wouldn't be able to function to get across the street—and there is the ability to flow together in some circumstances. I think many of us share consciousness deeply and frequently. So in one sense, I was part of Don, and Don was part of me, especially during that time.

When I work with patients, it is my preference to teach them physiology and biology as well as how to work with imagery, but I don't do that all the time. For some, it just isn't necessary. But for me, it is a potent aspect of my inner reality; it shifts and generates images. My own research is that if you image certain cells, those cells change. So I try to give a heavy dose of health education and medical information.

But here's a story that absolutely contradicts all this business about needing biologically correct imagery for healing. Shinichiro Terayma, who became the director of the Japan Holistic Medical Society, is a remarkable survivor of cancer. Andrew Weil also describes him in his book *Spontaneous Healing*. I had an opportunity to meet this beautiful man at a training I led on imagery in 1988 at Esalen Institute. Shin offered to tell his story and play his cello for us.

In 1984 Shin was diagnosed with metastasized renal cell carcinoma. In Japan, patients are often not told their diagnosis if it is cancer and often don't know what their treatment consists of. He was told he would get injections and ray treatments that were artificial sunlight just as "prevention." Naturally, Shin got even more violently ill. He was actually being given chemotherapy and radiation. One night he had this tremendous urge to get out of his room—the smells reminded him of death. He rushed to the roof of the hospital and was bodily retrieved and discharged—to his delight—because of the commotion.

Shin said that when he awoke the next morning at home, he went again to a rooftop on the 18th floor of his apartment building. When the sun rose he felt the rays enter and send energy into his body. He saw the sun as God, and he saw auras around his family, and he thought everyone was God. He started to cry, he was so happy to be alive. He realized that he had to love his cancer—it was a part of him, it was not an enemy. He wanted to love the whole of himself.

What healed Shin—the image of God or God? I think both. It's difficult for me to be specific because I think God is in everything. God is in a white blood cell. God is in an image. What I believe is that we are all part of this source. None of us sentient beings are lesser or greater parts of this source.

Ritual

I don't separate the imagery material from the ritual material because imagery is done as part of a ceremony. Once that became clear to me, I went back to every culture I could find to see what they were doing. I found that it was always ceremony, and it was always symbolic. That is just what medicine is; only the ceremonies vary greatly.

In traditional Navajo healing ceremonies, healers create exquisite sand paintings, especially for the patient or whatever ceremony is being held. They take days and days. Generally the community joins in the ceremony, so it is costly in terms of labor and everything else involved. Tibetan sand paintings are done with the intention that the various images are doorways or representations of symbolic forms. They have something to do with other worlds.

In the Navajo system, the patient is first diagnosed by someone who has special skills. Gazers or hand tremblers are very common cross-cultural diagnosticians. Once the patient is diagnosed, he or she sits on the part of the painting that was created with a particular doorway or the appropriate image in mind. Then the patient is asked to begin to imagine the nature of the problem and the nature of the healing—what it might be like in its symbolic form. The chanter chants for about three days, which is the equivalent of the memorizations of the Old and New Testaments. It has to be perfect. And so the patient is sitting there and, as the community is sitting around, he or she is imaging, and the chanter is chanting, and the villagers are holding some intentions for the healing. It is pretty classic—you see pieces of this in most cultures.

There is a lot of imagery and ceremony in conventional medicine. We hold symbolic meaning in things and events and maybe don't even realize it. I still laugh when I see advertisements with a picture of these guys in their white coats with stethoscopes around their necks. These are ceremonial costumes they're wearing. When I worked in the burn unit, the "sterile" suits were stored outside the unit. They would sit there for days. People would sneeze on them and touch them, but before we went into the unit, we would put them on—booties, masks, gowns. They weren't cleaner than anything else—we were just putting on costumes before going into the burn unit. So we still have the costume, and we still have foreign language or the invocations in magical words. Prescriptions still involve Latin words. There is still the formality of making rounds on patients, and there is a huge amount of protocol even in the admissions office. It's just a changed form. But what is it that stays constant as the forms change? The symbolic process—the ceremonial process—is the only constancy.

People make pilgrimages to the hospital. You take off your ordinary clothes—as you would in any other ceremony—and you put on a new set of clothing, the hospital gown. When you do this, you become a different person. You leave the old world and enter the new one. People treat you differently; you go into an altered state of consciousness. Usually you are on drugs, you are hurting, and you are frightened.

I look at the specifics of rituals in some cultures—such as the direction the Lakota Sioux must enter a sweat lodge, the taboos associated with menstruating women in many ceremonies, and the highly contrived litany and formal ceremony in many religions—and I wonder, "does this really matter, and if not, who made this up?" What I believe to be true is that the ceremony cannot dishonor one's beliefs. If one believes in the healing power of a person decked out in feathers instead of balloons, it might be best to leave the balloons home. There are many rituals found all over the world—heat or the use of a sweat lodge or sauna, the vision quest, the use of common symbols such as the circle and the cross—and I am convinced that the form is important at some basic level.

We talk about the need to respect the individual's belief system as well as to give due respect to any ceremonies that might be adapted from other cultures. This is a touchy area right now. Many cultures are sensitive to having their ceremonies coopted, but others are compelled to share their ritual heritage with the world. Many rituals are self-generated—we invent them out of our own special needs.

I teach shamanistic techniques such as drumming and vision quest, whether it involves going out and spending the night in your backyard or having a more formalized situation. But, again, it must be done in such a way that people are not offended.

I do a rattle journey that traditionally is intended to call the ancestral spirits and am careful to use language that people can understand, such as, "let's do a meditation and honor the ancestors who went before you." Much of this is done under the guise of social support. This has become a kind of mainstay for the cancer counseling groups that O. Carl Simonton and I do in Germany. Right before we teach the social support session, we do an ancestral journey in which people are allowed to spend about 20 minutes to see who shows up to be there for them.

People are often shocked at who shows up in their imagery. There is a tangible feeling of the room being full, just absolutely full. Angeles Arrien says that in her tradition, which is Basque, they line up behind you, saying, "I hope she is the one who breaks the pattern." So sometimes I give the participants that suggestion—that they might be the one who breaks the pattern of disease or family, gender, or culture. People are also amazed by who doesn't show up, but it is always powerful to spend 20 minutes and imagine your support.

One of the key rituals I do in my workshops with women involves the idea that we don't take a step until we let go of something. There is usually a door to close or a bridge that has to be crossed. We just don't take it all on; that is not how life works. The first stage of a spiritual journey is usually a release. I say, "Write down what needs to be released, and I will take it home with me if you want." Sometimes they keep their papers of release. If not, I take the papers home and, in a ceremony by myself, burn them. It is the intention of saying, "This no longer serves me, and I give it to somebody I trust to take it away." So that is a nonsecular ritual that is steeped in many traditions.

Any healthcare practitioner who wants to try a ceremony with patients could start with the release ritual. Any physician, nurse or therapist can say, "I can see that you are really worried. I can see that this concerns you greatly. Would you consider letting me take the worry for a time so you can go on with your healing?" Have the patients write it down. I use raffia and rice paper because they are organic and you can burn them. Other cultures would use a piece of cloth wrapped around tobacco or a bag filled with herbs. Just say, "Let me keep it for you." You don't have to read it; you don't have to know what it is. It is the idea of symbolically giving away something that is no longer serving you.

Scientifically, what happens is that less time is spent in worry mode. Worry is destructive; there is no question about that. Worry is an obstacle. Even if you can release it for a short period of time, you've facilitated a balance to the biochemicals that continue to get churned up when you are worried and sad and sick. It clears the way for more productive thinking, more productive activity.

One of the wonderful things that happened when Planetree, a special hospital unit, was opened in San Francisco was that people were asked to choose their surroundings. This is ritual. When patients were admitted to the Planetree unit, they were asked to choose their own sheets. There were places where you could make an altar. But you don't have to call it an altar. You can say, "Why don't you bring some things with you that are dear to you, that you would like to look at and have close to you?"

The founder of Planetree, Angie Thierott, was sensitive to architecture. She told me the doorways in Chinese healing temples are so glorious that when you walk through one you know you are entering a healing place. So she wanted hospitals to have portals. Healing architecture. Other hospitals have gardens made from all the plants that have been used to make medicines; that is also ritual. You don't have to put on a headdress and stomp around a room. That's not what it's about. It's about creating the symbolic environment that speaks to connection and healing.

Relationships

Another subject I have spent time researching and writing about is human relationships. These are the heart of ritual and imagery. If I imagine medicine, what I think of is this picture that I use in my talks on the healing web of community. It is an ancient clay form of people in a circle who have their hands touching. That is what I see as the manifestation of the ritual in imagery; I see people coming together. Obviously, people don't need people, necessarily, to get sick or get well, but most of the time that is how we do it.

Many New Agers would scream at what I just said and argue that we make ourselves sick and well. Perhaps that is true, but I also think we are made ill by our relationships in some way. For instance, we all can list a bunch of characteristics about relationships that are toxic. I can become physically and emotionally ill in relationships that are unkind or when I am around people who do not tell the truth. Others may thrive on these relationships. I think we know to whom we should not be connected; it is probably a survival mechanism and might be inherited to some degree.

We get a signal from our bodies that health, even life, may be at stake. I think those who are sensitive to such impressions are also fabulous survivors. Because our ancestors also read these signals, they knew when to put shoes on and run.

What is more interesting, though, is the healing that is fostered by relationships. One of my great interests now is in sustaining the nurturing relationships I have, because we are not going to stay healthy forever. We are not going to be young forever. So I am interested in creative, wonderful, loving relationships in an environment in which we can live until we die. I am also interested in being very conscious about how we are starting to plan for that. Most of us have made a decision that we want to live in a different kind of environment from that of our parents or grandparents. So my attention is on thinking of healing relationships that will sustain me through the latter part of life.

To describe a healing relationship, I'll borrow the definition from several bodies of wisdom, especially the Cabbala, which is used by mystical traditions in both Christianity and Judaism. A healing relationship is one in which individuals come together in some way that is essential for the evolution of their particular life paths or souls. The relationships might last an hour or a lifetime and be with parents, lovers, children, teachers, or even healthcare professionals. They may be ecstatic and they may be difficult. An image frequently used is that in healing relationships we are diamonds polishing one another's rough edges. Healing relationships seem to have a purposive, transcendent quality about them—a luminance. I especially like the imagery given by Ba'al Shem Tov, one of the founders of Hasidism, who said that from every human being there rises a light that reaches straight to heaven, and when two souls that are destined to be together find each other, the streams of light flow together and a single brighter light goes forth from that united being.[1]

---

[1] Isreal Ba'al Shem Tov (1700-1760) was the founder of the Hassidic movement. His principal teaching was the priority of emotion over intellect and the cultivation of joy.

CHAPTER 3

CANDACE PERT, PhD

The Science of Mind-Body Healing

Modern medical research has shown that brain function—and, consequently, body function—are modulated by chemicals. Many of these chemicals are neuropeptides, short strings of amino acids that are produced by the nerve and glial cells. When neuropeptides lock into their receptors, which are attached to cells throughout the body, they cause physiological reactions.

Candace Pert first described the opiate receptor as a graduate student. She then directed extensive neuropeptide/receptor research while working as the chief of brain chemistry in the clinical neuroscience branch at the National Institute of Mental Health. Her findings led her to conclude that neuropeptides and their receptors form an extensive but very flexible information network that the human body uses to communicate with itself. A further observation—that emotions come first and the communication second—has led her to believe that this is the biochemical substrate of emotions and the scientific explanation for mind-body healing.

Pert, who received her undergraduate degree from Bryn Mawr and her doctorate in pharmacology from Johns Hopkins University School of Medicine in 1974, works at Georgetown University in Washington, DC, as a research professor in the department of physiology and biophysics. She is the author of *Molecules of Emotion: The Science Behind Mind-Body Medicine.*

I interviewed Pert in 1995 at her home in Potomac, Maryland, where she lives with her husband, Michael Ruff. But rather than sit, as I do with most people, Dr. Pert and I walked along the Watts Branch of the Potomac River. And step by step, word by word, she drew a picture of a new paradigm.

In the early 1980s, Ed Blalock and Michael Ruff, two key scientists, made two shocking discoveries. The discovery was that the same neuropeptides and their receptors found in the brain could be found in immune cells. Now everyone believes that the immune system is not only responsible for fighting against infections but that it does the actual healing, so that if you cut your finger, certain immune cells rush in and secrete peptides and make everything work. Blalock discovered that immune cells have peptides in them, endorphins being the first one. Then Ruff discovered that the immune cells had receptors, too. Not just biochemical receptors, but functional receptors that affect which way the immune cells work.

Then, in 1985, Ruff and I and several other scientists published a pivotal paper in the *Journal of Immunology* called "Neuropeptides and Their Receptors: A Psychosomatic Network."[1] In

---

[1]Pert CB, Ruff MR, Weber RJ, Herkenham M: Neuropeptides and their receptors: a psychosomatic network, *J Immunol* Aug 135(2 Suppl):820s-6s, 1985.

this paper we talked about the psychoimmunoendocrine network. We said, "Look, there's this common language. It's got to be a network. It's sending information through peptides that are being released by cells all over, and they are receiving information." Based on the distribution patterns of these receptors that I had been studying for 10 years, we said, "Look, they're in the amygdala; they're in the hypothalamus; they're in the parts of the brain thought to be important in emotions. This is obviously the biochemical foundation of emotions." And that's where we started to bridge into the spiritual, if you will.

There were a lot of jokes, because, let's just say that emotions, ironically, are not dealt with in Western science.

But as it turns out, we not only experience emotions; they run every system of our bodies. These neuropeptides, receptors, run your physiology, your health, and your tendency toward disease. We have a culture that's in complete denial, not just about their importance but almost their very existence. Certainly in medicine, there's no time for it. Psychiatry theoretically deals with emotional pathology, but there's not much emotion, is there, in mainstream medicine?

That's a key difference (between mainstream and alternative medicine). Alternative practitioners are almost going in the other direction. They explain, "Well, I was trying to get rid of her virus, and I was using energy medicine. It was working, but she had unresolved issues with her mother." I'm not making fun of that because I can see how there could be a connection. I think that's the void that alternative medicine is filling because it has an emotional approach.

For instance, when you get mad, your brain releases neuropeptides. Angry ones. Now, most people would think that these neuropeptides find their receptors throughout the body and then trigger physiological actions. But that's wrong. It's not a brain-centered system where everything—thoughts, mind, emotions—comes from the brain and then peters down to the poor second-rate body, which is just this dangling appendage. The truth is so weird that I've only recently come to believe in it and experience it. And the truth comes out of Eastern thought in which molecules are secondary. The spirit, the subtle energy—which is the human body and the emotions that change the energies in it—that comes first and then things are manifested.

Emotions are not in the head. There's a cellular consciousness. There's a wisdom in every cell. Every single cell has receptors on it. The emotional energy comes first and then peptides are released all over. It's not that they're just coming out of the pituitary gland and diffusing down and hitting cells.

For example, there is a peptide that, when dropped into the brain of a rat, causes the rat to start drinking water and acting like it's thirsty. Drop it into the receptors on the lung; the lung will conserve water. Drop it onto the angiotensin receptors on the kidney; the kidney will conserve water. So it's happening everywhere. Everywhere simultaneously the molecules are manifesting. This gets almost into—I don't want to call it the metaphysical—but it goes beyond reductionist Western thought. Somehow the feeling is there first and then the molecules manifest themselves.

Consciousness precedes matter. It's not like a peptide creates the feeling. The feeling creates the peptide, on some level.

Here's an anecdote. Deepak Chopra went to India, and he was saying, "Ah, Candace Pert, the peptides, the receptors, this is such good stuff; it's wonderful." And the sages all scratched their heads and said, "I don't get it. What's the big deal?" Then he told it to a few more and they all said, "I don't get it." Finally, one man, the oldest sage, said, "Oh! I get it. She thinks these molecules are real."

We have it backward. We have a denial of the consciousness realm. We ignore it. Isn't that interesting? So it's a whole reorientation. In the beginning I could glimpse it for 10 seconds, but more and more, I feel like I'm experiencing that other perspective.

We're at a funny time. There is this amazing cross-cultural explosion. It's a reconciliation of Eastern and Western thought in medicine, in physics, in everything. Back in the 1960s, Fritjof Capra wrote *The Tao of Physics*. That was the beginning. He basically said, "Isn't quantum mechanics like Eastern thought? Here's how the two are similar." I said, "Whoa!" I didn't want to think about Eastern thought; it was totally repulsive. But quantum mechanics—that was something I was allowed to think about.

We can use this knowledge to heal ourselves and to heal each other. I think it gets used all the time except in classical Western medicine. Stanley Krippner studied cross-cultural healing and in every single culture they have emotional release, emotional catharsis. In our culture, there is a denial of it. So the first thing is just to recognize that emotional changes or releases can be part of a culture. But I have a whole rationale for embracing many aspects of alternative medicine based upon the fact that they would be expected to perturb peptides and do things to them.

As we published in 1980, there is clear scientific evidence that acupuncture and analgesia are mediated by the release of endorphins. However, acupuncture does a lot more than analgesia, and we suspect that it also releases some of the other 60 or 70 active peptides. But everybody's into biochemistry. It's reductionist, and that's okay. But emotions are in two realms. They're in the realm of the physical, the molecular, the material, and they're also in the realm of the spiritual. It's almost like the transition element. It slides back and forth. That's why emotions are so critically important.

Take breathing. Breathing is used in almost every alternative modality to which I've been exposed. People talk about breathing through, or projecting your consciousness and breathing into an injury, exhaling through it. Now, hundreds of scientists have mapped the location of the neuropeptides and any one can be found in the floor of the fourth ventricle, which is where breathing is controlled. Peptides are released into the ventricular fluid, and they affect how fast the breaths are—how shallow, how deep.

Breathing goes on automatically, but you can instantly take control of it without any training. For example, if I say, "Hold your breath!" You can do it. "Breathe faster." You can do it. So it's a way you can interface. You can take your will, change your breathing, change your peptides, and change your emotional state. Breathing is very powerful.

The AIDS Research

In 1986, my lab at NIH discovered that the brain and immune system have the same receptors. Every time we would take any receptor found in the brain and look for it in the immune system, it would be there. We'd take any immune system receptor, look for it in the brain, and find it there. Then we heard that the AIDS virus used a molecule called CD4, which is a receptor, to get into cells. We said, "Well, let's look." And sure enough, we tested it and found it in the brain.

So we started to study it. That led us to hypothesize that if you could find the peptide that usually uses this receptor. . .This was the thinking: Here's the opiate receptor. God didn't put the opiate receptor there so we could all get high from opium, and so we found the endorphins. The marijuana receptor has recently been found, and there's a substance that binds to it. It's actually not a peptide, but it appears to be a very important cellular communication molecule. So I said, "Hey, if we could figure out what peptide uses this receptor, this would be a great drug, because it would block the AIDS virus from getting in." That was the rationale. And then through some determination and a little magic. . .

The magic occurred on Maui. That's where Peptide T was actually mentally invented—hiking up Haleakala with Michael Ruff amidst lots of rainbows. But magic isn't in the realm of the science, and that's what I want to address here. The straight part of the story is that we used a computer-assisted database search, and we looked for peptides that were shared in common between the known database and the AIDS viral envelope, which is the part of the virus that encircles it and holds the nucleic acid. This is the part of the cell that sees. So we figured out this structure and we had great faith and hope and optimism on this.

I was very lucky. I was at the NIH, so I didn't have to write grants. I got to just do it. And it was unbelievable. The peptides came back in the very first experiments. It not only blocked the binding of GP-120, the virus envelope, but it blocked the binding of GP-120 to the CD-4 receptor in both brain and immune cells. And it also blocked the virus from growing, just as we had predicted. Then came the hard part.

The easy part was discovering the AIDS peptide. The hard part was convincing people I had discovered it.

I had spent my entire life being a mother and a scientist. Nobody had educated me in politics, political science, how the world works, money, economics. It's amazing how naive I was. There is tremendous politics in the AIDS arena, and unfortunately, AZT had been invented 3 months before Peptide T. And unfortunately, I worked for the National Institute of Mental Health, as opposed to the National Institutes of Health. Now it's part of the NIH, but at that time they were disconnected, so politically, they had separate budgets. And the people who controlled the AIDS budget were not the least bit interested in a discovery that was coming from outside.

There was a lot of weirdness that happened almost immediately, culminating in the fact that I learned that the drug would never be tested at the NIH, even though it was invented at the NIH. All of the research money went to AZT. And for many years, every study being paid for—and we're talking millions of dollars—was: AZT, plus or minus; AZT before breakfast versus AZT after breakfast; AZT delivered this way versus AZT delivered that way.

But early on I had sent a sample of the drug to Dr. Wetterberg, the head of the Karolinska Institute's psychiatry department. They have a rule that, in a fatal disease, the chairman, at his prerogative, can give a new drug. He gave it to four terminally ill men, and they all had surprising rebounds.

Well, that was enough for me to dedicate my life to it after that. But not enough to convince anybody that it was important scientifically. It worked in the test tube; it worked in people, but there was this major AZT shadow, which we are just coming out of. But right now we're doing trials with Peptide T.

The trials are being conducted by a start-up biotech company that was originally financed by one extremely brilliant, extremely forward-looking individual. He put up the initial money for the trials. He's not a scientist, but he had a number of friends who had AIDS, and the ones who got Peptide T several years ago are still doing great, and the ones who never took it—they're dead. So in his mind, it's proven.

Now, one of the myths is that it normally takes 8 years for a drug to be developed. But we went through an unbelievable saga with this. It's way too long to go into in the interview, but I just can't believe it's normal at any level for a drug that was invented at the NIH.

Let me say one thing: Peptide T isn't a cure. A cure in my mind would be: you give the drug, and the virus is gone. I think Peptide T may be *part* of a cure, but it's going to be in conjunction with a second drug.

At this point there's no doubt that Peptide T alleviates many of the symptoms of AIDS. It reverses the dementia, reverses the weight loss, reverses the fatigue and many of the symptoms, and seems to stabilize people's conditions so that many of them seem to live much longer. But *cure* is, as yet, too strong a word. However, the question of what it says about our culture—that we have politics surrounding medical research—is very important. And as you can imagine, it's hard for me. I went through a lot of self-searching, personal suffering, and personal disillusionment over this. I grew up on Walt Disney, and I really felt that science was truth-seeking.

So what's going on philosophically? Well, for me, great disillusionment. It has to do with money and power. There is not pure science going on at the NIH. A lot of what is done in medicine has not been proven by science, but it's economically supported. What I saw happen in AIDS is that overnight there were a bunch of AIDS experts. It didn't take any particular brilliance; it didn't take any dedication; it was just basically economics. And whoever got funded went up to the top.

So I began to open my eyes more and more. The very first trial that got AZT launched was a trial of death as an endpoint. There were only 60 people, I think, and after just a few weeks, more had died in the placebo group than the other. Instantly, they stopped the trials and declared it a hit. But it was not a true placebo-controlled study, because the side effects from the AZT were so bad that half of the people were having blood transfusions. The whole test was not well controlled. Then I started to realize, "My God, this isn't just AIDS; this is cancer drugs, too." Every study that validated cancer chemotherapy—did they have a truly controlled experiment or did the people who were throwing up and having their hair fall out have a placebo effect because they thought they were getting something really powerful?

There was a bias against Peptide T because it proved to be virtually entirely nontoxic. There was a prejudice: "How can this be anything if it's nontoxic?"

But I've got a big mouth, and I've already talked too much. I'm not against drugs. Drugs can be great. Hey, if you're dying and you need penicillin, penicillin can be great. And I'm not anti–mainstream medicine. If you are pregnant, it's now possible to determine if your baby has normal chromosomes. That's pretty high-tech stuff, and it's very worthwhile. I'm just anti-greed. It's very sad for me. I'm a bit isolated now, because the people I worshipped—not all of them—I see how compromised they've been. They're not really free to look at what works and what's good.

I'm speaking very frankly, but that's where I'm at today.

There have already been clinical trials with Peptide T, but now it's going on in earnest, particularly for some other uses as well. It turns out that this may well be the first effective treatment for psoriasis, and it also may be an effective treatment for chronic fatigue syndrome. It's still unbelievable to me, but it turns out that the AIDS virus is a member of closely related retroviruses that may be the cause of many human diseases. It hasn't all been discovered yet. Retroviruses were just invented by Dr. Gallo in the late 1970s. Of course, I mean discovered. I'm teasing.

We should have results about a year from now. And assuming I haven't irreversibly offended some of the companies that make these other drugs, there is a plan to team up Peptide T with some of the other treatments in combination because when you can hit a virus at two completely different points of its life cycle, there's a synergistic effect. It's called "combination therapy."

(UPDATE: I have had a "frame shift" and am less into blaming the politics of AIDS for the delay in Peptide T development and more into admitting that the science was so ahead of its time that many were incredulous. Also, I must take responsibility for making choices that did not permit needed funds for continuous Peptide T research. We now know that Peptide T blocks chemokine receptors, which the HIV uses to enter and infect cells. These receptors' role in HIV cellular entry had not yet been discovered in

1986. The October 2001 issue of Anti-Viral Research *proves that Peptide T is a potent anti-viral through chemokine receptors (Ruff et al). An ongoing clinical trial in collaboration with the National Cancer Institute at the National Institutes of Health (NIH) using low, intranasal doses of Peptide T is show- ing immune system restoration, and a new trial using high doses of intravenous drug—as was done for the Peptide T-20 AIDS drug—is being planned by Advanced Immunity, Inc., Peptide T's sponsor.)*

Religion

I grew up with religion being taboo. For most people, sex was taboo. In my house, religion was taboo. I think it was because my parents came from such diverse religious backgrounds. My mother was Jewish and my father was the son of a Congregationalist organist. So I never knew what I was. It was never discussed.

My religion has been science, and then through the science, I've seen more and more evidence of the spiritual. Now in my old age, I have a very strong spiritual inclination. I feel very spiritual but not in any traditional form.

I would define consciousness by saying that it's hooked up with God. It's ultimate knowl- edge and wisdom. In my mind, it's about communication and the information realm. It's like there's more and more information in the universe. We're all getting smarter; we're all getting wiser. Critical mass of information is happening. On some level, all the information in the universe is available to all the other information in the universe, and that, to me, is God.

There's a theory that Jesus learned from the Buddha. Buddha preached compassion and love, which is Jesus' message. This is a theme in all the world's religions, so obviously the love vibration, which is an emotion in the information realm, is pivotal. It's key. It makes us feel better; it's healing. And one day when we have totally worked out the physics of it, when we've gone beyond the biochemistry of emotion and gotten to the physics of emotion, there's no doubt that the love vibration's going to be some fundamental tone and we're going to understand why it's so healing and why it's so good. Perhaps this is the magic.

I talk about the informational aspect of God a lot in my lectures. The psychosomatic network is an information network of all my cells talking to my other cells. And when I talk to you, that's extracorporeal emotional peptide reaching. I'm not literally spreading peptides out at you, but I'm doing it with the receptor vibrations.

So when you pray, for instance, when you send thoughts out to the universe and pray for someone to get well, you are sending a peptide vibration. Remember, the mind is not just in the head—the mind is nonlocal. It's throughout the body and moves around in the body. We've all experienced consciousness being in different parts of our bodies. The next step is nonlocal, about which I'm no expert. I don't even have any real experience with prayer, but you know, I'm starting to see a lot of weird things.

Synchronicities are a piece of this. When I'm in the groove, they happen five, six, seven a day. I'm at the point where I walk into my office, the piece of paper that falls off my desk and flutters to the floor is the phone number I call first. And the guy on the other end says, "I was just thinking of you," and it will turn out to be really important that I called him at that moment. There's something going on with this connectedness among people who are plugging in. The illusion of being isolated; it's all an illusion, and I'm starting to experience that.

You really need mathematics and physics to prove it. There are experiments on subtle energies and how consciousness determines reality and how you can change mechanical events with your mind. It's not going to be a hundred years before that's all worked out. We're going to see that in our time. And there will be some young person who's been exposed to the biochemistry of these things and has the experience of it, and he'll work out how it's happening.

My intuition is there's something wonderful and exciting and promising about alternative medicine. It's sorely needed. And I think it's really frustrating for alternative practitioners right now. It's important to seek scientific validation for what you do, but I have the feeling sometimes that maybe we are holding alternative practitioners to a higher standard.

So I think alternative practitioners are too humble. They should be more proud of what they do and more assertive because I believe that they have something very valuable that helps people.

CHAPTER 4

MARTY ROSSMAN, MD

Imagery: The Body's Natural Language for Healing

Martin L. Rossman, MD, is the founder and director of the Collaborative Medicine Center (a private, holistic medical clinic that uses mind-body medicine, acupuncture, nutrition, body-work, and herbal medicine), and with David Bresler, PhD, is the cofounder and codirector of the Academy for Guided Imagery, both in Mill Valley, California. He is also a clinical associate in the Department of Medicine at the University of California Medical Center in San Francisco; chairman of the Department of Mind-Body Medicine at the University of Integral Studies in Sonora, California; and an adjunct faculty member at the California School of Professional Psychology in Alameda, California.

Dr. Rossman received his medical degree at the University of Michigan Medical School in Ann Arbor, Michigan. In addition to his conventional training, he is a diplomate of acupuncture with the National Commission for the Certification of Acupuncturists.

The author of *Guided Imagery for Self-Healing* and the tape series *Healing Yourself,* Dr. Rossman speaks and teaches nationally on the subjects of guided imagery, mind-body medicine, and self-healing. He and Dr. Bresler created a self-care series (CD and workbook) that uses guided imagery for 36 different medical and lifestyle applications, which was released in 2002 as a case-managed benefit by American Specialty Health.

In January of 2002, I interviewed Dr. Rossman, who I found to be both gentle and powerful, at his clinic in Mill Valley, California.

I have always been interested in questions like "What's our real nature?," "Why are we here?," and "What happens when we die?" I actually went to medical school with the idea of becoming a psychiatrist, but in the 1960s I was very socially motivated, and the zeitgeist I resonated with was more, "how do you bring good-quality medicine to the poor and disadvantaged?"

I graduated from the University of Michigan in 1969 and interned in Oakland. After that I practiced part-time in the Oakland County Medical Clinic and worked in the various free clinics in Berkeley and the surrounding area. I also worked with a house-call practice in east Oakland for a couple of years. During this time, I became interested in the problems of chronic illness because in a county clinic or free clinic you deal mostly with chronic illnesses. You deal with "diseases of civilization or lifestyle," as they're sometimes euphemistically called. It's the diabetic who weighs 300 pounds and still eats donuts four times a day or the chronic lung patient who smokes three packs a day and is mad at you because you can't get rid of his cough.

I've always enjoyed interacting with the people in my practice, but after a couple of years the practice of medicine seemed like a futile dance. I would put patients on medication and they'd feel better for a while, but a few months later they would have side effects. Then I'd either put them on another medication to treat the adverse effects of the first medication, or

I'd take them off the medication. They'd feel better for a while and then they'd come back feeling bad again.

What happened is that in caring for these people and trying to help them, I got burned out. Many doctors can relate to this. You're working hard to try to help people get better, yet it seems like they're working hard to keep themselves sick. You can end up being mad at your patients and then what have you got? Nothing, because a practice is really a series of relationships with people.

So that's how I became interested in the question: How do you get people to care for themselves?

It's why I call my practice "Collaborative Medicine." It's my attempt to encourage my patients to participate more in their own healing.

But to get back to the original question: imagery started doing me before I even knew anything about imagery. I remember the day when I knew I couldn't do it anymore. I literally had a vision. It was like a theater marquee with lights around it, and it said, "I quit."

I told myself that if this was what the practice of medicine was about, then I had to find something else to do. I didn't know what it was, but I knew I couldn't spend my life practicing medicine the way it was practiced at that time.

As fate would have it—you know what synchronicity is—the very next day at a medical staff meeting they showed a videotape of the American Medical Association's first visit to China in 1971. In the videotape, people were having major surgeries with acupuncture anesthesia. One surgeon was cutting a man's ribs open and lifting a section of his lung out and the man was awake and talking to the nurses who were feeding him little sections of mandarin orange, litchi nuts, and sips of tea. The top of my head just about blew off. It was so beyond anything that I had ever seen. At the end of the operation, the surgeons sat the man up and bandaged him. Then he put an arm around each surgeon and they walked him out of the operating room.

The head of the delegation was a surgeon from Columbia University named Samuel Rosen, who happened to be one of my medical heroes. Rosen invented an operation that restored hearing for some people by replacing one of the little inner-ear bones. On the videotape he said, "We don't know what's happening here. We saw a hundred of these operations and there's something very real going on that deserves immediate, serious investigation." So I took that as my cue.

I was able to spend three months with two Chinese psychiatrists who were doing the first research study on acupuncture for pain relief in this country. They were treating intractable pain patients—rejects from the Mayo Clinic, Case Western Reserve University, or the University of Michigan. I would examine them and go through their histories and then the two psychiatrists performed some straightforward acupuncture with electrostimulation. It was very clear to me that acupuncture was able to help a lot of those people.

When I came back to California, I opened a practice in Stinson Beach. I was the only one in Marin County doing acupuncture at the time. You couldn't get any training then, so we were all just reading books and talking to other people. And that's what brought me in touch with a physician in Bolinas, California, named Irving Oyle.

Irving is one of the unknown fathers of holistic medicine. He was a general practitioner from New York—a very sharp clinician with the gift of gab—who retired in Bolinas. He was interested in mind-body, and in the early 1970s he went on a number of trips to Russia and Czechoslovakia with people like Stanley Krippner and Stanislav Grof to study psychokinesis, extrasensory perception, and things of that nature.

There was a big oil spill close by, so he and a few other local doctors opened a clinic to help treat the volunteers. Then they stayed open because they had a mutual interest in what was emerging at the time. They were interested in acupuncture, biofeedback, meditation, the relaxation response, visualization, massage, and nutrition. Oyle was quite visionary, and the thing he was most excited about was consciousness. He was very big on Carl Jung, and he is the one who got me to study Jungian psychology and imagery.

The Language of the Unconscious

The reason I'm interested in imagery is that it seems to be the natural language of the unconscious. I've been referring to it lately as the Rosetta stone of the mind-body-spirit.

Imagery is a coding language of the nervous system. It carries information in such a way that what we call the body and the mind and the spirit are able to communicate through and respond to it. It seems to be a language or vehicle through which we can explore whatever it is that we are.

I'm not sure anybody has ever talked about this in terms of the history of the mind-body holistic movement, but one of the things that introduced many of us to imagery was a funny little course called Silva Mind Control.

Silva Mind Control was developed by a man named José Silva, and it is taught all over the world. It's a basic self-hypnosis course. You are taught to go to a sanctuary inside where you have controls that you use to call up pictures and images of anything you want to know more about. Part of the process is that an elevator comes down into your room and two guides come out. You can talk with the guides about anything. Silva Mind Control also teaches healing methods such as a visualization in which a person focuses on an area of the body—one's own or somebody else's—and changes the image to one that is healthy. It also teaches people how to diagnose at a distance through the images.

It was a wild time. Murray Korngold, Efrem Korngold's father, taught us the Silva course. Using what he had learned from Silva and Jung, Oyle would work successfully with patients day after day after day in the clinic in Bolinas. I was his devil's advocate for about 3 years, trying to punch holes in his logic. But after he demonstrated to me over and over and over again how much people could know and do if they used their minds in a certain way, I finally stopped fighting it.

In many ways, imagery is probably the oldest medicine there is. Every ancient culture had imagery-based rituals. They might have been called prayer or sacrifice or ceremony or taking a journey to another world, such as a shamanic healer might say, but however they explained it, the methods are similar. For instance, with shamanic healing you go looking for help and call up power animals or guides. You might encounter and negotiate or do battle with a spirit that is believed to be involved in the creation of the illness in question. But if you take away the elaborate ritual that the shaman participates in—the days of fasting and the rattling and the dancing and the sacrifices and possibly the psychedelic substances—the process looks pretty similar to guided imagery in terms of what actually happens.

So I tell people that I don't know if we're dealing with angels or spirits or power animals or guides or if it's just a part of the mind; I'm interested, but as a physician, I don't care. I care about what effect it has on you and whether it makes your headache go away. Do you feel more powerful in relation to dealing with your tumor or your arthritis? That's really what I'm looking for.

Some of the Western roots of imagery go back to the ancient Greeks. Aristotle said that imagination was a window to the soul, and the Greeks actually considered the imagination to be an organ. Their schema was that you took in the world through your senses, and your senses subtracted the matter.

It's true that our senses are data-reduction systems. Scientists tell us that we live in an energy soup of every possible frequency. But our eyes only see a certain frequency, so they select out the vibrations of that frequency, and now we have you and me sitting here in this room. The ears select out another frequency and the olfactory nerves another, and when we put those frequencies together, we construct a perception of the world.

So, the Greeks said that the senses take in the world, subtract the matter, and form an image in the psyche, which was their term for soul and which they believed lived in the heart. Now some of those images stimulated emotions, either positive or negative, and the emotions are what drove the circulation of the humors. Their model of the universe was that there were four different humors, four different kinds of substances or energies that, once combined, made all of physical reality.

It was the physics of the time, much like the Chinese five-element system. But the Greeks had a four-element system. The humors circulated around the body, and it was the balance between the humors and circulation of the humors that either supported your health or, through their imbalance, deficiency, or excess, made you sick. What's interesting about this model is that if you substitute the word "hormones" or "peptides" for "humors," you get a very up-to-date model for what we think are the mechanisms of mind-body medicine.

Treating the Whole Person

Sometimes—at least when you're dealing with stress-induced illness and maybe far beyond that—we have perceptions of consensual reality that make us sick. We all have our own perception of what's going on, and our own worldview is, in a very real sense, an image. We have an image of who we are and the world we live in and our relationship to it. It's a complex image that you can tease out of somebody if you pay attention. Most of the time we don't pay attention—it's simply deeply unconscious. But our images of who we think we are, what we think the world is, how we relate to it, and what we think we deserve are the basis of how we care for ourselves on a day-to-day basis.

So I have a perception of what's going on around me and some of those perceptions will lead to the stimulation of emotions. Emotions are normal, but sometimes we're overwhelmed by them, or we get stuck in one emotion, or we never feel a certain emotion. Our society is relatively emotionally illiterate. We handle our anger and anxiety very poorly. We handle compassion and joy pretty well, but we have difficulty with sadness, grief, fear, and anger. We either stuff them away or express them destructively. The drinking, smoking, drugs, violence, depression—I think all of it is evidence of an epidemic of unresolved emotional pain.

Chinese medicine, like all ancient medicines, teaches us that seasons cycle. Things are supposed to keep moving. We're not supposed to stay stuck in one place. We're not supposed to be angry all the time or never be angry or always be scared or never be scared or always be sad. If we get stuck in an unbalanced position, we tend to develop behaviors that are bad for our health, and somewhere along the line something breaks down. It's very often a direct or indirect consequence of how we're handling emotions.

The emotions are physiologically different from each other. We're finally getting to the place where scientists can physiologically characterize one emotion from another by measuring your breathing rate, your muscle tension, your levels of catecholamines in the blood, and so forth. The emotions are chemically different from each other, which is why they feel different. They have different patterns of muscle tension, of vasodilation, of endocrine output, of peptide output, and so on. And, again, if it's temporary and it flows and the situation resolves, it's no big deal. But if we live in a highly aroused state for a long time, eventually something breaks down.

Then, as far as I'm concerned, we make another error and call it a disease and try to make it go away without addressing its origins.

Let's say the oil light is on in your car. What you do is that you find out what's going on. Maybe you need to top off your oil or maybe you need a ring job or maybe the fuse is stuck. But there aren't 10 people in America who would take their car into a gas station and say, "Would you please rip the wires out? The oil light being on is making me nervous."

If we treated our cars the way we treat our bodies, that's what we'd do. We'd take it into the station and say, "The light's on and I've got a lot to do, so can you tape over it? Can you rip the wires out? I've got to be on my way."

But that's how we practice medicine. It's all "anti": it's antihypertensive, antidepressive, antianxiety, antibiotics, antiinflammatory. Largely it's because we don't really understand the nature of more than 90% of all the diseases we diagnose. We may know what the body looks like with the disease, or what people who had it look like after they're dead, or we might know some data about the pathology of it, but it's very rare that we step back and say to somebody, "Hey, the oil light's on. What do you think is going on?"

We don't ask what's happening with the whole person. What's happening in your life? How are you feeling? What's your stress level? How have you been taking care of yourself lately? This doesn't mean we shouldn't look for serious diseases for which we may have life-saving interventions, but, truthfully, only a small percentage of people who go to the doctor are that sick.

Imagery and its Uses

A symptom is a signal, so for me, one of the most striking uses of imagery is to answer the question "What does it mean?"

As doctors, we're taught to look for patterns of symptoms and signs that we classify as diseases and then try to treat, but in doing this, we've cut the patient out of the equation. I think this is one of the big things that is wrong with our whole medical system, and it's one of the potentially great things about the new influence coming from complementary and alternative medicine (CAM) therapies. But it's also one of the dangers that must be addressed so that we do not degenerate into a focus on the separate modalities. Yes, modalities are important. Extensive knowledge and skill are required to do good acupuncture and Chinese herbal medicine; nutritionists need knowledge and skill; and homeopathy is a lifelong study. All these things are important. But what's really alternative about alternative medicine is that it goes back to the understanding that you have a whole human being who has innate healing abilities that are built into him or her by nature or God.

People have a mind that can influence their health for better or worse, and they can learn how to use that mind to participate in the process of healing. The choices and decisions they make every day will affect, to some degree, whether they are going to heal or not.

I don't think it's all under our control, but you can certainly move it in one direction or another and sometimes to a startling degree.

Western medicine is the only medicine I've ever studied or heard of that doesn't appreciate that life is different from anything else we know. Whether you call it *life force* or *qi* or *prana*, it's self-repairing. Who knows where it comes from, and who knows where it goes, but it's capable of incredible healing. And it's totally ignored. Not only do we ignore it; we look down our nose at it because it's not scientific. Our attitude is very bizarre, and it's painful to everybody, including the doctors, because it's disempowering.

The Process

The first thing I do is spend time with a patient and complete a good medical workup. I'm not going to train someone to do imagery without knowing if he or she has a brain tumor. But the history I take is very expanded. I try to get to know the person and understand what his or her life situation is like. We call it a psychosocial history, and I may even get a spiritual history, depending on my sense of the person. Imagery is not something that you do *to* somebody; it's something that you do *with* somebody, so you have to have a sense of rapport and trust. You're not going to reveal intimate things about yourself, even to yourself, in the presence of somebody you don't trust.

So you've got to take however much time it takes to establish rapport. Say I have a patient with migraine headaches who's new to imagery. First I make sure she's had a good diagnostic evaluation and that we're really dealing with migraines. Then we may go through the physiology of migraines and how stress and relaxation play into that. For some people it's useful to know that there is a physiology behind it or that being stressed doesn't mean they're crazy or bad. And I usually share some of the research studies that show that regular, good relaxation practices prevent migraines just as effectively as the common drugs but with no side effects.

If the patient is willing, I'll also guide her through the body scan or a simplified progressive muscular-relaxation exercise. You know: paying attention to the feet, the ankles, the shins, and then each muscle group up through the body. I'll either do this myself or give her a tape to take home, depending on the time factor.

The first imagery I introduce patients to is a kind of ubiquitous image of a beautiful, safe place that they love to be in. I just ask them to imagine themselves in some beautiful place where it's peaceful, safe, secure. It could be a place they've been to or an imaginary place or a combination. It doesn't matter as long as it's beautiful, peaceful, safe, and secure.

Once they are there, we usually do imagery in an interactive mode. I'll ask them what they imagine seeing there and they'll describe whatever they see. I'll say, "What else do you see? What do you hear?" And they will say things like, "The birds are singing and there's some breeze in the trees." Some people tell me that it's very quiet or that they hear the sound of the stream. Then I'll ask about an aroma or fragrance. Some people will smell and some people won't. Either way is fine. I'll ask them what the temperature is like, what time of day it is, and what season of the year it is.

Basically, this is a hypnotic technique called *sensory recruitment*. You ask people to pay attention to each of their senses and describe what they perceive, because imagery is sensory-based thought. Imagery is thoughts that you can see or hear or smell or feel or some combination. And it's different from abstract thinking in words and numbers because it's based on senses.

For example, do you have a sensation for the number four? Do you have a sensory-based equivalent of four? You can imagine patterns of four things, but the number four is an abstraction just like liberty is an abstraction.

The kind of thinking humans are able to do with words and numbers that allows us to make calculations so we can send a rocket to Jupiter that will circle around the planet and come back to earth and land somewhere in the ocean is amazing. But they are abstractions. There's no sensory-based reality involved. And, for the most part, we mentally live in that world, while our emotions and bodies are much more highly attuned and responsive to the world of the senses.

We've all had a lot of education in linear, logical thinking. It's verbal and mathematic. Some people call it left-brained. Our whole educational system is based around it, and almost no one has had formal education in using the imagination as a thinking tool. So when we train professionals through our academy—the Academy for Guided Imagery—we're doing remedial education. We're teaching people how to use an incredible mental faculty that few of them have ever learned to use purposefully.

There is a physiological difference between sensory thought and abstract thought. We've learned from research with devices like magnetic resonance imaging (MRI) that you can actually watch which parts of the brain are active at any given time. When you ask people to visualize something, the parts of their brains that process visual information get active. Their occipital cortex lights up on functional MRIs. When you ask them to imagine their favorite tune or passage of music, their temporal cortex, which processes sound, becomes active. If you ask them to imagine doing something physical like walking, their premotor cortex gets activated. So when you imagine things, the part of your brain that processes that sensory information becomes activated.

So what we now think is that if you imagine yourself to be in a quiet place that looks beautiful and sounds peaceful and smells good, then you're activating all these different parts of the cortex. Your cortex is sending messages down through your hypothalamus to the rest of your body, and so your body goes into a relaxation response. A lot of reparative, restorative, and renewal processes happen more efficiently in the relaxation state than when you're battling the dragons, real or imaginary, of daily life. It's also a state of which most of us are deprived.

Back in 1968, Benson and Wallace published "Physiology of Meditation" in *Scientific American*, and showed that certain repair processes, like the cleaning of lactic acid metabolites from muscles, happened four and one-half times faster in a relaxed state.

I think that for many people, imagery is the easiest way to get to a healing state. Many of us almost never experience this state because we're either sleeping or trying to sleep or we're up and we're busy and we're stressed and we're focused on the outside world. But by nature we are probably meant to spend some time in each of those states. Natural-living humans, even though I wouldn't want to trade places with them, aren't always busy. They have down time. They've got their hunts and occasional wars and natural disasters, but in between they spend a lot of time hanging out in hammocks and playing with their kids and just doodling around.

What I tell my patients with chronic illnesses is that even if you do nothing else, do this because your body knows how to heal. I really believe that you don't need to direct your body on how to heal. What you need to do is get out of the way. You didn't have to sit in your mother's womb and visualize your arm and your eye sockets. That's carrying responsibility a little too far. The thing that knows how to make you knows how to heal you. What you do need to do is give it a chance.

So I tell my patients to go to their healing place and hang out. And if you want company, invite somebody in. It's your imagination, so you can have anybody there you want. You can do whatever you want. And if your mind wanders, use that place as your focus of attention. So it's in place of a mantra. Not that there's anything wrong with a mantra, but use that place of peace, that place of healing, to come back and focus the mind. Then, I think, a lot of healing happens by itself.

This is the first step, and almost everybody's successful in it.

Active Guided Imagery

About 30 years ago, the Simontons theorized that by visualizing—symbolically or anatomically—an active and vigorous immune system attacking the cancer, a person could stimulate his or her immune system. We now know that's correct. There are about 20 studies that show this. When people image their immune system stimulated, they not only increase the number of circulating natural killer cells, but the thymus gland actually puts out more thymic hormones that put the cells on a higher state of alert and responsiveness when they encounter an intruder like a virus or cancer cell.

There's enough evidence now that if this were in pill form, every patient in America who had a situation that needed immune stimulation would be on that pill or doctors would be guilty of malpractice. There is mind-body literature showing the benefit of imagery in all kinds of medical situations and events. Imagery doesn't cure everything, but there is tremendous benefit to people in everything from reducing anxiety and depression to increasing comfort, making surgeries go smoother, stimulating the immune system, and relieving pain. We just need to get the information into the medical schools so it becomes part of standard care.

But just because we can stimulate immunity with visualization doesn't mean that we don't need to treat people who have cancer with chemotherapy or surgery or radiation. But it does mean that we can effectively augment their treatment in a way that has no toxic adverse effect.

If I have a sore throat then I'll stretch out and let whatever image is happening at the time emerge. Once again, using the oil-light theory, there's something going on that I haven't had room to pay attention to, so I want to do that. But I will also imagine that all the blood vessels in my throat are open and that all the blood is coming into the area, because the body brings all its healing elements through the blood. The blood also washes away all that nasty inflamed material. Then I will imagine that the white cells are coming and gobbling up all the goop and that there are little guys in there with brushes who are painting my throat with soothing anti-septic liquids. All kinds of things have worked over the years and it's amazing how different you can feel in 10 minutes.

So that's healing imagery, and it's often the second thing we'll teach somebody, though it's very often the first thing I'll teach somebody who's had a life-threatening illness diagnosed.

Very often when people with cancer come to see me, they're in shock. Their bodies have been invaded by something strange and foreign that they never expected and don't understand. They feel frightened because it's not under their control, and the messages they too often receive from medical encounters tend to reinforce their sense of helplessness. That's why the model I like best for cancer treatment now is the integrated model. The purpose of radiation and chemotherapy and surgery is to reduce the number of cancer cells. CAM is about changing the terrain where that cancer could occur and nourishing the body, mind, and spirit on whatever levels are needed to create a stronger organism. So as you're reducing the cancer cells, you're also improving the immunity and vitality and livability of the organism, and that combination, I'm sure, is going to pay off with better cancer treatment.

Guides

The third and often most powerful use of imagery is its ability to connect people to both information and resources they have inside. If you look at my book or tapes or the way we teach professionals at the academy, the order in which we introduce things is relaxation, directive imagery like the healing imagery we've discussed, and then receptive imagery. If you use the oil-light model, receptive imagery is looking under the hood. And very often we'll use an imaginary intermediary that we call the inner adviser.

People have a lot of different names for this: inner guide or guardian angel or spirit guide or the God within. What we do is characterize the inner adviser as a figure who has two specific qualities: wisdom and compassion.

So I'd have you relax and go to your special place, and then invite an inner adviser—an image that's both wise and loving—to appear.

We encourage people to let that be however it comes, just so long as it's wise and loving, for several reasons. One is a safety issue. Generally when you have a life-threatening situation, there will be emotions and issues that are hard to deal with. There may be anger, or rage, or sad feelings that we've walled off. There may be fear or even terror. And we instinctively know that if we open the box it could be painful. So instead of going to that box directly, let an image come that is caring and wise and have a talk with that image about what to do with what's in the box.

If you were going on a safari in Africa, it would be nice to have somebody who knew his way around who would help you stay out of trouble. The inner guide is the same thing. It provides a safety buffer.

Then, my job as an imagery guide is to help you connect with your own imagination and to support you in asking the questions that are important to you. I will also help you hold the space where you can let the information come to you. My function is to be relatively free of content and to act as a facilitator in the process.

Your unconscious mind speaks in images and symbols, and that's a language your conscious mind may not have learned. So my function is to facilitate a conversation between your conscious mind and your unconscious mind.

This goes back to what we started talking about in the beginning, which is how to get people to care for themselves. One thing that truly doesn't work is telling people what to do. It just mobilizes resistance. Rachel Remen puts it in a beautiful way. She says, "The doctor could fall into the trap of becoming the voice of the disease," because you're telling people to take their insulin or not eat the donuts or so on. So here's this person diagnosed with diabetes. He hates it, and he doesn't want to have it, and he doesn't want the label, and he doesn't want to think about it. And now the doctor or diabetes educator or nurse keeps telling him about behaviors he should do, and he's getting more and more resistant. It feels like you're working against each other, and it's very confusing to the practitioner. But by learning some different communication skills and a different way of being collaborative and helpful with people, you can actually help them come to terms within themselves in a way that lets them take care of themselves.

When information comes from a source that is wise and loving and is inside the person, the information often has a power that it doesn't have when it comes from the outside.

Case Reports

Here is a story. A fellow in his late 50s was diagnosed with diabetes. He was a bright, successful guy with his own company and a wife and four daughters. Everyone loved him. But since he was diagnosed, his doctor of many years could not get him to take care of himself, eat right, exercise, or lose some weight. The man was on a couple of medications that he took erratically, and his blood sugars were way up. The doctor tried to scare him: "You're going to lose your eyes; your heart's going to go bad; you're going to lose your feet." The diabetes educators couldn't get him to take care of himself, either. And this is a really common story.

Finally the doctor sent him to me. We talked about the imagery and he was willing to try it. So he relaxed and went to a quiet place. I said, "Focus on diabetes—the word diabetes and the whole idea of diabetes—and let an image come to mind that represents the diabetes."

After a few minutes, he said, "It's like a big, heavy, black ball chained around my ankle."

I asked him to tell me about the ball and he said, "It's heavy; it's black; and it's chained to my ankle so I can't move. I drag it around and it's interfering with everything I do."

I asked him how he felt about it and he said, "I want it to go away. I absolutely hate it."

I began facilitating a dialogue between him and the image by asking him to tell the ball how he felt about it, which he did. He told the ball that he hated it. Then I told him to let it respond and to tell me what happened.

He was quiet for a minute and then he got a funny look on his face and said, "You know, it's sad. This is crazy, but it's got a little face on it, and it's frowning and looks sad."

I asked him if he felt any differently now about the ball, and he said, "Now I kind of feel sorry for it." After he let the ball know that he felt sorry for it, he got into a conversation with it. The ball told him that it was really sorry for interfering with his life and for making him carry it around. It told him that it didn't mean to hurt him, but it was just exhausted and couldn't move or go any further. It started telling him that while he had tons of energy, it couldn't keep up with him anymore.

So I said, "Ask the ball what you can do about it."

By this time he said, "This ball is not a ball anymore. It's a dog. It's this little black poodle." So then he gave the dog something to eat.

To make a long story short, he began to like the dog. As he was having a further conversation with it, he asked what he could do about the dog being exhausted. The dog told him that it just needed the usual things that any dog needs. It needed water and good food, to be walked twice a day, and to sleep when it was tired. The dog said it also appreciated a scratch on the back and time to play.

So I asked him, "How do you feel about that?"

And the man said, "That makes sense, any dog needs that." Then this man got a big smile on his face because he realized he was actually promising it to himself. After that, the man started doing all the stuff that everyone had been trying to get him to do because he finally realized that there was a part of him that couldn't go on unless he took care of himself.

I think it's one of the best examples of how you get yourself out of the middle. As a compassionate person and a physician, I wanted him to take care of himself, but there was no way I could do it without his participation. And making him feel bad or bossing him around wouldn't work. That's why I'm so excited about this. This process is a life changer for doctors and patients alike.

Here is an example of the difference between the directed or active imagery and the receptive.

I took a year off to write my first book about 15 years ago. I wanted to see what was possible in terms of healing with imagery, so during that year I conducted a private study with a dozen patients. They had to have a serious, incurable disease and be willing to see me 12 times so we could get deeply involved with imagery to see how much healing could be done. And I did not charge anyone.

One of these patients was a young woman about 31 years old. She had been diagnosed with a serious autoimmune disease called *polymyositis*, a disease in which a person's own immune system eats away at the muscles. The characteristic symptoms were pains in her arms and legs, and her upper arms were wasting away. It's a serious disease, usually fatal, and there's no known medical cure. She was on super-high doses of steroids when she came to see me but was getting progressively worse.

As we talked about her history, she told me that she had been working for this guy as his right-hand person. He produced television commercials and became very successful very fast. At first, they were making a lot of money and having a great time. Then all of a sudden he started disappearing for days and then weeks at a time, and she found herself as basically a secretary in charge of a multimillion-dollar television production business. When he came back, he would sometimes be full of praise, and other times he'd come in raging and yelling and screaming and throwing tantrums. It turned out that this guy had developed a bad cocaine habit and was getting crazy. She was stressed to the gills and after 8 months of this, the disease started to develop.

In our first session, I taught her to relax and to go to a quiet, peaceful place. The next week she came back with a new symptom. She had a burning stomach pain she'd never had before. Medically it was probably from the steroids, because that is a common side effect, but I suggested that it might be a good opportunity to see if there was something she could do with her mind or with imagery to give herself some pain relief.

I told her to put her attention directly on the pain and let any image come to mind that represented the pain, and she saw her stomach lining as a fire.

I asked her what she would do to help heal it or relieve the pain if the fire was the symptom. She came up with water, so I said, "Imagine you have a source of water and you can spray it on the fire." She told me she was imaging that she had a garden hose and was spraying the fire. Then she told me that it was fizzling and smoking. About 2 minutes later she said, "I actually feel as if it's cooling off."

I reminded her that it was her imagination and that she could have as much water as she wanted. So then she began to soak it with fire hoses.

Her pain was completely gone in about 10 minutes, and she was delighted. As she was leaving, I reminded her that she could do this any time she wanted. She canceled the next week's appointment and told me, "I get the burning once in a while, but I can always put it out. I've got a cold mountain stream going through it now and everything's healing up nicely." But the next week when she came in, she was crying. No matter how much water she put on it, she could not put out the fire.

We went through the relaxation process and I had her focus on the pain again. I asked her to let another image come to mind. After a minute she said, "There's this hand and it's pinching the lining of my stomach." I asked her what she wanted to do about it and she said, "I want it to stop."

I told her to tell it to stop, but she said, "It won't stop. It won't let go."

I had her ask the imaginary hand why it was pinching her stomach. When she did that, the hand let go of her stomach and turned into a fist that began shaking at her. When she asked it why it was angry with her, it turned into a finger that was pointing up into her heart. So I said, "Look where it's pointing and tell me what you see."

She grew teary and said, "My heart's in this big burlap bag and there's all kinds of sharp, pointed objects in there with it and everything's zooming and buzzing around. The hand is angry because I'm letting my heart get pierced." When I asked her what she wanted to do about it, she said, "I don't know."

Now normally if I'm doing a good job of being an interactive guide, I don't suggest anything, but this time I said, "How about opening the bag and letting it out?" Well, she almost had a full-blown anxiety attack. So I quickly told her that she didn't have to open the bag.

At this point, I introduced her to the inner adviser. An archetypal, wise old American Indian woman with beautiful, soft, brown eyes comes to her in buckskins and braids. She was a very wise earth mother and said, "Very slowly and carefully untie the bag and just let one thing out and then close it up again." She also said, "There's no one thing in that bag that you can't deal with."

So she slowly and carefully untied the knot, let one thing come out of the bag, and then tied the knot. The thing that came out of the bag was the face of her stepfather.

Her parents were divorced when she was young and her mother married a guy who was quite nice except when he got drunk. As things progressed, he became more and more alcoholic. One night she heard a big ruckus from downstairs. She went downstairs and her mother was lying on the ground. So she ran up and jumped on her stepfather, hitting him on the back and screaming at him to leave her mother alone. He turned around and grabbed her by her upper arms and screamed in her face, "If you ever hit me again, I'll kill you."

So here she has developed a disease in which her own immune system has started taking away the muscles on her upper arms, right where her stepfather was holding them. And it started in the context of her not being able to control a difficult situation and being at the mercy of an unpredictable and intermittently rageful addict. The parallels between her illness and her imagery memories were absolutely startling.

It doesn't always work like this, but it's an amazing story. After that session we worked on two levels: we worked on physical healing where we had talks with her immune system and her muscles, and then we worked on her life situation. She realized that she kept getting in relationships with the same types of guys, so I referred her to a good therapist and she did a couple of years of therapy. Her disease was rapidly progressing beforehand, and while it did not go away, it did stop progressing. Over a 2-month period we were able to get her down to five mg of prednisone every other day from more than 80 mg a day. I have since lost track of her, but she was in remission for at least 12 years that I know of.

This is a great example of what can happen when doctors include the patient in the equation. If I had left her out of the equation, she would have been dead. But she is the equation. And the cure isn't in the disease. The cure is in the person.

Helping people to mobilize their healing abilities—that's really our academy mission. My partner David Bresler and I believe very deeply in bringing the whole person back into the healing equation and empowering people to learn more about their own healing abilities. We feel that teaching professionals and the public to access their innate abilities is the best thing we can do to improve public health.

CHAPTER 5

KEN PELLETIER, PhD, MD (HC)

Mind-Body Medicine

Ken Pelletier, PhD, MD (hc) is a clinical professor of medicine at the University of Maryland School of Medicine (UMMC) and the University of Arizona School of Medicine. He is also a medical and business advisor to the National Institutes of Health; the World Health Organization; and many major corporations, including American Airlines, Medtronic, Disney, Merck, Ford, Microsoft, and Blue Cross Blue Shield. Dr. Pelletier received a doctoral degree in clinical psychology from the University of California at Berkeley in 1974.

Now the director of the Corporate Health Improvement Program (CHIP) at UMMC, he was previously the director of the Stanford Corporate Health Program and clinical professor of medicine at the Stanford University School of Medicine. Presently he is the chairman of the American Health Association and a vice president of Healthtrac, Inc.

Dr. Pelletier is the author of 10 books, including *Mind as Healer, Mind as Slayer; Sound Mind, Sound Body; Holistic Medicine: From Stress to Optimum Health; Longevity: Fulfilling our Biological Potential;* and *The Best Alternative Medicine: What Works? What Doesn't?*

I interviewed Dr. Pelletier, whose lifelong passion is ocean sailing, in the summer of 2002 at his home and horse farm in northern California.

After I graduated from my undergraduate years at Berkeley, I had a 2-year fellowship, during which I traveled through Europe, the Near East and North Africa. At one point, I ended up on the Greek island Ios. Ios is to the Greek Orthodox Church what Lourdes is to the Catholic Church—a place of miracles. I happened to be there during a pilgrimage to a church on that island, and I saw changes in people that defied explanation.

People in wheelchairs would stand up; people who were obviously in excruciating pain would then seemed to be relieved of pain; and people who had terribly deformed hands, probably due to arthritis, would suddenly flex their hands and move their limbs. I was astounded. The things I was seeing didn't conform to any understanding I had of neurophysiology and anatomy and how the body is supposed to work. That experience has stayed with me, and I've had an abiding curiosity ever since.

In the early 1970s, when I was conducting research at the University of California-San Francisco (UCSF) School of Medicine, there was a huge controversy about whether or not people could voluntarily regulate or control autonomic functions such as brain waves, heart rate, pain perception, and blood pressure. I remembered the incidents in Greece and felt that something about a person's beliefs could influence his or her physiology beyond the boundaries we normally think possible. But it occurred to me that you couldn't address this issue or solve the problem if you studied the usual 50 sophomore research volunteers. My idea was to study adept meditators or people who had practiced and developed demonstrable mind-body abilities.

So that's what we did. At that time, Dr. Charles Yeager, a professor of neurology at UCSF and the head of electroencephalography, conducted all the EEG analyses for me. We needed about $5000 to finish the experiments, so I asked Charles if he knew of anyone who could help us. Charlie said, "My brother-in law is interested in seeing strange things. I'll see if he can help us fund this study." And, sure enough, he did.

When we finished the research, Charlie said, "My brother-in-law would like you to come back to Michigan and give a presentation." Well, Charles' brother-in-law turned out to be John Fetzer. At the time, Fetzer owned the Detroit Tigers and the largest radio network in the Great Lakes area, though he is best known today for founding the Fetzer Institute. So I went to Michigan, made the presentation, and John and I stayed friends throughout his life. In fact, one of the last interviews he ever gave was at age 96 for my book, *Sound Mind, Sound Body*, since he embodied that platonic ideal.

The results of the research were fascinating. We tested three individuals—a karate expert, a drug smuggler, and a meditation teacher. We started with the karate expert, who would take a sharpened bicycle spoke and put it through his forearm. Then he'd suspend a heavy weight from the spoke and focus the qi using karate. We monitored 24 multiple EEG channels and other neuropsychological indices, including muscle tension, respiration rate and pattern, and heart rate and regularity.

Somehow, a writer from *Playboy* found out about the research and wanted to interview me. So I said "fine." Except I never realized how many people in the military and in prisons read *Playboy*. I was inundated with letters after the article came out. One prisoner in San Quentin wrote and claimed, "I can do that" and sent me some clippings of when he worked a circus sideshow. It took months of negotiations with the California Department of Corrections, but we finally got permission for him to come to the laboratory. So we had a heavily armed highway patrolman with a man in an orange prison uniform in the lab, which lent a whole new dimension to the idea of saffron meditation robes.

This convicted drug smuggler would take three bicycle spokes and put them through the cheeks of his face—in one side through his oral cavity and out the other. He'd learned to do this because he had been shot or wounded a number of times while smuggling and had taught himself how to control bleeding and pain in order not to be discovered or die. He also performed feats like breathing fire and eating light bulbs. We learned a lot from him.

Then the final person we studied was Jack Schwarz, a Dutch meditator who also taught meditation for many years. I knew that Jack had been studied by Dr. Elmer Green at the Menninger Foundation, so we contacted him. Within the course of an intensive 1-week study, Jack took a large-diameter knitting needle and pushed it completely through his biceps and out the other side. We filmed it and meticulously addressed every single objection that there had been to the prior research and tried to answer each one. Researchers said, "Maybe these people don't respond to pain normally," so we conducted standardized pain response tests. They said, "Maybe these people don't bleed normally, maybe they clot unusually quickly," so we did standard bleeding time and clotting time tests. From very rigorous testing, we established that Jack's physiology in a nonmeditative state was absolutely normal. But when he meditated and went into a deep meditative state, his neurophysiology altered profoundly such that he did not experience pain, did not bleed, did not experience infection, did not even experience the normal immunological response. We demonstrated this absolutely and definitively.

We also explored what happened to a person as he or she learned such mind-body disciplines. We wanted to know what happened internally, not just what was evident. Jack had been in the Dutch resistance. After being captured by the Nazis, he was put in a concentration camp, beaten regularly, and starved. At one point when he was being beaten, he passed out. Now, Jack grew up as a Dutch Catholic. When he passed out while being tortured, he found himself at the foot of the cross of the crucifixion at Calvary. He always thought that when Jesus said, "Father, why has thou forsaken me?" that he looked upward toward the sky. By contrast, in Jack's vision, he said that Jesus looked into the eye of every person and said, "Why has thou forsaken me?" When he came out of his reverie and from that time forward, he said to the people who had been torturing him, "I love you." From that point on, the Nazis thought Jack had gone completely wacky, and they left him alone. But also from that point forward he found that he could control pain and bleeding. Jack taught other people in the concentration camp how to survive by controlling bleeding and pain and resisting the torture.

The cumulative paper we published about these three individuals was heretical. Essentially, it was the first definitive demonstration that individuals could regulate multiple autonomic functions, such as the brain, the heart, respiration, and the pulse. At first it was rejected by the *Journal of Clinical and Experimental Hypnosis.* They didn't believe us. Their editor was Dr. Martin Orne, of the University of Pennsylvania, who was an outspoken critic at the time. That is why we submitted the research to this journal. We had to submit our original data tapes for external review before the article could be published. But in the end, it had many profound consequences because we demonstrated unequivocally and with absolute rigor that it was possible for trained individuals or adept meditators to regulate multiple autonomic functions, and that opened up a whole field of work for people.

What happened next was that the Montreal Neuropsychiatric Institute in Canada and the Canadian Broadcasting Company (CBC) series called *The Nature of Things* taped a documentary film about our research with Jack. Most recently in 2001, when *48 Hours* produced a program focused on pain, they discovered the CBC footage and contacted me. They said, "We have a man who self-mutilates, and we want to know is this a real phenomenon, and if it is, what does it have to do with pain control?" It was an interesting perspective from my 1974 research to a *48 Hours* documentary in 2001.

As a result of all this, pain is now considered to be the fifth vital sign; pain is now recognized as a major syndrome, and the fact that people can self-regulate certain aspects of pain has become accepted. This has applications with many clinical conditions like chronic arthritis pain, phantom limb pain, and intractable back pain. Patients don't report that the pain disappears but rather that their perception of the pain is profoundly altered. Like Jack Schwarz—he said that if he stuck himself with the needle without meditating it would be very painful, but when he does it while meditating, it feels like his own finger pressing against his arm. You can alter the perception of pain.

So the practical applications of mind-body interventions in pain syndromes really grew out of this and other pioneering research. Today, the use of biofeedback and the ability to self-regulate certain autonomic functions, the use of meditation, yoga, the Asian martial arts, and many other mind-body techniques are mainstream.

The Efficacy of Mind-Body Interventions

When I was writing *The Best Alternative Medicine,* I took my usual agnostic view and completed extensive literature researches. Much to my surprise and delight, mind-body interventions turned out to be, on a scientific basis, the most extensively documented area of alternative medicine with efficacy for the largest number of people with the largest variety and range of conditions throughout the world. That's remarkable. We tend to focus on herbs and chiropractic and acupuncture and Chinese medicine and Ayurveda, but if you look at the evidence you find that our ability to focus consciousness or human attention on the inextricable mind-body interaction actually has the most profound effect on disease states and health states, at least in the scientific literature, than all of these other areas. I did not expect to find that.

Collectively, mind-body practices have a very profound interaction and you can move that interaction toward states of health or toward states of disease. What occurred to me, even in that early research, is that if the mind-body system can regulate heart rate and bleeding and pain, then how many times do people unconsciously regulate in a dysfunctional direction, and how many times do they self-regulate in a functional direction? That still is an unanswered question.

Use of such mind-body interventions has a profound effect in heart disease, in cancer survival, and in the quality of life. There was an article about 2 years ago in the *Journal of the American Medical Association (JAMA)* that looked at mortality rates before and after Christian and Jewish holidays. They found that just prior to Christmas, Easter, and Yom Kippur, there was a decline in mortality incidents and then subsequent to that, 1 month to 2 months afterward, there was a spike. So people who were going to die held off and then died 4 to 8 weeks later. They were temporarily able to stave off death. Historically, you have people like Thomas Jefferson, who died on the anniversary of the Declaration of Independence, and Mark Twain, who was born and died when Halley's comet returned. These were very conscious desires. This "anniversary phenomenon," where individuals live beyond terminal-diagnosis stage to see a child graduate or a religious holiday occur, doesn't mean that mind-body interactions overcome death. But it does mean that even death itself, to some degree, is malleable. It means that the human consciousness and will has the ability to alter, even if on a temporary basis, the inevitable end of life, which is astounding.

In his writings, Paramahansa Yogananda pointed out that we tend to believe that we are material beings having occasional spiritual experiences, but in reality, we are spiritual beings having occasional human experiences. During those times of transcendence—however they occur, during crisis, during meditation, when faced with life-threatening disease or death—the spiritual core of the human being actually experiences that which is beyond space and time. Taken simplistically, these events last seconds, and the fact that an event lasting seconds in duration should profoundly alter a person's entire live makes no sense. That, in and of itself, seems to be *de facto* evidence of a higher order of reality.

I don't understand it, but it's profound and real. And the fact that these types of spiritual experiences have a subsequently transformative effect on the person's life is undoubted.

As another example, Lourdes has a medical review board that determines, independently of the church, whether or not an event constitutes a miracle. The criteria are extremely rigorous and very scientific. Basically, the cure has to be virtually instantaneous or within a very short period of time. There has to be unequivocal evidence of the diagnosis; the person cannot be under any kind of conventional treatment at the time; it has to be a condition for which there is no known or effective treatment at the time; and the person needs to remain in remission for at least a year. Ten years ago when I wrote a chapter in my book *Longevity: Fulfilling our Biological Potential* on this, there were 64 cases of miracles, or what we might refer to as profoundly transformative mind-body events, which is rather astounding.

This shows that under these very stringent criteria, something occurred completely outside of the normative boundaries of what we know about healing and medicine. Whether we call it a miracle, spontaneous remission, or mind-body reaction, the vocabulary is less important than the fact that these events are profound in their own right. What they indicate about our capacity as humankind is even more profound because if it happened to these individuals, it means there is the same potential in all of us.

The Corporate Health Programs

My interest in working with corporations started in 1980. At the time, IBM was developing the first programs in health promotion and disease management for their employees. They were the first to recognize that a company should have a vested interest in the health and well-being of their employees because if someone is disabled or sick, then the company has a direct loss. Although this seems obvious, it has still not yet been realized on a worldwide scale.

In 1980, Robert Beck, the senior vice president for personnel and human resources for IBM, brought together five experts in prevention to help think through and design what then became the basis for IBM's "Live for Life" program. As we were working, I realized that the largest sector of our society with an inherently vested interested in health is the private corporate sector. They need vital, productive, involved, motivated employees to be effective and competitive in the world marketplace. I thought to myself, this is great because I've always been more interested in health than disease and there is a huge population of companies with access to individuals who have the same interest, which is to improve health, well-being, and human performance. So that's how my interest in corporate programs began.

When Bob left IBM and assumed the same position with Bank of America in San Francisco, he kept asking me if there were any data about the clinical and/or cost efficacy of these programs—do they really improve health? Are they really cost effective with a return on investment? I didn't know, so through the Bank of America Foundation, he provided me with a 3-year grant. So we created a corporate health program at UCSF School of Medicine that brought together 15 companies to research these issues.

Actually, the first research project we conducted—this would have been in 1985—was with Levi-Strauss. At the time, mammography was an excellent technology but it was underutilized. Levi-Strauss was concerned because they had an inordinate number of female employees. Coincidentally, UCSF had one of the first mobile mammography units. We worked with the marketing group within Levi-Strauss and developed a campaign and brought the mobile mammography van to the workplace. Instead of a woman having to take half a day or more from work to go to a doctor's office, which is a loss to the company and a loss to the women, we brought the van to the worksite. It now seems incredibly obvious, but at the time it wasn't.

We wanted to demonstrate that, one, people would use it, and two, that the screening was as accurate as a full screening in a clinic. So we developed a campaign called the three Cs—Concern, Convenience, and Cost. Concern was the internal educational program about mammography and low-dose radiation. Convenience was that a woman could go downstairs for 15 or 20 minutes instead of taking a half-day off from work. And Cost was the fact that it went from $200 a screening to $20 because you brought it to the worksite. Levi-Strauss was so happy that they paid for anyone who wanted to be screened.

Seven hundred women went through screening, and, in fact, we had a predictable number of cases that were found, some of which were benign and others that were early malignancies. We demonstrated that you can take a useful medical technology, bring it to a worksite, and have something that's both clinically useful and cost effective. That was our very first study.

We've conducted interventions in work sites for carpal tunnel syndrome, low back pain, major heart disease prevention programs, cancer screening, and AIDS awareness. The consistent theme has been to work with companies at their worksites so you can interact with people in an efficient way. We've had a very transformative influence because it has helped companies think differently about how they spend their medical dollars. Rather than spending it after people are disabled, if you spend some funds before, you get a much higher payoff.

In 1990, I transferred the Corporate Health Improvement Program (CHIP) from UCSF to the Stanford University School of Medicine, where it became the Stanford Corporate Health Program. Its mission continued to be the same, which is to develop and evaluate innovative interventions with the focus on work sites for both clinical and cost outcomes and to touchstone the success, especially in the corporate world, meaning a positive return on investment for a company investing in the health of its employees.

During the 1980s, health promotion was our focus. By the 1990s, health promotion had become a commercial product through companies such as Johnson and Johnson, Healthtrac, and Healthwise. Since we wanted to be on the cutting edge of research, we focused on disease management. So our work was about the early detection of a symptom of illness and rapid intervention—like detecting an increase in blood pressure or cholesterol levels or a pain from carpal tunnel syndrome before it progressed to a disability.

Research published predominately out of our Stanford research indicated that a telemedicine intervention or a multifactorial intervention for reducing heart disease was more effective than usual care in reducing hospitalization, subsequent heart attacks, and those types of clinical and cost outcomes. It was also extremely cost effective, because you reached out electronically, in what we termed *electronic housecalls*, to the person rather than having the person come to a clinic or a hospital.

When Blue Shield of California saw those results they said, "That's interesting; could we apply that in a worksite?" At the same time, the General Electric Nuclear Energy, or GENE, in San Jose, has about 2500 employees. They service virtually every nuclear power plant in the free world. These people travel 80% of the time on troubleshooting missions. It's a stressful, high-demand job, and they were having a very high incidence of heart disease and sudden, nonpremorbid history fatal heart attacks. So Blue Shield funded the intervention at General Electric with our staff at Stanford providing the training and intervention. At the end of the study, we were able to demonstrate a major reduction in risk and a major reduction in incidence of heart attacks.

Subsequently, GE has implemented this program in six sites nationwide that use this same model of intervention in their clinics. Also, Blue Shield of California covers such interventions as part of the benefits within their plan for California.

This kind of intervention works for a number of reasons. One is convenience. People have instantaneous access. If you have a niacin or other adverse drug reaction, you don't have to make an appointment and go to the clinic to get a simple answer. You get the answer within seconds. Second, all of the interventions delivered by the nurse case managers focused on state-of-the-art behavior change. How do you get a person to modify his or her lifestyle? Third, we continued to use pharmaceuticals but we were able to reduce dosages, which decreased the frequency of side effects. Lastly, we taught them to how to live. They learned each step of the way with regard to stress management, sound diet, exercise, cardiovascular risk factors, appropriate use of medications, and social support. They learned along with us how to improve their health choices and freedom. That was a big factor.

If people want the source material on this work, there are a series of five articles that I have published in the *American Journal of Health Promotion*. In each one is a table in which you can see for a 2-year interval where the study was conducted, which companies were involved, what type of workers, what was done, how it was analyzed, what the clinical outcome was, and what were the cost outcomes. Most recently, the last article covers 1998 to 2000. And all of them are also available on Medline.

CHIP, the Third Generation

Part of what I am doing right now is rethinking the program. We're calling it CHIP (Corporate Health Improvement Program), the third generation. The first generation was about basic health promotion, when that was an innovation. The second generation was disease management—early detection, cholesterol screening, hypertension screen, diabetes, and similar conditions. Now, the third generation will focus on integrative medicine, because when we talk to our medical directors—and again this is American Airlines, Bank of America, IBM, Merck, Medtronic, United Health Care, and Ford—they tell us that the major areas that their employees are asking for is alternative medicine. So they want to know what to include on what basis? Should they cover chiropractic? Should they cover acupuncture? What about Chinese herbals? What about homeopathy?

So CHIP, the third generation, will focus on creating and implementing integrative medicine intervention and demonstration projects in worksites. Our delivery models are, by and large, telemedicine-based. As soon as someone leaves work and goes to a clinic or a hospital, it's inherently more expensive. So increasingly I'm interested in using nurses, doctors, and psychologists over the telephone, using computers and mail, and interacting with people very conveniently to manage their conditions. Once you do that, geography is no longer an issue. You can have a bank of nurses anywhere in the country or anywhere in the world that people can access for care.

Essentially, we are creating a virtual CHIP that will have ties to two or three medical schools. The actual delivery of the clinical interventions will be from remote sites. Again, we're trying to push the envelope both in content and model of delivery. But I like the challenge of making something work at least as well if not better than what is done conventionally and at least as good as, if not better, in regard to practical economic return on investment because we have an incredibly inefficient, wasteful medical system. Companies understand this because they pay the costs. If you can make a difference in low-back disability for a major automobile manufacturer, they don't question why are you using acupuncture or yoga. They care about both clinical and cost results.

Also, I always enjoy the challenge of producing a better, practical result. That's always what I've done in all of my clinical research over the last 30 years.

Here's a current project we are implementing. In 2000, one of the big three automobile companies spent about $70 million on direct medical reimbursement for low-back pain only! That's not absenteeism; that's not lost productivity, worker replacement, or down time. It was straight medical payout for low-back pain. They have 12 clinics nationwide that do nothing but low-back pain disability management. We met with their medical directors as part of our corporate program and looked at the protocols used in their clinics. It was primitive pain management.

They happen to have three manufacturing sites located in one city. The demographics were perfectly matched. At one clinic, selected at random, we will train the nurses and physicians to deliver an integrated medicine model for low-back pain. This protocol includes stress management, mind-body techniques, yoga, acupuncture, and education about what low-back pain is, what nonsteroidals can do and not do in terms of medication management, and information on reasonable alternatives like boswellia as an antiinflammatory herb. We will support them via a telemedicine model so that when they have questions they can call us and we will interact directly with patients and staff.

The study is still ongoing, and our hypothesis, if you will, is that even though the intervention is inherently more expensive initially, that over the 3-year time period of the intervention, people will go back to work sooner, have less recidivism, be more pain free, make more appropriate use of medications, and be more productive. We are looking at medical outcomes as well as cost outcomes. If and when this works, it's likely to be a model intervention that will be adopted systemwide. But this is an example of this convergence of my two interests—alternative or integrative medicine and the private corporate sector. In the past, they always seemed like parallel paths with a Grand Canyon between them. But in the last four years they've begun to converge, mostly because of the demand by the employees for alternative or integrative medicine and the absolute need for companies to resolve exploding medical costs that don't return productivity.

Another current research project of mine is that the word "presenteeism" has become the buzzword in the corporate sector. Absenteeism is one thing because a person is present or absent; it's measurable. But what does it mean if a person is present but not functional? How "present," how functional, how focused is a person at work if there's a condition or concern that's preventing optimal performance? So we conducted a 2-year study funded by Merek that focused on three different worksites and developed a scale called the Stanford Presenteeism Scale (SPSG). It's very sophisticated—we used rigorous statistics and biometrics, and developed a brief, six-item scale that measures how functional and how present a person is when at work. It bridges the gap between the purely medical, health issues that the personnel department is interested in and the performance and productivity issues that the finance and business people are interested in.

We published the scale in the *Journal of Occupational and Environmental Medicine* in January 2002, and I have never had as many responses to any article. Right now, the SPSG scale is being used in about 30 different companies, including Eastman Kodak, Dow, and Sprint. Also, the American College of Occupational and Environmental Medicine (ACOEM) is developing a white paper on new metrics, and our scale will be the cornerstone.

In September of this year, I am going to Singapore and Hong Kong for 9 days. There is a major collaborative effort between the private and public sectors in Singapore, the entire focus of which is to determine how the Singapore health and medical systems can make their corporations more effective. I'm going to meet with government, corporate, and foundation individuals for a series of consultations and lectures focused on clinical and cost outcomes as well as presenteeism. Again, you can influence presenteeism by conventional methods or alternative methods. To me, the interesting thing is how you can fuse these and create an integrative medicine approach that produces greater presenteeism.

The Snowball Effect

These types of things can cause a cultural "snowball effect." A good example is the study we conducted on cardiovascular intervention for General Electric, which we discussed earlier. It has now been adapted systemwide throughout General Electric. So from a single demonstration project that is clinically useful and cost effective, the company then turns to its health plan providers and says, "We want a cardiovascular risk-reduction program." So all of the health benefit providers who want to access these hundreds of thousands of employees during open enrollment then have to add cardiovascular risk-reduction programs to their offerings. Similarly, this occurs when people suddenly have access to a new service like acupuncture or herbal medicine or chiropractic. The ripple effect continues in that the clinical practitioners out in the community who provide the services through the health plans have to be trained, which ties back to education. So this is an incredibly critical leverage point for the kind of transformation of healthcare that has to occur as we evolve from a disease management industry to a true healthcare system.

Successful Aging

Stanford Medical School was one of the first centers funded by what has become the National Center for Complementary and Alternative Medicine (NCCAM) at the National Institutes of Health (NIH). At one point we conducted a study focused on who was using alternative medicine and why. It turned out that it was older adults who were more affluent, better educated, and who had a life emphasis on obtaining optimal health as opposed to recovering from illness. So we shifted our plans and now the entire research focus is on successful or healthy aging.

We wanted to find out if behavioral and/or pharmacological interventions could halt or reverse the malleable aspects of aging. One of our research projects within that program— many of them are still ongoing—focused on t'ai chi as an intervention to reduce or restore inner ear equilibrium for older adults. There is literature from China suggesting that, although they tend to have smaller bone density and mass than Caucasians, elderly Chinese experience fewer falls and fractures of the pelvis, which is the major cause of disability for older adults in the United States, especially women. Using a very sophisticated assessment that tells us whether someone is inclined to become disoriented and fall, we selected individuals on that basis. They either went to usual care or to practice t'ai chi. (It is an interesting note that our t'ai chi instructor is actually a professor of physics at Stanford.) We found that when people practiced balancing, which is one of the physical essences of the martial arts, they could restore and maintain equilibrium into advanced age.

SAGE is an acronym for the Successful Aging Growth Experience. This research project was really inspired by Michael Murphy and George Leonard's book *The Wisdom of the Body* and they served as consultants to us. They developed a group participation program based on the principles in their book that they believed would keep people healthy, functional, and disease-free. It had never been scientifically evaluated, so we took their basic ideas and information, modified and added to it, and developed a program called SAGE. It is still running, and again, it is one of those studies that promises very positive outcomes.

We deliberately selected people between the ages 65 and 85 and enrolled them in groups of 15 to 20 individuals. The question was: Could we develop a structured intervention consisting of educational modules like appropriate use of medical care, education about pharmaceutical use for adults, training in martial arts exercises like t'ai chi, stress management, diet and nutrition, imagery and visualization, and building a social support network? So if you created this in a structured environment, could you halt or reverse the aging process? Could individuals become more healthy than they had been even though they would be between 3 and 5 years older?

We also developed a very sophisticated battery of tests to determine the actual phenomena of aging. It turns out that measuring aging is an extremely difficult task. How do you know how old you are other than by having one more birthday? How would you measure if someone is moving in a positive direction rather than just maintaining or even prematurely aging? So we developed new metrics, which we are testing right now, that measure functions such as increased wisdom, or a broader, more global spiritual perspective on life, in addition to accuracy and rapidity of their memories.

What is unique about this program is that for the first 3 months a therapist runs the group. For the next 3 months, the members select someone from their own group to become the leader-therapist of the program. Then, in the final stage, from 6 to 12 months, the individuals are on their own. They can call on us for help and advice, but they are no longer actively participating in an externally structured group. Basically we wanted to see if we could transition the teaching from a therapist to the person and get people to carry the lessons and practices into their daily lives. Again, this is self-empowerment and enhancement of individual choices.

So far, our preliminary evidence suggests that, yes, we are absolutely able to do this. People in the study did halt or reverse a number of aspects of what we term the aging process. We'll have the final results probably in about 2 years.

Reversing the Effects of Aging

There is an indication from the study that when an individual engages in the balance-related martial arts such as t'ai chi that he or she is able to halt or even reverse the age-related tendency to have an impaired ability to balance while walking or climbing stairs. Another effect the study suggests is an improvement in short-term memory recall and accuracy. Again, we have objective evidence that through this program—though we can't say whether it was exercise or the diet or the stress management or the meditation that is the active component—that an individual's ability for short-term recall of specific information is improved both in terms of speed and accuracy of that recall. And not only in the specificity of the recall but the time lag between the question posed and the response was decreased. So they're remembering quicker and more accurately.

Those are two examples. Although we have not fully analyzed the data yet, we are seeing improved overall health status, reduction of specific risk factors, improved productivity, and improved connection to other people.

Federation Guidelines for Use of CAM

In the U.S., the Federation of State Medical Licensing Boards (FSMB) is the national entity that represents all state medical licensing boards. They are charged with issuing guidelines or recommendations to state boards that cover every conceivable aspect of medical practice. About 4 years ago they issued their first white paper on alternative medicine. It was dubbed the "search and destroy document" because it was extremely negative toward alternative medicine. I've forgotten the exact wording, but it had fraudulent and deceptive in the title and alternative medicine was synonymous with fraudulent and deceptive practices. The thrust of it was that any practicing physician who was using alternative medicine ought to have legal action taken against him or her.

A little over 2 years ago they decided to revisit this, so they invited Dr. Russ Greenfield, Dr. David Eisenberg, and me to be their advisors. The task was to come up with a new set of guidelines or decide to have the old ones stand. So for the last 2 years, we met regularly with their committee and provided them with documents, evidence, and information at their request. The composition of the committee covered the whole spectrum. It went from people who were open-minded toward alternative medicine, though not actively practicing, to not necessarily supportive but at least open-minded to negative, and I mean really negative. It took an enormous amount of time and effort, but the result was that a document was approved by the full FSMB House of Delegates on April 27, 2002, and is now actively disseminated as a model guideline to all 50 states.

States' actions will vary—some of them will take it as is; some will just disseminate it; and some will modify it. But it's very, very positive in the following way: the definition of alternative medicine they used was taken from the NCCAM web site. One of the points of our advocacy was that unless there was a compelling reason to deviate from the NIH and NCCAM norms and standards of definitions, then that was what should be adhered to, which

was different from the earlier document that defined alternative medicine as inherently negative. The most significant change, however, is that the new guidelines contain an explicit line
that a physician will not be subject to disciplinary action solely on the basis of using alternative medicine.

In the first paragraph and in the conclusion, the document acknowledges that patients have
the right to seek any and all methods of care. Period. So it recognizes the right and power of
individual choice, and it recognizes that the practice of alternative medicine is not *de facto*
fraudulent or deceptive.

Also, the document provides for referral to alternative practitioners. In the previous document, just the act of referral to an alternative medicine practitioner could have been grounds
for disciplinary action. Now it states explicitly that if you refer to another practitioner of
alternative medicine that that person should be licensed and certified in whatever discipline
he or she is practicing, but that it is an acceptable practice.

Literally, each word and each phrase in that document was gone over and debated and
tested. It was astounding. So I'm really pleased.

Our thrust was that you should have conventional and alternative medicine function with
parity. In other words, the standard is good practice, not whether it's identified as conventional
or alternative. Before there was a disproportionate level of burden, if you will, placed on the
alternative medicine practice. Now that's no longer the case. It's either good practice or bad
practice. What they realized—and we asked them to consider this—was that the vast majority
of disciplinary actions nationwide are not because of the use of alternative medicine. They are
because of the abuse of conventional medicine, such as excess surgeries, inappropriate prescribing,
dangerous prescribing, or self-prescribing. This was from their own database, and the point was
that using alternative medicine did not constitute grounds, *per se*, for disciplinary action. Again,
there will be a ripple effect because these guidelines will stand for a number of years.

Self-Care

Self-care is a vital issue. We need to differentiate between informed and empowered consumers,
and those who are misinformed. Self-medication when you are uninformed or misinformed is
potentially dangerous. To me, the promise of integrated medicine is when you have an informed
and empowered consumer-patient who works with a clinician who has special skills—be it
medicine or nursing or nutrition or exercise or meditation or whatever—to help that person
make the most informed decisions. It's very difficult to take general nutritional guidelines and
decide on the optimum diet, especially if you have a chronic illness. But that's what nutritionists can do. So to me the future is really an enlightened self-care in which the patient and
provider mutually interact in a model of integrative medicine using best practices from both
conventional and alternative medicine.

Here's what I mean. I remember after one lecture, a woman came up to me and said how
very conservative my approach to herbals had been. I said, "Conservative?" I mean, I'm used
to being called all kinds of things but never conservative.

She said, "It's because you were talking about all those precautions and contraindications."

So I responded, "That's not conservative, that's just being agnostic." So I would like to
advocate that people use St. John's Wort appropriately if they have a mild to moderate depression, but I would not want them to use it with other drugs, such as Prozac or other SSRIs,
with which it has an interaction, and I would certainly not want them to use it for major
depression because there is no evidence for that. So it's not a wholesale endorsement but
evidence-based advocacy.

As we become more sophisticated about the appropriate use of alternative medicine, we realize that the question really is: which of the 650 practices identified by NCCAM work for which persons for what condition under what circumstances relative to all the other factors about their biology from their genotype to their particular familial history? That's the challenge. Self-care is an inherent part of that and it is vital.

Surgery is surely the most extreme end of the continuum where the person is most absent and the practitioner is the most active. Yet surgical outcomes are equally dependent in many ways on the self-care involvement of the person pre- and postoperatively than on the skill of the practitioner. We've had some fascinating discussions about this with Medtronic Corporation, which makes implantable defibrillators and arrhythmia devices. What they have found is that the behavioral context of the surgery—how well does the person understand the unit and what do they do by way of exercise, nutrition and stress management?—is more predictive of a successful postoperative outcome than the skill of the surgeon. You see an enormous difference in patient outcome with the same surgeon, and when they look at what makes a difference, it's all these self-care dimensions. Even when we have very high-tech medicine or pharmaceuticals or genomic-based interventions, when you use medicine appropriately in a self-care model, you have much better outcomes. So it's not high-tech versus self-care or pharmaceuticals versus herbals. It's really to find the best evidence-based, integrative approach.

The Future Looks Bright

Presently, I'm more optimistic now than ever. If you look into the not too distant future, more corporations will be developing integrative medicine services for their employees, and we'll have better evidence that it really does improve health for the individuals and productivity for the companies. We'll see more medical schools with this kind of training and more collective practices where you really will have nutritionists, ministers, physicians, nurses, and psychologists all working together. Virtually every insurance company in the country now has some aspect of alternative medicine that's covered under their health plans.

It's not so much to advocate for alternative medicine but to advocate that people have the access to the full spectrum of choices they need to main their health, to manage illness and disease, to live to their optimal life span, and that they have access to the best knowledge we have as practitioners. We are getting closer to realizing this vision, and that is very exciting.

Part Two

Conversations About Death and Dying

"When we allow ourselves to be with dying, it will change not only how we die but also how we live."

—JOAN HALIFAX

CHAPTER 6

JOAN HALIFAX, PhD

Being With Death and Dying

Joan Halifax, PhD, is an anthropologist and Buddhist teacher. Her academic teaching credentials include faculty appointments at Columbia University, the University of Miami School of Medicine, the New School for Social Research, and the Naropa Institute. She is the author of numerous books, including *The Human Encounter with Death* (with Stanislav Grof), *Shamanic Voices, Shaman: The Wounded Healer, The Fruitful Darkness, Simplicity in the Complex: A Buddhist Life in America,* and *Being With Dying.*

Since 1970, Dr. Halifax has worked with individuals suffering from life-threatening illnesses, and she currently conducts a national teaching and training program on contemplative work with dying people. She has worked with indigenous healing systems in Southern Florida through the University of Miami School of Medicine and with indigenous peoples in Asia and the Americas around environmental and health issues. In 1979 she founded the Ojai Foundation and The Foundation School, where she lived and worked until 1990.

Dr. Halifax is currently head teacher and abbot of Upaya Zen Center in Santa Fe, New Mexico, where she practices, teaches, does social and environmental work, and works with individuals suffering from catastrophic illness. She has practiced Buddhism since the late 1960s and was formally ordained in 1976 by Dae Sahn sa Nim. She received the Lamp Transmission from Zen Master Thich Nhat Hanh in 1990 and Inka from Tetsugen Roshi in 1998. She is a Dharmacarya in the Tiep Hien Order.

I interviewed Dr. Halifax at the Upaya House in Santa Fe, New Mexico, in the winter of 1977.

Upaya is a Buddhist study center, part of the White Plum Sangha of Maezumi Roshi. As a Buddhist study center, we are very focused on engaged spirituality. How can we bring a spiritual perspective into our work of service with people? How can our work of service with people engage a contemplative frame of reference? Upaya has a number of different dimensions. It is a community of practitioners—people who are doing Zen Buddhist practice. It also offers educational courses and retreat programs that make it possible for people from all over the country and all over the world to come here for study and practice in three areas: contemplative work with dying people, contemplative environmental inquiry, and engaged spirituality.

In 1979, I started a community called the Ojai Foundation in Ojai, California. I left there in 1990 and began Upaya shortly thereafter. I did it because I wanted to bring Buddhist practice forward. Buddhism has so much to offer Western culture today, particularly in working with dying people and in engaged spirituality.

I was born a Christian, and I feel I'm a Christian still. I feel very much in touch with my Christian roots. But for laypeople, Christianity does not—or has not in the past—offered contemplative practice. When I read Buddhism in the 1960s, I felt, "I'm a Buddhist." This is not so much a religion as a philosophy and a psychology. Contemplative practice combined with the philosophy and psychology has been very important in my own journey.

Death and Dying

I began working with dying people in 1970 at the University of Miami School of Medicine, where I was a medical anthropologist. I saw that most conventional medical systems were not prepared for dying people. Death was looked on as a failure of medical expertise. It was a subject of great concern for many people because, at that time, they didn't have the kinds of pain management and palliative care that we have now. Moreover, there was a tremendous denial of death. The disclosure of a person's terminal diagnosis was still not that common in the 1960s. So death has come a long way, if you will, in the past 30 years—but it still has a long way to go.

I left the University of Miami to work with Stanislav Grof doing LSD-assisted psychotherapy for people dying of cancer. It was very edifying work because it was a contemporary rite of passage. The people with whom we worked were suffering from intractable pain, difficulty with medical management, depression, or severe anxiety, and were referred to us by physicians. They were carefully screened, carefully prepared, and then, in a very special setting with support, they were given LSD as an adjunct to psychotherapy. As a result of the whole context, these people went through profound experiences that often made it possible for them to approach and encounter death in a way that was very open, conscious, and even enlightened.

I was very grateful to participate in that project. It helped me realize that I was not well prepared, that what I was seeing and being with was so revolutionary—the vision of dying and death in America was so circumscribed—that I had to turn to my practice of Buddhism and a direct exploration of shamanism to deepen my relationship with the dying process. When the work with Grof came to an end, I continued to be with dying people. I had a gift for it and felt a sense of mission. I believe this is one area of human life that must be deeply addressed.

When the AIDS epidemic hit in the 1980s in this country, it affected a population that was very intelligent and self-conscious. And because it was the male homosexual population, they were motivated to transform the experience of dying for their brothers. So, early in the 1980s, I moved from working with people who had cancer to working with people who had AIDS. And the AIDS patients I have worked with have been important teachers for me. These men have such a profound motivation to explore dying and death in an active way and to create a context for dying that is meaningful.

I began practicing Buddhism in the 1960s, but my practice really deepened in the mid-1970s, when I started working with a teacher. I became ordained in 1976 and then ordained to teach in 1981. I took refuge with Thich Nhat Hanh in 1986 and was ordained to teach by him in 1990. It was then that I left Ojai and began to reorder my priorities. In part, the move was stimulated by the death of my mother in 1990. There was something I wanted to do with my life that I felt I couldn't do at Ojai. So I went to the Crestone Mountain Zen Center and was in retreat and wrote for 6 months. Then I went to a hermitage in Abiquiu and was given Upaya here in Santa Fe, New Mexico.

After moving to Santa Fe I began to sit with dying people. Some of the local caregivers were interested in what I was doing and asked to be taught. So I began the "Project on Being With Dying," which has several different areas. The first is education; we educate professional caregivers—physicians, nurses, social workers, clergy, and others—in teaching contemplative care of the dying. We offer retreats and courses to caregivers who are volunteers, community people, and dying people on contemplative aspects of being with dying. We also offer specialized, intensive courses on contemplative practices including various types of advanced meditation practices, sand-tray work, music thanatology, the arts, dream work, and calligraphy.

Second, we have a training and service program called "Partners," which is given over a 10-week period. In this program we train local people, both professional caregivers and what I would call "villagers," to bring contemplative care to dying people. The third area is the production of educational materials: instructor manuals, resource books, audiotapes, and videotapes that make it possible for people to teach others how to do this work for themselves.

The last area is my own travel around the country to medical centers, conferences, and educational centers, bringing forward this teaching of contemplative work with dying people. Although the teaching and practice areas are based in Buddhism, I think we have done a skillful translation of Buddhism into something that feels more nonsectarian. People from other religions who have been through our programs feel comfortable with it. There isn't any proselytizing; it's more that we have adapted Eastern contemplative strategies and a view of death to a Western perspective.

Buddhism as a contemplative practice of several thousand years has brought people to an understanding of the importance of seeing and realizing the impermanent nature of the phenomenal world. Not just contemplating death, but dying consciously is very important in the Buddhist tradition. The vision of death in Buddhism is not of annihilation or finality. During our life, we ride the waves of birth and death with each breath that we take. When we pass through the gateway of death we may experience awakening, freedom, true liberation.

This is quite a different vision of death than we have in Western culture. We had this perspective in the Middle Ages. There was a vision of death that involved coming home to God as a path of liberation. We are trying to bring this vision back into Western culture now because we feel that this perspective can have a profound effect on the medical care of people who are dying and on the lives of the living as well.

I don't get so involved in accounts of the hereafter. Past incarnation experiences are interesting, but I am interested in people who have gone through near-death experiences, or the observation of people who have died, where in the last phase of the dying process, and at the moment of death, there is a quality of luminosity in their passing.

One of the most important texts we use in our training work is Tolstoy's *The Death of Ivan Ilyich*. Tolstoy, without any Buddhist background, came to a very interesting perspective on pain and death. His protagonist, Ivan Ilyich, actually drops to the level of mind referred to in the Buddhist world as the natural mind ground, where natural luminosity appears. I like to use Tolstoy's text because it is an insight about the nature of death from a non-Buddhist source.

Some of the most interesting insights for me come not so much from scientific evidence or literature, but from my own observation of and work with dying people. Through this, my own vision of death has been transformed. That's what is fundamentally important. It's nice to have third-person accounts, but it's much more profound for us to bear witness with a dying person and to be there at the moment of death. Fundamentally, death is a release from suffering and perhaps even the moment of awakening of great liberation.

We've marginalized dying people. We've pushed death out of our sight and characterized it in a very negative way. I'm hoping, through my own experience and the experience of many colleagues who currently work with dying people as a contemplative practice, that we can foster a new vision of death in the 21st century that will transform the context of dying in the West.

This could have a tremendous effect on healthcare and palliative care of dying people now and in the future. The economic implications of contemplative care—in addition to its psychological, social, and spiritual implications—are tremendous. So often, costly technological interventions are brought in during the last days or last hours of an individual's life. This can be quite disruptive for people. If we accept death as the natural consequence of birth, then we may have a completely different possibility open to us—one of creating a context for dying that is very inclusive of human values and spiritual elements, which can make dying a victory, not a defeat.

Preparing for Death

My feeling is that we should practice dying now. We should not wait until the week before we're dying. This is a very fundamental part of our work. In tribal cultures, people begin rites of passage at the moment of birth, then at adolescence, marriage, aging, death, and so on—all the different rites of passage that happen are opportunities for people to encounter death and experience redemptional rebirth. There are two fundamental Buddhist practices: the practice of kindness and *Maranasati*, which means "being with dying." And if you do these two forms of meditation, liberation is possible.

My feeling is that we shouldn't wait until the last minute. I was raised in Florida. When we received a hurricane warning, we always stocked up on food, filled the bathtub with water, opened all the windows. Then, when the storm hit, we were prepared. Well, death is the inevitable outcome of birth. We know this most extraordinary event is going to happen to us. Why don't we prepare for it? I remember this Woody Allen joke: "I'm not afraid of dying. I just don't want to be there when it happens." Well, most people aren't there.

Preparing for death is not morbid. Many people think, "I don't want to think about death" because the fear of death underlies so much of Western culture. We don't know when we're going to die or how we are going to die, but we should prepare for it, because death is inevitable. In terms of preparation, now is the time—not only because the moment could be this afternoon but also because the actual preparation for death releases you into an appreciation for life and living.

Being prepared for death means that not only have you explored the obstacles around confirming that death is part of life—such as fear of death, depression about death, sorrow around loss, or a dispersiveness in trying to escape from death and other forms of denial—but you have also explored the experience of release and what it means to let go of control, to surrender.

The body goes through various stages in the dying process—a dissolution of the elements of the body in which it withdraws its vitality from the world and from itself, and then death happens. The exploration of those stages is important because it helps you practice releasing— not only at the moment of death but also in terms of your daily life.

Jonas Salk once said to me, "We have to learn how to cooperate with the inevitable." This opens up the sense of cooperation—loss is inevitable, sorrow is inevitable, death is inevitable, and we learn how to be present with the change that happens. We live in a culture of fixations. We resist change. We are a society in grief at the flow of inevitable losses. Meditation practice allows you to explore the fundamental experience of letting go. In certain states of meditation, one's concentration is so deep that it actually moves to a place that is below the discursive mind, below the level of psychological content of cause and effect of personality. Christians have had mystical experiences of luminosity, seeing the true nature of their mind as God. In Buddhism, it's very well described. At the moment of death, your primordial nature appears, and it is so brilliant that instead of turning away from that luminosity, you learn to recognize that luminosity as who you truly are. Learning that is a skill, and that skill is one we endeavor to cultivate in people.

It's learning to recognize the true nature of our minds. From this perspective it means that when we are with a dying person, we are able to perceive through their suffering to the point where we see who they really are—not just the identity that's constructed by psyche, culture, and genetics, but the identity that's already free—and to see that same element within our own nature. In other words, we see each being's capacity to be free from suffering.

Part of this work is learning how to develop what we call "bearing witness." Bearing witness is a practice that allows us to be present for whatever is happening—relatives who are exorcising grief, a dying person who's experiencing extreme pain, feelings of desperation, sorrow, or anxiety—and to accept it deeply and not try to manipulate the person. Going to the depth of our feelings, we can come out the other end to the mind ground. One comment that we hear so often is, "You have modeled my awareness for me, how my awareness needs to be, in how you have sustained presence during my suffering."

So what we want to do is to help sustain a quality of being present and to accept whatever is happening, like a string that's resonating sympathetically. It's not that if the person is in a state of hyperanxiety, you're in a state of hyperanxiety. No. We feel that anxiety—that's called "compassion"—but at the same time we have perfect equanimity. So we're working with the balance between compassion and equanimity. These are the two primary qualities that we try to cultivate in the work of caregivers. And it is those qualities that we try to bring forth in dying people.

There are many different meditation practices or contemplative strategies that we use— everything from mindfulness practice to compassion and loving-kindness practices to visualizations and guided meditation to prayer. Frank Lawlis, Larry Dossey, Jeanne Achterberg, Elizabeth Targ, Steven Levine, Ram Dass—these are some of the people who have worked with contemporary strategies and ancient techniques for working with suffering and the transformation to freedom from—or to the acceptance of—suffering. I make a distinction here between pain and suffering. Pain is a feeling of extreme discomfort; suffering is the story about that discomfort.

We are not always able to transform actual pain. Buddhism's approach, however, is to transform suffering into wisdom, compassion, and understanding.

If you were dying, and I was working with you, I'd sit with you quietly and say, "What will serve you?" Our number one guideline in this practice is to be led by the needs of the individual. If you're a Jew, Christian, Sufi, Hindu, pagan, atheist, or agnostic, we try to find out what will help your sense of spiritual values to come forth. What will help your heart to open? What were the meaningful experiences in your life? How can we help to heal relationships that have been disrupted? You would give us the context.

Opening the Heart

When we say "heart opening," what we mean is bringing forth the experience of love or nonduality, nonseparation, nonalienation in the relationship, whether it's the relationship between the physician and the patient, the hospice worker and the dying person, or among family members. What the dying person frequently experiences is marginalization, the experience of being pushed aside. The person is anticipating being separated from his or her body, family, material objects, and identity. So the fear of those kinds of experiences of separation lead an individual to feel he or she is in a loveless state that is alienated or divided.

We try to enter into a relationship that is unconditional, no matter how the person is with you—whether he is mad at you or rejects you or is indifferent to you. We try to hold a good heart in our presence with dying people. Very often what happens when people are dying is that they withdraw; they pull away; they cut the ties. We're trying to make it easier for them to cut the ties, to let go, to experience release, and, simultaneously, to do so on a pathway that is wholesome and meaningful, that is endowed with beneficial qualities that bring forth their own intrinsic goodness.

Sometimes people don't want to meditate, but they want to hear music. Sometimes people want to sit in silence or simply to weep. Sometimes people have enough energy to participate in putting together a family album so they can remember all the good moments of their life. The telling of their life history is a precursor to the life review, which happens in near-death experiences. Having people talk about the experience of their life is a means of helping them let go of their life. Let them give the story of their life away, so that they have the feeling that they are going to live on, that their story will be part of our lives in the future.

There are other possibilities that can be offered. For example, in Missoula, Montana, at the Chalice of Repose, there is training and practice in music-thanatology. (*NOTE: The Chalice of Repose and the School of Music-Thanatology has since moved to Mt. Angel, Oregon.*) The clinician artists go into the rooms of dying people and play prescriptive music, which is specifically prescribed for the experience of dying. For people who are in the earlier stages of dying, sand-tray work, working with symbolic objects and images, can help them begin to locate and bring forth very deep dimensions of the psyche related to their personal history and to the vision of how they want to die.

Everything I learned in shamanism is present in Buddhist practice for me. Practices of compassion, practices of presence, the willingness to encounter death, the story of the wounded healer—my work and practice with shamans has been very important.

Some people want to bring shamanic elements like smudging with the sage into their work. Whatever they want is fine. But there has to be a fundamental quality of authentic presence and compassion. At the University of Miami School of Medicine, I'd watch one doctor walk in and everybody on the ward would feel bad; another doctor would walk in and everybody would feel good. It had nothing to do with the person being a Christian, Jew, Buddhist, or Hindu, or being a shaman or an atheist. It has to do with a quality of steadiness and openness in the heart of courage and compassion.

Dying Well

People think mostly about material inheritance, material legacies. But I think about spiritual legacies. How you observe other people dying, or how you help them die, very much shapes your own experience of dying. How you live very much informs how you die. If you are willing to be with living and dying, then when dying happens to you, you are willing to be with your own dying. Death is a mystery; we cannot really know it. There's no scientific evidence of anything after the physiology stops. It's all in the realm of supposition. But if you see a death that has a quality of consciousness or peace about it, that will shape your own experience—not only of dying, but also of living.

Sogyal Rinpoche called his book *The Tibetan Book of Living and Dying* because death and life are inextricably intertwined. Our very experience of breathing, our inhalation, and every exhalation we take could be our last. There's contraction and expansion, whether it is in lovemaking or giving birth or in the flow of our lives. There are times of great opening and times when you need to be very internal and to heal.

So learning how to move through the inevitable change of our lives is important.

Being open to what is coming toward us—we call that "receptivity"—and being able to release—we call that "generosity." Being with that opening and closing, contracting and expanding, the movement of the life continuum, "riding the waves of birth and death," is about being present with the mystery. Being present where there is suffering brings one a sense of deep gratitude in one's own life. One is able to be much more in the here and now and to say, "Oh, this blessing that is this life" and then when pain does arrive, to know "Well, everything is impermanent. Now I'm having a difficult time. But this too will pass. Everything is subject to change."

This has to do with a worldview. We ask ourselves: what is this life really about? When we allow ourselves to be with dying, it will change not only how we die, but also how we live in terms of our patterns of consumption. So much of our life is addictive, running away from the mystery of the unknown and unknowable. We project our fear into the unknown. We seek pleasure at levels where the pleasure isn't about peace, stability, and true joy—where, inevitably, the end result is a disappointment.

Rituals for Dying and Death

I have a basic belief and it's very simple: even though we can't prove it, it's always good to cover your back. I can't say with any degree of certainty that ancestors exist as entities apart from my own mind. But I can say that upon my mother's death I realized that if I did not tend to her after-death state, I would be ignoring a precious opportunity to create an ancestor. Going through that process helped me move through grief in a very fundamental way.

In Buddhism there is a 49-day period after the death of an individual, during which it is supposed that the individual goes through various experiences. I tracked my mother during those 49 days. A good deal of that time I was in Asia, but just before returning to this country, I participated in a Tibetan ceremony with lamas in the Kathmandu Valley, during which my mother was called back to this world.

Let me explain. I had a dream about my mother when I was in the mountains of Nepal. It was during a shamanic ceremony and I had a strange vision of her bound up in dark cobwebs, completely confused, and her face bloated. I was so shocked that I didn't do what I wish I had done, which was to reach through the veil separating life and death and tell her that, yes, she was dead, and she should let go completely. I was shattered by not being able to do that. When I went back to Kathmandu, a ceremony was arranged during which my mother was called back into an effigy and recreated. It was a powerful experience to go through.

As the ceremony was happening, I experienced waves of uncontrollable weeping. The lamas would say to me, "Don't cry. That will make your mother want to cling to this side, to cling to her old life. She needs to let go."

I controlled myself and released her continually. I was happy at the end of that ceremony. I went back to California and on the 49th day of my mother's *bardo* journey, my community and I entered into a ceremony, speaking to her across the threshold separating life and death. In the course of this experience—it was in the evening—there were many falling stars and a strange erratic wind blew out every candle on the altar. It was quite eerie. I felt that my mother moved into space at that point; she was free. And it completed my period of mourning.

It was important to go through. Whether or not it happened for my mother I cannot say, but the actual process and practice was healing for me. It was also probably instructive for those people who participated with me. What happens so often upon the death of a loved one is that people are caught up in the arrangements, and the mourning period is truncated. Often lacking are the support and ritual processes that allow for people to go through a mourning that is deep and rich; that scours out the heart and makes an ancestor.

This is what I've learned from tribal cultures: do not ignore the dead. They are there to inform us about the mystery of death—not to expose death, not to reveal the mystery of death but to allow us to consider how the mystery of death can bring depth into our lives. It's a profound opportunity. There is a line from the poet R. M. Rilke that has been very important for me: "Love and death are the great gifts that are given to us. Mostly, they are passed on unopened."

When love and death come together, when they can join, you have the opportunity for going into an even deeper dimension of the mystery, of the unknown.

There are so many strong stories. This is a story told to me by a friend. A woman and her husband were standing at the bedside of the woman's mother, who was dying. The old woman was semicomatose and had not been communicating through her semiconscious state. Then she seemed to come out of it, and said, "Oh, this is beautiful!" The man and his wife were very surprised. Then she cried, "Oh, wow!" This woman was in her eighties and she was saying, "Wow! This is beautiful!" And then she died with this look of absolute joy on her face.

Now, this old woman had never practiced meditation. She just lived a life, a normal life, like most of us. But she died luminously. I tell that story just to show that death is a normal part of our lives and may be an experience of liberation. And it is also a way that we can awaken now.

CHAPTER 7

THERESE SCHROEDER-SHEKER

Music-Thanatology and Spiritual Care for the Dying

Harpist, singer, and composer Therese Schroeder-Sheker has maintained triple careers in music, medicine, and academia. After formative time in Stuttgart, Paris, Oxford, and Chichester, she studied composition in Colorado with Dr. Evan Copley and the distinguished Prix de Rome winner Normand Lockwood (Academie des Beaux-Arts in Paris). She made her Carnegie Hall debut in 1980 and has performed in solo concerts across eight countries and three continents.

As a musician-clinician with 29 years of experience in the care of the dying, Therese Schroeder-Sheker founded the palliative medical field of music-thanatology, the Chalice of Repose Project, its ancillary School of Music-Thanatology, and most recently, the Vox Clamantis Institute and Clinic, all located in Mt. Angel, Oregon, an hour south of Portland. Her work has been distinguished with a number of cultural, humanitarian, and media awards, including a shared Emmy, a shared gold record, a Gabriel, a Christopher, and a first place in the Palm Springs International Film Festival documentaries section.

As an educator and scholar, she publishes frequently in the areas of musicology, monastic medicine, contemplative musicianship, medieval music, music thanatology, and the women mystics. As a recording artist, she has to her credit five major titles *(The Geography of the Soul, In Dulci Jublio, Rosa Mystica, Celebrant, The Queen's Minstrel),* numerous television and film scores, the music to 30 radio documentaries, and ten guest-artist performances on American and European labels. Her scholarly work has been translated into seven languages. She has been the academic dean of the School of Music Thanatology for a decade, and the monograph *Transitus: A Blessed Death in the Modern World* was published by St. Dunstan's Press in August of 2002. I interviewed Therese Schroeder-Sheker in early 2001 at The Chalice of Repose offices where I also had the privilege of hearing her students sing.

Music thanatology is a contemplative practice with clinical applications. The sole focus of our work is the physical and spiritual care of the dying using prescriptive music. Everyone we see or attend is actively dying.

We are concerned about the alleviation of pain—both physiological pain and interior suffering. These pains can be worlds apart; they can also overlap. Sometimes the sheer amount of sleep deprivation that may come with a given illness (not to mention mechanical noises and routine disturbances that are part of a hospital) triggers anxiety and nervousness. Sometimes an analgesic can "get" the physiological pain but not always the interior suffering. So elements like anxiety, fear, anger, rage, and abandonment can be taken into consideration and be addressed, because they too can and do show up physiologically in heartbeat, pulse, countenance, gesture, respiratory patterns, and temperature. A person could, on a 1-to-10 pain scale, be living with physical pain at a two or three, but his or her spiritual or interior suffering could be much higher, especially if that person has been rejected or abandoned. (Think of a broken heart: no broken bones but an abyss of despair.) So we are concerned about the alleviation of both physiological pain and spiritual or interior suffering.

Music-thanatology is a palliative medical modality. Sometimes people say very loving and simple, uncluttered things to us, such as "We love your ministry." That's an honor, though we are very clear that we're a medical modality. With very few words, they are acknowledging a vision of healthcare, that is inclusive of healing and wholeness and that even now within hospital systems is all too often relegated to the domain of pastoral care. Saying that, my colleagues and I are unashamed to make room for body, soul, and spirit in our epistemology, our anthropology, and in the clinical practice. So I'm sure that when people stop us and say, "I love your ministry," it indicates relief that their loved one was able to be seen, met, attended, and cared for as a full human being, a unique human being, the core of whom includes sacred mystery, not just disease or disease process.

We work with elements that can be objectively observed and measured: the vital signs. Before the vigil begins, the resident music-thanatologist will note pulse—qualitatively and quantitatively—respiratory patterns, temperature, countenance, gesture, skin color, and so on. After notating the starting condition, we document the changes. We document vital signs before, during, and after each session and include both subtle and at times dramatic changes beyond those parameters.

But we distinguish between healing and curing. We often see deathbed healing without curing. We are trying to manage pain relief to the extent that a person will have energy left over to enter into the process of dying, of leave-taking, as deeply and meaningfully as possible. This is the place where mystery and the measurable penetrate. From my point of view, efforts to keep them separate come from some illusion of determinism or a need to control that might best be morally questioned. A good sign of deep peace would be indicated simply through the changes of pulse and heartbeat, the calming of tremors and the softening of formerly intense facial grimaces. If there is very rapid, nervous breathing and then a calmness sets in—for instance, if the person goes into a deep restorative sleep without morphine—that is a very strong indication that we have had a beneficial effect at that vigil.

The way we do this is to work with synchronizing the tempo of the music to a person's heartbeat and breathing. That is why it is very different from concert music. We actually synchronize the music with the heartbeat and the pulse of the individual who is dying. We link up with them and accompany them, physically, right down to heartbeat and breath, leading up later to entrainment.

Dying

I'd like to say something about what I've seen and experienced personally—things that aren't in a book. The process of dying isn't so much a loss of life as a particularly intensified living in which quickening, acceleration, alteration, change, and intensification occur physically, mentally, emotionally, and spiritually. Boundaries shift, roles are reversed; we separate the essentials from the nonessentials, and many distractions fall away. In dying, it's possible to lose and to gain simultaneously. Dying, particularly intensified living, can accommodate every fullness we can bring to it, the fullest presence of being, from both the dying one and the caregivers, familial and professional. This intensity can be all-consuming and draining, and/or it can be particularly rich and generative. Living and dying can benefit from bringing the fullness of consciousness, awareness, love, and creativity to the fore. Then, too, we have several descriptors: a blessed death or a peaceful death or a conscious death. We are trying to manage pain and suffering to facilitate something more, something beyond—a conscious, blessed, or peaceful death, if that is the desire of the individual. These deaths are more than medical statistics and they are certainly not failures; they are essential parts of a human biography.

We have been very moved by some of the people with whom we have worked. Of course, there are stages in which a person fights and is reticent to die. This places sacred value on life and love; it affirms life and loved ones. But then, after certain events and conditions, we come to terms with the fact that our time is drawing close. To many comes what I can only call a blessed acceptance. When this happens, we see how they work with their own leave-taking, as a woman does in labor. She works with the contractions, not against them. They have a rhythm and an awesome power, and she benefits from assistance and partnering. Many in childbirth need painkillers, but often, if a woman is supported, she needs less medication.

The parallel between childbirth and *transitus* can teach us a lot. In the last 20 years, in every thanatology practice, we have seen more and more people (probably like the constituency who read *Alternative Therapies*) who anticipate and welcome the possibility of a good death, be it blessed or conscious or peaceful, because consciousness of mortality is one of the things that makes us truly human. If we meet it fully and truly, and resist the temptation to remove it from culture and life, it can be a deep, multilayered, transformative individual and collective process. I'm not talking romance; I'm not talking prettifying. It's so similar to childbirth: pain, yes; new life, yes; and beauty, despite the blood and viscera and agony. Some mothers in childbirth want zero pain medication; others need a local or even much more. Every request reflects self-knowledge; everything on this pain-medication spectrum is available, for the good, and unique to each person.

Besides all this, there are still many people who have never thought about dying at all, but we're in a time of change. Often the patient wants to work consciously, deliberately, and lovingly with his or her own process, and the doctor and/or nurse discover that the patient's sheer presence of being, at the end of life, constitutes the single most powerful medicine the caregiver can offer. From my point of view—and this may appear as hopelessly misplaced idealism—there's a deep and effective practicality that accompanies this hope. It comes from many years of experience and thousands of deathbed vigils. I hope the day will come when love and compassion are brought into every department of medicine as a healing agent long before the onset of dying. But this is a vision that depends on the intentions of individual practitioners, not the duty of autonomous systems.

A few other thoughts. The delivery of prescriptive music live at the bedside is not a touch therapy, though we speak about holy touch. Monastic medicine even spoke about the holy kiss! That compassionate touch—patients know if the provider touches them with loving respect, a mysterious combination of strength and tenderness. The surface of the skin functions with the sensitivity of a drum head, a stretched membrane, when we are extremely vulnerable, so we are very careful regarding the volume of the music and the kind and quality of the tonal substance we deliver at the bedside. For this reason, the harp is particularly effective. We have a great opportunity to do effective pain relief that allows a person to have some energy left over to cross the threshold wide awake, with his or her eyes open, to do the finishing-up pieces with loved ones consciously, to prepare for the next stage with love and awareness. For many believers, this is a time to prepare for meeting their Creator. It is like a crowning. A conscious or blessed death is something that can and does crown the entire human biography. A good death is intensely personal, but the effects are not private. A good death affects the whole community, including the medical culture, for years to come. It doesn't mean that suffering has been eliminated, but if meaning has been found—ultimate meaning—we are surely, for all time, crowned, restored, and regal even in our vulnerability and dissolution. It's the life and/or the death that has been stripped of meaning or reduced to statistics that is tragic. The life unwitnessed, unremembered, is demoralizing to us all.

That's another contribution that monastic medicine made; the Benedictine Cluniacs quite consciously linked the communities of the living and the communities of the dead, not through séances and the like but by witnessing, by doing vigil, and by full participation at the death-bed, followed by memorials and prayer activities, sheer love, celebrated in special rhythms: a week later, a month later, a year later, 7 years later.

And maybe a word about the noninvasive aspect of music at the deathbed. Although music thanatology is a medical modality—a palliative medical modality—we also know that not everything prescriptive music brings or does or facilitates is measurable. Music can effect some changes and states of being that simply are not measurable in that setting (it would be inappropriate—our work is to help them die well, not to get data), and some-times even in another setting, the effects would remain immeasurable. We're at peace with that, even if all the physicians are not. We document the changes of vital signs; we note the softening countenance, the opening of formerly contracted hands and legs, the changed heartbeat and pulse, the calming of tremors, and the miraculous reconciliations that occur between individuals following years of painful separation. But that is enough—more than enough.

Then there is the element of the sacred, which fills us; we observe and participate within it but have no longing to measure it. Sometimes dying persons come out of a coma and are without any indication of psychosis; they have one foot in each world, they're on the threshold and begin clearly, quietly, simply relating to the presence of a being whom no one else can see or experience in the same way. I've seen their eyes shine and fill with a directed gaze. It's clear that they are in deep converse—their lips are moving silently; their hands are reaching out for or toward that which is unknowable in my cluttered heart, in my distracted everyday self. But the room is filled with such a palpable burning stillness and reverence, a quietude, an indescrib-able depth, witnessed by all present, clinicians and loved ones, that I cannot avoid or deny, and any desire to measure this picture would actually defy the experience. Aren't we talking about grace? This kind of peace and holiness isn't meant to be measured or analyzed; it's meant to be treasured.

It never crossed Moses' mind to measure the heat or transformative brilliance exuding from the burning bush, but the heat melted and illumined his heart. Nor did the apostles coming back from Mt. Tabor try to prove the Transfiguration took place, yet those experiences occurred, and changed everything and everyone. The proof of those events is this: they continue to bear fruit forever. Like those wisdom elders before us who made room for what is holy and immeas-urable, it seems like we're called to protect the sacredness of some events, and death is one such sacred mystery. Me? I want to live a practice that bows before mystery and remains content to measure the mundane.

Music Thanatology

Our historical inspiration is really monastic medicine as it was practiced in the late Middle Ages. There was a Benedictine monastery in France at Cluny that, during the 11th century, had an infirmary, and their customaries and primary documents have been invaluable to us. The monks had a twofold medical regimen that was "care of the body, cure of the soul." They had an epistemological humility about what they could or could not do. That is the historical inspiration for our work: monastic medicine. Our contemporary inspiration is from palliative medicine and all the great advances it has achieved in the past 30 years.

As a field, music-thanatology is now starting its thirtieth year, so our history goes neck and neck with the birth and development of palliative medicine as well as the various English and

American hospice movements. I would also say we get inspiration from the Gospels, especially those beautiful lines from Matthew in which he says, "In as much as you have done it unto one of the least of these my brethren, ye have also done it unto me."

The story of the Chalice of Repose is this: I was very shy when I was young. You might have called me a church mouse. Now, as an undergraduate student in music, you either get a part-time job playing in churches and synagogues and at weddings, funerals, and liturgies, or you play in a bar. I didn't have the chutzpah for the latter and though I played at the liturgies, I didn't get paid, so I got a job working in a geriatric home as an orderly. I think orderlies can have a profound effect on the daily lives of the residents in those homes, but I have to be honest and say that I was plucked off the street and given a job without any training.

I had zero background. Over time, I became incredibly uncomfortable with the deaths that I was witnessing in the nursing home. Most of the elderly people were dying alone, unaccompanied by family and friends. Their accompaniment was the television; I would walk in and find people in the death rattle with an I Love Lucy rerun playing in the background. But I didn't have the intellectual or philosophical or spiritual tools to articulate what was wrong. I was so shy that I couldn't even articulate it emotionally. So I actually wondered if I should quit my job. I wondered if I was doing something bad in helping people die this way. I talked to a minister. I am Roman Catholic, and he was from a Protestant tradition, but he made himself deeply available and I trusted him implicitly. I said, "What should I do? Should I quit?" And he said, "Oh no, this is a spiritual opportunity. Go back and be there in a new way. Protect them." So that was the beginning.

It was almost three decades ago. He also said that if a person were to go back and be there in a new way, the spirituality of that presence of being would be essential medicine, even if it were invisible. He was talking about moral courage, too. He said, "Deepen and broaden your religious identity until it becomes a true spirituality. Grow and learn and love; love them." That was new.

So I went back. Then one morning I was assigned to a man who was dying from emphysema. That was the turning point. I was told that there was nothing more that could be done for him medically. This was not a case of malpractice. Everything had been done for him that could be done. His lungs were just disintegrating.

When I walked in the room, he was in the death rattle. I was in my early twenties at the time and many of my young women friends were pregnant with their first children and had been speaking about Lamaze natural childbirth. So I got into bed with him and assumed the same Lamaze midwifery position I had learned when I accompanied one of my friends to her class. I had learned about this posture and this way of holding and supporting the breathing. So I got into bed with him and stayed there until he died. I sang a Gregorian chant, only because I didn't know what else to do and because it was filled with beauty.

At the time, I didn't understand that because his spine was next to my heart-beating chest, there was the bone conduction, and my singing was coming through to him in an amplified interior way. I didn't understand that the process that occurred, even though he was disintegrating, was one of synchronization of breath. I didn't understand all the clinical physiological pieces that were going on with just holding, touching, breathing, and singing these prayers. Of course, it wasn't curing. It was deathbed healing. And he trusted me. He leaned into my body just the way a woman would do in labor, and he held onto me until he died. I was able to hold him and could experience the exit of the life. The other orderlies allowed me to be alone with him for many moments, for a long time. It was a completely life-changing experience. None of us spoke about it, but from that moment on when anybody was approaching death, we all dealt with it in a different way.

Prescriptive Music

I had wanted a harp since childhood, so after I graduated I put a down payment on a harp with one of my first paychecks. Then I studied in Europe. When I came back to the United States, I began being present at deaths. Friends would call and say, "My husband has been in a horrible wreck; he is at Denver General; would you please come." Of course, I always brought my harp and played. I hadn't thought out all the nitty-gritty clinical and practical details of success and failure, what is effective and what is detrimental, what is binding, and what supports loosening—the use of warm tones, low tones, noninvasive tonal substance. That came in the following years, through trial and error.

From the beginning, I knew that what I was experiencing was as real as any aspect of my life. I had my concert and recording career, and I had my professorial appointment, chairing the music program at Regis University and later a master's degree program at St. Thomas Theological Seminary, but I knew that this other work was as vital and as substantive as anything anywhere.

So the work with the harp in the medical setting developed gradually and slowly. At a certain stage, I had many harp students from all over the world. They would say, "Therese, we know you are doing something. What are you doing?" They would say, "Would you give us a small seminar on what you are doing?" Now, not every musician has the constitution or temperament for a concert career, but there are many musicians who have it in their heart and soul to serve in another way. So I began to bring one or two of the students with me.

William Hynes, who was the academic dean at Regis University in Denver at the time, was a real visionary leader. We shared a meal one time and he said, "Therese, don't you think that you should work on a curriculum? There are musicians out there and people who are suffering who need this. There are musicians for whom this would be a vocation. Let us help you work on developing an undergraduate curriculum, and we'll bring it before the committee." At first, we had a BA music-thanatology program at Regis, and later on I brought Chalice to the seminary at St. Thomas and developed a master's degree through the School of Theology. In that program, the work was understood under the rubric of pastoral care. That was beautiful, but we weren't yet as fully effective in the world as I suspected we could be, and I knew that until we found a way to be working right in the heart of medical settings we would not have come to our full stride.

By the mid-1980s I had worked in every hospital and hospice in Denver. One of the big breakthroughs was when the chief of staff at Rose Memorial Hospital invited me to deliver medical grand rounds. I remember one physician turning to me and saying, "Therese, I have been practicing medicine for 30 years, and I've never been asked to do grand rounds." (I hadn't known enough to be scared until he said that.) There had also never been an invitation for a nonphysician to teach medical grand rounds up until that point, so it was a big threshold. Then there was a very strange period when a number of different hospitals in several cities approached me and said, "We want your program in our hospital." But they really wanted it for marketing purposes and it came with a caveat that the program could only be at such and such a hospital, and we couldn't do it anyplace else. They didn't understand that it was a medical modality, and as a medical modality, it would be against any spirituality and against the moral foundation of medicine to make it available to only one constituency. So I had to find the courage to say, "Thank you very much, but no." I held out a few more years until the right kind of medical invitation came.

The next visionary person was Lawrence L. White, Jr., the former president of St. Patrick's Hospital in Missoula, Montana. Through his invitation, I relocated the Chalice of Repose Project (clinical practice and school) from Denver to Missoula in July 1992. By then I had had 19 years to fully develop the curriculum and had a distinguished faculty for the school. Chalice always remained a separate legal entity; we never became a department of the hospital, but by having an institutional relationship and by being initially located within the hospital, we were right where we were needed. It was an incredible transition to be so close to patients' needs, and we received wonderful support from the hospital board of directors.

You need a polyphonic instrument to deliver prescriptive music. A monophonic instrument such as a flute will not be adequate. Polyphonic means "many sounding." The major polyphonic instruments are the piano, organ, lute, guitar, and harp. You can't move a piano or an organ in and out of an intensive care unit. The harp that you see here in the corner of the room is the size we bring into the medical settings. It is light enough so that you can carry it easily, put it in the car, and go up and down stairs with it, but it is also big enough. It is not a lap harp. The length of the deep strings is similar to an average-size human being. We are heavily reliant on the deep, rich tones because it would be a contraindication to stimulate the person, which occurs with high-pitched sounds and metallic strings that might be found on the wire-strung harp or on dulcimers. We try to soothe the person. The use of the harp is not a qualitative judgment against other instruments. But at the deathbed the way tonal substance is created is very important. You can have an equally beautiful instrument, such as an oboe or a French horn, but the way the substance comes out to a vulnerable person in a very small space would be far too invasive in that particular deathbed setting.

We work with the entire human being: body, soul, and spirit. That the sound accumulates in the room is pure physics. Our vigils are always done with two harpists, one on either side of the bed. Internally, we refer to it as anointing or bathing or surrounding the person in sound. The reason ushers close the door once a symphony has begun is not only a matter of courtesy to the musicians and listeners, as most people think. If the room is still, the overtones collect in the room, and as more and more overtones collect, the more the listeners experience the tonal color of the music.

So when we do a deathbed vigil for somebody, we coordinate with the nurses and physicians. Our vigil might last an hour, and they suspend routine medical activities for the duration of the vigil. The room is still, a harpist is on each side, right and left, and we have a chance to let sound accumulate and penetrate to body and soul.

It is almost like an arbor of sound. If you are the nurse or doctor and you have been in another place, when you go in the room the contrast between the room with music and the room without music is palpable. Most of the time our patients fall asleep in a vigil, and that is a good sign. We don't want them to be sitting up saying, "Oh, thank you. That music is great." We want them to be able to receive the music and go into a more silent place so they can hear themselves and the voice of their own needs, so they can hear what their own soul is telling them or what is rising up in their own lives.

There is a fabulous resurgence of spirituality today, yet while people are dying with spirituality, they are not necessarily dying with a religious identity. People know when they are allowed to be who they are and people know when they are allowed the privilege of being in their own experience instead of having to meet the criteria of somebody else's needs. We help facilitate this in a nonverbal way—music-thanatology is not a talk therapy. We get in the front door with beauty, intimacy, and reverence, without any preaching, without any dogma—and, bingo, they have an entrée into their own deepest selves. Oftentimes there is a reconciliation with family after the vigil.

Stories

This could be anybody in America. Mary is dying. She has four brothers and sisters between the ages of 50 and 60 who had a fight 20 years ago and have not spoken to one another since.

Nevertheless, when the telephone calls are made across the country to tell them that Mary is dying, all the brothers and sisters board planes immediately, even if they don't exactly know why. It's the first time that they have been in each other's presence since the big family fight, and the hospital room is bristling with tension. Without any talk therapy at all, with no psychological therapy, no religious doctrine, and no preaching, the depth and the peace of these low tones has an effect. The reconciliation piece is a very high-stakes gamble. People have cherished an anger or hurt for 20 or 30 years, and they suddenly get that Mary is dying and they can't go on fighting right now because they need to be present for her. People separate the essentials from the nonessentials. This is her time, her threshold. It is about Mary first and about the others second. We have many clinical narratives about family members who had hatred who, within an hour, experienced a profound shift. Tears also accompany that warmth. I always consider tears to be a sign of health. They can flow and cleanse. It is intense work.

Only once did someone experience a complete cure after a vigil. It was absolutely remarkable. We have had people who experienced such tremendous interior healing from the burdens of their life that they got a second wind and lived beyond any expectation for 6 months or a year. But, eventually, they do go. But I have had one absolute cure, though I don't know that it was the music.

There was a little girl who was 6 years old, the youngest harp student I had ever had. At the age of 3 she was a tomboy and was always trying to do everything her brothers did. One day, while her mother was in the kitchen, she was upstairs with her brothers on the second floor of their house. The boys were playing Superman and thinking she would one-up them, she leapt out of the window. She sustained severe cranial trauma and was raced to the hospital.

There were all kinds of surgeries. She lived but was plagued because she had a condition that wasn't diagnosed for years. In a matter of minutes, she would go from spunky to listless and spike a fever. She had spinal meningitis, but no one understood that she had a rip in her meninges. By the time she was 6 years old, she had had 27 spinal taps. When her mother called me, the little girl had had a vicious onslaught of fever and had gone into shock. By the time I got there, the doctors had already said to her mother, "Let go of this child. She won't make it through the night."

Her mom called me to do what she thought was the deathbed vigil. The little girl was in a coma, and I played and played and played. I played for her mother as well because this little girl was her only daughter. Then, all of a sudden, the little girl came right out of the coma and started bossing us all around. It was incredible. To this day (she's a young adult now), she has perfect pitch. She lost all of her olfactory senses, but suffered no other neurological damage. There is no explanation for it. I expect her to become the president or the pope or something because whatever that biography is about, she has a reservoir of strength. She is going to be a leader.

The Music

I compose a great deal. But much of the music we use in the deathbed vigil comes from monasticism, such as the Gregorian chant, and from the lullaby repertoire—there is so much important gentle rocking in the 3:4's, which is used in many lullabies. The music I use also comes from Jewish and Hebrew cantillation. So we draw heavily upon the sacred repertoire and lullabies and some new twentieth-century literature. Also, a few composers are emerging from the school here—contemplative musicians and musician-clinicians. And that's as it should be.

The reason The Chalice of Repose exists is for the care of the dying, but to see the students whom I teach come into their own voice as composers is very rewarding. That voice has a validity for the living as well as for the dying. You don't have to be in one condition or the other to benefit. So I feel like this curriculum equips people for life and a vocation.

Also, I'd have to say—and I hope this makes sense—that the music comes, most deeply, from the practice of silence. Stilling the inner tumult, letting the small but nagging voices die down, listening deeply to a voice much more important than the relentless and limited voice of our personality. Listening into the beyond. Real compositions, real living streaming music creates and recreates, brings a world into existence that didn't exist an hour ago. That means that the music comes from the places that are new and wholly unknown. I'm not describing improvisation; I'm attempting to name awareness, risk, inner emptiness, trust, and radical receptivity.

So the music is different for each patient and the singing is different for each patient. If someone listens to a piece of music, their heartbeat will end up being in the same pulse as the music. It doesn't take much. In clinical terms, the external auditory stimulus is stronger than the person, so the body converts to the extra stimulus. Can you imagine if someone was vulnerable and horizontal? People need to understand that it is nothing less than a *materia medica*. It isn't this feel-good, sentimental, distraction-therapy vagueness. The music and the singing are like compound medicines that we can administer wisely. Musician-clinicians the world over and medicine in general are still at the infancy of learning what can and cannot be done with sound—and to, for, and with the body and soul.

The Curriculum

The music-thanatology curriculum has always been rigorous and for the last 10 years, only a graduate level program has been available. Traditionally, there are 17 different kinds of subjects in five different tracks over five semesters, plus a 1-year internship. Generally, the different tracks are a musical track, an academic track, a clinical track, a medical track, and an inner-development track. We use the language of an infused curriculum. In most schools, each subject is taught as a separate modular unit. We all took courses in college from great professors who didn't know one another, and didn't know the content of each other's discipline. Our curriculum is completely infused so that every lecture series interfaces with every other lecture series. For instance, our students practice as a *schola cantorum*, which is the Latin term for "school of singing" and is considered a sacred and learned activity.

In college, we could get one or two semester-hour credits for signing up for choir, and we knew that we would get an A just for showing up. This is a very different activity. From day one, while you are learning your repertoire, you are also learning how to live inside your body. You are developing stage-one bodily awareness, starting to work with your own metabolism. You are taught clinical phenomenology. "This is F minor. Now, where is your heartbeat? Your pulse?" We are linking the clinical and the music in every single situation. You don't just learn the notes; you begin to understand, among other things, that your body has to transform to hold pitch.

Students with pitch problems come into the program with two tendencies. If I am vocally aggressive and I am pushing in my sound, I go sharp. If I am reticent and holding back, I tend to go flat. Pitch is actually a diagnostic tool. But it is not a personal moral judgment if my teacher turns to me and says, "You are flat today." He or she is also teaching me that to heal myself I have to step forward. And if a teacher says, "You have gone sharp," then I know that to heal myself and heal the community, I have to pull back. It is a matter of soul; it is a matter of psychology. I can grasp the intellectual concepts of sharp and flat and pitch and also experience it in my body. What am I doing when I am pushing and going sharp? Is it diaphragmatic? It is entirely coming from my feelings? Did I just have a fight with my husband this morning?

So you are teaching the vocal technique; you are teaching how to read the score. You also are teaching the psychological component of sharpness or flatness, the spiritual condition of sharpness or flatness, and the diagnostic tool of sharpness or flatness. It is very different from having a spiritual director say, "Bonnie, you are wrinkled and sullied." You now have a diagnostic tool to say, "I am sharp today." That is a *schola cantorum*, and it differs so much from university choir. It is educational and it is transformative; that's why a *schola* has always been described as a sacred singing school. And transformation from absolute point of entry is our goal.

Now, at the end of our tenth year here, after completing five cycles of classes, we have decided to completely restructure the educational program again for several reasons, and one of them is to better meet the needs of the kinds of students who are drawn to this work. A second is to look at our faculty load. The curriculum as it is now has been structured on the medical model—if you want to be a physician, you go through medical school, but then you do your internship and your residencies and become board-certified.

Some of the students singing downstairs have graduated and are finishing up their clinical internships. They are writing professional papers, and they will sit for their comprehensive exams, which are 3-day events in music, medicine, academics, inner development, diagnostics, and finally the written and oral exams. In the new programs that will become available in 2003, at the Vox Clamantis Institute and Clinic, we're going to be able to offer a series of apprenticeship programs that will allow musician-clinicians to "do" rotations in several places across the country, and to proceed at different paces according to their unique needs. I am simply thrilled about the new developments. The deeper aspects too, the contemplative nature of the work, including the clinician's inner development and transformation will be able to flourish and be supported very differently through the apprenticeship programs. Some people need more time for the musical formation; others need more time for the medical formation. And the dream of opening a free-standing clinic that is a genuine sanctuary has come true now, with Vox Clamantis in Mt. Angel. The work of music-thanatology will be able to deepen and expand and especially, continue to nurture the spirituality of the practitioner.

Personal Growth

Our conversation opened with a couple of words that often times go right by people: music thanatology is contemplative practice. What that means is that I don't see death as only a biological event. In the history of Christian monasticism, in the ancient Jewish ascetic tradition, in Buddhist monasticism, there has always been the call to die to something every day. That is really hard work. It is inspiring when you are reading about it in a book, when you are healthy and life is going well, but to actually meet the tumultuous experiences of life, to face adversity and struggle, betrayal, hypocrisy and deception, and to die to the events that occur in our lives—including institutional struggles and collisions with values and meanings—to when you are confronted with your own smallness, or to the huge events, such as when your own child has died—this daily dying is hard work, and a core practice for music thanatologists.

To actually meet the events of life and work with them consciously, to let them transform me and then let go—which means to go all the way through an experience rather than avoid it, to enter it fully and deeply with my body and my soul and my spirit and go all the way through—becomes increasingly more challenging every year. And yet I think the dimensions of my soul are larger and deeper than they were when I started this 28 years ago. Oh, and much more joy! The capacity for joy is alive and well.

In some ways I have more spiritual strength than I ever had before, but pioneering work *is* hard, and protecting a vision asks for faithfulness, vigilance, and sacrifice. People say, "Don't you get depressed? Don't you have burnout?" First of all, in my experience, the administrative work, the corporatization of medicine and the politics of medicine kills the spirit and guarantees burns you out; I never suffered from burnout over patient or student load. People work is life! It's great and fills the soul. With the inner work, it is almost like a postmodern monasticism. We are laypeople in the world, and we come from every different background—Jews, Christians, Buddhists, and so on—yet we share this deep inner call to the vocation. We know it is the spiritual underpinning of our own participation that allows us to get out of bed and come back again tomorrow. It's not procedures; it's participation.

I have changed a lot over the years. I had to become more courageous. I was born a church mouse, so I had to change to found a graduate school. I was born naturally to the arts, so to study internal medicine has been difficult. I have intelligence, but in youth I had pigeonholed myself in the arts rather than the sciences, so to be confident and articulate about my clinical capacities is tremendous growth. It is spiritually challenging to die, to grieve, and to live through disappointment and loss, competition, resentment, confusion, longing, and yet it's part of the assignment, over and over. To come to terms with the politics of medicine, the frustrations and challenges of fund development, people's private agendas, and the relentless corporate demands—aggressive and often diametrically opposed to mission and values—and not to let myself become greedy for my own time, my own space. This is all real work. But work with the dying and working in palliative medicine has asked me to change 100 times over. I'm grateful and filled with awe, even if I've howled along the way.

Asking yourself to be open to other people's pain makes you more, it doesn't make you less. But learning how to share the pain and be open without taking on the pain takes wisdom, not naïveté. I think I have become more compassionate, more patient, and persevering, especially in conflictual situations. Your eyes change; how you see changes. Doing this work is a school of humility. You play a jillion wrong notes; you err. Leadership is humility if you are working under a servant leadership rubric rather than being "the boss." Committing to this work has brought certain virtues to my consciousness that I might not have developed or even known about had I pursued a purely academic career at a university or pursued only my concert recording career.

I want to be closer to God. When we are present to people in their suffering, there is God. Certainly elsewhere too, but at the threshold, for sure. Sometimes it is the students as they are going through transformation that allows you to see God. It is not always the patients and their families. It is the doctors—they are broken-hearted. It is the nurses—they are so overworked. Hospital administrators become very hardened after fighting for every domain. You see people's pain and it makes you more humble. So this work has deepened my life of prayer like nothing else. In those ways, I think it has helped me grow and become a better person.

Here is a story. There was an elderly man who had been a famous historian and a journalist. He had been articulate, extremely successful, and highly published. By the time I met him, he was a senior citizen in his early eighties. He was not dying, but he was crotchety as hell, ran a very famous bookstore, didn't ever have to worry about money, and didn't hesitate to bark at anybody about anything. I was his next-door neighbor, and there was a door between his bookstore and my studio. I suddenly realized that he wasn't going to live forever, so for his next birthday I organized a bunch of the students to fete him in the old royal way, the way bards would play for a king or a queen. I played the harp for him and gathered my students around him in a *schola* formation. I said, "Mr. Bloch, we want to do and to be for you to celebrate all of these decades that you have been on the earth."

When he saw what was going to happen, he pulled himself up to complete full stature. This is a man who weighed 98 pounds on a good day. He wouldn't sit down but insisted on standing, received the music standing, though he leaned heavily on his cane. We played this late medieval, early Renaissance Benedictine music from the monastery of Montserrat in Catalonia. The music was tender and beautiful. The voices surrounded him, and you could see the crown coming on his head. He stood there receiving the music, and without ever letting out an audible whimper, big tears rolled down his face. We were very moved, and he was very moved, and his wife was moved.

A couple of weeks later, overnight, he had an all-systems failure, and everything started to go—kidneys, liver, heart, everything. I would go every day to visit him in the hospital. His demise was very quick, and he turned away from the world in the last three days and refused to face anybody. When I entered the room he was on every sort of apparatus—wires, hooks, catheters, inserts, and invasive technologies. I came late at night one time to visit him, and the nurse, who had had a really hard day, was irritated and tired and said, "I don't know why you are doing this. He is comatose; he can't hear a thing; and you are in the way." I guess I ignored her and kept playing. She left the room and I kept on playing. He was completely turned away from me with his face to the wall, but he began conducting with his left foot exactly in rhythm to the music to let me know that he was receiving while he was dissolving.

So those are my kinds of didactics. The sources of learning are plentiful, ever-present, and break the boundaries. The patients teach us. I have the great texts on internal medicine—Harrison, Husemann and Wolff, and others—but I learn so much from people, from patients and students, from the Book of Nature, inner reflection, all relationships. Learning and conversion come from many sources. Although I seek the Golden Mean everywhere (music is proportion and luminosity), I never let anyone tell me there is a limit to learning.

Part Three

Conversations About
Alternative Medical Systems

*"Healing involves opening what we have closed
down, remembering what is or was once sacred
to us, and honoring our connections with our-
self, others, and the Transcendent."*

—BARBARA DOSSEY

CHAPTER 8

MICHAEL MURRAY, ND

A Natural Approach to Health

Natural medicine has been steadily gaining respect for the past 15 years as research reveals its efficacy and people experience its benefits. Michael Murray, ND, is regarded as one of its leading authorities. In addition to his private practice, Dr. Murray is currently a professor of botanical medicine at Bastyr University in Seattle and the director of product development and education for Natural Factors Nutritional Products. He received his doctorate in naturopathic medicine from Bastyr University in 1985.

A prolific writer, Dr. Murray is the medical editor of the *Natural Medicine Journal* and author or co-author of many books and publications, including *Textbook of Natural Medicine, The Encyclopedia of Natural Medicine, The Healing Power of Herbs, The Healing Power of Foods, Natural Alternatives to Prozac, The Encyclopedia of Nutritional Supplements,* and *5-HTP—The Natural Way to Overcome Depression, Obesity,* and *Insomnia.*

As a consultant to the healthfood industry, Dr. Murray was instrumental in making many natural products—including glucosamine sulfate, St. John's wort extract, ginkgo biloba extract, silymarin, enteric-coated peppermint oil, and saw palmetto berry extract— broadly available to the American public and medical community.

In 1999, I interviewed Dr. Murray at his home in Issaquah, Washington.

The key point about diets and nutrition is that people need to move away from foods that are full of empty calories—junk food loaded with too much fat or too much sugar—and on to foods that are more natural. Specifically, people need to increase their consumption of plant foods, such as vegetables, fruits, nuts, seeds, and legumes. I believe our bodies were built to digest primarily plant foods, but we are getting away from what nature intended.

There are volumes of scientific data supporting the notion that diet is the major underlying factor in most chronic degenerative diseases, such as heart disease, cancer, stroke, diabetes, arthritis, and various colon disorders. Just about every chronic disease you can name owes its origin to diet.

We now know that disease can be reversed by changing people's diet, but I take a more holistic approach. I believe there are four cornerstones for achieving good health that cannot be ignored. First, you need a positive attitude, including the mental, emotional, and spiritual aspects. Second, you must have a health-promoting lifestyle—that is, you need to get enough sleep and exercise and avoid bad habits like cigarette smoking. Third, you should eat a health-promoting diet.

The fourth cornerstone is something I call "supplementary measures." Included in this category is anything that supports a person's basic level of health. Some of these supplementary measures are essential; others are more ancillary. For instance, I believe that everybody in America needs to take a high-potency multiple vitamin and mineral formula, antioxidants, and one tablespoon of flaxseed oil per day. These recommendations go a long way toward addressing some of the nutritional deficiencies and imbalances from which most Americans suffer. I also include medicines in the fourth category. For example, if you are a type-I diabetic, insulin is an essential supplementary measure. But for most chronic conditions and nonemergency situations, people should avoid drugs and try a more natural approach—nutritional supplements, herbal medicines, acupuncture, homeopathy, bodywork of all types—that is less invasive and more natural to the body, helping to promote the indwelling healing power of every person.

I recommend supplementing the diet with fish oil or flaxseed oil because Americans are low in omega-3 fatty acids. Supplementing with omega-3 oils, in addition to avoiding the omega-6 fatty acids so prevalent in our diet and eating cold-water fish once or twice per week, goes a long way toward restoring a proper balance of essential fatty acids.

In their book, *Pathological Basis of Disease*, Robbins and Cotran state that every disease has its origin at the cell membrane level. How can people expect to have healthy cells and tissues if their cell membranes do not contain the proper structural components? They can't. Most Americans have cell membranes packed full of saturated fats, cholesterol, and trans-fatty acids. Essential fatty acids play a crucial role in membrane structure and function. A lot of evidence has shown that low levels of omega-3 fatty acids are responsible for many common health conditions from depression and agoraphobia to heart disease, cancer, and diabetes.

Detoxification

A person's ability to detoxify harmful compounds from the environment, as well as harmful compounds that we manufacture, helps determine his or her overall level of health.

I usually rely on symptoms. People in need of detoxification are usually fatigued, have a general malaise, and typically exhibit low immune function. They may have been previously diagnosed with chronic fatigue syndrome, fibromyalgia, multiple chemical sensitivity disorders, or a number of other conditions. One of the simple things that should be done when these symptoms occur is to ensure that the patient drinks enough water. Everyone knows that. All my patients know they need to drink 6 to 8 glasses of water per day, but very few follow that simple recommendation.

Another element of detoxification involves eating a diet consisting primarily of plant foods. Plant foods are rich in fiber, which helps to flush out many of the fat-soluble toxins that are excreted in bile. Plant foods are also rich in antioxidants. We get our antioxidant nutrients from vegetables, nuts, fruits, and legumes. There is very little antioxidant nutrition offered in milk or dairy products, red meat, or poultry. So eating more plant foods is a good, simple way to enhance detoxification.

There are also many natural approaches for enhancing liver function. We can use lipotropics to increase the flow of fat to and from the liver. We also can use compounds such as choleretics to increase the flow of bile to and from the liver. The liver's response to injury is to incorporate fat and bile, a process that leads to cholestasis or fatty infiltration of the liver. Therefore one of the basic recommendations of naturopaths is to get the liver moving. This process involves using lipotropic and choleretic substances such as choline, inositol, methionine, milk thistle extract, or artichoke extract. These compounds have demonstrated an ability to improve hepatic function and promote proper detoxification.

Depression

The naturopathic remedy for depression again involves looking at those four critical factors that contribute to a person's mood and health. We don't get depressed because we are deficient in Prozac (fluoxetine hydrochloride). A naturopath tries to identify the factors that contribute to the depression.

One of the hallmark principles of naturopathic medicine is to identify and treat the cause. The application of this principle involves looking not only at biochemical factors but also social, emotional, and psychological factors. What is a person's dominant explanatory style? Is he or she a pessimist or an optimist? I believe we have to use psychological and cognitive therapies to teach people life skills. We have to get it across to them that every thought, every emotion, and every image they project makes an impression on the subconscious mind. The quality of their life is directly related to how well they control what is being imprinted on their subconscious mind. Because of this connection, I work a lot with affirmations, positively framed and empowering questions, and other techniques.

There is a great book on this subject that I think every healthcare practitioner should read: *Learned Optimism* by Martin Seligman, MD. Seligman is the man who developed the learned helplessness model for behavior.

In one classic experiment, Seligman took two groups of dogs and put them in shuttle boxes (boxes divided by a barrier). The dogs were then exposed to a shock. The first group could avoid the shock by jumping to the other side of the box. These animals quickly learned that they had control over their environment. The second group of dogs was in an identical shuttle box. However, for this group, it didn't matter what side of the box they were in—they were going to get shocked intermittently no matter what. After a while, the dogs in the second group gave up, crawled into the corner, and curled up into a ball. They had learned to be helpless. If you were to analyze their brain chemistry, you would find it parallels what is seen in human depression.

In the second phase of the experiment, the first group of dogs was put in a new environment. However, instead of having to jump over the barrier, they simply had to press a lever to stop the shock. They quickly figured out what they needed to do to avoid the pain. The dogs in the second group were placed in an identical box. They, too, could turn off the shock by putting their paws on the lever, but these dogs just crawled in the corner again. They had learned to be helpless.

You could give those dogs an antidepressant drug, and they would eventually unlearn their learned helplessness, or you could physically teach them that by pressing their paws on the lever they could stop the shock. Psychological therapies for humans are analogous to teaching these dogs how to turn off their pain. Taking drugs avoids the pain, but it doesn't really teach a person anything. In our society the message we receive is that if you don't feel good, you should take a pill. But as physicians we should be teaching people basic life skills that will point them in the right direction for the long term.

In my practice, time is an important element—we don't have enough of it. So I often prescribe reading materials to bring my patients up to speed. Or, if necessary, I refer patients to an appropriate psychotherapist. Most of my patients, whether they suffer from depression or some other illness, remark that I really listen to them. Listening, touching, and being there for the patient are extremely helpful in the healing process.

The prevalence of depression in America is astounding. Here are some other interesting statistics. First of all, 17 million Americans are taking antidepressant drugs. Of these patients, 80% are women between the ages of 25 and 50. Based on estimates using strict blood test criteria, 20% have hypothyroidism. The percentage of women afflicted with subclinical hypothyroidism is probably much higher than that. Depression is the first symptom of low thyroid function. We also know that many women between the ages of 25 and 50 have nutrient deficiencies of vitamin B_6, folate, vitamin B_{12}, magnesium, and zinc. Those are all common nutrient deficiencies in this population, all of which could lead to depression or hormonal imbalances. We also know that many women suffer from premenstrual syndrome (PMS), of which depression is a common feature.

Another astounding statistic is that 90% of prescribing doctors spend less than $3\frac{1}{2}$ minutes with their patients. In conventional medicine, practitioners are not addressing the underlying cause of PMS any better now than they were in the past. Previous therapies used were things like hysterectomies and then later tranquilizers—Valium (diazepam) and Halcion (triazolam)—that basically pacified the patient or shut her up. Those methods were barbaric.

Breast Cancer

Most women I've seen with breast cancer have come to me with the diagnosis. They had been somewhere else and were frightened but were doing a wise thing by consulting someone who was knowledgeable about nutrition and herbal therapies. Naturopathic medicine has a lot to offer in these cases, regardless of the decisions a woman makes in terms of conventional treatment. Much can be done to support the woman in her process, but there are no guarantees. I have seen women who elected to have lumpectomies continue to fare well 15 years later. I have also seen patients who had lumpectomies and did everything right but whose cancer came back. I have seen patients who underwent the most aggressive therapy and are doing great, and I have seen those who had the most aggressive therapy and have not done great.

We—and I mean the entire medical community—do not have all the answers right now on breast cancer. We can only talk about statistics. I try to help patients arrive at a decision they are comfortable with—not one that I am comfortable with. I will give them my opinion and my experience, but I won't try to influence their decision. Once they make their decisions, we focus on supportive therapy with nutritional supplements and herbal medicines.

If I knew 100% that the natural route was the way to go, I would push my patients in that direction. But we don't have the statistics. We don't have the studies. At this point, it is just an odds game with the goal being to give the patient the best odds for a positive outcome.

Human Immunodeficiency Virus (HIV)

I wrote a chapter on HIV for the *Encyclopedia of Natural Medicine* and was harshly criticized by some colleagues because I dared to suggest that if T-cell counts dropped below a certain level, the patient would be a suitable candidate for retroviral drugs and protease inhibitors. It is hard to argue against the statistics, and we just don't have the statistics yet with natural medicines. Hopefully, research being conducted at Bastyr University will show some benefits, but right now I am going to put philosophy aside and be pragmatic.

That being said, what appalls me about AIDS and HIV treatment in conventional circles is how prevalent nutrient deficiency is and how there is a lack of basic nutritional and immune system support. It baffles me. I don't understand it. Take vitamin B_{12}, for example. Vitamin B_{12} deficiency is apparent in roughly 35% of all HIV-positive patients. The degree of B_{12} deficiency is correlated to how fast the virus replicates. The greater the deficiency, the faster the replication. There are good studies demonstrating this, so why aren't these patients being given vitamin B_{12}?

In my lectures I am always amazed when I ask medical doctors whether they have heard of a particular study involving a nutritional supplement or an herbal remedy, and they say no, even if the article appeared in a journal like the *Journal of the American Medical Association*, the *New England Journal of Medicine*, or *The Lancet*. There is a tremendous blind spot and a lack of awareness by the entire medical community regarding natural medicines that definitely should be addressed, preferably within the medical schools. Natural medicines should be included in medical textbooks to a much greater extent than they are now.

I gave a lecture last year to a very large ophthalmology group. Before I spoke I was in the lobby browsing through the bookstore. I picked up some textbooks on macular degeneration and cataracts because I wanted to see what they had to say about nutrition. I was amazed to discover that the main pathology book had no reference to the role of nutrition in either cataract formation or macular degeneration. A lot of this information is not being taught in our medical schools. That must change and probably will change when the old guards retire.

Some of the older doctors out there suffer from what I term "the tomato effect." You see, 100 years ago people said, "Tomatoes are poisonous; don't eat them." Now we know that there are good things in tomatoes like lycopene, which prevents heart disease and prostate cancer. Likewise, a lot of these doctors were told in medical school that alternative therapies, nutritional supplements, and herbs don't work, and they are still suffering from those teachings. But just like we learned that tomatoes were okay, many of these doctors are learning that many of these natural therapies work.

Let me give you an example. A 52-year-old man who had severe osteoarthritis of his left knee and could barely walk came to see me. Two weeks before, he had been hospitalized for an acute bleeding ulcer that was caused by his nonsteroidal antiinflammatory drugs (NSAIDs). So he had to get off the NSAIDs and, as a result, was in pain. He said, "I read an article you wrote, and I want to give glucosamine sulfate a try." I put him on 1500 mg of glucosamine sulfate daily and 6 weeks later he came back ecstatic. He was jumping up and down, doing deep knee bends, and showing me how well the treatment had worked. He said, "I felt so good that yesterday, when I went to see my medical doctor, I told him I was taking glucosamine sulfate. Do you know what he told me? He told me that it was nothing but a placebo. You know what I told him? I said, 'Doc, if it was just a placebo why didn't you give it to me 10 years ago instead of those damn drugs?'"

The use of NSAIDs is a classic example of a drug that suppresses the symptoms while actually promoting the progression of the disease process. NSAIDs inhibit the ability of cartilage to repair itself. I think it is going to be one of the drugs that doctors in the future will remember and say, "Boy, what were we thinking back then?" Anyway, I sent the doctor a cover letter explaining that glucosamine sulfate is an approved drug in more than 70 countries and has been used by millions of people effectively and without side effects. I also sent him some of the double-blind studies in which glucosamine sulfate demonstrated better results in osteoarthritis than did NSAIDs such as ibuprofen or piroxicam. A few days later I got a great letter from the doctor thanking me. He was actually excited. He wrote that he had no idea glucosamine sulfate was so well researched. He was excited because he had a new tool that was not only more effective than his old one but also much safer.

Patient Stories

One of the first patients I saw in my practice was a 41-year-old man who had been diagnosed with ulcerative colitis. He was having six to eight bloody bowel movements a day, was on prednisone, had rectal implants, and was in bad shape. He had had this condition for 24 years, ever since he was 17 years old, and had always taken the drug sulfasalazine. We did tests for folate levels, and they were nondetectable. Sulfasalazine interferes with the absorption of folic acid, and one of the side effects of folic acid deficiency is diarrhea. Because the cells that line the intestinal tract never get the nutrients they need to replicate, they are not repaired as they are sloughed off. This leads to chronic diarrhea.

I felt that the folate concern was a major area of focus. But I also wanted to rule out food allergies. I found out he had spaghetti for dinner the night before, so I asked, "Did you have any cheese on that?" He said, "Yes, I had a pint of cottage cheese with the spaghetti."

I thought that was interesting. Carrageenan is present in cottage cheese. I had just read a study on ulcerative colitis in animals, in which the researchers used carrageenan to induce the colitis. Carrageenan comes from red seaweed and is used as a thickening agent. So I started looking at the link between carrageenan and ulcerative colitis. Some human studies have also been done to determine whether carrageenan is a problem. The researchers fed very large quantities of carrageenan to healthy human subjects without any noticeable side effects. It turns out rats have a different intestinal flora, and the reason carrageenan was so harmful was that the rats have high levels of a specific species of *Bacteroides vulgatus*. Healthy people don't have Bacteroides in their intestinal flora, but the researchers found high levels among patients with ulcerative colitis.

Suspecting that carrageenan might be a factor, I told my patient he had to stay away from cottage cheese. You would have thought I was asking him to give up his right arm. He loved it and was eating a quart of cottage cheese a day. To make a long story short, he went into complete remission. It is likely that he never had classic ulcerative colitis. He either had a milk allergy or it was the carrageenan. He didn't care—he was cured.

Another interesting patient, a 38-year-old man who suffered from insomnia for 20 years, came to see me. He had a file three inches thick because he had been to sleep laboratories. The doctors finally threw up their hands and said that he had an inherited sleep disorder and the only thing they could offer him was benzodiazepines. Well, he became addicted. He eventually worked himself off the drugs, but his insomnia was terrible so he came to see me. I started taking his history and asked him about his coffee consumption. He said, "I have two cups of coffee a day, sometimes a little more, but nothing after 3:00 pm."

I asked him how long he had been drinking coffee. "Twenty years," he said. I asked him when his sleep disorder started. "When I was in college, staying up all night." I asked him if he ever quit drinking coffee at any time. He said, "No, I have not gone a day in 20 years without drinking coffee."

So I said, "There are a lot of things I could prescribe for you, such as natural sedatives, but the very first thing I want you to do is give up coffee."

We got him off the coffee, but things weren't good right away. He had caffeine-withdrawal headaches, and his sleep was disturbed. But after a week he was sleeping better than he had in 20 years, and after two weeks he was completely cured of his "incurable hereditary insomnia." Then his wife came to see me. She was 42 and going through an early menopause.

She was complaining because her gynecologist had put her on Premphase (conjugated estrogen and medroxyprogesterone acetate tablets), and she was gaining weight. But the gynecologist also did a good thing. He did a bone density study and found that the patient was 1.8 SD below normal, which meant she already had significant bone loss. So she went on Premphase and, in the six months prior to seeing me, gained 12 pounds. She also said that her moods were erratic, she had breast tenderness, and she felt bloated all the time. She asked me if there were any alternative treatments. I said sure and did an Osteomark test, which is a urine test that measures bone loss, and discovered that even though she was on the hormones she was still losing bone. Her Osteomark measure was about 48; anything more than 30 is not good for a woman of her age. She was already taking calcium, high-potency multiple vitamins, and some extra antioxidants. I added flaxseed oil and a black cohosh extract called Remifemin, which is probably the world's most popular approach to menopause. We also took her off the Premphase. Three months later, we repeated the Osteomark test, and her level was 21. It has been more than 3 years now, and we have kept the level between 21 and 24.

I feel strongly that regardless of what therapy a woman chooses to help her through menopause or beyond, she should be properly monitored. I think that includes Pap (Papanicolaou's) smears, mammography, and baseline bone density studies along with periodic urine assessment. I think there are a lot of women on hormones being lulled into a false sense of security. There are also a lot of women who are choosing to go the natural route who aren't paying attention to how their bodies are responding. Bone density studies and rate of bone loss assessments are absolutely critical whether a woman is using a conventional or a natural approach.

Evolution of Medicine

There is an evolution occurring in medicine of all fields. If you look at what has happened in naturopathic medicine in the last 10 years, you will see that a lot of new therapies and new medicines are melding with some age-old practices. For me, this is a very exciting time.

Before I graduated from Bastyr in 1985, I had been collecting information on natural medicines, but many of them—ginkgo biloba, St. John's wort, glucosamine sulfate, and Remifemin—weren't available for practitioners to purchase. The state of the herbal medicine marketplace back in 1985 left a lot to be desired, and I wanted to see high-quality standardized herbal medicines in America. So I started talking to various companies about importing some of the more popular standardized extracts that were starting to emerge in Europe, but my efforts weren't met with a lot of success. Then I had the good fortune to meet Terry Lemerand, president of Enzymatic Therapy/PhytoPharmica. We established a professional and personal relationship that has lasted over 15 years, and we were instrumental in bringing many of these natural products to the marketplace. For instance, we were the first to introduce standardized extracts of ginkgo biloba, St. John's wort, saw palmetto, and bilberry. We were also the first to introduce glucosamine sulfate in America.

We are labeling many of these therapies and medicines right now as "alternatives," though I believe they will be incorporated into conventional medicine. I'm always amused when people introduce me as an expert in alternative medicine, because that is not what I'm about. What I am about is promoting what I like to term "rational medicine." There are many things that are done in conventional medicine that make absolute 100% good sense.

All of us have had our lives touched in some way by conventional medicine—someone close to us may have benefited from antibiotics or surgery or may have been kept alive because of the latest wonder drug. In those situations, modern medicine is quite good. Where modern medicine doesn't make much sense is in the treatment of chronic diseases. In many cases, the drugs induce the very thing they are trying to treat, or they cause other problems. That isn't rational. We look back at medical practices from 100 years ago, such as blood letting and the administration of mercury and other poisons, and we think, "Oh, that was crazy, what were they thinking?" Well, I'm sure some of the drugs, therapies, and surgeries used now will one day be viewed as similarly barbaric.

There is an evolution in natural medicine as well. We are going to see some things get discarded because they will be proven ineffective or because they're not based on sound principles. So I tell people that I am a proponent of rational medicine. I view the future as incorporating the best of both worlds.

One of the most valuable parts of my education was precepting with other doctors. I got a sense from this one old-time naturopath that it really didn't matter what he prescribed or what he gave people—he possessed the ability to heal. People would get better by being in his presence, or by his touch, or just by the faith that they had in what he prescribed. I think some people have that innate ability to heal. We have all been around people like that. Probably the best healers on this planet don't have any formal education.

But more than having things fall away, I think there will be an opening up and an acceptance of some of the technological advances by practitioners of alternative therapies. I view some of the high-tech advances as being natural. For example, I think gene therapy is the ultimate natural medicine. Imagine a child with cystic fibrosis. You perform gene therapy and cure the child—I am all for that. We can't do this now but I think it will happen in our lifetime. I also think we will continue to see the development of natural biological drugs and compounds that are inherent to our bodies. A good example of that is erythropoietin, which has been a great advancement both in patients who are undergoing hemodialysis and in some cancer patients. Other examples are interferon and some of the interleukins. I view these substances as natural medicines because they address the underlying cause.

Biology is important in the healing process, but clearly we need to look at all factors in a patient's life. When I was a student at Bastyr I came across an article that described what it was like to be a patient of Hippocrates and detailed his interview process. Hippocrates was interested in diet but more so in the person's social environment and dreams. There is much to be said for focusing on these areas. How empowered are people at work or in their life? How loved are they in their home life? What do they dream about? I remember a great quote from the Talmud: "An unexamined dream is like an unopened gift from God."

What Naturopathic Medicine Does Well

I think naturopathic medicine is exceptional in preventing disease and in the treatment of most chronic degenerative diseases. Specifically, I think we do very well in treating osteoarthritis, benign prostatic hyperplasia, high cholesterol levels, depression, peptic ulcers, and various functional disturbances of the gastrointestinal tract such as irritable bowel syndrome and nonulcer dyspepsia. In addition, I think naturopathic medicine is exceptional in building up people's health when there is no real disease state yet.

In my years of practice, I've found that patients are very good at knowing when something isn't quite right with their bodies. Often they feel discouraged because other doctors tell them there is "nothing wrong." That is because our medical system is based on diagnosing the presence of disease rather than promoting health and the proper function of body systems. If we view disease at one end of the spectrum and health at the other, we see that anyone can benefit from naturopathic medicine because it provides the guidance to move away from disease by focusing on the promotion of health. The earlier we see a patient in the disease process, the better the results will be with naturopathic medicine. Natural therapies may not be as effective for an end-stage disease like cancer, but certainly naturopathic medicine can play a huge role in prevention.

Future Directions

I have taken a little time off from my practice right now, and I am looking at some different options. I have always had a strong sense of mission and at times have either fought the direction my life was going in or have not understood it. I think that as you get older you become more receptive, so I am letting things unfold, and we will see what opportunities present themselves. I see myself as someone who can inspire and influence people to take more responsibility for their own healthcare.

When I graduated from Bastyr I thought that there was a big division between the intent of a medical doctor and the intent of a naturopath. But the intentions of both practitioners are identical. Both want to see people healthier, happier, and enjoying life more. I think that naturopaths as well as medical doctors have tools that can help achieve that goal, but the patient has to meet us in the middle.

One of the first patients I had in my practice was brought to me by his wife. This guy was 5 feet 6 inches tall, 230 pounds, diabetic, and had diabetic renal disease, hypertension, and angina. He was a strong candidate for hemodialysis and was probably on 20 different drugs. His wife wanted me to get him off the drugs and on to a more natural approach, but no supplements or herbs that I could recommend to him would ever overcome his diet and lifestyle.

I called the nephrologist he was seeing and introduced myself. I said, "I want to talk to you about this patient and get your input because I don't really understand why he is not willing to make any dietary and lifestyle changes." The nephrologist said he was just as frustrated as I was in dealing with this guy. If the patient made dietary and lifestyle changes, there was a possibility that he would not need dialysis. But he was unable to make those changes. The doctor told me that the only reason he was prescribing those drugs was because if he didn't, the patient wouldn't be alive.

I learned a lot from that patient and that doctor. It's a cliché, but I learned that you can drag a horse to the water trough but you can't make it drink. I was seeing many of these types of patients and getting frustrated that they weren't making the changes they needed to be healthy. So what I realized was that I needed to learn how to inspire people to want to change. I read somewhere that real leadership involves getting people to do what they want to do, and I think being a good doctor is similar. We have to inspire our patients to do what they really want to do, which is to be healthier. I think the desire to be healthy is innate in all of us. Sometimes the pain of living may cloud that picture, but I think this is only temporary. People want to live and be healthy, and there is great satisfaction in helping them do so.

CHAPTER 9

THOMAS RAU, MD

Biological Medicine and the Dynamics of Regulation

Thomas Rau, MD, received his medical training at the Medical School of Berne University, Switzerland. After graduating in 1977, he took the U.S. Final Medical Examination for foreigners. Rau then completed postgraduate clinical education in general medicine, rheumatology, and internal medicine at different hospitals in Switzerland, France, Spain, and the United States. From 1981 to 1992, he conducted a general and rheumatological practice and began formal education in homeopathy, isopathy, complex homeopathy, darkfield microscopy, thermography, neural therapy, and Chinese medicine. It was during these years that Dr. Rau began to develop his signature concept, biological medicine.

In 1992, Dr. Rau began serving as chief medical director and part owner of the Paracelsus Klinik in Lustmühle, Switzerland, the first center in Europe for integrative European biological medicine and holistic dentistry. The center specializes in chronic and internal diseases; colitis; lupus; rheumatoid arthritis; allergies; and neurological diseases such as multiple sclerosis, neuralgias, and tumors.

The author of many articles on biological medicine, darkfield microscopy, isopathy, homeopathy, and holistic dentistry, Dr. Rau has conducted educational seminars for physicians and nurses in Germany, Austria, Switzerland, Spain, and the United States since 1993.

In the spring of 2002, I interviewed Dr. Rau at Fox Hollow, an affiliate Paracelsus clinic, in Louisville, Kentucky.

The expression *biological medicine* is used very differently in the United States than in Switzerland. For me, biological medicine is the integration of different traditional healing methods such as Chinese medicine, homeopathy, Ayurveda, and the ancient European traditions like druidic medicine. We integrate these different methods into a way of treating patients individually. Biological medicine is individual and solely alternative. But alternative is the wrong expression; it's a natural way of healing patients.

I was a rheumatologist—you would call it internist—and I ran a rehabilitation clinic. I came to this different approach because my patients seemed to get sicker and sicker over the years, especially the rheumatoid patients. Many diseases don't respond to conventional treatment, and our patients proved that the orthodox model didn't work because they got worse.

Now, all my colleagues and I are open individuals—open to new and other thinking. So after a while we had to ask ourselves: Is it just the fate of nature that people with these diseases don't get well, or do we think wrongly?

Some patients came to me and said, "Listen, Dr. Rau, I was in your treatment for my arthritis for 5 years, and I just got worse. Now I have tried homeopathy or I began a diet or this and that, and I am better." Of course, at first I got angry because all doctors get angry when they are shown that they are not right. But after several patients said things like this to me, I began to ask myself: shouldn't I integrate all these other methods?

I realized that orthodox medicine has a wrong thinking behind it. It doesn't work on the real dynamics of life. You see, everything rebuilds in the human organism. For this patient who comes now, in 7 years, not a single cell will be the same cell as it was before. For example, blood, which is the energy stream in the organism, renews within 1 month. The white blood cells, which regulate the immune system, renew within 4 weeks; lymphocytes, 3 weeks; granulocytes, 2 months. So it's all renewing.

But what creates the character of these cells that renew all the time? What we give as nutrition—what we give as minerals and proteins and amino acids and so on—determine how a cell rebuilds itself. So in biological medicine we work on the dynamics that change the organs.

Conventional medicine always wants more immediate results. I know this very well because as a rheumatologist you do fast methods. You give antiinflammatories; you give antiimmune drugs; you give anti, anti, anti. And it's only treating the symptoms and never treating the cause. So we began to look for causes and ways to remove those causes. The new cells rebuild differently when the cause that made them bad is not present.

So I run my patients on different tracks. I may have to remove a tumor, or whatever, but we also work on the story of this patient. Why did the cells or the tissue go wrong in the first place?

Multiple Sclerosis Patients

We see multiple sclerosis (MS) patients who have myelin-sheath decay and who no longer have nerve functions. In orthodox medicine, this is called a *nonhealable disease*. But nobody thinks about why the myelin sheaths decay. They just say we can't repair the myelin sheath. But that's not true. So we try to find the cause. The patient has different causes, not one single cause, but together the causes can destroy the neural sheaths or diminish the rebuilding of myelin sheaths.

I am open to new ideas, one of which is that MS is caused by neurotoxicity. *Neurotoxic* refers to the influences that can bother the nerve cells of the myelin sheaths. When we look at this, we begin to see more and more possible causes that could affect the nerve system. For example, and we see this again and again, root canals are very toxic. The material goes into the mesangium, into the lymphatic system, and from there it goes into the blood and then to the neural sheaths. Boyd E. Haley, PhD, professor of medical chemistry and biochemistry at the Markey Cancer Center, University of Kentucky in Lexington, has proven that you find the same toxins in a root canal that you find in the myelin sheaths that decay. Exactly the same toxins are there. So the dynamism of an organism that changes all the time is that these substances get into the whole body and they fix on the weak organs. That's one cause.

The other possible cause is hepatitis B vaccination. In Paris, 450,000 children were vaccinated against hepatitis B. Five hundred eighty got MS within 2 years. When I got this information, I asked myself: shouldn't I look for this in all my MS patients? I have over 100 patients; shouldn't I look for antibodies to hepatitis B? And, in fact, I found them. So now, when an MS patient comes to the clinic, we look for hepatitis B, underground antibodies, root canals, and for mercury or palladium. We look for a deficiency in unsaturated fatty acids because rebuilding a good myelin sheath needs a lot of unsaturated fatty acids. If the renewal process is not working correctly, then the myelin sheaths will be of a lower quality.

So it's a multilevel approach, but it's also logical. That's why biological medicine is called biological, because it's about bios and it's logical.

Energy and Information

We have frequently found chronic viruses in degenerative nerve diseases such as Parkinson's or fibromyalgia, which is a negative nerve system disease, as are MS and amyotrophic lateral sclerosis (ALS) and all these horrible diseases that lead to a decay of nerve cells. We found that viruses sometimes create diseases that don't come to the surface. They make an underground load. It's an underground disease that destroys slowly without being noticed. And for these patients, we activate their immune systems specifically against this type of virus.

So we make the organism work against the virus. This is done with a nosode, which is a homeopathic remedy made from idle viral cultures of patients who were infected by this virus. We take the blood or the serum or the lymph of the patient and make the nosode. You destroy the virus or the bacterium in whatever you want to use for the nosode. There are no living viruses or bacteria in the homeopathic solution, but the information is still there. Then you give this information to the patient, and it begins to cause a reaction so that the unnoticed underground virus now gets noticed.

How does the information get transferred? Well, the answer to this would be enough for two books. This is a deep and difficult question. What is information? There are different approaches. You know, I am not a scientific person; I am only a very open person, and I can't explain everything. But you have to see that homeopathy works purely on information and not on material.

It's arrogant to say that homeopathy doesn't work because it works extremely well, and it's been proven over 200 years that it works. But we still can't explain why. There are some tendencies that can be explained and some hypotheses on which to base new scientific research. One is that energy makes a change in the organism and is above the material part of the cell.

A good example of what energy can change is a seed. When you look inside a seed you will find amino acids, carbohydrates in the wall, and some fatty acids and cells and so on. This material is in the seed, and the seed produces a wonderful tree—for example, a nut tree. If you heat the seed up, if you cook it, and then look at what material is inside, it is still cells, amino acids, proteins, fats, and carbohydrates. It's the same composition. But while the seed looks the same, it will no longer produce a tree. So what is the difference? What is the energy, the upbuilding force within the material, that is changed by the heat? So you see, there is some dimension that is above the material that is in a cell or an organism or a human being. And that is the energy.

Researchers ask: What makes the homeopathy in the homeopathic solution? And now they have found that even though you have a homeopathic dilution above a potency of 23—if you have a DX30, for example—there are no molecules left of the original substance. So what can make this substance that is not present still have an effect? The answer they found is that the homeopathic remedy changes the water that it is in. So the water molecule changes.

Water is the main part of a human being. Sixty percent of what you see here is water, and water works through every cell and through everything in your body. So the water molecule is changed by the homeopathic solutions. The 17-degree angle of the H_2O molecule is changed.

A water molecule is not a single molecule. They are in clusters; 10 to 20 molecules are together. And the homeopathic solution changes the number in the cluster of molecules.

Professor Fritz-Albert Popp, PhD, biophysicist at the Technology Center in Kaiserslautern, Germany, works on test methods to measure how the spectral analysis changes. When you look at water and make a spectral analysis, homeopathic remedies change the water. It makes another spectral field, and it makes another photon emission.

If you feel sympathetic or antipathetic to me or to somebody else, that's something you can't see or describe, but you still feel it. This energy field is caused by photon emissions. As yet, we don't have test methods to prove this photon emission exists. At some point we will develop such tests. Professor Popp was able to prove that photon emissions change when you give homeopathic remedies or biological remedies. So slowly, slowly, there is proof that all this natural medicine can work.

It's amazing how intensive the effect of these nosode treatments can be. First, we build up a person's milieu so that the organism can react better. We make the patients stronger with antioxidants, vitamins, alkaline treatments, and infusions. We make them more reactable, because most patients are severely blocked. And then, if we give them a nosode or very specific stimuli, they really notice how intensively it works. Sometimes, in very happy cases, the virus or the toxins get removed.

Chemical Sensitivity Patients

This disease is actually more rare in Europe. Many of our chronic chemical-sensitivity patients come from the United States.

But let's speak about chronic chemical sensitivity. Some patients are sensitive to everything and they are really disturbed fundamentally, so much so that they can't go outside. But we have to ask ourselves: why do some patients react so badly while others who are exposed to the same chemical don't react at all? On the one side, there must be the bad chemicals that they are sensitive to, but on the other side, there must be some individual weakness that makes these patients susceptible.

So we have to work on two levels again. We have to work on the detoxification levels and bring out the toxins, the heavy metals. Those are simple to detoxify. But the organic toxins—the ones that bind to the organic substances in the organism, such as preservatives, fertilizers, and insecticides—they are very difficult to eliminate.

It's a different process. Somehow these patients have metabolic pathways of detoxification that are blocked. So we work on detoxification and on the changed metabolic pathways, trying to rebuild the patients' detoxifying pathways. This is one track.

The other track is that we try to remove all the things that lower the ability to react and reduce the healing tendency in this patient. We try to change the individual situation of the patient that is making him get sick while others do not get sick from the same toxins. And that's very often due to totally different things, such as energetic imbalances or chronic viruses, which affect the reaction capacity of the patient, or trace-element deficiencies, mineral deficiencies, and so on.

Then there's another item, the meridian imbalance, which is whatever energy is not in balance in the patient. So we work on the individual energetic situation and on the detoxification pathways. And it's amazing. These patients get well or at least much better within 6 to 12 months.

So I take this individual and say to myself: every cell will be renewed in 7 years. The important parts—liver cells, white blood cells, red blood cells, thymus, thyroid—all these organs that meddle with the chemical sensitivity patients or chronic fatigue patients, rebuild within 2 years normally. If there were no more rebuilding force in this patient, he would die now. So the fact that the patient is alive proves that there is still a rebuilding capacity. Every dynamic in the human being is based on rebuilding and renewing. But these patients renew more slowly or in a wrong way.

So we have to create better conditions for these cells, and we do this by giving trace elements, vitamins, and rebuilding forces. In the anthroposophical way of thinking, we try to give them whatever it is that makes the upbuilding forces. We try to give that back. And that force is based on internal bacteria, which are the rebuilding elements in the organism. You understand, the bacteria in the small intestine rebuild in 2 days, so they have a giant rebuilding force.

Very often we see that the rebuilding forces in the intestines and in the bacterial layers are diminished because of preservatives, because of antibiotics, because of antiviral substances, and so on. So this rebuilding strength and force has to be given to patients again.

Heavy metals, however, don't leave the organism unless you do a drainage treatment. I would say that nearly all chronic fatigue patients or chronic chemical-sensitivity patients have heavy-metal toxicity. Palladium, mercury, zinc—these metals can be drained, and it's not difficult. There are chelation agents; there are vitamins; and there are amino acids that bind with the heavy metals and eliminate them through stools and urine if you do it correctly. So that's not so difficult. It can be done with all patients, but sometimes it's very difficult to remove the organic toxins that bind deeply into the tissue.

Diagnostic Technologies

We have to find out about the dynamics and regulation capacity and compensation capacity of an individual. Anatomic investigations like positron emission tomography (PET) scans and magnetic resonance imaging (MRI) don't work for functional diseases, for diseases that are based on a disturbance in the dynamic process of renewal. Orthodox medical diagnostic methods don't show this. It's like a fisherman who wants to catch sardines. He doesn't use a whale net. And that is what we do in medicine: we take the wrong nets to diagnose a disease. Since these diseases work on a totally different level, we have to have diagnostic methods that cover the other levels.

The main one that shows the dynamic processes is darkfield microscopy. We also have the dried-layer test that shows us about toxic products and the need for antioxidants. We have a special bioterrain assay that shows us the redux potentials, the membrane potentials, the vitality of fluids, and the amount of free electrons and protons. Then we have the thermal regulation test that shows us the disturbance foci and the disturbance fields in the organism and the connections between different organ systems.

For example, the meridian connections are very important in chronic diseases. In human beings, the thyroid and breast belong together, and the stomach and ovaries belong together, and these connections and their regulation capacity can be found in the thermal regulation test. So these are the main tests.

Then we have a new test method for the autonomic nerve system. Until now, orthodox medicine didn't get into these dimensions of autonomic regulations. Everything that regulates and that adapts itself internally couldn't be diagnosed before. But now we have methods to diagnose the functions of the autonomic nerve system.

The heart rate variability test is based on the rhythmic functions in an organism. While a patient is standing, we lower the temperature and give him small stimuli. Then we look at how the rhythmic regulation changes, at how well the organism can react to small stimuli. That is what we want to find out.

We are successful with prostate cancer and with the early stages of breast cancer, much more so than orthodox medicine. But we are not successful with pancreatic cancer, and we are only slightly successful with kidney cancer. Therefore the only patients we try to attract to our clinic are those for which we are sure we can do better than orthodox medicine. That's chronic fatigue, chemical sensitivity, breast cancer, prostate cancer, colitis, Crohn's disease, asthma, and allergies. These are functional diseases that deal with a disturbed reaction ability.

Darkfield Microscopy

Darkfield microscopy shows a lot. We take one drop of blood and look at it under a very large-scale magnification. The blood is life under the glass. Once it's on the glass, there isn't oxygen or light or heat. This is a giant stress for the blood. So we see how, over a time, the blood reacts to this stress, and how the blood cells tolerate the stress. You can see the changes. So we take a drop of blood that represents the organism and put it under stress and look at how the cells react to the stress, and then we can see the tolerance and the resistiveness of these cells. Do they have a good cell-membrane face? Do they have good energetic behavior? Do they clot together? Is there a chance for degenerative diseases? Is there a cancerous tendency in this blood? We see tendencies. And that's what we are interested in—tendencies.

For instance, a cancerous tendency is a change in the cells. They get rigid, so to say. They don't react very well.

Blood can live for several days. But after 1 hour, the blood is already seriously changed. For example, a leukemia patient came to my clinic for another disease. But when we did darkfield, I found the leukemia. We saw that his white blood cells were atypical. Look at this slide—the fact that there are so many white blood cells together is absolutely unusual, and the fact that there are atypical white blood cells. This shows me that the patient has myeloid leukemia. The patient had been diagnosed as having rheumatoid lung pain, but it was absolutely not true. The real cause of his pain was an infiltration of the spinal bone by these lymphocytes.

Biological Medicine and Dentistry

Toxic dental materials are the main factors for decreased regulation. The materials that are used for dentistry for replacement and for root canals create a large amount of toxicity. The most common and best known is the mercury in amalgam fillings. This knowledge is now established in the medical world. It has been proven that mercury is very toxic. But there are other materials, such as tin and copper and palladium, that are used in many filling and crown materials. Even titanium, which is used for implants, is oxidating and can make a lymphocyte transformation and be the cause of autoimmune diseases. Another point is that when you root canal a tooth, it dies off, but this dead organic material is still inside the canal of the roots and can decay. This can be the culture for bacterial overgrowth. So in the apex and the bone around root-canalled teeth, you always find toxic material. And this material can create other diseases.

There is very interesting book by George Meinig called *Root Canal Cover-up*. He talks about all the research around this. So, from this viewpoint, I said to myself: I can't create a holistic or biological medicine and honestly detoxify the patient if I don't integrate biological dentistry.

It's amazing, but not a single MS patient—and I have more than 100 in my care—not a single one was ever tested for toxicity. Parkinson's patients and ALS patients and patients with neuralgias or polyneuropathy—all these patients were never tested for dental electricity, for dental focus-disturbance fields, or dental toxicity. And in many cases it was the major cause of their diseases.

For instance, we have many neuralgia patients, and when we remove these disturbing factors—for example, a toxic root canal—the trigeminus neuralgia goes away. But we don't do miracles. We just do other approaches.

So in the Switzerland clinic, we have five dentists who work with our patients. They are not only taking out fillings and teeth. They are testing if the teeth are disturbing the regulative capacity of the patient or if the teeth release toxins. And if there are these toxins, they remove the filling or the tooth or whatever is needed.

The biological dentist is an important instrument. After the toxins are released from the person's body, I can better work to rebuild the dynamics of the metabolic pathways. I will give you an example of patient regulation. You have an inside temperature of 37° C. When you are in the desert and it is much hotter outside, then you have to cool down to maintain your inside temperature. When you are in the arctic and it's very cold outside, you have to heat up to maintain this internal temperature. So what makes you recognize if you have to heat or cool to maintain the inner temperature? This only a very simple example, but it shows how you have to recognize the needs of your organism and be able to react. The relationship from outside to inside, we call this adaptation, and the reaction, we call regulation.

Another example: Who tells you that you don't have enough water and that you need to retain fluids or that you have to produce urine? What tells the organism what to detoxify and how to detoxify to maintain the internal milieu? That is what we call regulation—the capacity to adapt to the needs of your organism.

Now comes the important point: there are agents that lower this regulation capacity—for example, heavy metals; hyperacidity; or overproteinization, which block the lymphatic flow; and other toxins, such as preservatives from food. Of course, our psychological backgrounds, our life backgrounds, can lower the capacity for regulation. And also very important, electromagnetic disturbances or loads from portable phones or television can lower the capacity. All these things can be tested for, and we can then begin to take away all the factors that block the regulation.

So we look to see how much blocking the patient has and what is it that fills the barrel of disease so that one day the patient will no longer have any regulative capacity. Then, as much as possible, we begin to remove these regulation blockages.

We never treat diagnoses. We never treat against symptoms. We always treat to make the regulation capacity better. It's a way of bringing back the organism to a state in which it compensates and regulates itself.

Cancer Patients

I have about 150 breast cancer patients in my permanent care. And if they come early enough after the diagnosis, we can nearly always stop the development of the cancer.

We look at why the cell degenerated, why the cell began to produce new cells in a wrong way. First, we remove the causes—free radicals, heavy metals, toxins, and so on. Cancer cells have a different metabolism from normal cells because cancer cells, as with all degenerative cells, have a low membrane potential. Their surface load is different; it's lower and therefore the cell can't change or interact with its surroundings. That's why cancer gets a node and only reacts to itself and not to the needs of the organism. It loses contact with the surrounding region. But we can work on this changed metabolism by increasing the cancer cell's membrane potential. And we try to put the cells back to a normal stage of membrane potential. We do this by changing the redux potential through an electrode treatment called *local hyperthermia* that builds up the membrane potential of the cancer cells so that they interact with the surrounding region again.

We do local hyperthermia on cancer cells. These cancer cells are thermically labile, so they don't support heat as well as healthy cells. When we heat them locally, they fall apart. But the healthy cells around them don't fall apart. We also use different methods—vitamins and antioxidants, for example—and we have special mistletoe preparations that work even better if combined with catalysts from citric acid.

Now, here is something very interesting. I made a study of breast cancer patients, and I found that over 98% had a disturbance on the stomach meridian. (The breast belongs to the stomach meridian.) These patients have a typical psychological background patterns, and they have disturbances of their stomach meridians. In about 150 cases of women with breast cancer, we only had three patients who did not have a root canal in a tooth that belongs to the stomach meridian. You see, each tooth belongs to a meridian, and over 97% had a root canal on the same meridian that belongs to the breast. It's very interesting.

Of course, when I brought this up in a medical congress, they simply said, "Well, in this day and age, all women have root canals." So we did a study of women in the same age range without breast cancer, without chronic diseases, and only 30% of that group had root canals. It's a significant difference.

I'm not saying that root canals cause breast cancer, but if you have breast cancer and you don't remove your root canals and the other toxic elements that bother the breast tissue, then you have a lower chance to heal.

The meridians I'm talking about are the acupuncture meridians from Chinese medicine, but I don't think you can heal breast cancer with acupuncture. It's only about the correlations of meridians. It's about the organs that belong together. The thyroid belongs to the breast and the upper molars belong to the breast, too. So do the ovaries. That's why so many breast cancers are hormonally related.

We do acupuncture, but it's only one minor instrument in the whole process. The mistake that is made in the biological field is that there are many practitioners who use one instrument. But you have to use several instruments, and you have to add them to one another very individually. There is no single method in biological medicine. There is no single remedy that works against this or that chronic disease. There is no cancer remedy. It's only an individual combination that works well against a disease.

So if you really want to do biological medicine, you have to get away from this materialistic thinking of organs and of single treatment.

Anthroposophy

I am a spiritual doctor, and I have some healing capacities. I feel what is wrong with the patient. That's my gift. So yes, I work with them spiritually, but there are also two healers in our clinic who do the same thing. I can't explain with an intellectual explanation what we do on a spiritual level, but I can feel it. When I see a patient and I interact with him in the examination, I simply can feel what the patient has and on which meridians I need to work. That's my healing gift. But I can't put it into words.

A healer just knows what patients have wrong with them. Nobody understands why he knows things that you didn't tell him. Why does he know about your mother or what happened to you five years before? He just knows, and nobody can explain it. But getting things out of the unconscious into the consciousness is, in itself, a healing act.

But a healer alone can't make a chronic disease heal. This might have been possible 50 or 100 years ago, but today, the healing capacity, the reaction capacity, is so decreased by toxins and different regulation blockages that we have to combine the healer's healing forces with detoxification and upbuilding of the regulation. A healer can only heal a person who is still able to react. We can't heal a stone.

CHAPTER 10

STEVEN WEISS, DO

Kneeling at the Axis of Creation

Steven J. Weiss is a licensed osteopathic physician, board certified in Neuromuscular/ Osteopathic Manual Medicine. Dr. Weiss consults in the field of chronic pain and treats sports and performing arts injuries as well as prenatal and pediatric problems. He practices in New York City, where, for more than 16 years he has devoted his work to clinical approaches that invoke and support the power of the human body to heal itself.

In 1973, Weiss graduated from Washington and Jefferson College in Washington, Pennsylvania and in 1985 graduated from The University of New England College of Osteopathic Medicine in Biddeford, Maine. In addition to this traditional osteopathic training, he has studied extensively with Rev. Rosalyn Bruyere, healer and founder of The Healing Light Center Church. He is founder and medical director of The Medicine Lodge Clinic and the creator and director of The Altar of Creation training program for healers and healthcare professionals.

I interviewed Dr. Weiss at his offices in New York City. During the course of our conversation, Dr. Weiss taught me to deepen my perceptual capacities by hanging my attention behind me on a floating hook and helped me sense the differences in vibrations between human and animal bones.

Where I am today and how I approach the challenges of healing is a weaving together of many different teachings and lineages. I often approach my patient's bodies more like an engineer than a doctor. But I am also a student of energy medicine and Spiritual Law, an ecologist, a child to the Zuni Bear Clan, a board-certified practitioner of osteopathic manual medicine, a student of Chinese internal martial arts, and a follower of the Bön religion of Tibet, to name a few of the different strands. Each has contributed to my evolution as a healer and on a practical daily basis, represents an important tool or piece of the map that I need to support my patients' healing.

I was raised to be a conventional doctor. The problem arose when I got to pre-med in college—I hated the lab sciences and the courses and the nature of many of the people who were studying to be doctors. But there's a saying that you'll know the right path by having taken the wrong one. So in my junior year, when I took my first ecology course, it was like coming home. The natural world had been a refuge and sanctuary when I was growing up, and the study of the interrelationships in ecological systems made perfect sense to me. So I switched from pre-med to biology. In 1974, I attended the University of Maine as a grad student in ecology and entomology and then two years later, I joined the faculty of the University of Maine at Machias under a grant from The National Science Foundation (NSF) and started my own environmental consulting company. And I loved it. But I was living from grant to grant and was having misgivings about my future in the academic world. Then the NSF grant ended and money for environmental consulting began to dry up. So I spent time praying and asking God for a sign about what I was supposed to do with my life.

About this time, I developed a painful ulcerative condition on my feet so I went to a local doctor. He treated it as a fungal infection, which made it worse. I went to someone else and he said no, its bacterial, and gave me another medicine that made the condition even worse. I went to five different doctors in three counties and no one could tell me what the problem was or how to heal it. Then, in the middle of all this, my football-injured left knee gave out, and I was unable to bear weight or straighten my left leg without pain. So I started going to orthopedic surgeons, none of who had any idea as to what was wrong with my knee.

I was crying in my beer one day when a friend told me to call a Dr. McIver at the Lubec Medical Center. He was a stout, grizzly sort with a salt-and-pepper beard who grunted more than he spoke. I was told to bring all of the medicines that the different doctors had given me so he could see what their presumptive diagnoses were and what they had done. He comes in, looks in the bag, looks at my feet, looks back in the bag, curses, and throws the bag across the room. "These guys are killing you," he said. "They have no idea what they are doing. But I know a case of trench foot when I see one."

He asked me what I did for a living and I explained that I worked as a marine biological consultant. He then asked if I had torn my rubber boots in the recent past. And, of course, he was right. Trench foot is a moisture-driven problem where the increased moisture leaches all of the lubricating oils from between the layers of the skin. The skin breaks down, ulcerates, and gets horribly inflamed and will continue to do so unless you treat the source of the problem. He spelled out a treatment program for me and within a few weeks the ulcers and pain were gone.

However, that same day as he was writing on my chart, I hopped across the room to get dressed, and he noticed that I couldn't put any weight on my left leg. After motioning me back onto the exam table, he evaluated my knee. While doing this, he told me that he was an osteopathic doctor. Now, I'd always thought that osteopathic school was where people went who couldn't get into "real" medical school. Yet here was this brilliant diagnostician telling me that he was an osteopath. Then he frowned and said, "I'm training to be a surgeon and don't believe in osteopathic manipulation, but I think your knee problem can only be successfully treated with an osteopathic manipulative procedure. I'm not very experienced but if it's okay with you, I'll get out a manual, read about what to do, and then do it."

After he read the manual, Dr. McIver completed a forceful procedure on my leg, and there was this loud crack. When the body suddenly gets what it needs to support its healing, there's often a dramatic release of endorphins and a huge shift in qi—the response can feel euphoric. All at once my whole leg and foot relaxed. The sensation I felt was one of warm oil pouring down through the knee into my leg and foot. And when I stood up, there was no pain!

I was overwhelmed—not only had this doctor made a superior medical diagnosis about my trench foot, but he had also made a correct structural/mechanical diagnosis and actually done something *with his hands* to support the immediate healing of my knee. Then Dr. McIver said, "I know who you are, Steven. Maybe you ought to think about becoming an osteopathic physician."

In that moment it felt like the hand of God was pointing in the direction of osteopathic medical school. To make a long story short, I moved to southern Maine and enrolled in the University of New England College of Osteopathic Medicine. There I had the blessing of being taken under the wings of the handful of luminaries who trained and mentored me in osteopathic manual medicine and healing—people like Dr. Ruby Day, Dr. Robert Fulford, Dr. Anne Wales, Dr. Larue Kemper, Dr. Carl Schoelles, and Dr. James Jealous. For the most part these practitioners are all dead now, with the exception of Dr. Wales, who will celebrate her ninety-ninth birthday this January, and Dr. Jealous, who is a still quite young. But before they passed on, these people crammed as much training and guidance down my throat as they could, and for that I am grateful. I am first and foremost an osteopathic physician. That is the glue that holds together all the different strands of my healing practice.

Engineering

At one point I had a part-time job in Maine rebuilding old houses with a lobsterman and retired civil engineer. Capt. Dwelley taught me about Physical Law and the supreme importance of structural integrity as an engineering requirement for all weight-bearing structures, which I later came to realize includes people. We rebuilt many foundations and jacked up many buildings to plumb-and-level as a prerequisite to any other work. It's funny and perhaps even prophetic that structural integrity work—focusing on how people bear weight and their relationship with gravity—has grown to be a huge focus in my practice.

Rosalyn Bruyere

In my early years in practice I found myself confronted with doors that my osteopathic training hadn't prepared me to go through. I kept having the feeling that I was treating the tissue side of an energy-tissue interface and that I needed to get to the other side. I also had the increasing sense that if I was going to truly support healing for my patients, I needed skills I didn't yet have.

A friend took me to a body symbology workshop on Long Island. The presenter, Rev. Rosalyn Bruyere, walked through the audience and said, "Who has a knee problem?" I raised my hand. She asked me which knee and then she asked what had happened? I explained that in 1966 I tore the anterior cruciate ligament, the medial collateral ligament, and the medial meniscus during a football game. She looked at me—actually, she looked through me—and asked, "What was her name?"

I gasped, "What?"

Rosalyn said, "The girl that you were in love with when your knee was hurt."

"Do you mean Debbie?" I whispered.

And she said, "Yes, that's in there too."

I received a treatment from her on a table in front of 225 people. As Rosalyn and her student assistant started working on me, they were whispering to each other. Then Rosalyn said, "Check out how much he's armoring, how suspicious and resistant he is." When she put her hand on my chest, I felt this huge electric shock that made me feel like I was being defibrillated.

Rev. Bruyere is one of the most studied minds in the world and a phenomenal healer who is capable of generating enormous amounts of qi. She is recognized by several native tribes as a medicine woman and has been enthroned as the living oracle of the Bön—the ancient, pre-Buddhist, indigenous religion of Tibet. The treatment she gave me changed my life and the things she has taught me have changed my capacities as a healer. I have been a student of hers for 13 years. She has helped guide me to a place where I look at the human body without the usual distinctions that separate tissue, energy, and Spirit, and she has opened my heart and helped me surrender to Spirit and its guidance.

There's a huge piece of human existence that pertains to energy. As Rosalyn says, "Energy is all there is." If we're spiritual beings inhabiting a physical container, then looking at Spiritual Law and energy (qi) is vital if we are to really address the needs of the whole being. So after many years of study with Rev. Bruyere, my approach to diagnosis and treatment includes considerations of the human energy field, the chakra system, and Spiritual Law.

Native American Traditions

Another thread of my work comes from the Zuni pueblo tribe. During my first year of osteopathic school, I began experiencing troubling dreams and had a strong feeling that I needed to go on a vision quest to the Four Corners region where Colorado, Utah, Arizona, and New Mexico come together. I wasn't prone to this sort of thing but the feelings were so strong I decided to take heed. I ended up at the Zuni Indian reservation in western New Mexico and before the day was over, was sent to the house of a medicine man. His mother-in-law, Mary, eventually adopted me as her son and as a child to the Zuni Bear Clan.

Through this experience, I met Jimmy Awash'e, a Zuni bone doctor and healer. Jimmy was struck by lightning in his late 30s when he was a sheepherder. He was in a coma for three days and left for dead up in the hills. He finally woke up, walked 11 or so miles to town, and said, "I guess I need to start doing healing because while I was asleep, Creator and the spirits of my ancestors came into me and filled me with the knowledge and power of healing and then put me back together."

One day, while I was on the reservation in one of the rooms of Mary's house, we heard a big commotion. A boy had been hit in the head with a baseball and was unconscious. But instead of calling an ambulance, they sent for the bone doctor. The unconscious boy, who had vomit all over his face, was convulsing lightly and had a lurid egg on his forehead.

Jimmy sat down behind this boy, closed his eyes, and started chanting. After a while, I became aware of a change. Something was happening—not in Jimmy's body, but in the air *around* his body. I'd never experienced anything like it. If there was a color around him, then the color was changing. If there was a shape to that space around him, then that shape was changing. As Jimmy kept rocking back and forth and chanting, I watched this glistening, gold cloud start to emerge out of the ground and wrap around his legs and then up his body. When the cloud had filled the space around him, it arced over around the boy's body, where it appeared as an imperfect shroud—it had holes and tears in it. Everywhere there was a hole or a tear, Jimmy used his hands to work on it until the tear disappeared and the cloud grew smooth. When everything was smooth and the cloud was circulating evenly, Jimmy stood up, spit in his hand, pulled an arrowhead out of his pocket, and put it on the boy's forehead. There was a sizzling sound and then the boy opened his eyes. The color had come back to his face and he looked around alertly. Jimmy said, "You can go." And the boy left.

As I was sitting there pinching myself and wondering what facet of reality I was in, I realized that I was alone in the room with Jimmy. Everyone else had gone. He leaned toward me and said, "I understand you're in a medical school where they teach doctors to heal. They (my Zuni family) thought you might have something you wanted to ask me."

So I asked him, of all things, "How do you protect yourself?" It was a stupid thing to say but it was such a part of my conditioning from first year osteopathic training that I just blurted it out.

Jimmy jumped out of his chair, got real close to my face, and started yelling at me at the top of his lungs. "Who do you think you are? Do you think you can heal? Do you think that any person can heal? What more is a human being than just a bag of mud brought to this space by the Great Creator to do the work of our ancestors? All you have to do is get out of the way and you'll never be hurt. There is nothing to be afraid of and nothing to protect yourself from if you only get out of the way." Then he sat back down. I had the same sense of electric shock in my heart that I had when Rosalyn "defibrillated" me several years later.

Jimmy died a few years after that, but before he went, I had a chance to spend time with him and watch him do healings. (I worked in the hospital by day and at night was taken around to do healings on the traditional people who wouldn't go to the hospital.) The director of the hospital told me that they had a file in the basement that contained x-rays of cases in which Jimmy had done inexplicable things, such as re-crystallizing bone fractures overnight.

Whenever I asked Jimmy what he did to heal, he always said: "I get out of the way. I told you. Spirit comes through me; the Great Creator comes through me; the spirits of my ancestors come through me and they heal."

Years later, Dr. Ruby Day, a wonderful older osteopath from western Maine, was teaching me an osteopathic procedure. I was having such trouble getting the technique right that we were both becoming frustrated. I asked Dr. Day how she originally learned to do it herself and she said, "Dr. Sutherland just told me to get out of the way." I felt an electric shock in my chest and Jimmy's words, "You just have to get out of the way!" reverberated through me like a freight train.

Dr. Day showed me a technique she had developed to "get out of the way." It was like some of the meditative techniques I had studied, but her approach was more practical and had a more immediate effect in deepening my level of awareness while keeping me present in my own body. After Dr. Day taught me "to get out of the way," the original osteopathic technique she was trying to teach me became easy. I have worked with and refined this "getting out of the way" practice for many years and on many different levels and now teach it to my students as a tool for listening to their patients' bodies and to my patients as a meditative practice to calm their minds and support their own healing.

The Bön Tradition

Another thread of my work comes from the Bön, the pre-Buddhist indigenous religion of Tibet. I came to study this tradition because of Rosalyn Bruyere. The Bön people teach, as do several other traditions, that the world is arranged on four levels: the literal level, the symbolic level, the irrational level, and the place where you break through to God. Not everything that occurs in the irrational always makes sense in the literal world and vice versa. I tend to appreciate the power that is in the irrational, but my work is about taking it back to the literal.

So all of these different threads are woven in my own journey as a healer. Many of the most potent pieces come from outside traditional osteopathy but they have helped give meaning and power to my work.

The Altar of Creation

Two and a half years ago, commuting home on my bicycle, I was hit by a taxi. In the moment where time stood still and I was bouncing first off his hood, and then off the pavement, there was this profound sense that it would be a violation of law if I were to die in this accident. I am the beneficiary of so many teachings, and so many people have transmitted their love and knowledge into me—there was this sense that I couldn't die before I wove it together and began sharing it with others. So I woke up from the accident with a drive to teach and share the lessons of my journey.

I have to make a point here that I am not training people to become osteopaths. To learn the practice of osteopathy one needs to go to osteopathic medical school, do an internship and residency, and obtain a license to practice medicine. But there are many things within the science of osteopathy that are really truths about the human body and don't belong to any one discipline. We have an obligation to share these with other healthcare professionals if it will help them be more successful in reducing the suffering of their patients.

Based upon the initial premise that the body is alive and therefore possesses the infinite capacity for self-healing and self-regulation, my goal as an osteopathic physician and healer has been not try to figure out how to fix my patients' bodies, but to figure out what is keeping their bodies from healing themselves. It's not about reductionism. In fact, it's the opposite of reductionism, which is the process of taking a complex, multidimensional being and reducing him or her to a symptom, which we call a diagnosis, and then coupling that to a therapy that treats the body like it's dead. This doesn't produce very good results. Instead, we kneel in reverence at the Altar of Creation (an expression I have taken from Andrew Taylor Still, the founder of osteopathic medicine), we get our egos out of the way, and we allow the inherent wisdom of Creation in the body to communicate to us how we can be of help. We find ourselves working with and in support of rather than against or doing things to the body, and the clinical results are dramatically better.

The curriculum for the training program, The Altar of Creation, begins with the simple process of getting out of the way and then keeps refining it. This fine-tunes the students' nervous systems as perceptual instruments, and, as it does that, guides them in beginning to construct a map of the body's health requirements.

Despite our uniqueness, there are a number of things that all human beings require to be healthy. On the Spiritual Law side of the equation, there is a Breath of Life and for us to be truly alive, it needs to ignite as a one-dimensional spark in us. The spark must then organize itself along a two-dimensional axis, which then stimulates a series of responses that create a three-dimensional being reflective of the original formation of the embryo. This process is built into the anatomy and into the nature of the human body on many different levels. If this process isn't happening, then the person is in shock, their perceptual clarity will be off, the person's consciousness will be defective, and there will be a deeply impaired capacity to self-heal and self-regulate or even respond to appropriate treatments.

Equally important is the Physical Law side of the equation. When a body is subjected to a violation in primary structural integrity and is forced to compensate for defects in structure, a whole avalanche of compromises and consequences will ensue: from direct mechanical problems to indirect diseases or conditions such as spinal problems and pain, balance problems or gait disturbances, arthritis, muscle spasms, tendonitis, headaches, shoulder and arm problems, and even tempero-mandibular joint syndrome (TMJ), visual problems, and hearing problems. How and where the symptoms actually manifest in the body is irrelevant. The *source* of the problem is the primary loss of structural integrity. So if we resist the temptation to treat the symptom and instead focus on digging down to its root, thus evaluating the symptom(s) in the context of the whole body and its engineering requirements, we break through to another possibility of healing. We engage the possibility of identifying and *curing* the underlying deficit in structure, and then observing the body actually beginning to heal itself spontaneously.

This is how people heal themselves and how we can begin to truly support them in their healing. When I have students in my office and I initiate structural integrity into a patient's body by raising their leg with a heel lift and thereby changing the shape of their primary weight-bearing mechanism, the students are always amazed to see how many spontaneous changes the patient's body accomplishes on its own, while we're just standing there watching. Things heal spontaneously. You see, it doesn't matter how many healthcare professionals you've been to, how many pills you've taken, how many acupuncture sessions you've had, or how many massages, physical therapy visits, or even surgeries you've had. If there is a primary loss of structural integrity, then nothing will change the violation except fixing the structure. You have to look at geometry of weight bearing and asymmetry, just as a structural engineer has to look at it in a building.

In my practice I see people who have fallen through the cracks created by this blind spot in both the healing and conventional worlds. There's a law that I jokingly call, Weiss's First Law. No one taught it to me. I got it out of engineering texts and my years of rebuilding old houses, and it represents a realization that saved me. And it is: *"The source of the problem is almost never where the symptom first appears. The source of the problem is almost never where it hurts."* In Chinese medicine it is stated: "He's such a bad doctor that when a patient comes to him with head pain, he actually treats the head." It's hard for me to train students to accept this because they're trained to treat the body like it's dead and "fix" the part that hurts or doesn't move right. And it's often hard to get my patients to accept this because they want me to attend to their pain in a literal way.

Getting out of the Way

In the beginning of the curriculum, I teach people the process of getting out of the way. Now, it is really hard to do this. Our egos defy the process. It took Jimmy Awash'e a lightning bolt to have the capacity to get out of the way to the extent to where he could re-crystallize bone fractures. And I think if we attain that same "out of the way-ness" then we will be capable of the same level of healing. But I am not putting my name on the list for lightning strikes.

Essentially, to "get out of the way," you remove your attention by creating a floating hook out in space behind you and then you put your attention on that hook. For the first course in the curriculum, I guide the students into a meditative state and instruct them to create a hook in space that floats about 18 inches behind the second sacral segment, creating a unique set of conditions in their bodies. Then I tell them to peel off their attention, like they're taking off a wetsuit or a heavy winter cloak, and hang it on this hook.

Once you have done this, the only really real work you have to do is to keep your attention there. It doesn't like to stay out of the way. It likes to slip off the hook and get into everything. So your job is to keep it there on the hook. So I have students devote a bit of their awareness to that job and then bring the rest of their awareness back to me or to the patient.

When you do this, the room seems to expand and you become more aware of your surroundings. Sometimes your body seems to get very small or very large. There might also be other perceptual shifts and perhaps a sense of losing boundaries. Students who usually don't feel much suddenly become aware of this enormous fire hose-type surge of qi running through bodies and out their arms and hands. I have come to call this surge of energy the creation wave. It seems to carry a broad set of frequencies of many different tones and vibrations. So we have nothing to do other than to get our attention out of the way in order for this massive flow of qi to spontaneously happen.

The Body as a Living Field

I start the first trainings by dividing the group into threes—I want one person on the table, one person at the head, and one person at the foot. Then I give a short discourse about how I was trained to contact the body as if it were the most exquisitely crafted eggshell porcelain globe on the planet, extremely delicate and containing a sacred elixir. We have to hold and support the head or the feet so as not to even dent the surface of the eggshell or create any distortion. We have to make sure our hands are relaxed and the placement is correct and that we are not getting in the way. It's about teaching people that they are entering a living field. There must be reverence. Every time you touch somebody, you're communicating a great deal. How we contact our clients cannot be underemphasized.

Then I teach the students to wait and do nothing, because the system will drive itself. It will come to completion by itself when it's done. It's an educational experience for both the people who are the operators at the head and feet, but also for the person on the table. It is almost like the people at the head and feet disappear, and the person on the table feels suspended in the air. There is a sense of being met and supported for one's own uniqueness.

The people at the head and feet are always astonished at how much happens without them. First, perceptions deepen. Then awareness expands and they start becoming aware of all the things that are happening. Of course, the first tendency is to jump in and start getting in the way, so I have to keep helping them pull their attention out and put it back behind them. But the whole process that takes place is a continual observation of how powerfully, incisively, exquisitely, specifically, and comprehensively the body will heal itself. My goal in my practice, and what I teach, is to do less and less and support this self-healing process more and more.

Some of the things that might happen are that the energy field will shift itself, but that's intangible for many people. More practically, spasms will release, tissue restrictions will spontaneously release, and joints will begin to move better. Muscles will relax, people may spontaneously shudder or their breathing will change, and they will often shift into a deeper state of relaxation or even experience emotional, auditory, or visual effects. Many get off the table after this simple exercise without the pains that have been plaguing them, or just changed in some way.

I perceive the human being as a continuum between energy and tissue, or energy and matter. There are lots of ideas about the human energy field—some people call it the aura—but there is an energy associated with our being, and it appears to have many different layers, each with a different function. The outer layer, referred to as the ketheric body, is more associated with the affairs of the soul than of the body. The innermost layer, the etheric body, is the energy most directly associated with the physical body. Interconnecting with and within the etheric body the tissues are formed, the chakra system exists, the meridian system exists, and there is this intimate relationship between structure and function. It's in the etheric layer of the energy field that you see the dissociation, which occurs as a result of structural abnormalities, or loss of structural integrity and geometry. We exist as a continuum between spirit and matter. And my job as an osteopath is to sit and work at the interface, to bring the healing from the energy back down and into the tissues themselves.

Sacred Geometry

Sacred geometry is about the Laws of Creation. It relates to the shape of how Spirit enters the body and how it lives there in health. In my practice and courses, I work with an aspect of sacred geometry called The Sacred Count of Creation. It is a powerful engineering tool that evaluates a person for their health and their capacity to self-heal and self-regulate.

The Sacred Count is not easy to explain, and students don't really begin to get an understanding of how to work with it until somewhere in the second or third course. But I'll try to explain and you'll just have to trust me that there is great clinical importance to this. As I mentioned already, there is a point that trained hands can find—literally a one-dimensional point—where Life is transmuted into the body by The Breath of Life. That is the "one" of the Count that immediately polarizes into two opposing sparks. These sparks then arc between one another and form the two-dimensional line or axis that is the body's midline. That's the number "two" of the Sacred Count. Immediately, the body then organizes around its midline in three dimensions, which then initiates a complex coiling and folding of energy. That's the "three" of the Sacred Count. As an event, this ONE, TWO, THREE, is the geometry of all that has to happen for Spirit to enter into the being and for the being to function in health. Any errors or defects in this count must first be recognized and corrected before we can expect the body to heal itself or before we should begin to intervene with any other treatments.

When you hold the body and observe it, and you're sensitive to the energy, what you see forming in front of you are discourses in anatomy, sacred geometry and embryology, organizing, configuring and driving the body to health. Much of what I teach about sacred geometry comes from the lessons my patients' bodies have taught to me. The movements and patterns of the embryo are how the sacred geometry becomes established in the anatomy and maintains the relationships that are preserved and maintained in the energy field. Understanding this guides you to where the healing power is, what the wisdom of the system is trying to do to heal itself, and how to support that process.

A Patient's Story

Here is an experience I had when I was a third-year osteopathic student and was at the Zuni Pueblo. One of the traditional religious people there used to be a tackle for the San Diego Chargers and a sergeant in the Marines in Korea. When he came back to the reservation, he became involved in the religions traditions and was a special kachina dancer for one of the big medicine festivals where he had to run enormous distances and plant prayer sticks all around the pueblo. But one year, he came up lame about three weeks before the celebration.

Many healers worked with him, but Paul wasn't getting any better. Anthony, my brother in the family and himself a medicine man, had some idea that I might be able to help. So I agreed. As I was working at the getting-out-of-the-way process, this voice comes into my head and says, "Steven, why don't you check out his foot?"

Because Paul had a knee problem, I disregarded it. I worked for a little while and said to myself, "Well, his fibula is twisted a bit, his patella is off a little bit, and he's got some swelling in the back of his knee with some tendon irritation, so let me work with that." But the other voice came back, this time a little sweeter and maybe even a little patronizing, and said, "Steven, really, why don't you check out his foot? Please."

So I looked at his foot. It seemed that Paul had dropped an important bone in the apex of his arch. As a result there was a strain in his foot and ankle that pulled straight up into his knee. As I held his foot, I was aware of the shape of the health in his foot and an axis of energy running right down his leg into his arch from his spine as part of the "Two of the Sacred Count." I was also aware of the straining motion present in the pathology and of the vectors that had formed around the pathology, representing the injury. Going to where the Sacred Count energy guided me, I put a thumb at one end of the axis of Health (under the bone of the arch) and my other hand at the knee at the other end of the Health axis. I held the bone in his arch and gently began to lift it until the Health and the pathology—not the tissues but the energy lines—seemed to line up. I did what I perceived the system had asked me to do. There was this wobble between the pathology of the displacement and the Health of the system, and I just held on until the lines lined up and the wobble went away and everything seemed like it was happier. I held it for a long time. When it tried to push my hands back, I just kept holding on to that bone in his arch and his knee. A force went up his leg and he shook. "Something is happening in there," he said. "I can feel it."

I felt a series of very profound tissue releases in the bones of the transverse arch that traveled up his leg, through his knee, and into his pelvis. The bone in his arch, the external cuneiform, suddenly lifted back up into place almost spontaneously. And the whole time I was probably putting no more than a postage stamp's worth of pressure on this bone, but his foot, ankle, leg, and knee reorganized. When I took my hands off to recheck his knee, he said, "That feels pretty good." He stood up and he didn't have any pain.

So that's an example of how the healing can work.

I talked to some healers and some people on the reservation about the voice and they said, "The Spirit world is communicating to you and guiding you. It's a blessing."

Then I called Dr. Jim Jealous and asked him. His opinion was that Spirit was essentially feeling sorry for me and trying to help out because I was so inexperienced. "It's grace for sure, and undoubtedly a real blessing, but they must realize you don't know enough anatomy, so they have to give you direct instruction. My advice to you is to buy a couple of anatomy texts and learn them from cover to cover. And maybe you should do another dissection or two. Then I suspect the voices will stop."

So I made it a point to follow his advice and learn more and the voices stopped.

They have been replaced over time by instincts. The voices have changed to understanding—a deep, knowing awareness of what's under and around my hands, and perhaps, on a good day, real wisdom about what my patients require to heal themselves.

Observations about September 11, 2001

I live in Brooklyn and on most days, ride my bike to my office, which is near what used to be the World Trade Center. On September 11, 2001, I was on my bike riding back downtown from an early morning homeopathic visit when it happened. By the time I got to my office, my first patient was there and she dragged me to the street corner. It was like a scene from a science fiction movie. People were screaming and shaking, and cars were stopped, and people were crying, "Oh my god, oh my god." As I struggled to move into observation, I became aware that everybody's energy field was completely blown apart. I stayed and attended the people who showed up for treatment over the next couple of days for the obvious shock that we had all undergone.

Weeks and even months later, former patients started showing up at my office complaining of old symptoms. The new patients had mostly the same story too. Even though these patients were coming to me with knee problems, or foot problems, or headaches, they also complained of irritability, sleeplessness, and difficulty concentrating. When I "got out of the way" and listened to their bodies, I realized there was a profound lack of any energetic integrity in their bodies and fields, and that there were disturbances in their Sacred Counts. I was also aware from that out-of-the-way place that their systems were hemorrhaging energy and that their second chakras were spinning in the wrong direction.

Their energy fields were warped and distorted. Their diaphragms were in spasm and the movement of qi that one should expect in the body was absent or very bizarre. Many of the symptoms improved when I released the diaphragm spasms, but within a couple of days and with the collaboration of colleagues, we pieced together a scenario that explained the phenomena we were observing and guided us to effective diagnosis and treatment. The magnitude of the tragedy itself shattered people's fields and sent them into shock right down to the level of the sacred Counts. The emotional data of the tragedy was more than the second chakra (the emotional center) could process, thereby causing it to essentially explode and begin to hemorrhage. It was being spun the wrong way to try to block the flow of energy through it to minimize the loss of qi. And the diaphragmatic spasm was there to shut the whole system down and reduce the flow of qi to the damaged parts. The patients were in shock and highly compromised, but they were still functioning on some level. What I first observed as pathology was actually a survival mechanism and an adaptation to the unthinkable overload that all New

Yorkers experienced. The symptoms were there as an indirect consequence of the fact that their pain thresholds had dropped as a result of the shock.

I realized that if I restored integrity to the Sacred Count and put energy into the second chakra and just held that, the patients would begin to heal and regulate themselves. When I did this, the second chakras started spinning correctly, diaphragms relaxed, the qi began to circulate in a healthy way, the hemorrhaging of energy stopped, and the symptoms mostly went away on their own as the patients' pain thresholds rose back up. It is amazing to witness how the body heals itself if and when it gets what it needs.

But if I hadn't studied with Rev. Bruyere and gained some understanding of the chakras, if I hadn't gone to Zuni, if I hadn't learned to get out of the way from Dr. Day, or if I didn't have an engineer's sense of how the body worked or hadn't learned the sacred geometry of the Sacred Count, then I neither would have had the ability to understand what my patients' bodies were trying to show me nor would I have had the capacity to do the work needed to support their healing.

What Medicine Needs

My whole journey has been to create a standard of care that is based upon the body's truths—that is, the body's own health requirements. First of all, we have never had a standard of care that is uniform across the board for all healthcare practitioners regardless of credential or specialty. What matters to a neurologist doesn't matter to an acupuncturist or doesn't matter to a homeopath or doesn't matter to an osteopath. It's like we are treating different bodies and contradicting each other all the time, which is not only silly but a crime against our responsibilities to our patients.

And we are therapy driven. I think of this as a form of reductionism that ultimately treats the body like it's dead and at its worst chases the symptoms around the body like a puppy chasing its tail. The difference between many complementary and alternative practitioners and allopathic practitioners is the therapies they use and not necessarily the way they think. Complementary therapies may be more benign, more herbal, with less morbidity, and fewer side effects but they are still often administered from an allopathic perspective. The therapies may differ but the thought process is often disturbingly similar.

We need to look at the body in a different way. What I teach and practice is not about the differences in *what* I do, but the different *way* in which I do it. When I recommend a surgery, it is the result of a totally different way of looking at the body that's brought me to that conclusion.

Patients say to me, "But my MRI that shows that I've a herniated disc. And my surgeon says that the MRI indicates that I have to have surgery." Yet there's a whole movement in medicine that recognizes that there is often no statistical connection between the radiologist's interpretation of the MRI and the patient's pain! So we need to solve problems at their roots.

We need a standard of care that holds us all equally responsible for working with a problem-solving algorithm based upon how the human body works: structural integrity, mechanical integrity, balanced muscular integrity, neuro-regulatory function, psycho-spiritual integrity, energetic integrity, metabolic and genetic factors, and occupational factors, to name a few parts. Whether you're an allopathic physician, acupuncturist, chiropractor, healer or osteopathic physician it is still necessary to look at all these things in order to truly serve your patients.

Medicine as a practice of Healing is about the person on the table in front of you who has come for help from their suffering. We have lost sight of that. What we mostly seem to do is impose our concepts and our egos and the therapies that we are trained to do on everyone we see. To get it right, I think we have to change something first in ourselves, in our hearts. We have to learn to listen—with our minds and our hearts and our hands. We have to let go of our concepts and really serve our patients and not our egos. We have to have the courage and faith and the training to allow our patients to show us how we can help heal them. Like Jimmy the bone doctor, I pray that we can begin to get out of the way and let the Creator and the Spirits of our ancestors come through and help us heal.

CHAPTER 11

LEANNA STANDISH, ND, PhD

From Neuroscience to Naturopathy

Most of the people I've interviewed for *Alternative Therapies in Health and Medicine* have come from conventional medical or science backgrounds. Then, at some point, each of them had a life-changing experience that opened their minds and hearts and made them pay attention to things previously ignored. Leanna Standish, ND, PhD, is no exception. Interestingly enough, for her, it was a deeply moving encounter with primates that changed the course of her life and led her away from neuroscience to become both a naturopathic physician and acupuncturist.

Now the principal investigator for the Bastyr University AIDS Research Center and codirector of the Bastyr Research Institute, Dr. Standish also serves as senior scientist at Bastyr University and as a staff physician at the University Health Clinic. She received her doctoral degree in biopsychology from the University of Massachusetts; completed a postdoctoral fellowship in psychopharmacology at the Yerbes Primate Research Center; codirected Smith College's neuroscience program; and served for two years as a visiting scientist/senior fellow in the University of Washington's Department of Physiology and Biophysics.

In 1996, I interviewed Dr. Standish at her office at Bastyr University in Seattle, Washington.

How did I get out of the box of conventional healthcare? I'll tell you what I usually say, and then I will try to answer more deeply. I was the codirector of the neuroscience program at Smith College in Massachusetts and was involved in the most reductionistic work you could possibly imagine, based on the belief that if I understood how the brain worked, then I would understand what it meant to be a human being and would understand human suffering and human passions. On a second sabbatical from my faculty appointment at Smith, I came to Seattle to take a position as a visiting scientist and senior fellow in the Department of Physiology and Biophysics at the University of Washington. I was studying gene expression in the monkey hypothalamus using computerized image-enhancement procedures, radioisotopes, and microscopes and was counting how many grains of audio-radiographic displays there were in the hopes of understanding how the primate brain goes from prepubescence to pubescence. So there I was. I had never heard of naturopathic medicine, and if I had, I would have dismissed it as a quaint, antiquated, irrelevant thing of the past.

A friend of mine came to visit me and said, "I want to go to this place called Bastyr College on 144 Northeast 54th Street. Do you know where that is?"

I said, "No, but I'll get you there." After we got in my car, I took a map out and drove to this small building. I went up to the third floor into the library and was amazed at their book collection. There were books about homeopathy, acupuncture, botanical medicine—books I'd never seen before. I was very taken with two disciplines: homeopathy and acupuncture. They were so implausible. For me—to whom human beings were nothing more and nothing less than complex, biological machines, composed of interacting molecules and synaptic clefts and whatnot—to encounter homeopathy, which claimed that there can be biological effects of substances with no molecules in them, was outrageous. But if there was any truth to it at all, it meant that the universe was really much more interesting than I had imagined and that what I had been thinking was really limited, something I had deeply suspected for a long time. I had the same response to acupuncture. How could it be that putting a small filamentous needle into a point here—Large Intestine 4, I learned five years later—could possibly affect the lungs? There are no nerves connecting the two spots. It violated everything I knew about anatomy.

I can't really explain to you why I did this, but at the age of 37, I gave up my tenure-track appointment at Smith College, where I had a beautiful house in the country and a wonderful salary, gave up my very nice visiting professorship at the University of Washington, and took a job as research director at Bastyr University, which was 5 hours a week, $11.33 an hour. That's what I did. I knew that if I was going to find out more about homeopathy and acupuncture, I had to immerse myself, so I enrolled in the medical program here at Bastyr. (The deeper story is that I'd had my PhD for a long time, and I'd published and was "going places," yet there was a desperately unhappy side to it all, but I will get to that later.)

When I started as research director, it was during the height of the AIDS crisis in Seattle when people still believed you could get AIDS from toilet seats. I thought the most important thing the medical community needed to know was whether natural medicine had anything to offer the AIDS epidemic. I knew nothing about AIDS and nothing about natural medicine, but I started working with some of the faculty members here. Jane Guiltinan, the chief medical officer, and I put together a study with 30 males who were HIV positive. We put together what we thought was the best protocol, combining botanical medicine, homeopathy, psychological counseling, support group, Chinese medicine, hydrotherapy, and artificial fever therapy. We treated people for a year. Even though this study was uncontrolled, the results looked promising. It seemed that a comprehensive program of naturopathic medicine had reduced symptoms, improved neuropsychological status, and produced some transient immunological improvements. Five years later, more people in our study were alive, and fewer had progressed to AIDS than in the general HIV-positive population in King County.

We began that study in 1988, and I became more and more fascinated by the challenge of AIDS. It wasn't just that we were in the middle of an epidemic; it was also a deep fascination with the virus hypothesis: is the HIV virus the single and sole cause, both the necessary and sufficient cause, of AIDS? What is the relationship between the mind and the body in this disease? AIDS is a very complex, multifactorial disease with immunodeficiency components and autoimmune, inflammatory components. It affects the brain, the gastrointestinal system, the spinal cord, the skin, the lungs—every organ is affected.

Now, all this didn't come out of the blue for me.

Themes of My Life

There are a few important themes in my development as an intellectual. First, I was trained at Mount Holyoke, which is a women's college in Massachusetts, a place that prides itself on educating the uncommon and scholarly woman. At a very young age I was taken seriously as an intellectual, and that had a tremendous effect on me. Another theme was that I was in the five-college area—Smith College, Mount Holyoke College, Wellesley College, Hampshire College, and Amherst College—in Massachusetts, when feminism exploded. It was a hotbed of the finest intellectual thinking. I studied object relations theory from a feminist perspective and became obsessed with the question of what would happen if women's minds did science. Would science be different? I was convinced it would be. I wrote a paper titled, "Women Work in a Scientific Enterprise," in which I talked about the important implications of object relations theory, feminist thinking, and how women are selves-in-connection, whereas the masculine psyche is described more as a self-in-separation, and the implications of that for science. That is now almost cliché, but 18 years ago it was a big insight for me to start asking those questions.

Theme number three is animal ethics. I've killed thousands of animals in the name of science, in the pursuit of "truth." Two years ago, I was asked to give a speech about women's wellness at the University of Washington to 500 women. I was talking about my experiences being a researcher and scientist and how I'd killed animals. I stood there and for about 7 seconds I was overcome with grief and couldn't speak. I couldn't hurt a living thing now. I can't even kill a spider. But I had in the past. When I realized what it had cost me to kill all those mice and rats and monkeys and cats, what I had to do to myself in order to see these beings as little machines that were there for me to figure out how they worked, and what that means to a person to have to do that. . .

Let me explain. My first sabbatical was at Yerkes Primate Center at Emory University in Atlanta. It has the largest collection of great apes in captivity. I was there for a year in 1979, during which time they had a huge, million-dollar conference on the issue of infertility in the great apes. They were looking at the protein coat of the sperm, analyzing the polysaccharide matrix of orangutan vaginal mucosa, and so on. People came from all over the world to try to figure out why these animals were not reproducing in captivity. But all you had to do was walk down the beautifully clean, sterile corridor of the Primate Center and look into the windows of each locked room. First you would see the infants in their diapers who were there without their mothers, because their mothers were so psychopathological that they either ignored their infants or killed them. If you went to the next room, you would see this beautifully clean area full of toddlers who were hitting their heads on the wall. If you went to the next room, you'd see the preadolescents masturbating or eating their feces. What you saw was a perfect succession of psychopathology. And nobody there got it.

One day during that conference I couldn't bear to be in the building, so I was sitting outside eating my lunch. I looked behind me at this big, green metal garbage container and there was this chimpanzee arm hanging out of it with a little tag. It just floored me. Here was this fancy conference with everyone wondering why the primates don't reproduce, and nobody got it. That was when I started running. To get through that experience I would run several miles several times a day in the raging heat of Atlanta to release the despair and self-hatred and immense conflict associated with my work, though I did not know then that it was conflict. It just felt like there was something terribly wrong—probably with me. I felt like a demented Artemis running through hill and dale.

So in 1979, I began asking myself how we could do science differently. I wanted to know how the cells of the brain were interconnected to produce emotions, thoughts, and actions, and I wanted to know if there was another way to know how the brain creates the mind besides chopping off the head, chipping the bone away, putting the brain in formaldehyde, and slicing it into 50-micron-thick sections so you could look at dead tissue under a microscope. Was there another way? I was sure there was, but I didn't know what it was.

Four years later I was here in Seattle and then, on September 6, 1986, I bolted upright in my bed and thought, "Oh! You're supposed to be a naturopathic physician." I didn't know what that was, but it was one of those few times when I felt that information was made available to me that didn't come from inside my head.

I didn't exactly know what a naturopathic physician was, but I opened the phone book and ran my finger down until I came to the first woman. I ended up going to see Dr. Ellen Goldman, who now happens to be the chair of Bastyr's homeopathy department. I was very impressed, mostly by the depth of her medical interview. (I will not reveal what polycrest she prescribed for me.) The next year I started as research director here. And that's my story.

The other thing that's strange, looking at my life, is that I've always had this secret fascination with science fiction, mysticism, and the occult. I'd be ripping open brains and reading *Science* magazine, but when I would get depressed, what would comfort me would be Piers Anthony's *Macroscope* or Suzuki's *Zen Buddhism*.

My mother was also extremely influential on me. When I was 13, she handed me *Existentialism Made Easy* and I just gobbled it up. She bought me two very important gifts: the first was a microscope. My favorite activity as a child was to get on my bike and go tearing down the country road to this pond. I would fill up a little glass jar with the pond water and then go home and put water droplets under my microscope. She also bought me a telescope. So being able to look really far away and see things that were big and to see things that were tiny, the macroscopic and microscopic—to be in the middle of this expanding, infinite tunnel—was great. That's where I developed my interest in what the universe was all about.

My Work at Bastyr

I often feel that it's my mission in life to figure out how to cure AIDS and cancer. I know how silly that sounds, but I just wish that as a doctor, I could simply, by some powerful but gentle medical art, make disease and pain go away. It's more than just wanting to help stop the suffering. I believe there's tremendous mystery, wisdom, and knowledge to be gained by understanding these two diseases that will take us to our next level of transformation.

I have a wonderful partnership with Carlo Calabrese, who is the codirector of the Bastyr University Research Institute. Carlo has created an infrastructure for doing research in natural medicine here. I sometimes say that I know what to do and he knows how to do it. Our missions are different, but without each other we wouldn't have done nearly as well.

John Weeks told us that there was an Office of Alternative Medicine (now the National Center for Complementary and Alternative Medicine) and that we should try to get appointed to their advisory committee, which we ultimately did. That happened in 1992. In 1990, we did a small study with 12 women to ask, does the naturopathic protocol that's been used for decades to treat uterine fibroids work? Does it shrink the tumors, and if there is bleeding, does it stop the bleeding? We did a 3-month study with 12 women, and do you know what? It didn't work.

We went to the American Association of Naturopathic Physicians and reported our study. I think it was the first time in the entire realm of alternative medicine that someone on the inside said, "It didn't work." There were some angry people, but my role is not to promote alternative medicine. My role is to evaluate and also to expand. It was an opportunity to point out the importance of communicating negative results. Most results in medicine actually are negative. We can't learn as quickly unless we tell each other our failures.

I believe that the answers to serious chronic diseases are going to come from minds trained in the concepts of natural medicine and that our responsibility is to develop those therapies, keeping in mind the work of people like Anne Wilson Schaef, who don't believe in "medical" solutions to problems like AIDS and tell us that we don't actually control anything. Maybe if I sat and wrote about it, I would be clearer, but it's a very important point. It seems to me like there are levels. In the first level, we just facilitate patients getting better. That's a strong naturopathic principle. Physicians do nothing. Then we go to the physician having but a single task: to cure. The next level is to relinquish control. We're worrying about dragging people back from the edge of the chasm of death, but we haven't answered the question of whether there's life after biological death. If you don't have that question answered for yourself, how can you possibly proceed with being a doctor? If you can't answer that question, how do you know if you should be dragging people from the abyss of death and uttering nothingness or facilitating the process?

Sometimes I feel like we're all just hurtling toward death at various velocities, and this whole edifice of medicine is laughable, but I can only get into that mode when I'm listening to somebody who's really jumped out of the box of boxes, like Ann Wilson Schaef. I consider her an important thinker of our time. The whole concept of trusting the deep process, as a medical principle—holy smokes. The implications are immense.

The Principals of Naturopathic Medicine

The principles of naturopathic medicine have been very clearly articulated, and we live them. Principle number one is *Vis medicatrix naturae*—the healing power of nature. All living organisms have a self-inherent principal property of homeostasis, healing, reconstituting, renewing. That's an amazing thing. And the physician's role is to remove the obstacles to cure.

Principle number two: find the cause *(tolle causam)*. Don't suppress the symptom, but find what's really the cause. Example: a lot of asthma is caused by gut problems. Conventional medicine typically treats the lungs, but usually that's not where the problem is. Another principle is the doctor as teacher, teaching self-reliance. Another is prevention, and, of course, what we mean by prevention goes beyond mammograms and immunizations. We mean real prevention. Diet, exercise, fasting, nature cure, sunlight, fresh air—the basics. One of my most common therapies now is short juice fasts. I'm getting much more into nature cure. In fact, as a school we are moving more in that direction. We went through a period of being pill-oriented. Instead of giving pharmaceutical antibiotics, we'd give plant antibiotics, and we thought that we were somehow morally superior. But now we see that we've moved away from our vitalistic roots.

What I mean by nature is everything that is. I do not separate humanity from nature, though sometimes I slip into that thinking.

It is plausible to me that nature is pure consciousness, that everything is connected with everything else, and that some part of our being does continue after biological death. Equally plausible to me is that the universe started with a big bang; natural evolution is what's going on; and when we die, that's it, period, because we're nothing more than biological machines. Those two views are now equally plausible to me.

When I started the naturopathic school, I was on a quest to experience the life principle, what we call the vital force. I would make appointments with people and say, "I hear that you're doing such and such kind of medicine. I would like you to show me the vital force." And I would actually go to visit them, but I would always be disappointed because I never saw it. I'm laughing. Why am I laughing? Because the vital force is either everywhere, in everything, or it's nowhere and in nothing. I just think that's so amusing that someone, *me*, seriously and earnestly went in search of the vital force.

AIDS Research

Two weeks ago a dream of mine came true, which was to draw the best minds together for a whole day and talk about what's really going on in AIDS. We had a think tank in alternative medicine and AIDS here at Bastyr: Candace Pert; Michael Ruff; Robert Root-Bernstein;

John James, the editor of *AIDS Treatment News*; Lark Lands, a nutritionist who works with AIDS patients; and Barbara Brewitt all came. We had a wonderful day because finally we could say what we really thought to an audience who could understand the significance of what we were saying and talk back.

I met Candace when I was a neuroscientist. In 1982, before I even knew about AIDS, I was in my lab at Smith College cutting open rat brains, and my colleague, Pat DiLorenzo, got a little note from Candace. Inside was a Polaroid picture of a section of monkey brain showing the location in bright red of CD4 receptor sites all over the cortex and in the limbic system. Candace was the first person to show that there were CD4 receptors in the brain. And there was a little note attached to it that said, "Pat, I'm really scared."

Candace has done some very important thinking. The concept of our emotions being distributed informationally throughout the whole body is deeply true. Of course, Candace is a committed feminist. Can you see how feminism has so profoundly influenced what's going on in science and medicine? I think it was Beverly Rubik who said, "It's not science that's leading this movement. It's medicine." Sometimes when I ask my neuroscientist colleagues what they are studying they say, "I'm looking at such and such synaptic connection in the CA3 area of rat hippocampus." And I ask myself, just for a moment, "Is this the work of a grown man?"

I must tell you one thing that's really important. Remember I was telling you before about how homeopathy and acupuncture seemed implausible to me? I decided I just had to study acupuncture, so I started eight years ago, and I'm just about ready to get my license. I'm fascinated by homeopathy. Now my research has moved to injecting homeopathic preparations into acupuncture points as a therapy for AIDS.

Let me tell you a story. It was 1992, and I had just finished writing an essay called "The Winter of Our Discontent." I'm sitting in my office, totally bummed, because everybody is saying, "AIDS is a chronic, manageable condition, but [there is] the mind-body connection, and you just have to love yourself." And it's not true. I'm in the trenches with these guys, and they're dying. They have diarrhea, they can't breathe, they have dementia, they are totally screwed up, they're in wheelchairs—and they're only 23 or 43 years old.

So I'm sitting there saying to myself, "I have failed. Natural medicine is not taking care of this problem at all." So this complete stranger, Barbara Brewitt, a PhD from the University of Washington Department of Biological Structure, walks into my office and says, "I have an idea, and I'm looking for a place to work to develop my idea. My idea is to develop growth factors and cytokines into homeopathic medicines."

Growth factors and cytokines are the molecules that the immune system uses to communicate between itself—sort of the "neurotransmitters" of the immune system. The brain and spinal cord communicate with the immune system with growth factors and cytokines. You've probably heard of them: interleukin-2, granulocyte-macrophage colony stimulating factor, interferon, tumor necrosis factor. There are now a couple of dozen that have been identified. We think the brain is the most complex thing in the universe, but the immune system is even more complex, because it's moving around. It's not fixed in three-dimensional space, and therefore it's even more dependent than the brain on those messengers, or the neurotransmitters or the cytokines that communicate to tell the cells what to do at a distance.

So Barbara says, "My idea is to make these growth factors and cytokines into homeopathics and treat chronic viral conditions with them." You know, there are times in your life when you think, "That's a *great* idea." I knew that some great truth had just been uttered to me. I said, "Yes, and let's do it in AIDS."

Some of our best thinking, our most innovative thinking about medicine, about the immune system, can be worked out in AIDS. It's a great model. Last year Barbara and I started a trial, and do you know what? This idea is actually feasible. We picked four growth factors, cytokines, to give orally in very, very high dilutions to a group of HIV-positive patients in a double-blind, placebo-controlled trial, and we got a difference in the two groups. We gave 10 drops of four growth factors orally to the patients in the study. Some of them got drops of fluid that were placebo. The CD4 count stabilized in the people who got the real dilutions. Viral load came down a third of a log unit. Their weight went up compared with that of the control group. Their platelets went up into the normal range. Things happened that surprised me.

Last year Barbara and I went to a local hospital's institutional review board here in Seattle to get permission for our patients in the study who were hospitalized to continue taking the medication. We presented our data and the people politely listened. Then, at the end, they said, "Thank you very much. The committee will get back to you," and we were escorted out of the room. The big metal door closed, and I heard a burst of laughter. I couldn't believe it. So I pressed my ear up against the door. I heard somebody—I think it was the chair of the committee—say, and I'm quoting because it stunned me, "This is nothing but spiritual science. We can't have this going on in our hospital." The medical bigotry amazed me.

The Arndt-Schultz Law

So this is the insight: when you go to medical school, you learn that when you study the relationship between the biological effect of a drug versus the dose of the drug, that the curve looks like this. [Draws on a piece of paper.] Low doses produce a small effect. Medium doses, now you're getting a good effect. And then as you get high doses, the biological effect starts to taper off. You get extremely high doses, you get inhibition because it's toxic. It's a sigmoidal curve.

What I realized from Benvenista's 1988 *Nature* paper is that this curve is actually a repeating sinusoid that continues into extremely low doses. We are now looking at a 10 to 30 to 10 to 2000 mol/L. There are essentially no molecules. Ten to 24 mol/L is beyond Avogadro's constant, so we know that there's only a tiny probability of even a single molecule being present, yet the data show that immunological and clinical changes were occurring in these patients in our study. The implications are huge. What this might mean is that the holographic, informational paradigm that Beverly Rubik talks about is probably true. Remote healing can probably really happen. You can have a biological effect with no molecules, and we demonstrated it. We probably didn't pick the exact right combination of growth factors, but it opens up the whole field of clinical immunology.

Last week I went to New Jersey to try to talk a small pharmaceutical company into making homeopathic everything, like homeopathic Taxol and homeopathic protease inhibitors. I said, "Do you realize that a microgram could treat the entire city of Seattle? Look, all I'm asking you to do is a tissue culture experiment and I'll tell you what dilutions to try." I think I have a sense of this from reading the literature now, which, by the way, is mostly European. This country is so behind in high-dilutional biologics and pharmacologics; it's pathetic. But I said, "Please, I'm begging you, please just try this."

Barbara and I have been criticized for calling these things homeopathic, because we are not using the principles of classical homeopathy in prescribing them. Our logic goes something like this: there's chaos in the immune system of the person who's HIV-positive, as evidenced by depletion of CD4 lymphocytes and serious illness. We can measure many things about an HIV-positive person's immune system in the blood. How can that be brought into some kind of order? It's by small, repetitive signals. That's been demonstrated in chaos theory to bring order out of chaos. Barbara and I presented this work at our conference here, and Candace Pert and Michael Ruff got it. They understood that we were talking about some kind of electromagnetic tweaking of the receptor site—something to do with electron clouds, with high-frequency Fourier domains. At the end of our talk, Barbara and I presented a slide on plausible explanatory mechanisms, which were resonance and coherence. We don't even begin to understand it because we're just beginning to think about the biophysics of it, but it is something like that, and it doesn't require molecules.

There's some important work being done, mostly in Italy, France, and Germany. The implications are profound. My dream is to have a whole research facility that will develop high-dilutional drugs, high-dilutional AZT, high-dilutional Taxol, high-dilutional poisons of the nth degree, growth factors, cytokines, interleukins, and interferons, and use them in doses well beyond Avogadro's constant, observing their clinical effects. And I don't want to do animal research. In fact, for this endeavor, it would be irrelevant.

The wave chart I showed you is called the Arndt-Schultz Law in pharmacology. One night I was lying in bed. I had read Benvenista's paper in 1988, and I had studied pharmacology and had been studying Fourier analysis. I spent a long time in my scientific career trying to figure out how the brain "sees." We know now that the brain does a Fourier analysis, a frequency analysis. It doesn't see lines and sticks. It does a Fourier analysis of the spatial frequencies in the two-dimensional image on the retina. Do you know that a square wave is made up of the fundamental, the third harmonic, the fifth harmonic, the seventh harmonic, and every prime number, and when you add all those waves together you get a perfect square wave? So your ability to see the edge of this is based on your brain's ability to see the fundamental frequency, the third harmonic, the fifth harmonic, the seventh, and so on.

What I'm proud of is that my brain was able to put these ideas from diverse fields together into something that might be clinically and conceptually useful. Figure 2 in Benvenista's paper shows that degranulation of basophils by immunoglobulin E, as a function of dose immunoglobulin E, is a repeating sinusoid. He shows that with tiny doses—homeopathic doses—white blood cells physiologically can respond. Nobody ever talks about this. I was lying in bed and went, "Oh, I get it."

I use homeopathy in my practice, but as a clinician, it's hard to tell whether anything really works. It's strange, because at some other level, I absolutely trust in homeopathy. For example, in my briefcase, which goes everywhere with me, I have only two medical tools: a set of acupuncture needles and a bottle of Arnica 12C. Still, I can't say definitively that homeopathy is real, except from that one experiment Barbara and I did in HIV and then reading this wonderful book by two Italian scientists called *Homeopathy: A Frontier in Medical Science*.

The thing that's extraordinary about a holograph is that if you smash it, every little piece, every fragment, has the complete image. It is so exciting. I want to scream: "Please, everybody stop." Perhaps everything—every poison, every drug, every neurotransmitter, hormone, cytokine, and growth factor—could be made into an ultra–high-dilutional medicine. But the thing is, you must choose the right potency, the right concentration. In classical homeopathic thinking, everybody acts as if the relationship between dose and response is a linear function and that if you use a 1M versus a 6C, the difference will be only one degree and depth of action. But it's not. It's like this: a 28C might be up here on the curve and be excitatory, or it could be down here and produce an inhibitory action. We don't know, but I think we could find out.

Does every substance on the planet have a different frequency? Probably not. We don't even know that. Could there be anything more important to know than that? For me, it would be one of the largest contributions to understanding the nature of reality. It means that the world really is kind of magical and, frankly, I think we should reclaim magical thinking from Sartre.

So right now I'd like a high-tech, molecular biology/pharmaceutical company that understands the implications of what I'm talking about and has the guts to go forth into this new venture, and [that will] put up the capital to do the clinical experiments to develop a new class of drugs, a totally new approach to medicine. Can you imagine? If there's any truth at all to what I'm saying, it means that you could effectively treat people in a nontoxic manner. We'll look back on the twentieth century and say, "Oh, my God, they used pharmacological doses of AZT or Taxol. How barbaric."

Here's the problem: you could take anything and make it into a homeopathic. There's no way to validate that it is done correctly. We don't have the technology. So a collaborative collective of people like Candace Pert, Barbara Brewitt, and myself, and far-reaching pharmaceutical companies that understand the concept need to come together. My dream is of a science collective, where everybody shares. It's difficult. This biomedical industry environment is competitive. A lot of people say, "Leanna, you're such a fool for even talking about this idea. You're giving away your and Barbara Brewitt's best stuff." But I don't buy it. I just want everybody to know it's important. I don't care about the business angle. In fact, for me, it's not the right way to go. I want to give away the ideas. I want the collectivization of the whole enterprise. I don't want anybody to make money off it. I want it to be a university endeavor, and I want Bastyr University to be the home of this research because we have the right philosophy.

Having the right philosophy is really important. We have no money. It's a ridiculous building. The bathrooms are built for third-graders, but I love it here. We make terrible salaries; we drive old cars; but we're happy. I look at many of my colleagues with their anxiety and rapid aging, and their cover-your-ass philosophy that seems to color everything in conventional medicine and science, and I say, "There, but for the grace of God, go I."

I've been in all kinds of environments, and they do kill a person. I was a wreck. Maybe I looked okay, but I was dying inside. When you're separated from what is really alive, you're slowly dying, but you don't know it because you think that's how it's supposed to be. It's a dreadful thing.

Science and Spirituality Course

Bastyr University is taking its first steps toward developing a spiritual component to our work here. I am very interested in the whole endeavor and I have offered to teach a course called "Science and Spirituality."

The class will focus on four questions. The first is: Is there life after biological death? Question number two is: What is the role of consciousness in the world? That question is important. Let me tell you a story: I was at the airport, on my way back from Philadelphia and had to change flights. I was at the gate counter to get my boarding pass, and the agent said, "I can't let you on the plane. These tickets are wrong, and you need to go back to the ticket desk, and you'll probably have to pay more money." The plane was about to leave. I was totally exhausted, sick with the flu. I decided that I was going to do an experiment. I just stood very calmly and decided to love this guy. I focused my awareness on the man's chest, his heart, and experienced loving him. All I did was love him and stay detached from the outcome.

A few seconds later, he looks up from his terminal and says, "You're right. You already paid that $50 and it's okay," and hands me the boarding pass. Now, there's no way to know, but if I keep doing experiments like this, then maybe someday before I die I will know the answer to that question about consciousness.

Question three is: What is the nature of reality? Sometimes I feel like the veil is about to be lifted. Like many people, I am increasingly interested in the science of mystical consciousness. I have a strong sense of that. Question four is: What is the purpose of human existence?

The course has been accepted as an elective in our naturopathic medical curriculum. I'll be teaching it next year in the medical school, not the psychology department, at Bastyr's new facility at the Saint Thomas Seminary.

I gave Carlo my course syllabus. He scribbled back a little note that said, "Science has nothing to say about these questions." I understand where he's coming from, and in a certain, limited sense, he's right. But I think that the mind of a scientist needs to grapple with these questions.

Is there life after death? I don't know. I believe that everything in the universe is interconnected and that I have an important destiny to fulfill, and part of that destiny meant becoming a naturopathic physician and doing what I'm doing now. I feel like I am on an important path headed toward something that is well beyond me and my little ego and my little self and my little body.

The claim that's made by a lot of people is that there are other ways to know besides the five senses. It's an interesting proposition, but I don't know if it's true. I haven't experienced it in my own life. Everything I know comes through what I've seen or heard or read or felt. I don't think there's anything that you can show me that I can't offer a plausible, mechanical explanation for within the bounds of neuroscience.

I know I said earlier that I woke up one night and said, "I have to be a naturopathic physician." But I could generate a neurobehavioral explanation for how I think that happened. However, I do believe that message came from elsewhere—from where, I don't know. I'm very taken with the holographic notion that everything is hooked together. One time, in an altered state, I looked up at a tree, and for about 20 minutes I actually experienced everything as one. It wasn't just an idea or a philosophy or something I read. I experienced it. That experience has kept me nurtured.

I've had some important teachers. Most recently I had a teacher come to me out of the blue, a British theologian named Dr. Richard Kirby. He came up to my office a year and a half ago and started talking about the Michelson-Morley experiments and consciousness. He could talk circles around me. He was a deeply spiritual man. I called him up at his hotel that night and asked if he would teach me to meditate. He said, "You think that you're just going to add another thing to your busy schedule, don't you?" I denied it, but of course he was right.

He said, "You have no idea where you are headed and how big this is." He started working with me. So every 3 or 4 months I go to see him, and he does a fearless spiritual inventory on me. The last instruction he gave to me was that I should go into intensive psychotherapy, three times a week. I did it, and I'm still doing it, and I am now learning how to be a fully autonomous self so that I can shatter ego boundaries, so that I can perceive reality as it truly is. I'm seriously engaged in this, and I am doing a most important experiment. I'm doing the experiment to see if I can perceive what every spiritual tradition since the beginning of recorded time has told us is there. I don't know if it's there, but I have to find out.

My burning questions used to be "Is it true? Is life after death real? Is there a continuation of consciousness?" Those are not my questions anymore. My question now is "Am I capable of perceiving it?" And that is a very different question.

The only way to answer that is to generate those experiences in which you are more likely to perceive such things. Psychotherapy and meditation are two techniques in Western civilization that get to the point I'm talking about. I would give a lot to have a transcendent experience, but you know what I've noticed about myself? All these years I thought that all I wanted was to have a true experience. But what I've noticed about myself is that I'm actually scared of it. When I get really close, I get scared, because it's ego-shattering. It's a frightening experience to get that close to the dissolution of the self. And I have this sense that I need to have a really strong self to be able to go bravely into that terrain and step through that door.

CHAPTER 12

BARBARA DOSSEY, RN, MS

Holistic Nursing and Florence Nightingale

Just as Florence Nightingale helped to revolutionize hospital care in her day, the Holistic Nursing Movement has helped to reincorporate "healing" back into the art of nursing. Barbara Dossey, RN, PhD, is one of the internationally recognized pioneers of this movement.

Dr. Dossey received her bachelor of science degree in nursing from Baylor University, her master of science degree from Texas Women's University, and her PhD from the Union Institute University in Cincinnati, Ohio. She is currently the director of Holistic Nursing Consultants in Santa Fe, New Mexico.

A prolific writer, Dr. Dossey has authored or coauthored 19 books, including the *American Holistic Nurses' Association Core Curriculum for Holistic Nurses,* which she edited; *Handbook of Critical Care Nursing; Holistic Nursing: A Handbook for Practice; Rituals of Healing; Cardiovascular Nursing: Bodymind Tapestry; Critical Care Nursing: Body-Mind-Spirit;* and *Florence Nightingale: Mystic, Visionary, and Healer.* The winner of many awards, she is a seven-time recipient of the prestigious *American Journal of Nursing* Book of the Year Award; was named Holistic Nurse of the Year in 1985 by the American Holistic Nurses' Association; was designated as a Fellow in the American Academy of Nursing in 1992; and was the recipient of the Healer's Award by the Nurse Healers-Professional Associates International, Inc., in 1998. She is certified in holistic nursing by the American Holistic Nurses' Association.

I interviewed Barbara Dossey in the summer of 1999 at her home in Santa Fe, New Mexico while she was researching and writing her book on Florence Nightingale.

Holistic nursing embraces all nursing that has as its goal the enhancement of healing the whole person from birth to death. It is a philosophy and perspective that addresses the body, mind, and spirit of not just the patient but the nurse as well. This philosophy or way of being serves the holistic nurse in her or his personal life, as well as in clinical and private practice, education, research, and community service.

I want to emphasize that holistic nursing is not a specialty in nursing, as I so often hear, but is the essence of nursing, reflecting the diverse nursing activities in which holistic nurses are engaged. Standards of practice in this field are well developed. For example, the American Holistic Nurses' Association (AHNA) Standards of Holistic Nursing Practice are used in conjunction with the American Nurses Association Standards of Practice as well as the specific specialty standards wherever holistic nurses practice. Holistic nursing also is derived from a number of explanatory models, of which biomedicine is only one.

The AHNA conducted a survey and documented 24 complementary or alternative therapies that are frequently used in holistic nursing practice and which are also referred to as caring-healing modalities. People often refer to holistic nurses as "those nurses who do those different kinds of therapies." However, it is important to remember that holistic nursing is not about complementary or alternative therapies. The finest contemporary holistic nurses have an integrative approach that uses the latest technology, procedures, and medications in addition to addressing the person's mind and spirit.

For example, when I was practicing as a critical care nurse, I was intensely aware that the emphasis was on the latest technology. A patient could have open-heart surgery or thrombolytic therapy to limit or stop an evolving heart attack and save his or her life. These technological interventions take only minutes to hours, but it may require years to bring about a fundamental shift in one's consciousness and reshape the thoughts, emotions, and behaviors that contributed to the heart disease in the first place. I'm referring to how patients choose to live their lives and create healthy lifestyle patterns that include their spirituality, meaning and purpose, loving relationships, emotions, and health promotion activities such as exercise, stress management, and nutrition.

This example is very personal. My family and I share a profound treasure—a single healing event that will be with us the rest of our lives because of a critical care nurse's holistic approach. This event occurred right before my father's death. Three months before his death, my dear Daddy was healthy, having celebrated his 81st birthday. He was so happy because he had a great day on the golf course, having "shot his age, an 81." One month later he was diagnosed with non-Hodgkin's lymphoma.

Daddy was started on oral chemotherapy and was doing fine but then had to be placed on intravenous chemotherapy. Shortly thereafter, he developed a bladder infection and within 14 hours was hospitalized in the critical care unit with septic shock. He improved for a few hours, but the drugs could not save him. The critical care nurse who was caring for my father was tall—6 feet, 4 inches—and he had Daddy's bed in the top position. But when my sweet mother, who is 5 feet tall, came in to visit, the nurse stopped what he was doing and adjusted the bed to the lowest position. Daddy promptly pulled off his oxygen mask and said, "You can't believe what they're doing to me in here." Mother said, "I know, but I hope that they're doing all this so I can take you home." Daddy looked at Mother and said, "You think I'm going home?" Mother said, "I hope so, but if not, I'll see you in heaven." At that point, she bent over and kissed him. Then he said, "I'm so tired. I'm going to take a nap."

Those were Daddy's last words, because as my mother left the room he went into cardiac arrest and could not be resuscitated. That same critical care nurse removed all the equipment from my father's body, cleaned up the room, and then went back to see my family. He asked my mother, "Would you like to see your husband?" Mother said, "I don't think I can go in there." So this nurse said, "I just want you to know that he looks very peaceful. He died with a smile on his face." So what did Mother and the family do? They went right back into the critical care room and stayed there with Daddy for 45 minutes. And that is holistic nursing at its finest—technically competent while being able to recognize the many underlying patterns within the lives of patients and their families.

In healthcare today the emphasis is on disease and pathophysiology. Of course it's important to identify these patterns, such as my father being in septic shock. But at the same time other patterns existed that were crucially important—my father's behaviors, words, and emotions, as well as the perceptions and meanings embraced by the family members who were involved. Because the critical care nurse recognized these coexisting, complex patterns and used his compassion and intuition, a healing moment occurred.

The Holistic Caring Process

Nurses use intuition in their work all the time. Intuition involves a perceived knowing of things and events without the conscious use of rational thought processes. It is using all the senses to receive information, including a gut feeling or hunch. The nurse in my story had a hunch that Mother wanted to be closer to Daddy.

Another example might be a critical care nurse who is using physiological monitoring equipment. She or he might sense something that is not reflected in the hard data. This may be nothing more than a feeling that something is awry. The nurse's cue may be the look in the patient's eye or the way the patient taps his or her fingers, indicating that there is a story embedded in the present moment that may need to be told. So the nurse asks with a profound presence of caring, "What are you feeling and thinking when you tap your fingers on your chest?" And then, all of a sudden, the story comes forward. But even if it doesn't, the patient sees, hears, and feels the concern of the nurse. These sorts of interchanges make up the holistic caring process. And the holistic caring process is that moral state in which the holistic nurse brings her or his whole self into relationship to the whole of another person and other significant beings, reinforcing this presence, this connectedness in the moment.

This doesn't need to take a lot of time. What it takes is an intention in the nurse's consciousness—which is instantaneous and timeless—and being totally present in the moment, not thinking about all the other responsibilities. It is being focused, the "being with" and "being there" as much as possible in that moment. And intention involves consciously creating an image of the person's spiritual essence and wholeness that is experienced as a sacred space of inner calm. It is also a volitional act of love.

My Own Story

In the late 1960s I began my own personal journey of learning self-regulation strategies. This began primarily because of a medical condition. I was in Mexico on a vacation and ate some bad food that resulted in a 24-hour fever of 102° F, diarrhea, and vomiting. Two days later I was home and feeling awful. Then my right eye became swollen shut. I was diagnosed with dendritic keratitis, an infection of the cornea caused by the herpes simplex virus. At this time antiviral medications were still experimental, and I was placed on topical ointment. It cleared up after 6 weeks. However, whenever I was under any type of stress over the next 8-year period I had many flare-ups, and with each flare-up I developed severe scar formation of my cornea and eventually had no vision in my right eye.

By the end of 1975, I had gone a full year without a flare-up, which was then the criterion for a corneal transplant. Six weeks after my transplant, I had two bouts of acute rejection that were managed by an injection of steroid into my cornea on each occasion. An eyelid stretcher was placed around my right eye to keep it open while I received the injection. My anxiety in seeing the needle coming toward my eye and the helplessness I felt has never left my consciousness. I can still remember holding my breath, bracing, and tensing. This event made me aware of the need to be more present with my patients before I poked, suctioned, and performed all the procedures and treatments on them that were part of caring for a critically ill patient.

I tried to relax, but my skills and knowledge were limited prior to my surgery. In 1976, my husband Larry and I attended our first biofeedback workshop. Larry learned to manage classical migraine headaches without taking medicine, which he still does very successfully. This was such a significant discovery for him that he began a biofeedback department in his group practice of internal medicine. I also began to realize that there was no difference in stress management for migraine headaches and stress management for my corneal flare-ups. So I asked myself: what am I going to do about it?

Around this time I began to read as much as I could find in the literature on psychophysiologic stress. It was clear to me that my recurrent eye condition was related to stress, as were both episodes of corneal transplant rejections. So I seriously pursued biofeedback, relaxation, and imagery. I learned how to play more and take personal time to do nothing.

As I integrated these new behaviors into my life, my clinical practice began to change. It became obvious to me that the self-regulation strategies I was using in my own life could also be taught to patients in the critical care unit, used in teaching nursing students and hospital staff, and could benefit me in my research. This was a turning point. I began to teach relaxation, imagery, and breathing exercises, and used music with critical care patients before doing procedures, during their recovery, and in outpatient cardiac rehabilitation programs. It was thrilling to participate with patients and their families as they learned to reframe their stories of fear into modalities and rituals for healing, to learn how to alter their own internal physiology, and to decrease their fear and anxiety.

For example, a postsurgical patient I took care of who had minimal blood flow to his severely injured left leg used relaxation and imagery skills to increase circulation to the leg and avoided amputation. By changing their attitudes, emotions, and thoughts, these patients could marshal their inner healing resources to facilitate rather than impede healing. These bedside experiences allowed me to understand the importance of rituals and the rich tapestry of the interconnectedness of body-mind-spirit.

These experiences started me thinking about how critical care equipment could be used in the biofeedback process. I realized that most of the physiological monitoring equipment in the critical care unit—heart-rate monitors, temperature monitors, and Doppler devices to hear blood flow—was much like that used in an outpatient biofeedback department. In the outpatient biofeedback department, patients with high levels of anxiety and fear often had cardiac dysrhythmias. With biofeedback they were learning to abort these problems and to manage hypertension, migraine and tension headaches, peripheral vascular disease, and many more conditions by increasing blood flow to their hands and feet. Many were able to decrease or discontinue their medications. If people could learn this in a biofeedback department, why not in a critical care unit?

The Art of Listening

Patients want to be heard and listened to, particularly when they are critically ill. In fact, my hunch is that deeper healing goes on in critical care units than perhaps in any other area of the hospital. It's not difficult for nurses to facilitate these healing moments. When a patient tells you about a dream, you don't merely say, "Oh, that's an interesting dream" and drop it right there. If you are really listening and value the story in the person's healing, you say, "Tell me more about that."

For example, a 42-year-old man told me about his dream of a skull and crossbones two nights before he was scheduled for open-heart surgery. Rather than saying, "Don't think about that"— because I knew he would—I responded, "Tell me about it. What do you think it might mean?"

He said, "What's going to happen if I die in surgery?"

So I asked, "What are you afraid of?"

And he replied, "I've got six investments my wife told me not to invest in. She knows nothing about my portfolio. She doesn't even know how to write a check. And I don't have a will."

Because I had listened to his story, I was able to say to him, "I can help you handle some of these things before you go to the operating room. Would you be interested?"

After he agreed that he wanted some help, I said, "Let's get somebody in here to write your will, and then you might think about that conversation with your wife about your investments." I also said, "You know, it is very unlikely that you will die in the operating room. You do need open-heart surgery, but there are many things that can help you prepare for surgery. For example, you are now exploring ways to eliminate an enormous amount of anxiety and fear, which will help you a lot."

I suggested that it was important for him to be aware of the ongoing story that he was telling himself. I shared some ideas on how to use imagery and relaxed breathing to help in his healing, and I asked him to focus on his successful surgery and recovery.

When I asked him what he liked to do in his free time, he quickly responded that his passion was sailing and racing competitively. So I suggested that he feel what it was like to be on his sailboat—not trying to win a race but imagining that it was just a normal day and that he was relaxed. I encouraged him to let that image be a ritual of healing, something he could invoke any time he wished. I also rehearsed with him what he could expect when he got back from surgery—for the first 12 to 24 hours and the next 2 to 5 days. Then he wanted to know about his recovery at 6 weeks, 3 months, 6 months, and a year.

So it turned out that the dream he shared with me was his wake-up call to get his act together, both before and after surgery. Sharing the dream permitted the story he was telling himself to change from one of fear to one of healing.

Our lives are made of rich stories that have the potential to block or facilitate healing. The joy in my work and the joy of being with others is listening and reflecting on stories. I always ask myself: How can I fully hear the stories of others and my own as well? How can I attend to the metaphors and shielded meanings that emerge in a way that helps me get closer to the story's core meaning?

Just last week, Mother told me a story about a couple who had been married 60 years and lived at her retirement village. Bea was 82 when she died from a heart attack. Her 83-year old husband Leon was heartbroken. Following the funeral Leon told Donya, the activity director, "I just don't think I can live without her."

Donya walked from behind her desk to hug him and express that there were many people to help him. But he died, right then, in her arms.

How often have we heard things like, "I can't live without him"? What does it mean to be unable to go on living without someone? These deep, bonded relationships are very real and can be a matter of life or death. So when we have the privilege of hearing someone's story, how can we be present in a way that allows us to appreciate the life-and-death potential of what we are hearing?

Standards of Holistic Nursing Practice

The standards involve a very exciting, evolving process with many levels of development over the last 5 years. We, the American Holistic Nurses Association (AHNA), recognized that it was important to more clearly define and refine the practice of holistic nursing, so an AHNA Core Task Force reviewed 10 years of literature on holistic nursing and related fields. From that review we created the IPAKHN Questionnaire (IPAKHN stands for Inventory of Professional Activities and Knowledge of a Holistic Nurse). Next, the AHNA conducted a national survey of its members by having them complete the IPAKHN Questionnaire. From the data analysis we were then able to establish the 24 most frequently used interventions in holistic nursing practice. We were also able to establish the content for the AHNA Core Curriculum as well as a blueprint to write the first national certification examination, which will be given this fall. And it was from this process that we were able to identify nine core values that recently have been refined and revised to five. (*NOTE: In 2002, the AHNA advanced standards were also adopted; see Box 12-1.*)

BOX **12-1**

American Holistic Nurses' Association Summary of Core Values

Core Value 1: Holistic Philosophy and Education

Holistic Philosophy: Holistic nurses develop and expand their conceptual framework and overall philosophy about the art and science of holistic nursing to model, practice, teach, and conduct research in the most effective manner possible.

Holistic Education: Holistic nurses acquire and maintain current knowledge and competency in holistic nursing practice.

Core Value 2: Holistic Ethics, Theories, and Research

Holistic Ethics: Holistic nurses hold to a professional ethic of caring and healing that seeks to preserve wholeness and dignity of self, students, colleagues, and the person who is receiving care in all practice settings, be it in health promotion, birthing centers, acute or chronic healthcare facilities, end-of-life care centers, or in homes.

Holistic Nursing Theories: Holistic nurses recognize that holistic nursing theories provide the framework for all aspects of holistic nursing practice and transformational leadership.

Holistic Nursing and Related Research: Holistic nurses provide care and guidance to persons through nursing interventions and holistic therapies consistent with research findings and other sound evidence.

Core Value 3: Holistic Nurse Self-Care

Holistic Nurse Self-Care: Holistic nurses engage in self-care and further develop their personal awareness as being an instrument of healing to better serve self and others.

Core Value 4: Holistic Communication, Therapeutic Environment, and Cultural Diversity

Holistic Communication: Holistic nurses engage in holistic communication to ensure that each person experiences the presence of the nurse as authentic and sincere. There is an atmosphere of shared humanness that includes a sense of connectedness and attention reflecting the individual's uniqueness.

Therapeutic Environment: Holistic nurses recognize that each person's environment includes everything that surrounds the individual, both the external and the internal (physical, mental, psychological, sociological, and spiritual) as well as patterns not yet understood.

Cultural Diversity: Holistic nurses recognize each person as a whole body-mind-spirit being and mutually create a plan of care consistent with cultural background, health beliefs, sexual orientation, values, and preferences.

Core Value 5: Holistic Caring Process

Assessment: Each person is assessed holistically using appropriate traditional and holistic methods while the uniqueness of the person is honored.

Patterns/Problems/Needs: Actual and potential patterns/problems/needs and life processes related to health, wellness, disease, or illness that may or may not facilitate well-being are identified and prioritized.

BOX   **12-1—cont'd**

Outcomes: Actual and potential patterns/problems/needs and life processes related to health, wellness, disease, or illness that may or may not facilitate well-being have appropriate outcomes specified.

Therapeutic Care Plan: A mutually created plan of care focuses on health promotion, recovery or restoration, or peaceful dying so that the person is as independent as possible.

Implementation: The mutually created plan of holistic care is prioritized and holistic nursing interventions are implemented accordingly.

Evaluation: Responses to holistic care are regularly and systematically evaluated, and the continuing holistic nature of the healing process is recognized and honored.

Courtesy of the American Holistic Nurses' Association *Standards of Holistic Nursing Practice.* © 2000, American Holistic Nurses' Association.

Self-Care

Self-care includes those activities that allow nurses to develop different levels of personal awareness so they can truly be an instrument of healing. Nurses can easily give to everybody else and feel drained at the end of the day. Our body has a built-in pattern called the ultradian rhythm, so that every 90 to 120 minutes it registers certain physiologic needs. For example, a nurse begins a shift at 7 AM. At about 8:30 or 9 AM, her or his body gives a signal to take a short break, to sit down, to eat something nutritious, or to empty a full bladder. But what happens? The nurse doesn't take a break and before long it is 11 AM with another ultradian pattern emerging. The nurse's body now registers hunger, thirst, and a fuller bladder, but work often is continued. Before long it's 1:30 PM and no break yet. And then the nurse wonders why she or he is chronically tired. Those nurses who engage in basic self-care activities such as good nutrition, exercise, and stress management are more productive and have more joy in life.

However, I think that the deeper level of self-care involves caring for one's mental, emotional, and spiritual well-being; spending quality time with self, family, and friends; and engaging in activities and work that have purpose and meaning. It also involves setting aside time each day for prayer, meditation, and quiet in order to be present with our self for our own reflection and healing. This takes discipline, but basically it's a matter of priorities. When we care for our self, listen to our own stories, and weave those pieces of our life together, we become more connected, focused, centered, and balanced. So when a nurse is coming from that space, the connection she or he has with others is more authentic. This is the art of nursing—being able to listen to others and recognize the threads and patterns that make up our patient's life, as well as those of our own life. This may sound ordinary, but it's actually profound.

Healing Rituals

For me, healing is a process, our lifelong journey. It's the weaving together of the threads of our life. When daily stress, illness, or a crisis occurs, there is an interruption, literally, in the fabric of our lives, and we have to weave those broken threads back together in a way that makes sense to us. When those patterns of fear, anxiety, and frustration come forth, we have to ask ourselves: What does this mean to me?

Healing requires engaging in self-care activities that have meaning for us. Healing involves opening what we have closed down, remembering what is or was once sacred to us, and honoring our connections with our self, others, and the Transcendent. For me, healing involves incorporating my personal rituals into my life each day.

There are three simple yet very profound steps in a ritual of healing. The first one is to separate—to disengage from daily activities and enter into a different state of consciousness so you recognize a part of yourself that is in need of healing.

The second step is the transition period. This can take a few moments or much longer, 10 or 20 minutes, to get into a quiet space within yourself—a completely different level from our busy, ordinary mind. This involves connecting with your inner self and an inner truth about your healing. In connecting in this way, we can remember how we have gotten through crisis before, and we can envision what heals us.

The third step is the return. After spending quality time with our self or with another, we can return to the day's activities and feel an inner peace that is special. This allows us to have more joy and meaning in our daily activities.

To me, generating self-healing rituals is the most effective way to manage our very busy lives. No one else can heal us, and each of us has to find our own way to create healing rituals to bring about that balance and connectedness. Healing rituals are different for each of us, and there are no formulas or rigid rules for generating them.

If we cultivate rituals of healing each day, then when we get pulled off center at work, at meetings, or at any other time, we have a way to get back to that place of healing. Rituals help us to show up, to pay attention, and to tell the truth, whether it makes sense to anybody else or not. They also help us to keep our ego out of the way, to not be so attached to outcomes and personal expectations. Healing rituals help us go to a deeper level of being. When we do so, we are clearer about what is important and what is not, and we learn to connect with our deepest core.

Consider the stories we tell ourselves about those times that we've felt uncomfortable or wounded in our lives. If only we'd done this or that, things might have been different. If we engage in this endless self-guessing, we can lose our center, our sense of self. If we can just go back to telling the truth, without judging our performance, we can keep touch with our sense of inner worth and who we really are.

Sometimes during these moments we see things about ourselves that aren't pleasant, aspects of ourselves that need change. These are opportunities to explore what mythologist Joseph Campbell and psychologist Carl Jung call our "shadow" side. Engaging in healing rituals can help us do this.

I'll never forget the first time Larry took me backpacking to a high mountain lake 25 years ago. To this day, Warbonnet Lake in the Sawtooth Mountains of Idaho is the place I go in my mind when I do my meditation practice or as I sit using relaxed breathing and imagery for several minutes to get to a place of healing. I step into the sounds, sensations, and feelings, and imagine sitting by this pristine lake, going below the surface of the water, going very deep down. Using the water metaphor, to have a deep sense of connectedness requires going below the surface of our busy, day-to-day activities and the superficial awareness we bring to them, and going deeper and deeper down. Each time I enter this image, I see if I can go deeper and see another level of images, patterns, and processes in my life.

For me it is from the deep level of the human spirit, the soul level, that there emerges that relatedness, that connectedness with our self to do the work we are called to do. The words seem so trite, but there is a profound feeling and inner experience that occurs. And the goal is to live life from that space.

It's like my Florence Nightingale project. I felt so connected and compelled to write about her that I had to ask myself: Why do I feel such a strong connection to undertake such a project? What could I possibly add about this remarkable woman, when hundreds of people have already written about her? So I just waited to see if I should proceed. Then one day, sitting by my lake in my mind, I was struck by the possibility of exploring Nightingale's life as a 19th-century mystic—to examine her profound sense of connectedness with God. Her God was not a white male who spoke only English but a Universal Truth permeating all the great religions—the God/Life Force/Absolute/Transcendent. Spirituality was the unifying force in her life. It infused everything she thought and did in her long life of 90 years. The more I researched, the more clearly I saw that she indeed appeared to be a genuine 19th-century mystic. Her life journey was similar to that of St. Catherine of Sienna, St. Catherine of Genoa, and Teresa of Avila. That's when I began to say, "Maybe this is what I can add."

Florence Nightingale

Nightingale was a profound mystic. Evelyn Underhill, one of the foremost scholars on Western mysticism, defined mysticism as an individual's direct, unmediated experience of God. A mystic is a person who has such an experience, to a greater or lesser degree. The life of a mystic is not focused merely on religious practice or belief but on what he or she regards as firsthand personal knowledge of the love of God or the experience of the Divine Reality of God. Nightingale received her first call from God at age 16, and she recorded three additional calls throughout her life.

Underhill's framework for the study of mystic spiritual development is well recognized. The first is "awakening," in which one hears the voice of God. This is so profound and true that it becomes embedded in that person's life story, forever changing his or her life dramatically. The second stage is "purgation." This is the period in which the person realizes that he or she is not good enough. How could they possibly be called to do this profound work of service? So they try to purge themselves of worldly connections, often through fasting and extreme acts such as giving away their material possessions. The third phase, "illumination," is when the person is utterly filled with passion for and a sense of God. The fourth phase, "surrender," typically goes on for a long time. It is a very profound period in which the person explores his or her inner, divine connection. This period of spiritual development often includes much suffering—as the person strives for perfection, she or he can never be good enough. Finally, the fifth phase is "Union," during which the mystic realizes that he or she has reached a level of deep inner connectedness with the Divine Reality.

Mystics seldom follow these phases in a rigid, linear sequence. They can experience the first phase, awakening, and then the fifth phase, union, but then they may fall back into purgation. Often purgation and illumination run parallel, and surrender and union go back and forth.

I found these patterns in Nightingale's life. In fact, her life represents that of a fully developed mystic. At an early age Nightingale had a serious religious and spiritual nature, and she always had the desire to nurse the sick. On February 7, 1837, when she was 16, she recorded her first call from God. As I mentioned, she also recorded three other occasions later in life when she heard the voice of God. Her purgation period lasted for 17 years before she was finally able to break free and pursue her interest in nursing. This long period should also be viewed in the context of Victorian life. Nightingale was from a very wealthy family, and nurses at that time were mostly from the uneducated and lower classes. Her family wanted her to marry into wealth and high society, but she refused, making a conscious choice to serve God through social action.

Nightingale believed that nursing was a very high calling—that nurses could be in service to others and to God without taking religious vows. She advocated that nurses not only receive proper instruction and education—including instruction in how to live a moral life—but also that they be open to treating people of all religions. She saw nursing as a complement to medicine—for her, nursing and medicine were two distinct entities. Because she focused on the science and the art of nursing outside religious vows, Nightingale is considered the founder of modern secular nursing.

When Nightingale was 34, she received an official invitation from her dear friend and Secretary at War, Mr. Sidney Herbert, to become Superintendent of Nurses of the Turkish Hospitals during the Crimean War (1854-1856)—an invitation that was later extended to the Crimea as well. At this time she had only received 3 months' basic instruction at the Kaiserswerth Institute in Dusseldorf, Germany, and had 1 year of experience as a superintendent in a small, 27-bed hospital in London called the Institute for Sick and Gentlewomen in Distressed Circumstances. Part of her success and fame while in Scutari, Turkey was due to her self-education in sanitation and the new science of statistics during her twenties and early thirties. In fact, by age 30 she was recognized as one of the most knowledgeable people in Europe on hospital construction.

Nightingale was blessed with monumental intelligence. She spoke five languages and knew advanced mathematics. Moreover, she was an organizational genius. She went to Turkey in service to God, which was the source of the legendary "Nightingale Power." She recognized that most of the major problems at the sprawling Scutari hospital, as well as at other facilities in the war zone, were not due to war wounds; rather, they were the result of poor sanitation, lack of proper diet, and the close contact of soldiers suffering from different kinds of fevers, cholera, typhus, and typhoid. Because of her knowledge and her keen, analytic mind, she identified these problems and wrote detailed letters to Sidney Herbert that included her observations and the best solutions to correct these problems. In early 1855 two different Sanitary Commissions were sent to the site of battle at the southern tip of Russia, the Crimea, and to Scutari. These two commissions had been given the power to implement the needed changes that Nightingale had suggested. The commissioners worked closely with Nightingale and, within 6 months, the death rate at the large Barrack Hospital in Scutari fell from 42% to 2.2%.

As a scholar and a seeker of Truth, she spoke and wrote about God, the Universal God, the One. For example, she wrote, "What do we mean by 'God'? All we can say is that we recognize a power superior to our own, that we recognize this power as exercised by a wise and good will."[1] She believed in the messages contained within Christianity and saw Jesus Christ as a great man who revealed the fundamental truths of God. She seriously studied and contemplated the words and parables in her Bible, heavily annotating her own King James version, which had a blank page between almost every printed page. She wrote her own ideas, meanings, and her interpretation in English, French, Latin, Greek, and Italian, which have been translated and analyzed.

She was extraordinarily tolerant and ecumenical in her attitude toward world religions. She wrote that "to know God we must study Him in the Pagan and Jewish dispensations as in the Christian." To her, this broad approach gave unity to the whole; it was the one continuous thread throughout humanity. She called for religious tolerance and she also asked others to be

---

[1]Calabria M, Macrae J: *Suggestions for thought by Florence Nightingale: selections and commentaries*, Philadelphia, 1994, University of Pennsylvania Press.

respectful of cultural diversity. This can be seen in her work with India for more than 40 years and her papers on the aboriginal races. She read world religions widely and was familiar with translations of early writings such as the Upanishads of Hinduism, works by Plato, works on gnosticism, and the writings of Jesus, to name just a few. She wrote her own liberation theology in three volumes of 829 pages, which she had privately printed.

She believed that nature heals and that it is the nurse's responsibility to put the patient in the healing hands of nature. She said that the first thing that should be done is to place the person in the best state for nature to work on him or her, because nature is a reparative process. Her writings are very relevant today. Her *Notes on Nursing*, published in 1860, are also profound because she wrote from personal experience as a person living with a chronic illness. She also integrated what today we refer to as complementary therapies such as pet therapy, light therapy, music therapy, aromatherapy, and much more.

Nightingale wrote about how a small bird in a cage is sometimes the only outlet for an invalid confined to bed. She commented that the effect of music upon the sick had been scarcely noticed, and that wind instruments, including the human voice, and stringed instruments capable of continuous sound, have a beneficent effect—while the pianoforte and other instruments that have no continuity of sound have just the reverse effect. She wrote about the effect of fresh flowers, good food, a healing environment, and the negative effect of noise and trivial conversation on a patient's healing. And we are only just beginning to integrate these areas into mainstream healthcare.

My hope is that people who read my book on Nightingale will reflect on their own healing journey and identify their "must," which is what Nightingale called her work. I hope they will explore what it means to be called to a work of service for the greater good of family and community.

Part Four

Conversations About Spirituality, Love, and Healing

"Not only can we witness Mystery; in some profound way we are Mystery."

—RACHEL NAOMI REMEN

CHAPTER 13

Rachel Naomi Remen, MD

Kitchen Table Wisdom: A Conversation That Heals

Rachel Naomi Remen, MD, is co-founder and medical director of the Commonweal Cancer Help Program, and founder and director of the Institute for the Study of Health and Illness (ISHI) at Commonweal in Bolinas, California. In addition, she is a psychooncologist and a clinical professor of family and community medicine at the University of California – San Francisco, School of Medicine. Dr. Remen received her medical degree from Cornell University School of Medicine in 1962.

A medical educator whose award-winning course in medicine and spirituality is now offered at medical schools nationwide, Dr. Remen's innovative work with people who have cancer was featured in the Bill Moyers PBS special *Healing and the Mind*. She is the author of *Kitchen Table Wisdom: Stories That Heal* (Riverhead Books, 1996) and *My Grandfather's Blessings: Stories of Strength, Refuge, and Belonging* (Riverhead, 2000).

Dr. Remen's unique perspective is shaped by the fact that she is both physician and patient. She is a 50-year survivor of Crohn's disease and has undergone several major surgeries. In 1997, I interviewed Dr. Remen in Los Angeles while she was on a book tour, and during the course of our conversation, I was struck by her compassion, her deep understandings, and her love of life. This wounded healer is, without a doubt, one of the most remarkable women of our times.

As a physician, I was trained to believe that the unknown is an emergency, like a hemorrhage. It requires action. You need to convert the unknown to the known as quickly and efficiently and cost effectively as possible. But I've learned that the unknown does not require *action*—it requires our *attention*. Often it is the unknown, the Mystery in life, that sustains and strengthens us. My colleague, Marion Weber, who is an artist, has taught me to relate to the unknown as an artist does, with patience. For her, the unknown is a blank canvas. It's a place of revelation.

Not only can we witness Mystery; in some profound way we are Mystery. Our lives may not be bounded by our history and may go on longer than we dare dream. If life itself is not fully defined by science, perhaps we too may be more than science would have us believe.

Here is a strategy. When Ahiro came to see me, he was in the final stages of prostate cancer. He had come to prepare himself to die. He was Japanese, a beautiful man who had lived with integrity and a certain elegance. His life had been his family and his work. From the beginning, he had a clear agenda for our meetings and took charge of them. He told me that he wanted to invite those who had blessed his life to come to our sessions, one at a time, in order to thank them for all they had given him.

And so we began. About halfway through this agenda, as were discussing the meeting we had just had with one of his sons, Ahiro suddenly paused in midsentence and looked at me.

"Rachel," he said, "I am an educated man. I must believe that death is the end. And you, as an educated woman, surely you believe that death is the end also. Don't you?" Caught unaware, I looked back at him. He was leaning toward me, smiling, but his eyes were serious. For the first time, I wondered if our meetings had a deeper agenda than I realized.

"I used to think that death is the end," I answered slowly, "but now I simply do not know. Death seems to me to be the ultimate mystery that gives life its meaning and even its value. I do not know if death is the end." He sat back in surprise. "Why, surely you do not believe in heaven with little angels flying about?" He looked at me and raised an elegant eyebrow. "Do you?"

"I don't know," I told him. There was a pause. Something shifted in his eyes, and I had the distinct sense that we had engaged each other on some level I could barely appreciate. Then he smiled at me and let the matter drop.

We continued to meet week by week with those on his list. But now in every one of our sessions, he would raise the topic, often when I least expected it. Each time, after listening to his carefully reasoned arguments in support of the finality of death, I would tell him, "I still don't know."

During our next to last meeting, he again raised this question. Hearing my "I don't know" once again, he began to laugh. "Rachel," he said. "I am an educated man. I must believe that death is the end. But just in case it isn't, I will come back as a great white crane and give you some sort of sign that I have lost the argument."

Only a few months later, this remarkable man died. Shortly afterward I was in the TransAmerica building, a large pyramid-shaped structure in the downtown business district of San Francisco, waiting for an elevator to take me to an appointment. The building is tall, and so the elevators are quite slow. This gives everyone a few minutes to themselves. In this brief time, I found myself thinking of Ahiro and how much I missed being able to talk with him, and what a delightful man he had been.

At last one of the elevators arrived. It was empty. And so with my heart and mind filled with memories of this relationship, I stepped in. The doors closed and the elevator started upward so abruptly that I was thrown slightly off balance. I glanced down hurriedly to regain my footing and there, lying on the floor of the elevator, was a single, large, perfect white feather.

The important thing is that Mystery does happen and offers us the opportunity to wonder together and reclaim a sense of awe and aliveness. The feathers that fall into our lives offer neither proof nor certainty. They are just reminders to stay awake and listen, because the mystery at the heart of life may speak to you at any time.[1]

We may need to know less and wonder more. If we can wonder together again, we may be able to recover a sense of awe about life and about death, which is part of life. I think if we can recover our sense of awe, we will go a long way toward healing the wounds in our culture.

Perhaps some things are meant to be carried with us, unexplained. This is a story from my book *Kitchen Table Wisdom*. It's called "The Question" and was told by a physician who attended one of the continuing medical education (CME) training workshops we have at Commonweal.

For the last ten years of his life, Tim's father had Alzheimer's disease. Despite the devoted care of Tim's mother, he had slowly deteriorated until he had become a sort of a walking vegetable. He was unable to speak, and was fed, clothed and cared for as if he were a very young child. As Tim and his brother grew older, they would stay with their father for brief periods of time while their mother took care of the needs of the household or went out with friends.

---

[1]Remen R: *My grandfather's blessings: stories of strength, refuge and belonging*, New York, 2000, Riverhead Books.

One Sunday, while she was out doing the shopping, the boys, then 15 and 17, watched football as their father sat nearby on a chair. Suddenly, he slumped forward and fell to the floor. Both sons realized immediately that something was terribly wrong. His color was gray and his breath uneven and raspy. Frightened, Tim's older brother told him to call 911. But before he could respond, a voice Tim had not heard in 10 years, a voice he could barely remember, stopped him: "Don't call 911, son. Tell your mother that I love her. Tell her that I am all right." And Tim's father died.

Tim, a cardiologist, looked around the room at the group of doctors mesmerized by this story. "Because he died unexpectedly in the home, the law required we have an autopsy," he told us quietly. "My father's brain was almost entirely destroyed by this disease. For many years I've asked myself, 'Who spoke?' I have never found even the slightest help from any medical textbook. I am no closer to knowing this now than I was then, but carrying the question with me reminds me of something important, something I do not want to forget. Much that is important in life can never be explained but only witnessed."[2]

In part, our CME training program at the Institute for the Study of Health and Illness at Commonweal, enables physicians to wonder more and to recover a sense of service and the personal meaning their work has for them. Medicine is in deepening crisis. In times of crisis, people instinctively reach for meaning. So we begin by remembering why we have chosen this work in the first place.

Service is not a technique; it is a way of life, a state of the heart. Service can't be taught but it can be remembered. One of the most powerful ways to remind physicians of service is to invite a group of doctors who have come to trust one another to talk about mystery: those things that we've all seen in our professional lives that simply don't make sense.

Someone tells one story, and then it's like a dam breaking. Everyone has one or more stories of things that cannot be explained, things they may not have shared with other doctors before. As they tell these stories, a sense of awe grows in a very natural way. Awe evokes the wish to serve. We serve life not because it is broken, but because it is holy. The meaning of medicine is service, not science. Science is just our most recent set of service tools.

Relationship-Centered Work with Cancer Patients

Years ago in 1980, I was doing research for the National Institute of Mental Health as the associate director of a program called the Collaborative Health Program, researching and designing curricula for collaboration between nurses, doctors, and patients. We studied their interactions and identified variables that prevented collaborative interaction—what perceptions, behaviors, and attitudes?—and built a curriculum for the five major hospitals in San Francisco. But then we couldn't get funding to implement the curriculum because of a change in administration. So we wrote grants for about 6 months. As I was writing grants and struggling to find a way to pay the rent, people would call me and say, "Do you counsel patients?"

And I would always say, "No."

Of course, I eventually ran out of money so when I got the next one of those phone calls, I said, "Matter of fact, I do counsel patients." I had not planned to work with people who had cancer. The area that I knew something about in depth was chronic illness, because I had lived with my own chronic illness for about 25 years by then, and I thought I might be able to help people facing that same kind of a challenge recover a sense of personal integrity despite it.

[2]Remen R: *Kitchen table wisdom: stories that heal*, New York, 1996, Riverhead Books.

By then I had been trained for years in psychosynthesis, which is one of the transpersonal psychotherapies, and in imagery, but I had never used this training in practice. So I took an office—it happened to be on a houseboat in San Francisco Bay—and opened the doors, and all these people with cancer rushed in.

I suppose I had inadvertently stumbled on an unmet need. I got many referrals from well-trained psychiatrists and psychologists who felt unprepared to deal with people who had life-threatening illness, with all their physical changes and the threat of death. I also got referrals from oncologists who did not feel prepared to deal with the emotional and spiritual issues cancer raised for their patients. At that time no one was doing this sort of work. So within about 6 months I had not only a full practice but an overflowing practice and had begun to train others.

I met Dr. Michael Lerner, the president of Commonweal, when he and Ken Pelletier invited me to consult with them. We met for the first time in a Chinese restaurant in San Francisco. It was an incredible meeting. He told me that he had a lease on some national park lands, and had thought about creating a retreat center for people with cancer out there at the edge of the Pacific Ocean. But he was not that comfortable working with people with cancer. Of course I was. So we talked about this for a few weeks and eventually he said, "Perhaps we could work together. When would you like to start?"

And I said, "How about next week?"

It's been quite an experience. Commonweal has now run 107 or 108 week-long retreats for people with cancer. The Institute for the Study of Health and Illness (ISHI) also runs the Tradecraft training, which is a 4-day retreat that allows us to share what we have learned in all this time with others who also want to do this retreat work. These people do their work in their own way, but we share all of our experience and expertise (and all of our mistakes) so people can do their own work perhaps a little easier or better.

My work is focused more on the person than on the cancer, enabling the person through the experience of having cancer to uncover a greater integrity and sense of direction than they had before the diagnosis. Sometimes healing of the physical body may occur in the setting of the healing of the whole person in ways that I find quite mysterious.

At 15, I, myself, was told "the facts" about my disease by my physicians and that I would be dead by the age of 40. So I should have died almost 25 years ago. There is a great deal of mystery in life. We each have our own story. Whenever there is a discrepancy between the facts and the story, you are in the presence of a mystery.

A diagnosis is a true confrontation with the unknown. This is often very difficult for people, and yet therein lies the great opportunity. It might be good to actually say to people, "Your diagnosis is cancer. What that will mean remains to be seen." But that would require that we, physicians, or family or friends have a much greater comfort with the unknown than we actually do. As a culture, we have such little tolerance for the unknown that we tend to fill it up with stories that may not be true stories, like, "You have 6 months to live" or "You will be dead by the time your are 40."

What I do with the people who come to see me in my practice is to accompany them in their meeting with the unknown and to help them open up to it rather than close down. I've frequently found that people are carrying some belief about their cancer locked in their hearts and unconscious minds that they've read or that someone has told them—a belief like "No one ever survives pancreatic cancer" or "People with ovarian cancer die in 18 months." Something that is not true.

Often, the first step is to help people let go of those beliefs. You would think it would be easy to release something that painful, but it's often not easy for people to release it and deal with their diagnosis as if it is the unknown, to accept that freedom.

I think we health professionals need to be much more cautious about what we say to people in the setting of illness. I was taught that when people have a diagnosis like cancer, they're so emotionally overwhelmed that they can't hear you, so you may need to tell them something over and over again. That may be true, but that is on the intellectual level. On the level of the unconscious, people take in everything, even their doctor's tone of voice and facial expressions. And they hold this frozen in the unconscious. It's difficult to free people of such beliefs.

So I help people explore the beliefs they may be carrying in their unconscious minds, the beliefs that have been placed there by either their reading, or by media, or by the words of someone else in the family, or a physician, or the person's experience with other people with cancer. I also help people explore any of the constraints they may have placed on their life and their survival. Beliefs they have about their worthiness to live, any guilt they have, any sense they have of not feeling entitled to take up space in this world or to be the sort of person they genuinely are. So many of us have made a contract with life that is conditional. We also examine their sense of nurture and self-nurture: are they worthy of attention? Are they worthy of care? We work together to free the will to live in them from beliefs that constrict it. I think the life, the vitality, in a lot of people is constricted, but usually it doesn't matter; you have vitality to spare when you are a healthy person. When you have a diagnosis like cancer, it requires that you pay attention to beliefs that you may have been able to live with for a long time. Now they matter. You may need to free yourself of them in order to fight for your life.

There are many tools for exploring these deeply held beliefs. Sometimes it's just about talking. Sometimes it's imagery. Sometimes it's sand tray. Sometimes it is a very careful examination of the person's behaviors and choices, so that they can see patterns that, alone, they might not be able to see.

We also explore meaning. Why is life worth it to them? What matters? And all the time we're doing this, of course, we're also dealing with the nitty-gritty, nuts-and-bolts stuff—the chemo, the surgery, and the radiation; the effects of these things; and the changes in their physical appearance, their sexuality.

Of course, I'm not their oncologist. I work with their oncologists. We often talk about integrating traditional approaches—like acupuncture, herbal therapies, homeopathy, or yoga—with the conventional treatment their oncologists are giving them so that they have the best of both worlds. We also deal with their kids and their job. We deal with the fact that maybe their boyfriend or husband or wife has left. I've accompanied people to surgery. I've gone shopping with people for wigs. I've smuggled their cats into the hospital. I show up for whatever is happening. So we deal with their concerns on many different levels at the same time that we uncover a genuine sense of the value and integrity of their lives. Often, things change.

Healing happens on a level playing field. It is a conversation. It isn't about my expertise or that my analysis of the situation is more important than yours. The level playing field model of interaction opens up enormous possibility and potential. If you and I were to sit down in the setting of cancer, we would put all our stuff—everything we brought with us—on the table between us. It turns out I've been trained as a physician and have 26 years' experience counseling people with cancer and those who care about them, including their doctors. I know how the medical system runs and the mechanisms of disease and treatment. And I had a grandmother from Russia. I've got a cat and do a lot of shopping at second-hand clothing stores. I once made stained glass windows and silver jewelry, and I have remodeled a house. I'm a gardener and a patient with half a century of Chrohn's disease. So I put all that and more out on the table.

You put your stuff out on the table, too. You know a great deal about yourself, your preferences, skills, fears, dreams. You have a deep unconscious sense of your direction and even your purpose in life. You have a 3-year-old son; you ski; you sail. You've survived the losses of your life, and we share these things generously with each other. You put all that out on the table. Then we sit there together, and we examine all this. What's important and what isn't eventually becomes clear: What is the helpful thing? What isn't the helpful thing? What is real and genuine—and what isn't?

My expertise is often not the most important piece on that table. The most important piece in your recovery may be that you know how to trust the unseen and follow the wind as a sailor does, and that will offer you the model for your healing.

I used to sit across from people at my desk with their disease between us. I was on one side of the disease, and they were on the other. Now I sit shoulder-to-shoulder with people. We look together at the situation and the patterns; we discuss what's there, what's happening, what's emerging. It's a subtle but important shift. We sit next to each other on the same side of whatever problem we are dealing with together.

Now, this is a funny story. I got new chairs for my office a number of years ago—one for my clients to sit on and one for myself. The day that they were delivered, a friend who is a psychiatrist came by and invited me to lunch. I said to him, "Come in and see my new chairs. I'm so pleased."

He looked into the office, and there were these two new identical leather chairs. He looks at them and says in this puzzled way, "But which one is *your* chair?"

The level playing field is not the way we physicians are trained to do things. Even the chair we sit in is supposed to be different from the one our patient sits in—it has to assert our difference. But a conversation between two human beings is more powerful than a conversation between an expert and a problem. It opens up a lot more possibility, more resources. Healing is not a function of expertise. At Commonweal, people with cancer heal other people with cancer. It's the wounded healer archetype.

Often, wounded people will offer each other the most profound healings, not from medical textbooks, but from experience. It's about a kind of fearlessness and trust of life. It's about presence and listening and respect and waiting and trust.

Healing is mutual, by the way. The interesting thing about healing relationships is that the work itself sustains you. It inspires you and fills you up. When I was curing, when I was doing all the talking and making all the decisions, I saw other people's problems and needs as something I needed to fix. The more I fixed people, the more I experienced myself as surrounded by weak and needy people. When I started receiving and listening to people, uncovering their way of doing things, their wisdom, looking to see how they made sense—because everybody makes sense—I found that the people around me were strong, often stronger than they had previously realized. But that's one of the problems with being a fixer. It's exhausting. Because if you don't trust life, you have to fix it and the more you fix life the less you trust it. Experts trust only themselves—their own expertise.

Learning to Trust Life

I was a patient long before I was a physician. That has been an invaluable experience for me. Whenever someone talks about illness, nearness to death, healing, I can often tell whether or not they are speaking from experience or from theory. Disease is brutal. It is not this benign teacher of wisdom. The fact that human beings can find authentic meaning in such experience says a great deal about human beings, not about the nature of disease. It's not that disease is the teacher but that human beings have the remarkable capacity to find authentic meaning even in the most brutal and painful of times. It's about the hidden greatness in us all. So my own illness experience has been very helpful to me.

Another factor that influenced my life was that I was lucky enough to be part of a program that Sukie Miller and Stuart Miller put together at Esalen Institute in 1972. It was called the Institute for the Study of Humanistic Medicine. These two visionary people had a small grant—it was only $10,000—and they took a dozen credible Western-trained physicians and brought us to Esalen for a weekend a month for 2 years. Each weekend we met with someone who was on the cutting edge of what was called the *human potential movement*. Our job was to look at their ideas and their work, to experience what they had to demonstrate to us, and to see if it had anything to do with the work of medicine.

This was at least a decade before holistic health was born, and it was an extraordinary experience for me. We met people such as Elmer Green, George Leonard, Joseph Campbell, Michael Murphy, and many others who expanded our way of seeing human nature and human resources.

I had been a philosophy major in college and had bought into the belief of my medical teachers that this was irrelevant to the practice of medicine. But it all came back—the comfort with uncertainty, the importance of having the right question, not the right answer. At the end of the Millers' program, most of the others went on with their medical work, and I quit my faculty position at Stanford and began my life work. It was such a powerful experience for me. Esalen was my first experience in education. Up to that point, I had been trained, not educated.

Educare, which is the root word of "education," means to lead forth the wholeness, the innate, hidden integrity in someone. So education and healing are related. Training, on the other hand, is about shaping one's self to be an expert, a process which encourages you to deny and repress certain parts of your wholeness in the belief that this will make you more useful to others. All those years ago, my training encouraged me to repress intuition, emotion, and even the soul. Anything that couldn't be measured, anything that couldn't be expressed in numbers, was not useful and was even seen as counterproductive.

Fortunately, I am basically a mystic. Do I think there is mystery in life? Certainly. I am aware, for example, that when we do a group sand tray, the collective unconscious will often speak in a way that is profoundly mysterious. The symbolic items that people have selected, often without knowing why, have meaning for everyone else at the table, not just for themselves. Every piece that's put on that table is part of a deep wisdom that is carried collectively in all physicians and has validity for us all. The deepest meaning is often carried in the unconscious mind. This meaning emerges as a sort of revelation as the group talks.

Finding the Meaning in Medicine

For the past 11 years, I have run a postgraduate training program at Commonweal for physicians who wish to recover the deep meaning of their work and practice medicine as a spiritual path. Part of the recovery of meaning is to recognize medicine as rooted in Mystery, as a calling and not a job. One of the many approaches we use to uncover a deeper meaning is to offer the physician study group the opportunity to do a group sand tray on the meaning of their work as doctors. This approach often evokes experiences of Mystery as well.

So during our 4-day continuing medical education retreats we often use a group sand tray technique to help physicians recognize that everything known is not in the conscious mind, and to evoke an experience of wisdom. Sand tray is a Jungian technique, but group sand tray was developed by my colleague, Marion Weber, as a way to demonstrate to people the power and wisdom of the unconscious mind. A group sand tray is a round table about $4\frac{1}{2}$ feet in diameter, filled with sand and separated into pie-shaped sections with sticks so that each person sitting around the rim of the table has a slice of the pie in which to do his or her own work. A group of eight physicians moves through the sand tray object room—a room filled with thousands of little objects that represent everything in our inner and outer worlds—choosing whatever magnetizes their attention. They are asked to take the objects they are attracted to even if they do not understand why the thing is attractive or how it relates to the topic.

Sand tray is a discovery process. Often they will not know why they've taken certain things until they put them into their sand tray and begin to talk about them. Then they each sit at one of the places at the table and put these things in the sand, making a little scene. It's all done in silence. They all put their selected objects into their segment of the table at the same time and in a few minutes the empty table becomes full. Then everyone listens as, one at a time, people talk about what they have put down in the sand. Often, of course, the unconscious mind has resonated with certain objects, made them appear attractive to the conscious mind, because they reveal meaning. Jung calls such objects "numinous." As each person talks aloud, he or she may suddenly understand that meaning, often for the first time. So there's a lot of revelation and a lot of discovery.

It's a very powerful exercise in deep listening to each other and to yourself. At the end, we have them take the stick that's at the right of their tray and remove it from the tray. So all the divisions come up and the sand tray becomes a single whole. It's a very powerful moment—a lot of our individual sense of meaning is part of a larger and more universal meaning, which we can now see for the first time.

We suggest a sand tray topic at the start, such as "healing" or "death" or "the meaning of being a doctor." We then tell the group they can forget the topic because the unconscious mind now has it. When they go into the object room, their unconscious mind will call their attention to things that have to do with their own sense of what healing or meaning is about. We suggest they take those things to put into their tray even though they may not know what they mean.

We did a sand tray once with eight elderly women, ranging in age from 75 to 95, who were part of a club. When they came in, they seemed very old, fragile, and uncertain. Vulnerable, even. The topic we suggested to them was "What's important now?"

So these fragile and frail older women went into the object room, chose their objects, and went upstairs to the group sand tray, very slowly. And they did the most powerful sand tray I have ever witnessed. They talked about sex and death and loss and taboos and the body and being women—about decades of living and what can be learned from life.

One woman had known her great-grandmother, and she had a great-granddaughter, so in her mind, there was the lived experience of seven generations. She said, "I look behind me; I look before me. And I have a sense that there is no beginning and no end." The power they brought to the discussion was truly awesome. And then they got up and, moving slowly and uncertainly, they left.

Marion and I still talk about this sand tray. Their power and wisdom was so dramatically different from the way these women appeared on the surface. The challenge is always to find ways to give human strength a voice, isn't it? When we don't see someone's inner depth or wisdom, it's because we have not found the right tools to give it a voice. People are usually stunned by what emerges in their tray and in the trays of the others. Everyone leaves the table with a deeper respect for what it means to be a human being and a wish to know others at greater depth.

In one of our workshops, we had just finished a discussion with eight physicians about managed care and the enormous invasion of the physician's integrity that it can represent. In the daily practice of managed care, someone who may not have gone to medical school may tell you how to practice medicine or what is being allowed is not the best that you could do for the patient but has a basic profit motive. Physicians may be forced to function at levels far below their own personal excellence. This is morally eroding, and some of the physicians were considering finding other work.

Soon after this discussion, we did a group sand tray on the meaning that the work of being a physician has for each of us. One physician had felt that she needed to leave medicine. She had run a statewide program for the care of premature infants, but the frustrations of managed care, with its bureaucracy and paperwork, had caused her to feel she couldn't go on. And she had said a couple of times, "I can't change the system; I have to leave and do something else."

Per the instructions, she selected items from the sand tray room, following her intuition and taking what attracted her attention, often without knowing why. Several of the items she chose did not make sense to her—she commented how difficult it was for her to risk taking items that appealed to her for unknown reasons. Witnessed by the other seven doctors in the group, she laid her chosen objects in the sand and began to talk about them. As she spoke, the meaning of each object became clear to her, all except the object in the center of her sand tray, which happened to be a tiny dried starfish.

She told us that in the object room, she had wanted to leave it behind but kept coming back to it again and again. Finally, she realized that taking it was a "matter of personal integrity" and so she had brought it with her. Somehow it seemed right to put it in the very center of the tray, but she still didn't know what it meant.

I suggested that she pick it up for a moment and hold it in her hand. She picked it up so tenderly that it was obvious that it was filled with meaning for her. Suddenly, she began to cry. She had remembered a story about an old man walking down the beach. The tide is low, and there are starfish all over the beach drying in the sun. When he comes to a starfish, he picks it up and throws it back into the water. He keeps walking, doing this over and over again. As he is doing this, a young man who passes him and says, "Old fellow, what are you doing?"

He explains that he's picking up the starfish and throwing them back in the water.

The young man starts to laugh. "How foolish," he says. "Don't you know there are thousands and thousands of starfish on this beach, and there are thousands and thousands of beaches in this world? What makes you think you can make a difference?"

But the old man keeps walking. Coming to the next starfish, he picks it up and holds it thoughtfully in his hand for a long while. Then he throws it back into the ocean. "Made a difference to that one," he says and smiles to himself.

But the woman said she'd forgotten that everything she did—the phone calls, the paperwork, the forms—"made a difference to that one." Everything. The doctors witnessing this were as deeply moved as she.

Isn't that interesting? If I had just asked her to tell me the meaning of her work or what strengths she needed to find to continue in medicine, I'm not sure she could have answered me. But her unconscious mind showed it to her and to every other physician in that room with great elegance and power. It wasn't just her starfish. It belonged to us all.

Meaning is carried in the unconscious mind. The deepest levels of meaning are not the meaning we deliberately seek or make up or construct intellectually. She almost left it behind, she said, because she didn't know what it meant. And then she decided to trust the unknown. The meaning of that starfish is there for every doctor alive—and every doctor who has lived medicine as a work of service not a work of science.

Many medical students are on fire with the spirit of service. It's true at every medical school in the country. Over the years of training, we eradicate it because the training requires people to go into survival mode. I think we're going to have to have a look at that. There is no reason for us to put those who want to be healers into survival mode for 10 years. It does not make any sense. There are other ways to create physicians. Thankfully, this is being rethought now all over the country. This is a very exciting time in medicine, as are most times of crisis.

The medical system is just the child of the culture. If you want to understand the strengths and limitations of a culture, look at its medical system. All of a culture's strengths, dreams, illusions, limitations, and wounds will be clearly reflected in its medical system.

We're a culture that demands instant gratification—a "just add water" culture. Yet we're offended when we turn to our doctors with our suffering and they add water and two pills. We want something different, something that responds to our suffering as the unique and personal thing it is. Medical training devalues what the culture devalues—the "soft" things, the intuition, the heart, the soul. But those "soft" things often turn out to be our strength and the source of our healing.

America is a frontier society. Self-reliance, independence, competence, self-sufficiency—on the frontier these sorts of qualities were highly valued because the nearest neighbor was 100 miles away, over very rough terrain. Now, living right alongside each other, we still admire these values. Yet living by them may not the best way to live a fulfilling and satisfying life. The shadow side of independence is alienation, isolation, and loneliness. Doctors are supposed to be so self-sufficient that they don't even need to eat or sleep or cry. But we have needs. They are part of our human nature. We have the need to communicate, the need to touch, the need to be seen by others, to be heard, the need to know our life matters to others. We have the need to wonder.

A medical culture is often a clear mirror for the larger culture it serves. Often the wounds of the larger culture can be most clearly seen in the limitations of its medicine. The present crisis of meaning experienced by American doctors may parallel a crisis of meaning in our culture. The need to recover Awe and Mystery in our medicine may simply point to a culture-wide need to recover Awe and Mystery in our lives. We may all need to know a little less and wonder a little more.

CHAPTER 14

STEPHEN WRIGHT, MBE, FRCN

Creating Sacred Space

Stephen G. Wright, who earned his master's degree in nursing at Manchester University in 1981, has published widely on nursing issues. In addition to being the editor of the journal *Sacred Space: An International Journal of Spirituality and Health,* his most recent books include *Therapeutic Touch* and *Sacred Space* (both with Jean Sayre-Adams). Wright was awarded a Fellowship of the Royal College of Nursing in 1991 and an MBE (a distinguished award from the Queen) in 1992 for his services to nursing.

With Sayre-Adams, Wright created the Sacred Space Foundation, a charity dedicated to the care of nurses and the teaching of the healing arts. Wright is associate professor in the Faculty of Health at St. Martin's College in Lancaster, England, with special interest in spirituality and health matters.

I had the pleasure of meeting and interviewing Stephen Wright in the spring of 1998 in San Diego, California, while he was visiting the United States on a speaking tour.

My story is this. A while back, I was somewhat of a "rising star" in nursing in Great Britain. My career was falling into place the way I thought I wanted. Of course, there was no doubt of my own unbridled ambition. I loved going to conferences and having people applaud me and tell me I was wonderful. I loved being on television and talking to government officials and so on. But one day when I was speaking at a conference in Ireland, I passed out as I came off the stage.

Of course, being a nurse, I knew it had to be something serious. I couldn't possibly have anything simple. So I went to my doctor for a full examination, but he said, "There's nothing wrong with you that 6 months on the Cote d'Azur wouldn't cure."

I said, "What do you mean? I'm not stressed. I'm fine. You've missed something."

He said, "No, you're simply going to kill yourself if you carry on like that."

About this same time, my father died. I'd had a difficult relationship with him since childhood, so when he died, I did my duty, supported the family, went to the funeral, and so on, but there wasn't a tear that fell. I was glad he was gone. Now, we had a "Caring for the Carers" program at our hospital to help the nurses deal with stress, and when I went back to work the day after the funeral, a colleague of mine said, "Who's looking after you? You're doing all this stuff for everybody else, but who's taking care of you?"

So I started seeing the psychotherapist in our program and that began a shift. About a year later, I met Jean Sayre-Adams, a nurse from San Francisco, who almost single-handedly introduced Therapeutic Touch (TT) and restored notions of healing into nursing in the United Kingdom. I took one of her classes and was so taken that I began working with her. Then my therapist introduced me to meditation. And Jean introduced me to Ram Dass, Stan Grof, Jack Kornfield, Michael Harner, Jeanne Achterberg, and so on.

So a number of experiences piled on top of each other and became ever more complex and powerful. Then, for whatever reason, I began to have one powerful mystical experience after another. I finally reached a point where a new path, both in nursing and in healthcare, began to unfold for me.

Sacred Space Foundation

Jeannie and I originally set up a charity called the Didsbury Trust. Its prime purpose was to provide a legitimate base for Jeannie to teach Therapeutic Touch and other complementary-therapy healing techniques. We had this sense that patients were often getting better in spite of—rather than because of—what was going on around them. There was also an overwhelming tendency by those in healthcare to think that everything could be solved with a drug or a treatment and that the relationship between healer and patient was relatively insignificant, if considered at all. Jeannie and I felt uncomfortable with this. So Therapeutic Touch (TT) became the medium that we used to help nurses and other healthcare professionals reexamine their caring, healing role.

A second phase, which paralleled my own spiritual path, was a sense that other work needed to be done. We became increasingly aware that when healthcare workers came to us, ostensibly to learn TT, they were saying things like, "It doesn't work for me anymore. I'm stressed and exhausted. I don't know where I'm going. I've lost faith in my work." So more and more of the people we were working with were in a spiritual crisis. Even nurses in relatively good work situations were uncomfortable. That's when we began to recognize the need to care for the carers. And that culminated in three areas of work we call the Sacred Space Project.

First of all, if people are in crisis you provide a safe place for them to be looked after and receive help. Secondly, when these people return to the wider world, they have to go into it in a different way, and they must be better able to take care of themselves. Part of that means remaining centered, where "going back" becomes an irrelevant concept that can no longer harm you because you are always "right here, right now." Third, the greatest task is to shift the organizational culture, the managerial style, and other factors in the workplace, so that none of this is created in the first place.

We have organized a series of international, multiprofessional conferences each year called "Spirituality and Health." The first was at Durham Castle and Cathedral—an ancient sacred site. It was so successful and the feedback was so significant that it was clear the Didsbury Trust had served its purpose in birthing this new phenomenon. We changed the name of the trust in 1998 to the Sacred Space Foundation, which crystallized around a range of projects that would be available to healthcare workers and those who employ them and grounded this in a wide range of emerging research that was underpinning our hunches about the "spiritual crisis" which causes burnout.

The projects range from teaching TT to bringing meditation into prisons, from cultivating sacred yew trees to developing the use of labyrinths. Currently, the most time-consuming one is the Sanctuary Project. It is based on the idea that people who are exhausted and burned out—nurses, doctors, therapists—can come and be in retreat. They can have a quiet place either to restore their energies by being alone or to participate in one or more of the programs. For instance, they might work with me on career counseling, or I might take them walking in the hills or canoeing on a lake. Jeannie or I might read the tarot with them or do TT with them. We also have volunteers locally who help out—aromatherapists, sports people, an osteopath, a t'ai chi teacher. People build their own programs. And, whenever possible, we feed them from our organic garden.

The idea is that you create a safe, sacred space where people can come home to themselves. We have two beautiful locations in the countryside—Jeannie runs one; I run the other. But the sacred space that people are looking for goes beyond a nice environment. It's deeper than that—to come home to yourself is to discover the most important sacred space of all.

Creating sacred space in a hospital setting is an extension of the Sanctuary Project. There's no point in providing a nice, cozy environment where people get in touch with themselves if they just have to go back and do the same things. It's pointless. So our program also works with organizations. A recent report by the Nuffield Trust in the United Kingdom demonstrated that there was a phenomenal loss of money in health services due to the number of staff who left sick, exhausted, or burned out. We tell hospital administrators, "Look at your sickness levels, at your absenteeism. This is telling you something. If we can help you care for your staff better and develop policies and practices at work that will make the environment a safe, sacred space, you may find your staff and your patients will be happier, and it will save you money down the line."

We've now got projects under way in various organizations to help them shift their culture to be more responsive to the needs of the staff. For instance, it's great to have a sanctuary out in the countryside, but why not have one at work?

We are currently seeking funds for a substantive program that would research sanctuary space in the workplace. At the moment, the only research being carried out is by a few staff from the College of Health on one particular project. However, the immediate feedback is highly positive.

But it's not that simple. When people get to a stage where they need sanctuary, they are in, or are very close to being in, spiritual crisis, and if the difficulty is one of a spiritual nature, then it demands spiritual solutions. The creation of sanctuary rooms is only a tool to help people shift their consciousness. The real work is inner work. The goal is to reach a stage where you can feel at home with yourself and the presence of the divine anywhere at any time. Puja tables, lovely pictures and icons, quiet rooms, spiritual music—that stuff won't change anything if people get stuck in spiritual materialism. So the sanctuaries or labyrinths in hospital sites are simply tools to get you to where you want to be, rather than an end in themselves.

Labyrinths

Jeannie was inspired by the work of Dr. Lauren Artress at Grace Cathedral in San Francisco. She and her colleagues had been to Chartres Cathedral and seen the labyrinth. I hesitate to talk about energies because it sounds like New Age gobbledygook, so let's just say that at Chartres, people report very powerful, transformative experiences when walking the labyrinth.

Dr. Artress subsequently set up a labyrinth at Grace Cathedral. We contacted them, got the design, and had one made—the first in the Didsbury Trust's grounds, the second a portable one of canvas. It's about 60 feet across. We take it to conferences, and it's available to local churches and so on. We hope to make them available on hospital lawns so staff and patients can walk them. There are reports of very beneficial effects from labyrinth-walking for patients who have mental health problems, for example.

The labyrinth is a tool like any other. Just as you might light a candle or walk into church or sit in silence when you go to pray, the labyrinth is a spiritual tool. It's built on the principles of sacred geometry, and it has particularly feminine characteristics. The phases of the moon are marked around the outside. In walking the path, which winds backward and forward, sometimes you seem to be going back on yourself and sometimes, when others are walking the same labyrinth, you know you're passing them, and they're passing you. So there's this sense of being on a winding journey until you eventually reach the center.

People tend to enter the labyrinth taking something with them—a problem, a difficulty, a need—or they may go into it saying, "I'm available. Tell me, God, what I need to do." So the person enters and walks and goes through a phase of what is known as *dissolution*. In the center, you might pause to pray or meditate. You stay there until you feel you've finished whatever you need to finish, and then you return through "resolution" as you walk out again. I've made it sound rather linear in my efforts to describe it. In practice, what happens is complex and interconnected—everyone has his or her own experience.

The labyrinth has many uses—as a problem-solving tool, as a meditative tool for deepening your connections, as a contemplative tool for feeling the presence of the divine. It is a tool for altering consciousness, for helping you to enter a state in which you are open, receptive, and available to whatever is right for you at the time.

Our work has been primarily with healthcare professionals. Last year, when we had the conference, almost everyone walked the labyrinth. Some had profound experiences. They were leaving with joy or in tears. Interestingly, the cathedral and university staff were initially tentative. But at the end they were walking it themselves, and several of them said to me, "I wish we could keep this here. I'd like to do this every morning before we start work." By chance, we did leave them a labyrinth. As we rolled it up and left, its outline remained on the lawn!

So it is a meditative tool to help you on your path, whatever your path is. Labyrinths have been used in all societies, all cultures, and all religions throughout time.

One thing that concerns me, however, is that the "new paradigm" or "New Age" is really a new age for a relatively small number of people: healthcare professionals, the well-educated, the white and middle class, often the powerful—the ones who already have it. You could argue that they are the ones who need it least. To great masses of people, the New Age is just an invisible train going by on another platform in another town. On one level, I can accept that if you are working with the caregivers—social workers, nurses, policemen, doctors—and they start to be different in the world, then there will be an effect in the environments they work in. And maybe that's what we have to do. But when I sit in my lovely rural retreat, a part of me still says, "What can we do to make this available to everyone?" I'm not sure of the answer to that—maybe it's less about doing and more about people "being."

I look at the world and think, "My God, it shouldn't be like this." I never bought into the kind of hunching-of-the-shoulders perspective of, "It's suffering. It has to happen." It is suffering, but I'm not so sure it has to happen. I don't have any ambitions to remove all suffering from the whole planet—I'm not quite that egotistical yet—but if things like the labyrinth can be more available to people, if they can be made ordinary to all those millions of people for whom churches have become meaningless places they don't go to, then it might help. Our planet is in danger as never before, and never has it been more urgent for more people to awaken spiritually. It is interesting that tools like the labyrinth are reemerging to help us at this time. It can't be a coincidence, and they may be part of the "better way." Who knows?

Am I a Healer?

Let me first say that everybody is, in some sense, a healer. It's more about recognizing one's potential for doing it and then deepening one's skills and practice to be more available to it. But nowadays, I find myself deeply skeptical of the healer-patient divide. It reinforces the old medical model and power structures. Healing happens, but I do not believe "healers" control it. It is a mutual process—no healer or healee—just a couple of people in search of wholeness.

When I first began TT, I simply added it to my practice. But, after a while, I noticed that while I was using the TT techniques, I felt myself getting to a stage where I didn't need to actually do it. I could just be it. So if you deepen your practice and work at it and learn from it, you may get to a stage where you don't need to do TT for people; just your quiet presence or the way you hold someone may be enough.

I'll tell you a story. I was working with a student nurse at the clinic and this patient, Mazie, asked to go to the toilet. Mazie was very, very sick. She was in her early nineties, had cancer, and was dying. When the nurse and I brought the commode to the bedside, Mazie was quite distressed. So I went behind the screens with the student nurse and told Mazie, "You can stand against me and then we'll clean you and help you back into bed."

While I was holding Mazie and she had her arms around my shoulders, she said, "It's been a long time since I've held a man like this."

Now, funny enough, as I held her I remembered when I was a little boy and used to go to the Tower Ballroom in Blackpool with my parents. My father wouldn't dance, but my mother liked to dance, so I danced with her. I was only up to her navel at this stage, so I would stand on her feet as we waltzed around. There was a very famous organist in Britain at the time named Reginald Dixon. So I said to Mazie, "Well, it's been a long time since I've held a woman like this. In fact, my mum and I used to go on holiday to Blackpool, and I would dance with her."

Mazie said, "Oh, I've been to Blackpool. To the Tower Ballroom. Reginald Dixon."

So I said, "Would you like to dance?"

And she said, "I can't."

But I said, "Don't you worry." I put both her feet on top of mine—she was only about four stone (56 pounds), God bless her—and we waltzed around the room. After we danced and got her back into bed, the student nurse said, "Where did you learn to do that?" Because nowhere in the nursing curriculum does it say you are allowed to dance around with patients. But I told her, "It just seemed right at the time."

It was a lovely spring day, and a few minutes later I brought Mazie some flowers from the garden and put them on a table in front of her. She was thrilled—beaming and smiling and happy. The other nurses couldn't understand what had happened. This woman who was in pain, suffering, miserable, frightened, was now happy. Blissful. Mazie died 2 days later—I'm told—with a smile on her face. For a little while, Mazie and I connected in a much deeper and more meaningful way than do the average "helper-helped." In that encounter there was healing and transformation for both of us—the place of mystery where we can both be made whole.

To me, that is how TT moves beyond the ritual of doing something with the hands to just being—that is, being a healing presence so you don't have to do anything except be with the person, and then whatever feels right, you do it. So your agendas go away, and it has nothing to do with your role or your training or anything like that.

I've worked with people who instinctively, intuitively, got to that point. I look back to those people who were able to move beyond the formalities and the structures and the training with great admiration. They were able to be a healing presence, and I think, "What a world we could have if more and more people could work in that way."

Alternative Medicine in Great Britain

In the early 1970s, HRH Prince Charles started promoting organic gardening and talking to plants. He was spending time with people who were mystics, such as Sir Laurens van der Post. Most of the British population ridiculed him, particularly when he said that orthodox medicine should be looking at complementary medicine. But then, of course, the world changed, and he has been proved right.

Now we are moving away from the paradigm in which orthodox medicine is here, and complementary medicine is there, and never the twain shall meet. A few interesting phenomena have occurred, one of which is public demand. Regardless of what doctors and therapists think, people are turning to alternatives. They are searching for something that has a deeper meaning and is more comforting. There is also a growing concern about many aspects of orthodox treatment, particularly drugs and their side effects. So there's a groundswell of public interest. There is also evidence of increased awareness and use of complementary therapies within the mainstream of medicine. Jeannie and I were instrumental in setting up one of the largest groups within the Royal College of Nursing—a specialist's forum for nurse complementary therapists. Many other such groups have blossomed.

I feel optimistic because I believe the movement is not dependent upon ego-driven, power-driven models. There's something else going on. Call it "the spirit of the new millennium" or "the new age" or "the divine intervening." I don't know. I just know it's changing.

I don't think it's something that we're entirely in control of, however. I can only loosely describe it as a shift in consciousness. We've gone through generations of disconnection and segmentation, of working in blocks and structures and systems, and now the word "integration" means more than integrating one system with another. It's about reconnection between people. You see it in the deep ecology movement and in spiritual revival. It's manifesting itself in countless different ways. When Princess Diana died, I woke up and thought, "What country do I live in? I don't live in England." To see millions of English people weeping in the streets at the death of a woman—we don't do that sort of thing. And it didn't happen because suddenly there was an outpouring of therapists working in Britain. I think there is a social, cultural, spiritual, psychological, and emotional shift taking place, and not just in my home country, but everywhere in different degrees.

My Spiritual Practice

I recall working with Jack Kornfield in Switzerland, and we were meditating. It was one of those meditations in which you meet a divine being. In this meditation, I was bargaining with this being of light about what I was prepared to give up in this life—what my spiritual practice should be to achieve enlightenment. So I said to God, "Okay, but I won't give up the five C's: I'm not going to be celibate, and I'm not giving up chips, chocolate, champagne, or Calvin Klein underwear. I'll work on these next time around—all the rest can go." And I came out of the meditation laughing myself silly because it was such a funny thing to do. One loses the attachment when it's laughed at.

I rise each morning fairly early; I go for a run and meditate; I practice t'ai chi. Recently I've gotten to a stage where I'm not sure when I meditate and when I don't. There is a point in the day when I sit down and my eyes are closed. I'm in a pleasant environment and may have some music on or some incense burning, but I'm not sure where it ends and begins any longer.

The other area of practice for me is in my relationships—my children, friends, partners, colleagues. Your practice is right under your nose all the time. However, when you're doing all this, it's important to be wary of spiritual navel gazing. Have the experiences, by all means, but then go out into the world and do something with them. Do good.

As far as teachers go, I see Ram Dass as often as I can when I'm in the States, and I see Mother Meera, a wonderful woman, when I'm in Germany. She is a young woman from a Hindu background who works in a village north of Frankfurt. Some believe she is an avatar. Thousands of people go to see her. You sit for 2 or 3 hours and meditate, then go forward and receive her blessing. She touches you on the head, looks you in the eyes. No words are exchanged. Then you go back and meditate for a while and then return to your hotel room. You can see her a maximum of 4 nights a week, up to 8 nights if you travel from the States. Seeing her is part of my spiritual practice. But my learning also comes from books, from my own mystical experiences, and from many different sources. One advantage of technology is the shrinking of time and distance—so many great teachers and their words are now so much more available to us.

A while ago it became clear to me that you don't have to go into retreat in a Buddhist monastery for 40 years. I became aware that everything I need for my particular spiritual path—and I believe this is true for almost everybody—is right under my nose. It's actually right there in daily life, in work, in relationships with people, in one's relationship with the planet, with God. Every second of the day something happens that teaches us. If we can become aware of this, in so many situations in which we might otherwise flounder, we could say, "What's going on here? What's this teaching me?"

So I guess my spiritual practice is a hodgepodge of all kinds of things—whether it's meditating in my garden or climbing into the hills, it permeates everything. There are many ways up the mountain.

I hesitate to tell any personal stories, first of all because words are such a limiting medium to express an inner experience, and second because they are just "my stories"—relevant to me and my deepening of life in the spirit. Perhaps they are also irrelevant and, frankly, odd to others. However, since you ask, one occurred when I was looking for a place to live. Before I arrived at this place, I had a strong sense that this was where I was going to live. So here I am in the middle of nowhere in England and I am outside in broad daylight in the sunshine where five or six hawks are wheeling over my head. As I stood outside, I heard this voice saying, "This is it. This is where I want you to work."

I've never been one of these people who sees God as someone "out there." To me, God is the inner voice you're hearing, which is out there and in there; it's one and the same. But I thought I'd check it to be sure. So I doused it. I do some dousing, and there was a lay line that ran right through the building at one end. That was where I instinctively felt the sanctuary room would be.

Some months later, I began to dream about spirals. Then I read this book about a spiral labyrinth, and it mentioned a pattern found in Hopi country. So I journeyed to Hopi country and traveled around in the desert buying silver brooches with spirals on them. This went on for ages. Spirals kept popping up all over the place, and still do. I worked through the tarot with Jeannie to discover I fit with the spiritual number seven, the Chariot—the changeling, the eternal, always spiraling through the universe, constantly changing.

So all these spirals are popping up all over the place. Then one day I was with my godson and goddaughter, both of whom were dousing. We were out in the field at the side of the house, which is where I usually sit and meditate in the mornings. My godson, who is a very sensitive lad, said that his rods were going crazy. But I just couldn't get the pattern at all. It was bizarre. Then Justin stood up on the bank and looked down. He said, "You're going the wrong way, Steve. I can see it. It's a spiral."

I said, "What do you mean, a spiral?

And he said, "I can see it. It's a spiral."

So we moved the directions around, and every time the rods went off, we put a stone down. Several tons of stones later, this beautiful, 50-foot spiral emerges that feeds into the lay line. So that was the culmination of all the dreaming about spirals.

We put stones around it so it appeared like a maze—a simple, spiral maze. Some months later, a group of people gathered for meditation work, and at the end of the session many of them were quite distressed. They had gotten in touch with something that was quite difficult for them. So I said, "Okay, everybody walk the spiral. Whatever pain and distress you've got, walk in to the center, leave it there, and come out without it." So people walked in in tears, but they walked out laughing. And I thought, "That's what you are for." It's a tool. People come and walk the spiral now, even when I'm not there, and just enjoy being in it.

So it is interesting how that whole symbolism of the spiral was going on all that time. Coincidence? Synchronicity? I'm left with questions. Was it there affecting me? Or was I creating it with my consciousness? Do we "create" sacred space, or is it already there? I think it's probably both. I think it's quite possible for people to create something through their consciousness if it's right or appropriate, if you're available to it in some way. But I suspect that the spiral had also been whirling around there for a while.

Another time, during October of last year, I was with friends in Walnut Creek on a visit to San Francisco. I went and sat outside in the garden where there was a little arbor with some bushes around it. I thought, "What a nice spot to meditate." The sun was shining down on me and I just sat and meditated as usual. I don't bother with a mantra nowadays. Sometimes I do, but mostly I just sit. I became intensely aware, after a few minutes, of not being solid, of seeing myself sitting, of hearing distant voices, movements, animals, cars, and felt an absolutely intense sense of not being separate from anything. I was profoundly and intensely connected with everything. The planet, absolutely everything, was connected, all vibrating, all full of life, all moving, and yet absolutely, perfectly still.

There was this intense sense of connection and no sense of time. Time was suspended, and even though everything was moving in time, it was also very still. Nothing was different; everything was the same; everything was changing. When I opened my eyes, the sun was shining through a dewdrop on the end of this leaf, and it was as though everything that was here went into that, and everything that was in that was here. It's like that old line "To see a world in a grain of sand."

So most of my experiences either have been this kind where there's a sensation of complete connectedness or just sitting in a divine presence, watching it, participating in it, and standing apart from it, both in it and out of it. Occasionally my experiences have been accompanied by a distinct voice that has said, "This is what you should do."

Now, this path has not always been easy. About this time 4 years ago there was an article published about me in *Nursing Times*. The editor interviewed me, and we talked about some of the things I've talked about now, but I was conscious of being afraid. Of course, people had interviewed me about nursing and healthcare countless times before, and I'd never hesitated to pontificate and tell the world how it should be. Never hesitated. Rampant ego. But I was sitting and listening to myself talk to this person, and thought, "Why am I afraid? What's going on here?"

I realized that, probably for the first time in a public arena, I was talking about something that was deeply personal that had affected me, changed my view of the world. I was reticent, too, because my experiences are my own and not necessarily generalizable to the rest of the world. Also, the "well-known professional" part of me was afraid that I would now be ignored or cast into the wasteland.

When the interview was published, a part of me felt at ease. I thought, "I don't mind if people tell me I'm completely bonkers. I've been genuine and honest." And then it started— the outpouring! The journal had never had anything like it. The letters and phone calls from people saying, "Wow, thank God someone, especially someone in his position, was willing to say this." It was as though I, the journal, and others had pressed a button that now said to people, "Okay, you can talk about this stuff now."

People have been waiting a long time to talk about this. It's been taboo for quite a while, particularly among healthcare professionals, because we've said, "You can't have religion mixed into it." And in a certain sense you can't. It's not up to healthcare professionals to proselytize or fix patients into their worldview or their view of God. That's totally inappropriate. But I think more and more healthcare professionals need help to integrate their spirituality into their work.

When I was a teacher in the College of Nursing, talking about God was something to be laughed at. "Nobody believes in God these days," I'd hear, or they'd say it was irrelevant to their work. The rationalist approach to healthcare has little time for that which is seen as irrational. Yet the divine, God, the universal spirit—however you see he or she or it—means an awful lot to an awful lot of people, particularly when they have a healthcare crisis. So nurses or doctors or therapists who can't work with that can't fully meet their patients' needs. Now this doesn't mean you tell them to pray to God to solve illnesses. But it might mean that you work with them much more sensitively or that you be aware that helping them bring meaning to their healthcare problems is as important as sticking on the plaster.

But, until recently, we have not had legitimate forums within the healthcare professions to talk about spirituality or its significance. My wariness about going public went beyond the personal effects on myself. It was more—and I can see it now—that somebody will start setting up courses in spirituality in medicine. If we do that, we run the risk of segregating it from everything else. But it actually underpins everything, pervades everything. You cannot avoid it. In the *Upanishads* it is said that absolutely everything that has ever existed is pervaded by the divine, which means the divine is as much in a can of Coke as in your eye. So I think there is a need on the part of healthcare professionals to find appropriate, legitimate means of expressing spirituality, and then to help their patients when necessary. Once again, that doesn't mean getting patients on their knees praying to God for forgiveness, but it might mean that when the patient wants to talk, you sit and listen because that's just as important as sticking in the needles.

For me, the most appropriate pattern is not to work with my patients by saying, "You can solve your problems if you take up meditation or change your diet or do this or that," but simply to live my spirituality. Just by being around them authentically—by being honest, supportive, loving, available—expresses spirituality. That's the way to help. That's the way to avoid falling into the trap of helper and helped. That's the way to be most effective as a "healer."

CHAPTER 15

EUGENE TAYLOR, PhD

Spiritual Healing and the American Visionary Tradition

In the Fall of 1998, when I first met Eugene Taylor at the Harvard Faculty Club in Cambridge, Massachusetts, (what a privilege to be in those hallowed halls) I thought I was going to spend the next few hours in an academic conversation about brain and mind and how the field of psychology came to be. Instead, I was swept away by conversation about the philosophy of William James, loyalty and how it became a form of psychotherapy at the Massachusetts General Hospital just after 1900, the psychospiritual revolution currently in progress, and the psychological symbolism of angels, who, profoundly, may be embodied in those we meet in everyday life.

Dr. Eugene Taylor holds a master's degree in general/experimental psychology and Asian Studies from Southern Methodist University. He attended Harvard Divinity School as a resident graduate in applied theology and history of religions before joining the faculty at Harvard Medical School as a research historian. He received his PhD in the history and philosophy of psychology from Boston University. Dr. Taylor is the author of numerous books, including *William James on Exceptional Mental States: Reconstruction of the 1896 Lowell Lectures; William James on Consciousness Beyond the Margin; Pure Experience: The Response to William James; A Psychology of Spiritual Healing;* and *Shadow Culture: Psychology and Spirituality in America.*

Founder and director of the Cambridge Institute of Psychology and Religion, Dr. Taylor is also editor of *Studia Mysticorum,* the newsletter of the Mysticism Study Group in the American Academy of Religion. He holds an academic appointment at Harvard Medical School as Lecturer on Psychiatry, is a Senior Psychologist on the Psychiatry Service at the Massachusetts General Hospital, and a faculty member at Saybrook Graduate School and Research Institute. He is also a longtime student (4th-degree black belt and shidoin, or instructor) of aikido, a nonviolent Japanese martial art.

Thank you for this opportunity to speak to you about my work. In order to set some kind of context, let me say first of all that I believe mind/body medicine and its offspring, complimentary and alternative therapies, owe a great debt to an era of medical psychology that has already occurred in advance of today. This is to say that, contrary to the scientific ideal, in the mental sciences, which have never been very well integrated with the physical ones, the evolution of ideas about the mind/body problem has not always been cumulative. Different world views have supplanted each other in such a way as to obscure earlier advances. Such has been the case in the history of depth-psychology, when Boston was at the center of developments in scientific psychotherapy in the English-speaking world between 1880 and 1920. The people involved were part of a larger international consortium of investigators associated with British psychical researchers, experimental psychologists in Switzerland, and neuropathologists in Europe who followed the lead of the so-called French Experimental Psychology of the Subconscious. This consortium drove the international development of scientific psychotherapy in the West for a 40-year period, before psychoanalysis became an international movement.

Their view was based on a completely different model of consciousness than that of psychoanalysis. Their model was one of dissociation. It was more akin to what occurs today within psychiatry and psychology in the treatment of posttraumatic stress disorder and the study of multiple personality. Because it was based on then-known advances in brain neurophysiology, it was more like the philosophical problems taken up in the neurosciences today, and because it dealt directly with the dialogue between psychology and physiology, it touched on principles of mind/body interaction now common to alternative medicine. Freud abandoned the physiological hypothesis and proceeded solely with the symbolic language of the unconscious, hoping that someday physiology would come back and verify what he had to say. But with the waning of the Freudian influence over the last 20 years, people are not only reinterpreting Freud, but also returning to the nineteenth-century model to reclaim the earlier lineage before Freud and bring it up to date.

As psychiatrist and historian Henri Ellenberger noted, depth psychology was one of the only major developments in Western science in the late 19th century that was not brought into the flow of scientific information to form the mainstream disciplines in science and medicine that we know today. Mind/body medicine and alternative and complementary therapies have been a direct historical reaction to this state of affairs. Their major contribution to the modern scientific discussion about the relationship between consciousness and healing, in my opinion, is their assumption, like their nineteenth century forebears, that, in addition to a pathological dimension to human functioning, as well as an everyday, waking, functional state of consciousness, there is also a growth-oriented dimension to experience that modern science and medicine consistently ignore.

Introduction to the Iconography of the Transcendent

Experimental science at least acknowledges the reality of the normal everyday waking state. Indeed, the history of Western science and medicine has largely been a colossal elaboration of the rational categories we create to understand the data of the senses. Depth psychology, and particularly psychoanalysis, at least, acknowledge the reality of the unconscious, opening us up to understanding the pathology of the emotions and the effects of repressed thinking on our motivation. In the late nineteenth century, certain expressions of depth psychology less well known then psychoanalysis injected into our understanding the possibility that we could experience higher states of consciousness—higher, deeper, and more profound than the everyday waking condition. Thus, any concept, word, or image that refers to these higher states in any theory of depth psychology I refer to as "iconography of the transcendent." When Freud presented his theory of the unconscious, a great debate ensued that still rages today as to whether or not psychoanalysis was a science. He had no iconography of the transcendent. The issue was confined to whether or not there was an unconscious.

Jung added the iconography of the transcendent, because he came from an earlier tradition— the period from 1880 to 1920—that had already demarcated the growth-oriented dimension of personality. Jung said in the unpublished version of the English translations of *Memory, Dreams and Reflections* that he believed the reason medicine thought Freud's theories scientifically questionable was not for his sexual theories—that was simply the terms of the public argument. They rejected Freud because he was confronting reductionist, positivist medical science with the reality of the unconscious. Jung suffered an even more ignoble fate. His theories were never even considered by mainstream medical science because he had injected the iconography of the transcendent into the discussion, even as his work has had wide popular appeal internationally within the psychotherapeutic counter-culture.

While Jung is most often seen as a mere acolyte of Freud by mainstream historians of science and medicine, in reality his tradition was the nineteenth century psychologies of transcendence around William James, Theodore Flournoy, and F. W. H. Myers. In the United States, for instance, after 1882, the British and European experiments on hypnosis and dissociation were replicated in the Harvard psychological laboratories. Once this laboratory material entered the American scientific literature through the professional journals, it became legitimate for physicians to employ light hypnosis, crystal gazing and automatic writing in the diagnosis and treatment of the ambulatory psychoneuroses. This occurred particularly in the outpatient departments at the Massachusetts General Hospital and the Boston City Hospital as early as the mid-1880s, partly based on William James's work on the physiology of the emotions. James was later a major influence on Jung. Science today is built largely upon a philosophy of reductionistic positivism— reductionistic because reality is always reduced to measurable numbers, and positivistic, meaning there is nothing to be assumed that exists beyond the senses. When he wrote *Principles of Psychology* in 1890, James had said that, in order to launch an experimental science, you need to begin with reductionistic positivism. But sooner or later all infant sciences have to be overhauled by philosophy. This is because, at its base, all science rests on philosophical assumptions.

The two reigning epistemologies at the time, aside from positivism, were spiritualism and associationism. James thought that these are not sophisticated enough metaphysics, so he decided to use reductionistic positivism to write his book. It took him 12 years, and when the *Principles of Psychology* came out, it became an instant classic, launching psychology as a new scientific discipline. However, by the time he finished, he had his hands on the beginning of a different metaphysics. He had begun with positivism. However, he soon repudiated that position. In his presidential address to the American Psychological Association at its second annual meeting in 1894, he reminded his audience of the problem he had had establishing the appropriate metaphysics to launch a scientific psychology. He declared then and there that he was overthrowing reductionistic positivism for a more sophisticated approach to the scientific study of human experience. That was the germ of his radical empiricism, which is a focus on pure experience in the immediate moment.

An analogy today would be the work of Amedeo Giorgi. Giorgi's claim is that experimental psychology and experimental science must be completely reconstructed because of their overemphasis on the objective at the expense of the subjective, which represents a special problem in psychology as nowhere else. This is the dilemma posed in the neurosciences with advances in the biology of consciousness. The more we move from the inorganic to the organic and from there to the psychological, the closer we get to studying the organ that produces science in the first place, and the more philosophical questions come to the fore. Once we begin to examine the way science is conducted, the key question becomes "What is the role of the experimenter?" This leads us to the very heart of the science-making process, which is the internal phenomenological worldview of the scientist him or her self.

Right now, the stance required of the scientist in psychology is to be objective, a viewpoint in which we believe we have eliminated the subjective. The subjective, however, continues to exert an unconscious influence, the more so because it is denied. Because of this, the experimenter not only confounds the psychological atmosphere of the experiment with his presence, his thoughts, and his conceptualizations, denying that he does so, but he also generates a science that excludes large amounts of human experience. This has created a crisis, where the methods of psychology do not fit its subject matter. The people in control of experimental psychology do not believe there is a crisis. Meanwhile, alternative forms of psychology, such as mind/body medicine, positive psychology, existential-humanistic and transpersonal psychology, even nonwestern indigenous psychologies, are breaking out all over the place.

Giorgi's position is that you do the same thing when running an experiment that you do when you engage in therapy. There is the phenomenological moment experienced by both the experimenter and subject and the therapist and client. To build a psychology on this kind of phenomenological science would be less manipulative and more descriptive of what is actually going on. There would still be the opportunity to gain control over conditions, but it would not be the exclusive focus of reductionistic science, as it is now. James took psychology as an example and appropriated the problem of subjectivity to refer to the larger problem facing science in general. Giorgi is doing the same thing.

There is another philosophical issue here as well—the idea that there can be no knowledge of any kind without the observer or the interpreter—that knowledge, nay the universe itself, is not independent of the observer. John Wheeler, Professor Emeritus at Princeton and a former student of Niels Bohr, is working on just this problem in the field of theoretical physics. Max Velmans at the University of London, a cognitive neuroscientist, has proposed a reflexive theory of consciousness in which the observer is calculated in with the observation, and what is observed. James was there ahead of them. He understood clearly that there is some integral relation between the knowledge we have that enables us to generate scientific information, and the fact that we are present, that we are the ones trying to understand the world of phenomena and articulate it as knowledge.

This is the focus of my work. I call it "psychology as epistemology."

Almost all the sciences are constructed on the idea that two objective observers can be switched with each other, as long as they both stay objective. In this way the causal laws that are found from their measurements are corroborated. This generates a body of data, however, that is easily elevated to the status of a world view. At most interdisciplinary conferences, for instance, the humanities people say, "I'm happy to look at the data, but I would also like to offer my poetry, which is a language beyond words." The scientists say, "Skip the poetry, let's just have the data." This implies that the only important reality is data driven. But science is only one form of useful knowledge. There are other forms—economic, political, social, but also visionary, numinous, and mythic. The point here is that traditional science is conducted by presuming that there is a world independent of the observer, whereas psychology as epistemology makes the claim that everything is a function of human consciousness somewhere. If you do not take that part of the equation into account, you are not fulfilling the criteria you originally established of trying to accurately portray the universe. This is because, right away, the subjective factors—such as the unconscious—enter in ways over which you have no control.

What is the ultimate nature of reality? This is the question our sciences and our religions seem to be asking. I hope it is the right question, since everyone seems to be coming up with a different answer.

In the Christian sense, there has to be an origin and an end. It is built into their cosmology. The Buddhist view of consciousness is that there is no such thing as a beginning and an end. It is all co-dependent and co-created in the immediate moment. In this view, the linear process of biological evolution is simply a statement that everything keeps going. The Buddhist concern has to do with consciousness and your relation to immediate reality. These are the same kind of questions, but they are cast in completely different forms. So we are no longer looking for an ontology—an explanation for being, and an eschatology—where it will all end—as we are conditioned to look for in Western thought. Rather, the here-and-now is the phenomenological moment in which we become grounded in the ultimacy of immediate experience.

Actually, the Buddhists talk not about human consciousness, but about sentience—or knowing. The issue is not where consciousness stops and matter begins. There is no such point, because there is no place you can go in matter where your consciousness would not be. This is the most important confounding variable for that particular question. You can be a fundamentalist scientist and pretend that you are being so objective that no subjective influence is there. But you are there, defining and manipulating the conditions of the moment, being a part of the creation of those conditions. To deny that this is so is not even logical.

So talking about the phenomenology of the immediate moment requires a major shift in thinking. But could you imagine the basic natural sciences grounded in psychology, rather than physics or biology? This is too fantastic for experimental scientists to imagine because psychology and psychiatry currently have such a dubious status with regard to the other sciences. But it is precisely because psychology and psychiatry are the lowest on the pecking order that I think they have the greatest chance of leading a person-centered revolution around the problem of consciousness in the basic sciences in the future.

The Consciousness and Unconscious

Understand that anything I say will be tainted by my epistemology, my unique, existential point-of-view about the world. This is true for everyone. The words "consciousness" and "unconscious" are examples. When you refer to consciousness, there are always several meanings. One is that consciousness and awareness are the same—that to be aware is to be conscious. That is a typical definition. In medicine, for practical purposes, consciousness ranges from coma, through the normal everyday waking state, to hyperactivity. In the tradition of depth psychology, however, the claim is that, at any given moment, there can be an expansion into all other dimensions of experience. To me, consciousness is both the totality of all experience; at the same time I often use it to refer to "waking consciousness." It is whatever state you are in when you are actually physically awake. There could be the waking condition we are experiencing now, but also at the same time, hidden from view, states of consciousness both less intelligent and more intelligent than the waking state could be exerting their influence. In this sense, consciousness and awareness do not necessarily have to be the same thing.

I parked my car six times this morning, trying to get in the space. And every time I got out, either I was not near the meter or my wheel was over the line. I was conscious, but was I really aware? I mean, why didn't I just park the car and get out and walk away? I had to make this issue out of it. I remained conscious, but I was not fully aware of what I was doing.

At the same time I think other states exist beyond the threshold of waking awareness. I think it is also possible for domains of the unconscious to enter into the field of waking conscious awareness. From a very basic standpoint, we try to educate ourselves so that waking consciousness is almost always operating under the control of rationality and logic. It has to be because that is the way individuals interact with the biological environment. That is how we ensure the survival of the bodily vehicle through which we can then experience different altered states of consciousness, even though those states might not have any relevance for biological, material reality.

But traditional biology, traditional psychology, and traditional science do not acknowledge that. They say there is only one state—the state we are presently experiencing, the biological state of the organism, the state of birth and death. But dynamic psychology says that there are other dimensions of consciousness swirling around us at any given time.

F. W. H. Myers's theory, which influenced both James and Jung, was that we have within us a broad spectrum of possible states, ranging from the pathological to the transcendent, and that waking consciousness, occurring right now, in the present, is only one among many other states. Because the purpose of waking consciousness is the biological survival of the organism, we spend a lot of time in that state, and tend to confuse the pathological and the transcendent because they come in through the same channels. But there is plenty of evidence, Myers says, that they are different, and that they have different fields of application and adaptation in their own right. Myers said there are what he called *dissolutive states*—states of psychopathology and personality disintegration, and there are evolutive states—states of higher consciousness. We know when we are in these higher states because of the spontaneous appearance of psychic abilities. The point I tried to make in my book, A *Psychology of Spiritual Healing,* was that the true function of psychic abilities discovered through interior exploration is not to find dead bodies and lost wallets. Their function is to indicate our progress on the path of self-realization, or what the monotheists would call God-consciousness.

We can know the higher path through the discovery of the interior symbols that guide our personal destinies. The function of these symbols is to give meaning to our lives, which is how we bring the will to live to situations of trauma and tragedy, where healing needs to take place. The true function of these symbols is preparation for the hour of one's death, which is a transition to the higher states that we are going to pass into, whether we know how to conceptualize them or not.

One of the claims that James and Myers made is that we can have states within us that are not present in the waking state, but still influence us. So we can have neuroses and complexes that make us act like idiots, or we can actualize our latent potential by tapping into these higher realities. We can also be changed just by being in the presence of someone who is in touch with such higher and deeper states. In these cases, there is the possibility of some higher dimension of personality operating behind the scenes that can inform waking consciousness about which direction to turn.

The unconscious is a different story. The word *unconscious* historically comes to us through Freud, who, in my opinion, did not discover the unconscious, so much as discover his own unconscious. But then he reified it by trying to study it objectively as a science. So there are parts of his theory that are definitely true, and parts that are definitely idiosyncratic to his own unique, existential and phenomenological view of the world and have nothing to do with anyone else. The enduring problem is that we still do not know which was science and which was his own idiosyncratic, existential language of interior experience.

Freud's linguistic conceptions, meanwhile, come from the specific traditions of Von Hartmann and Schopenhauer. The French used the term *subconscious,* but they were not just different terms for the same thing. Historically, they refer to epistemologies so radically different that you cannot really compare them point for point. You cannot say, "Let's interpret the work of Pierre Janet from a Freudian point of view." It does not mean anything, because you are not getting Janet, you are getting Freud. You have to reconstruct Janet's own historical context, his frame of reference, at which point you see that it has got nothing to do with what Freud was talking about. It is a totally different way of conceptualizing consciousness.

This has not been done yet, except that the task was begun by Ellenberger and has been carried on by his most avid readers, such as Sonu Shamdasani, Mark Micale, and myself. When you study the history of psychotherapy, historians start with Charcot and jump to Freud. There is a big 40-year gap in there that we know little about because it is not the story of biological psychiatry or Freudian analysis. But a whole new generation of scholars is working to reconstruct that period so that we can now see it as it was.

The American Visionary Tradition

My very small contribution to this bigger picture is reconstruction of the Boston School of Psychopathology, which also draws its origins from a generic kind of spirituality in the folk-culture which I have called the American visionary tradition. My book *Shadow Culture: Psychology and Spirituality in America,* is a selective historical look at a psychospiritual visionary psychology; that is, a visionary language of interior experience that has been part of American popular culture since its very inception. It first came out in 1999 through CounterPoint Press.

It is not widely acknowledged that this country was founded not only by pilgrims, politicians, and soldiers but also by mystics. Contemporary spiritual seekers have wept when they realized that they are not alone in the direction they have chosen in their life, but that they are part of a much older, uniquely American visionary tradition.

I once published an article called "The New Science and the New Medicine: Do They Have a History?" in which I made the claim that there is nothing you can show me today in psychotherapy that I cannot show you a better example from 100 years ago. Of course, people point to some new technologies, but are television and the computer improvements? Beyond that, what are we talking about? Even William James used the image of the Marconi wireless in his Ingersoll lecture on immortality in 1898 to challenge the biological view of the transmission hypothesis—that the brain only transmits consciousness and stops at death. James's theory was that the brain could equally well be a conductor. So, like a wireless, it picks up consciousness and funnels it through a unique individual, whose effects live on after death.

Physical, Psychological, and Spiritual Healing

In one sense, all healing is miraculous, no matter what kind it is—whether you attribute it to a pill or a doctor. But we tend to think of healing as all physical. With physical healing, you cut your finger, you put iodine on it; you have a brain tumor, you go to a surgeon, and they take it out. It is the attitude that says, "It's all physical reality."

Psychotherapy, on the other hand, is about using a good idea to fix another, distorted idea. It is about how ideas can cause physical symptoms and how such symptoms can also be cured by ideas. For instance, imagine you have a young child who is the product of a divorce, and who took the main psychic blows of the family's separation. The therapist gets the child, now a grown person with all kinds of nonspecific physical and emotional problems, to recreate the trauma that he has never talked about. When he comes to terms with it, he is healed both physically and emotionally, and can go on and lead his life, and get into a decent relationship without recreating the problems experienced by his parents that he had internalized. That is an example of psychological healing.

The central point here is that ideas can also have physical effects. But the psychogenic hypothesis, which says that trauma and conflict can lead to physical symptoms, also implies the developmental hypothesis—that things that happened to us early in life can influence what happens later. According to this thinking, parts of us can become fixated at a certain level while the rest evolves. Consequently, you can be perfect or at least normal in all aspects of your life except one, because something happened to you when you were young. Psychodynamics can take you back and recreate that situation and help you resolve it.

This is the developmental hypothesis within the concept of psychogenesis and the history of dynamic psychotherapy. It has some credence. But it is not the whole answer to what is actually going on. It is a functional working model of how we can deal with the flow of things, however.

The more I am talking about refers to the higher dimension of personality within. Aldous Huxley has a wonderful essay about this called "The Doors of Perception." Swedenborg called it "an opening of the interior spiritual sense." It is like the difference between seeing things in three dimensions in the natural world and realizing that everything is infused with the dynamic of the spiritual—literally, a fourth dimension. This gets back to the conversation we were having before about consciousness because there is a certain logic in the idea of sentience—that humans have consciousness but rocks do not.

But at what point in nature do we make the leap? In animistic religions, everything has a soul. Even in the West we have examples of what's called *pan-psychism*—the idea that the universe is everywhere alive and conscious at all levels. Let us say you had not thought about your dead father in a long time, and then, all of a sudden, as soon as I say something about your father, all these images and feelings about him rush into your field of awareness. That is an example of the opening of the doors of the unconscious, where the field of consciousness is flooded by unconscious contents. You find that when someone comes up to rob you, all of a sudden the unconscious invades the field and you are paralyzed. As opposed to when, in those all-to-familiar moments of complete numbness in the midst of deep pain and anguish, you realize you do not feel it. Temporarily, you are numb to all the pain and the suffering you have been going through, but this had not occurred to you before. Before, you were the victim of these waves of pain alternating with feeling numb. But then there comes that moment when in the midst of numbness you develop the capacity to call the pain forth with your intention.

This realization is the beginning of the first moment of healing. Self-healing takes place when you realize you are in the middle of something really terrible, and you do not feel a thing. So the question concerning consciousness becomes, "Where is it? Can I call it forth?" Before, it always came and grabbed you and threw you on the ground. In this particular case, you say, "I'm now ready to meet it. Where is that pain?" The next minute you could still be picked up and thrown against the wall again, but now there is a big difference. Before, you were the victim of it. Now, you called it forth. So the first step in conquering pain is to learn how to call it forth.

But what happens with systematic confrontation of serious conflict? Well, there is a desensitization that takes place. That is just straight behavior therapy. But with self-healing, you are doing it yourself. You are saying, "I'll take it in little doses. I'll go sit down and meditate each day and ask where it is and why it happened." With that kind of questioning, you are actually rebuilding your cognitive ability to traverse two states that are radically different: your waking state and wherever that larger experience of pain is being held within you.

An interesting thing is happening in the field of psychotherapy now. There is a psycho-spiritual revolution going on that focuses on the nonpathological, growth-oriented dimension of our experience. In this way, the techniques of dynamic psychotherapy are becoming more well known in the population at large. Everyone and their neighbor seem to be seeing clients. The language of depth-psychology is becoming common knowledge. Everyone is finding out what these mechanisms are all about, whereas before they were the unique province of a special group of professionals.

I am not talking about psychotherapy for neurosis, but education for transcendence. The evolution of mind-body medicine is rooted in this attitude. Thirty years ago there was the collective opening of the doors of perception—remember my point about psychology as epistemology—that led to a science with this kind of alternative worldview. Since then, we have seen the development of biofeedback, meditation, yoga, hypnosis, guided mental imagery, psychoneuroimmunology, and so on. People began to risk their entire scientific careers to study the expansion of consciousness. So the opening of the doors of perception is the conscious, voluntary willingness to turn within and traverse the interior domains, whatever the risk.

I think there is a certain experience of higher consciousness that, once seen, leaves you with only two choices: one sees that there is death or there is responding to the call. You can deny it, but then you end up sick, you start getting more traffic tickets, your mortgage is foreclosed, your spouse leaves you, and so on. Your world starts falling apart. Not that one cannot think positively. It could be a world that needs falling apart. But all the signs point to the moral necessity of finally acting on the vision of a higher reality that was earlier denied.

Jung says that when a person is sitting in a room having the right thought, he or she will be heard a thousand miles away. He says the interior journey is so profoundly personal that it can only be taken by one's self; but soon, unknown friends will appear. There are also the beautifully painted *thankas* in Buddhism in which you see the Buddha and then a thousand Buddhas in a halo around him. The idea is that within these deep interior states, eventually you make contact with other souls.

But then you have to ask, depending on how far in you go, "Is there a collective unconscious? Do we participate in it? What is our identity once we get there?" And another question: "How is individuality preserved in such a domain?" It is like asking, "Do we still live in the physical body after death?" We just cannot conceive of it. You only have the glimpse from here, where we stand in external material reality.

The Laws of Spiritual Healing

When I first wrote my other book on healing, the companion volume to *Shadow Culture*, I called it *The Psychology of Spiritual Healing*. Then I remembered an episode I had with the Harvard psychologist and physician, Henry A. Murray. I sat with him four hours a day, five days a week, for seven years, talking about Jung, Erikson, Skinner, in addition to all the other things we were working on, like Melville and personology. One day I said to Harry, "What do you think about Erik Erikson's eight stages of development?" He said they were fine but that he thought it was a problem that they were presented as *the* eight stages.

When I remembered that, I changed the title of the book to *A Psychology of Spiritual Healing*, which actually made a better point, because I was trying to say, as Jung had, that it was applicable to no one else but me. If you glean something valuable in what I wrote, that is strictly something you got out of it. I am just revealing my map. It is up to each person to discover the symbols of his or her own personal destiny and to construct his or her own interior map.

The section of the book in which I go into that idea is patterned after a book William James recommended called *The Souls of Black Folk*, by W. E. B. Du Bois. Du Bois was the founder of the NAACP and a former student of James's. In the middle of the book, Du Bois says, "But these are all words and ideas and have nothing to do with what I am really talking about, because if you really want to know the soul of the Negro, you have to turn to the sorrow songs." The sorrow songs are the tradition of black music that links the African tradition to the American tradition. When he was young, his mother used to sing him the songs that he selected. He listed 12 of them. Anyone would choose a different 12, he had said, but these are the ones that meant something to him.

Of course, scholars have come along and criticized them, asking how Du Bois's songs could be the basis of a musical tradition. But that is not the point. It was a mix of slave songs, tribal folk songs, gospel tunes, Christian hymns, and music that was a syncratic mix between them. When you get down to that deep inner level, you are talking about the vehicle that connected a people who were forced to live in the white man's unconscious. They had a culture, but it was not allowed to be visible. They were fully conscious, but of realities beyond the ken of whites. DuBois made that internal spiritual consciousness visible. In that chapter, by revealing his own meaningful songs, Dubois becomes a living conduit that defines the Afro-American religious experience.

In James's terms, the point of my book is that we have within us the potential to actualize either the good or the bad at any minute. It is our moral duty to actualize the best in the face of the worst, which can also spring into existence at any time, just through our apathy. Actualizing the good is not something you do and then are finished with. It is a continual struggle to maintain some level of decency, aesthetics, and meaning. It can slip away from you at any time. You have to keep renewing it. James called the goal "the continued renewal of the moral and aesthetic sense of life."

I thought if I could codify some of my intuitions they would be easier to remember. They are like psychic laws because if I disobey them something awful always happens. One of my laws is that "Spontaneity is an important key to recovery." It is not original. It is the idea that you have to believe there is a parking space with your name on it, with time on the meter by the front door of wherever you intend to go, for there actually to be one when you get there. And if there is not one there, then you drive around the block, and it will be around back. This intuitive law further suggests that if it is not there either and you have to park 10 blocks away, on the way back you will find a $10 bill. You have to trust that the space will be there, and if not, open yourself up to other possibilities in the universe.

It goes back to the basic theme we touched on earlier about phenomenology: you have to be able to suspend your categories of how the immediate moment is defined to let other dimensions of consciousness rush in. In some cases it is functional to do so; in other cases, we call it irrational, or even a definition of the psychopathic. But the creative person knows how to manage analogies, cultivate the flooding in of the universe, and float in the pool. The insane person cannot manage these forces and feels as if drowning.

Similarly, the *Brujeria,* or Mexican Indian healer, at the end of the trance ceremony smokes a cigarette. The purpose is to come back, to pollute oneself deliberately so he or she can return to the world of others. The chain smoker has no such control over the unconscious.

It is what Jung calls *synchronicity*. James called it *tychism* or *synechism*, and in Jung and James's hands it was a wonderful idea. They believed the universe is tychistic. It is spontaneous. It is synchronous and alogical, which means that in a total world, as part of the possibilities, there must also be some spaces somewhere that are logical. Too bad science sticks to only that small part, they said, when there is a much wider world out there.

Jung and James were struggling with the basic philosophy of causality, upon which scientific research is normatively based. This is the philosophy of positivism. But James's ideas of positivism, though they influenced the early development of psychological science here at Harvard, have been overtaken by European, continental definitions, which are completely counter to that. James's idea, following Chauncey Wright and C. S. Peirce, was that reality is defined by conditions. It is like the weather, where forces come together at one particular moment to create a situation. This is very Buddhist, so there are some interesting analogies between William James's conception of consciousness and the Buddhist conception.

Another one of my psychic laws is that one should always remain loyal to something. This is important. Josiah Royce was a Christian philosopher at the turn of the twentieth century, a close friend of William James, and a believer in the Absolute. Of course, James was a pluralist, so his great retort was "Damn the Absolute!" Even so, Royce eventually had a profound influence on symbolic logic as well as the evolution and development of the philosophy of science. He wrote *The Philosophy of Loyalty* in 1906, which had a huge influence on the way scientific psychotherapy was being conducted at Massachusetts General Hospital. Following his ideas they developed what they called *social therapy*.

Royce said that healing is based on harnessing the will to live, and that to be committed to something is to have a reason to live. To be committed to something is also what brings meaning to us. We must live for our ideals because they give us a goal to strive for. The whole point of the book is to say that it is not the number of our days, but their quality. In this way, even the sick bed can be an arena for personal and planetary transformation.

It is in commitment that we find the ability to harness the will to live, but the real function of loyalty and commitment is the actualization of values, which then transcends the physical. That was why I put that chapter in *A Psychology of Spiritual Healing* on the obligation of the healed.

There is actually a fundamentalist aspect to that idea that is frightening, however. Suppose it is the wrong commitment? Suppose it is the commitment of the Hatfields to wipe out the McCoys? One must be wary of an element of spiritual fascism here. Then again, you can find fundamentalism everywhere. There is fundamentalism in religion, certainly. But there is also fundamentalism in science. That is an unrecognized issue I think we have been struggling with unconsciously throughout 20th-century science.

As far as the responsibility of the person who is healed—it is as though you have caught a glimpse of eternity, finally understanding the path you were supposed to take. And you realize, as we have said, that all else is death. In the moment of seeing it, you realize that if you do not make a promise to follow that path, then you will die. I think all of us at some point have profound moments during which we make promises to ourselves, whether consciously or not, that then influence everything from then on—how we speak, how we dress, who we are. It is in those promises that we have a duty, an obligation, to be fulfilled. We would like to believe it has to do with the good and the best of our highest ideals, but it is something that can also be narrowly interpreted. Each person takes the experience of ultimate reality in a different way. The task is to actualize what we have seen. This is the only definition there is of authentic living.

This also brings up another interesting problem: should we all ascribe to the same belief system, or should we cultivate individuality? Vivekananda once said that he hoped someday there would be as many religions as there were people. But what is religion? My answer is that it is this idiosyncratic, fearful understanding of our own place in the universe and the awesome realization of our responsibility to keep ourselves in the best shape we can so we do not infect others with our incompleteness. The issue is not whether we should all believe in the same catechism, but how we can cultivate a rich and diverse spirituality that leads to a consensually validated way of behaving, so people of different viewpoints can live together. To me, that is the true meaning of America as a spiritual democracy.

Angels

If you take Swedenborg literally, he says that we live in a physical, human world, but that there are other celestial and spiritual worlds inhabited by angels, which are spirits of those who have died and departed and who have a direct relation to God. These angels are intermediaries between God and men and they live in Heaven in societies. This is not a new idea, by any means.

Instead of interpreting Swedenborg literally, however, as I was saying, think about it from the standpoint of depth psychology. When you go within, people appear to you in a physical sense. If you can see into their interior, spiritual domain, you realize that the drunk passed out in the doorway could be the one person whose teachings, nay, whose very being, may transform your life. If you are open and ready to receive, you may see that he is the vehicle for profound learning. So what does that make of each person except a conduit for the Divine?

If you believe in angels but then undervalue your human relationships, you are missing the point. It is not beings with wings who come down from heaven with a lamb in their arms and the Mormon Tabernacle Choir singing in the background. It is somebody who crossed your path this morning, or someone who is just about to drop into your life from the past. It has to do with Divine energies, and you cannot imagine where they came from or how they entered your reality. These things are profoundly mundane but in an instant can also become deeply mystical.

Back in the 1960s, I was very much against many of the elements of mainstream culture, and thought all conservatives were Republicans and all Republicans were from another planet. Take anyone with short hair and a Banlon shirt—there was something wrong with them because they were engaged in power and acquisition, and not engaged in the process of self-knowledge. Then, one summer, I was touring the United States with a friend of mine. We drove to British Columbia from Dallas, and then back.

At one point, we were coming down from the Northwest into Colorado through Utah. It was about 4 o'clock in the morning and my friend was asleep. Near Salt Lake City, there was this unusual sign that said "Tourist's Spring." I was tired of driving, so I pulled off to the side of the road and walked up the path where there was a beautiful, natural spring. I got our water jugs and filled them all up, for no reason, really, except I was a tourist and this was a tourist spring. Then we drove on. We made it to the Colorado border and were having breakfast in a diner. The place mats were maps of Colorado, so we looked to see where we were going. The map showed a road that would save us 50 miles, so we decided we would take it.

Well, it turned out to be a dirt road over a high mountain pass. It was like a Laurel and Hardy movie, but once we were committed we could not turn around. We just kept driving and driving. The road kept going higher and steeper. Suddenly, the Travelall we were driving stalled. We were on a hill, so I put the brakes on and put a stone under the tire. I did not know what to do. There was no one around, no phone, nothing, only mountain mist and thin air. I opened the hood and looked in, but I could not see anything wrong with the engine.

All of a sudden, this young man comes out of the fog, jogging *up* the mountain. He had short hair and was wearing a Banlon shirt and shorts and running shoes—your typical conservative Joe. I had no idea where he was going or where he came from. I was sitting there, scratching my head, trying not to notice him.

As he jogged by, he looked over and, without stopping, said, "Vapor lock. Just pour some cold water on the gas line." And he kept running. So I thought, "I've got some cold water. I got it this morning." The car started right up and we kept right on going. But it showed me that the person you perceive as being your complete opposite may, in fact, have the information you need, which no one else can give you.

The point of my discussion about angels was to talk about experiences in which you have superficial perceptions of individuals in everyday waking life, but then find that there is an interior, spiritual reality to them. The moments when you need people are extraordinary moments. That is when the doors of perception open. That is when you know that even though you are conscious and awake, you are not actually in the normal everyday waking state. Some other state has captured the field, and the people who come and go now seem to have a completely different function. It is the waiter or the person taking your money in the taxicab. They are performing their regular functions, but what they say and do synchronistically appears to have more to do with the larger spiritual reality presently engaging your attention.

The Psycho-Spiritual Revolution

My book on American visionary psychology, *Shadow Culture*, is an attempt to state that there is a psychospiritual revolution going on around us that is not in the churches but is out there in culture and is popular in nature. To the dominant culture, it appears to be superficial, insignificant, and inconsequential. But take a second look. It is not new; it is old. It is part of the uniquely American tradition that has been around since the founding of the American colonies, and it is gaining strength for various reasons and influencing everything that is now happening in the heart of mainstream culture.

You cannot walk into a Star Market today here in Boston without seeing a whole-foods section. You see new bike paths in Cambridge. Think yogurt, whole wheat bread, organic foods, clean water, and health consciousness. In other words, everywhere you turn, you see signs of this revolution. The question is: Where is it coming from and what is driving it? My book is an attempt to say that there is a uniquely American visionary tradition that is part of a larger alternative-reality tradition in the West that also links us with non-Western cultures in profound ways. This alternative reality tradition is a shadow culture of Judeo-Christian Protestantism. It is still largely Anglo-Saxon, but it has deep affinities with the various American subcultures of Afro-Americans, Native Indians, Asian Americans, and Latinos in ways that the dominant culture does not. As a visionary shadow culture, it is a force still to be reckoned with.

I trace the mystical communities from the founding of the American colonies, then go through the development of the early spiritual communities such as the Shakers, Quakers, and Mennonites. Then I look at the evolution of Transcendentalism as the overarching psycho-spiritual philosophy of the 19th century. Within that over-arching framework, I examine the development of homeopathy, phrenology, mesmerism, spiritualism, mental healing, Christian Science, theosophy, and New Thought. That leads us to the late 19th century and the development of scientific psychotherapy, when scientists actually began studying the mediums and the mental healers. Although science, medicine, and psychology take a completely different turn at that particular point, heading off into reductionistic positivism, depth psychology nevertheless continued to flourish, but was pushed out into popular culture and to a large extent went underground. As I have said earlier, these are the roots of the alternative-reality tradition today, which is now generating a new kind of science.

Three things are happening: there is the dominant science and medicine of the mainstream, which remains reductionistic; there is the counter-culture tradition of folk psychology, which remains experiential; and then there is a new science of mind/body medicine. The new science is emerging not from the experimental laboratories, but at the interface between consumer demand and the delivery of clinical services.

With it, a new breed of scientists is also emerging. If you look at the experimental literature on meditation, for instance, you will note that 40 years ago, few studies of meditation were going on. No scientist practiced meditation and no studies in the subject were being funded. Today, scientific studies on meditation are being funded by the government in the millions of dollars and are being conducted by scientists who are meditation practitioners who can pass peer review in science. That represents a new generation of thinking and a new kind of scientist. This is the way the cultures of objective science and personal experience are converging. In this way, the counterculture tradition is having a profound influence on the mainstream at the level of a popular revolution. It is challenging the old top-down model, in which the laboratory is the only place true science goes on. The new revolution insists that science actually goes on at the level of personal experience. This is a whole new way of thinking to which we must now learn to adapt.

CHAPTER 16

JEFF LEVIN, PhD, MPH

The Power of Love

Known for his pioneering research on the epidemiology of religion—how religious involvement and spirituality are related to health—Jeff Levin, PhD, MPH, was trained in religion, sociology, public health, preventive medicine, and gerontology at Duke University, the University of North Carolina, the University of Texas Medical Branch, and the University of Michigan. From 1989 to 1997 he served on the faculty of the Department of Family and Community Medicine at Eastern Virginia Medical School in Norfolk, Virginia. Dr. Levin now devotes himself fulltime to his research and writing.

Dr. Levin, who has been funded by several National Institutes of Health (NIH) grants totaling more than $1 million, is a research consultant to the Institute for Research on Unlimited Love at Case Western Reserve University, and a past president of the International Society for the Study of Subtle Energies and Energy Medicine. Dr. Levin is the author of more than 130 scholarly publications and the author or editor of five books, including *God, Faith, and Health; Religion in Aging and Health; Essentials of Complementary and Alternative Medicine; Religion in the Lives of African Americans;* and *Faith Matters.*

In the spring of 1999, I interviewed Dr. Levin at his home in Kansas, where he lives with his wife, Dr. Lea Steele Levin. I was prepared for a fact-based discussion, the "statistics of spirituality," if you will. But like so many of the people I have interviewed, Dr. Levin's personal experiences with the mysterious and the mystical provided for a conversation of refreshing honesty and depth.

I am trained in social science and epidemiology and have always been drawn to the writing of a sociologist named Pitirim Sorokin (1889-1968). Dr. Sorokin was Alexander Kerensky's secretary and at one time was under sentence of death from every side during the Russian revolution. He escaped to the United States and ended up founding the sociology department at Harvard. In 1949 he received a grant from the Lilly Endowment to create a center at Harvard for the study of what he called creative altruism and began writing about love. His writing was unusual for a sociologist. He would often quote the *Vedas,* the *Upanishads,* Jesus, and the masters of all the great traditions. I encountered this work when I was a graduate student, and it interested me.

A few years ago, as I began rereading Sorokin, it struck me that social scientists and epidemiologists have pet constructs—things like type A behavior, social support, stress, coping, locus of control—that we study a lot. These are all wonderful concepts and they have helped us understand how human beings and their minds, emotions, and social relationships interact to affect health. In fact, we have tens of thousands of studies on these concepts. But there are also basic personal resources, such as love, hope, forgiveness, gratitude, and so on that we never study. There's literally no research literature in epidemiology or the medical, social, or behavioral sciences on the impact of these concepts. It's as if they don't exist.

What especially interested me about Sorokin's writing was that he had devised a typology or taxonomy of love. He talked about the various dimensions—he called them *aspects*—of love. Being a typical left-brained scientist, I was struck while rereading Sorokin's work that here was a scale waiting to be made. That was my reaction. Of all the ways I could have reacted to this material, my first thought was, "This is a scale waiting to be made."

But this was problematic for several reasons. For one, Sorokin had been dead for 30 years. If you are going to create a measurement instrument based on somebody's theoretical writing, it helps if you are able to chat with him about it, but I couldn't do that. The other problem was that Sorokin was very much against quantitative social science. He despised the idea of developing scales and indexes to measure people's attitudes about things. So wherever he is now, he probably doesn't approve of the idea of empirically studying love.

I sat down with a colleague, Dr. Bert Kaplan, emeritus professor of epidemiology at the North Carolina School of Public Health, and we spent several days reading through Sorokin and ended up writing about 70 questionnaire items based on his different dimensions of love. About this same time I ran into Dr. Marilyn Schlitz at a research conference and told her that I was interested in studying love and health. The Institute of Noetic Sciences (IONS) had its "Inner Mechanisms of Healing Response" funding program going at that point, and I ended up with a small grant.

So we developed a questionnaire and distributed it to the patients who came into the family practice clinic in the department where I was a professor.

Sorokin proposed seven dimensions of love. These were religious love, ethical love, ontological love, physical love, biological love, psychological love, and social love. Religious love, as Sorokin defined it, was about the giving of love to God or the Absolute or the Higher Power and then receiving it in return. We wrote a number of items to assess this, such as "I love God," "I feel loved by God (or a Higher Power)," and "God's love is eternal." Sorokin also spoke of ethical love, by which he meant the identification of love with other concepts such as goodness, truth, or beauty. So we took statements like "Love makes things better" and "Love is the essence of goodness" and asked to what extent people agreed with them.

Sorokin had another concept that he described as ontological love. This is an affirmation of the ability of love to unify, harmonize, and enrich people's lives—the ability to empower and elevate people. Sorokin also talked about physical love, which was an unusual concept that he described as encompassing beliefs—for example, that there is a loving energy permeating all things, that the earth is alive, and that the physical universe is loving and conscious.

Psychological love he defined as love that was given and received at the interpersonal level; it had to do with empathy, kindness, goodness, and friendship. Biological love was his term for the sexual and romantic relationship dimension. And social love, as Sorokin described it, might be construed as analogous to altruism.

Except in the cases of physical and social love, we were able to create and psychometrically validate good, reliable scales to measure these constructs.

There are more sophisticated types of psychometric analyses that I didn't include in my final report to IONS. At some point I will go back and do this so it can be published. But for now we have good, solid measures for five of the dimensions that other people eventually will be able to use and that we can use in data analyses of health and well-being.

The Outcomes

I've completed several analyses and found some very interesting things. For instance, people who are more loving—at least according to the ways we assessed it—tended to be in better health, have greater positive emotional well-being, and have significantly less negative or depressed affect. These folks also had higher self-esteem and a higher sense of self-efficacy or personal control. *(Note: These results have now been published.)*

We also found that people who scored highly on the religious love dimension—folks who affirmed that they loved God and felt loved by God, however they conceived of God—and who had a two-way loving interaction going on with this higher power, rated their health better. What was fascinating about this—and for me is still inexplicable—is that we controlled for more objective measures of health status such as current and lifetime prevalence of chronic disease, a measure of functional limitations, and an indicator of symptomatology. We controlled for various religious and spiritual items as well because we knew from my work and that of others that spirituality has a positive effect on health. So what this means is that feeling loved by and loving God or the Eternal or the Divine has a statistically significantly positive impact on people's ratings of their own health—above and beyond whatever their actual state of health is—in ways that have nothing to do with the positive health effects of religion or spirituality. In other words, the association between a loving relationship with God and one's own health was not explained by what we know about spirituality and health and was not accounted for by people's actual health status. Something else is going on here.

I have some ideas on that, but they are things that I don't know whether I can study as a medical scientist or a social scientist. I can talk about them as a person, but in doing so I am really leaving behind empirical epidemiologic research. My wife Lea and I were talking the other day about what would be a good definition of love. She said, "Qi with intent." In other words, the natural life force backed with intentionality. I thought that sounded pretty good. As I reflect on how I have experienced love in my own life, the thing that comes to mind is the love I feel for Lea and the love I receive from her. It is an essential part of my life and sometimes it is hard for me to differentiate loving God from loving Lea. We also joke that sometimes we feel so much love it is hard to tell if it is love I am giving her or love she is giving me. It all blends together.

I think love is the most fundamental human experience and expression. It is the stuff out of which reality is made. It is the actual substance, if you will, from which all of creation is manifested. I think that when we activate it, when we feel it or think about it or express it, we call into being the same forces that lovingly created the universe and created all of us. It is like a positive feedback loop. The more love we give out, the more love there is and the more we feel.

Love is also probably the one thing that humans can actually create. The Jewish mystics believed that the germ of everything was present at the creation and that God lovingly willed these things into physical form and manifestation. I believe that, but I also believe that one can always create more love; there's an inexhaustible supply. There are so many arguments and intellectual disagreements about whether consciousness or energy or intentionality describes the basic building block of reality. I think, ultimately, that love is at the foundation of all of these metaphors. It is some sort of life force with harmonious intent behind it.

I also think that something akin to love underlies the findings in the epidemiology of religion that I have written about for so many years. There are studies that show, for example, that if you go to religious services you are at less risk for hypertension. Much of that is explainable by biobehavioral or psychosocial variables. For example, people who go to religious services, on average, are more likely to receive social support and experience positive emotions. These factors, in turn, are known to promote health and well-being. But what underlies *that*?

I suppose through our research methods we can eventually become reductionistic enough to explain the health effects of human emotions and social relationships on the basis of the behavior of molecules. Sadly, molecular biology and genetics are quickly becoming the paradigm of explanation for most epidemiologists. But I believe there is something that underlies all of these findings and that it cannot be captured in a specimen dish—the idea of some type of loving spirit or consciousness that created and permeates everything. This could ultimately explain why people who love God or feel loved by God would also be less depressed and healthier.

But I suspect that there are limits to how fully we can understand this through the methods of naturalistic science. I'm not sure that social or epidemiologic research will ever really get us there. The best way to tap into universal truth is probably through meditation and intuition.

Why Study Love?

Another thing that drew me into this area was trying to understand why we found that people who were more religious or spiritual also had better health, greater well-being, less depression, and the like. Epidemiologists are good at providing evidence of associations—answering the "what" question—but less anxious to tackle these sorts of "how" or "why" questions. The way a social epidemiologist is trained to answer the *why* question is to ask a bunch of additional questions about other concepts—called *mediating factors*—and then control for their effects statistically. That provides one sort of answer to the question of what underlies a spirituality-health link, but it is not really all that satisfactory.

The problem, of course, is that if we don't think up a concept, create a measure based on it, and ask the questions and analyze the data, we can never find that part of the equation. So if we never ask people about their feelings of love or whether they love God or other people, for example, then obviously we can never include that information in our logistic regression models of religious effects on mortality, morbidity, or whatever we are looking at. And until that changes, that is why we can never find that love plays a significant part.

The way the epidemiologic research establishment works is that if there is no evidence that something is part of the equation, because no one has ever looked at it before, then it is difficult to justify including it in a study protocol. What's worse, no one will fund you to include it because there is no evidence that it has anything to do with the topic at hand. So someone has to be the first person to say, "We ought to study this link." Of course, if that happens, you aren't going to get any NIH [National Institutes of Health] money or any other big grant. So I really lucked into the IONS funding. And, in the end, we found that love indeed has everything to do with our health and well-being.

My goal with this pilot study is just to get love on the table, so to speak, the same way that religion and spirituality have finally been put there. My desire is that some day scientists will ask people about love and that it will be sought in medical history-taking and included in clinical study protocols and other research designs along with social support and cholesterol and everything else. It will just be one of the things we normally think of as having to do with our health and well-being.

Can Love Be Increased?

This was basically a social survey and not a clinical intervention study. The respondents were people who came in for routine preventive visits at the primary care clinic. But to answer the question of how to increase love in someone's life, I can only reflect on what has occurred in my own life and in terms of what we found in the study. People who responded that they had more love in their lives, that they gave and received more love and perceived more love in their lives, were people who were more likely to be part of functional and wholesome networks and who had positive interpersonal relationships. Does one thing cause the other? I don't know, but it is interesting that people who reported less satisfactory family relationships, for one, didn't score as high on the psychological love dimension. People who had an active devotional life, however defined—whether they prayed, read the Bible, or watched religious television—and who had a personal spiritual life, also reported that they experienced more love in their lives.

Now, the effects of social relationships and spirituality on health make a lot of sense to me. We have tons of evidence that being integrated into supportive social networks is a very important factor for health. Having an active spiritual life is also very important. It doesn't surprise me that the relationship between love and health might be understood in those terms.

However, we didn't find a difference between people who were married or not or in a relationship with a romantic partner or not. High scores on the various other dimensions of love seem to correlate well with health, well-being, and self-esteem, but scores on the biological dimension—the romantic, sexual aspect—sometimes went in the opposite direction. So it appears that if our only conception of love has to do with the relationship between sexual partners, then we are missing many other types of human experiences that could be called love. These dimensions may even be inversely related to each other, in terms of the level of importance people attach to them and their salience for general well-being.

According to Sorokin, the "physical" aspects of love are beliefs such as "the earth is a living organism." At first it was difficult for me to see why he considered these beliefs to be a subdimension of love. It didn't seem to fit with the other dimensions. But the questions we asked do make for an interesting scale. You might call it a scale of belief in consciousness. The respondents rated statements like "When I look at nature I see harmony" and "Earth is a living being" and "There is an energy or force that runs through all things." These statements seem to tap into the Gaia hypothesis, the belief in a subtle bioenergy, and belief that the earth itself is conscious. I did a preliminary analysis, and the people who endorsed these beliefs experienced, across the board, more love according to virtually every other dimension.

They also had better health, less psychological distress, greater self-esteem, greater feelings of mastery, greater spirituality, and, interestingly, they were less likely to be publicly religious. Looking at it from the flip side, people who didn't endorse these metaphysical views had lower self-esteem, were not as healthy, were more depressed, and were less spiritual but were more active in organized religion.

I would call these beliefs part of an emerging worldview. What I found was rather encouraging—endorsing this worldview seems to be a factor that predicts greater adjustment emotionally and a deeper sense of spirituality. It also suggests that organized religious activity may tend to "inoculate" against both a greater experience of love and a belief in seeing the earth as a living, conscious being. This is rather disconcerting to me—I'm very involved in and supportive of organized religion—but our results seem clear.

For sure, many other studies have found that people who have personal devotion and are intrinsically religious as opposed to extrinsically religious are better adjusted and have a greater sense of self-efficacy and self-esteem. But if somebody's religious expression comes exclusively through a once-a-week participation in which they sit passively and are dictated to, then it is not surprising that, on some of these measures of love or new paradigm worldviews, they might not score as high. But I don't wish to bash organized religion. I would score high on any scale of "organizational religiousness."

Clearly, these findings do not mean that if people stop going to church they will be healthier. In fact, all the research I've done shows just the opposite. But we found that people who have a more holistic or multidimensional approach to their spiritual lives do the best. There are some health effects that accrue from simply affiliating with a church or synagogue, but just because people go once a week doesn't really tell us why they go or what they do when they are there. It doesn't mean that they actively take part in worship. There are so many other dimensions of spiritual expression such as active participation in religious groups, worshiping God, prayer, devotional practices, affirming certain religious beliefs or spiritual worldviews, and actively having a sense of faith or commitment to a set of values. Then there are experiences like the *siddhis* spoken of by Patañjali in the *Yoga Sutras,* the gifts of the spirit that some charismatic Christians are blessed with, and numinous or mystical feelings of grace or union with the Divine accessible through spiritual practices such as meditation. My sense is that there are ways people can engage the spiritual domain of life much more completely than by simply showing up at a building. By complementing public worship with other forms of expression, people can derive much more benefit in other aspects of their life.

Science and God

Science is afraid of God because God is the adversary.

To many scientists, science *is* their God. That is a very disturbing thought. I think it is important to distinguish between what many scientists believe as part of their own worldview and this idea of science with a capital S. There is no reason that science can't engage God, think about God, or investigate what people feel about God or anything else. But people who call themselves scientists and who are trained in the physical, natural, social, or behavioral sciences typically exclude God. My experience from being in academic medicine for many years is that many physicians and scientists do not believe in God. Moreover, they think that belief in God or in a spiritual reality is pathological, that it is something to be eradicated and perhaps even treated by drugs.

In the years when I was actively researching religious and spiritual factors in health, I encountered various responses. The first response was that there is nothing there—that there is no evidence that any of this is connected. Then, when clinicians began to discover that these things were very important in their patients' lives, the sense was, "Well, maybe this is important to my patients, but it is not important to me, so it probably doesn't really matter." I think that is still a commonly held sentiment among physicians.

But I like to think it is changing. The general public believes that their physical, emotional, mental, and spiritual lives are intertwined. And because so many scientists and doctors still don't believe this, ultimately people are just going to start ignoring them. We scientists are very self-important. We think that what we as scientists believe is of the utmost importance and has the highest meaning. But, really, most people couldn't care less.

For science to begin to acknowledge and appreciate the potential contributions of spirituality, love, hope, and similar concepts could have a tremendous impact on the world because it would eventually change the way physicians and other practitioners go about investigating health and illness and practicing healing. Because of the work of Dr. Larry Dossey, Dr. Herb Benson, and others, and books like Dr. Dale Matthews's *The Faith Factor,* some healthcare practitioners who do believe that these concepts are important in people's lives now feel that they have permission to inquire about them with patients. Some scientists are now asking these questions, and studies are showing that these things are important for health and well-being. As a result, new generations of medical, nursing, and allied health students will be taught that these things are important. Slowly, perceptions about the determinants of health will change and thus what it means to be a human being will change.

Right now the prevailing scientific view is that humans are just a sack of bones jangling about in a chemical soup. Most people I interacted with in academic medicine probably don't even believe that there is such thing as a mind. They think it is just an epiphenomenon of neurochemicals. But for people who came of age in the last 20 years, the idea that the body and mind are interrelated and that our emotions, thoughts, and beliefs affect our health is becoming noncontroversial. I think the same thing will happen with the idea of a body-mind-spirit nexus. And I would include things like love under that rubric as well. But it will take some years, because, as Max Planck once said, "A new scientific truth doesn't triumph by convincing its opponents and making them see the light, but rather because its opponents eventually die, and a new generation grows up that is familiar with it."[1]

Subtle Energy

The International Society for the Study of Subtle Energy and Energy Medicine (ISSSEEM) was organized to promote the study of the basic sciences and medical and therapeutic applications of subtle human bioenergy. This work draws on research at the interface of consciousness, spirituality, complementary and alternative medicine, parapsychology, psychophysiology, bioelectromagnetics, and other fields. In a nutshell, subtle energies and energy medicine is a very multidisciplinary field. I doubt there is a common worldview among members, though I imagine the membership would endorse the idea that body, mind, and spirit are all components of a human life and that all these factors interrelate with what Elmer and Alyce Green have called "extrapersonal" and "transpersonal" factors to affect our health and well-being.

A survey was done of the membership several years ago. If I recall, it asked individual members whether they had ever had a massage, been to a healer, had an out-of-body experience, done biofeedback, and on and on. Out of three dozen questions like that, I remember checking yes to about 33 of them. I thought, "My God, I'm really out there." When I mentioned this to Penny Hiernu, the Society's CEO, she said, "What are you talking about? Ninety-nine percent of our members checked all of them." So maybe there is a common worldview after all.

My one concern has always been that the concept of subtle energy is rather limiting. My feeling is that it is a useful metaphor but that ultimately the idea that everything can be explained by or understood in terms of some type of physical energy—as opposed to, say, consciousness or spirit—will hold us back.

According to Jewish tradition there is one God, a supernatural being or presence who created the universe *ex nihilo* and who transcends its creation. This Oneness created consciousness, and then consciousness went out and manifested as matter by radiating energy. So here you have a perspective that encompasses a supernatural God, consciousness, subtle energy, matter, and physical reality, and all of these concepts get along just fine and interconnect, interrelate, and emanate from each other in all sorts of ways. And energy is certainly part of the picture. So whereas it's not the whole story, the subtle energy metaphor is certainly useful. And for understanding things like proximal noncontact healing, it seems to be a reasonable explanation or model. We know through both instrumentation and the experience of mystics and intuitives that we have—or rather are made up of—energy fields. Intuitives can perceive them, and people who do healing can feel them. But I don't think it's the best or most parsimonious explanation, for instance, for the kind of nonlocal healing that Larry Dossey talks about.

---

[1]Planck M: *Scientific autobiography and other papers* (Gaynor F, transl.). New York, 1949, Philosophical Library.

How Much Do We Need to Understand?

Trying to understand every single type of healing or every single thing that occurs in nature by any one particular model really screws us up. In a sense, I think this is where the allopathic biomedical model has gone wrong. Its presumptions cannot help us understand things like distant prayer or even why love of God influences health status. Its tendency is to just deny that these things happen. My concern is that in the complementary and alternative medicine field, a paradigmatic worldview is coalescing exclusively around concepts like qi or prana or consciousness. We should not try to fit everything that we encounter into a single conceptual straitjacket. We would be better off maintaining a little humility and not thinking that we can come up with perfect models or equations to understand all things.

For instance, this has led to problems in acknowledging the success of homeopathy. We know that homeopathy works in certain situations, but because there is no single understanding of the mechanism involved that everyone can agree on—no consensus—the skeptical response is just to say there is nothing happening, even though something most certainly is. It is the same with prayer. We have double-blind trials that show that distant prayer works, but we can't completely explain it or account for all the variants in it on the basis of mechanistic theories—even "woo-woo" theories. So until there is some type of explanation that suits everybody, people who choose not to believe will simply not believe.

Of course, people don't typically believe because of a study; they believe because of an experience. There have been hundreds of studies showing the relationship among religion, spirituality, and health. And there is this evangelistic sense among a lot of my colleagues in this field that if we just keep publishing more studies, others will finally believe. I have long contended that there could be an infinite number of studies, that almost every scientist in the world could do nothing but publish on this topic, but there still wouldn't be enough evidence for some folks because they would have to rethink their entire worldview, and they're afraid to do that.

If I hadn't had experiences in my own life that involved spiritual questing and physical healing, I probably wouldn't believe it either. I read somewhere that in many cases the specialty choice of doctors usually has something to do with issues in their own lives. People who have heart disease in their family often become cardiologists, and so on. For me, my own experiences no doubt drove my choice of a research focus.

My Personal Journey

I had an experience when I was working on my comprehensive exams for my PhD. I was living in Galveston, Texas, attending the University of Texas Medical Branch, and the day I began my comps there was a big storm. I was wearing flipflops and running to grab a bite to eat. I had just been given my exams and had a week to complete them and turn them in. I ended up slipping down a set of concrete stairs and hit my back on every step, landing on the ground with my elbows. I was numb for a while but eventually was able to move my legs. I had broken my ribs and the bursae in both elbows.

The doctors told me it would take 6 weeks to heal. I called my mom, who is a healer and part of the Spiritual Emergence Network. She mobilized a group of people—Jews, Christians, Buddhists, New Agers, yogis, psychics, nuns, you name it. Some prayed; some visualized or sent energy; some loved me; some did ritual work; some left their body; and God knows what. A day and a half later I was better. But I was afraid to go back to school because I thought they would see me without the slings on my arm and think I had faked the whole thing to buy more time on my exams. So I devised a plan to wear the slings and then, after a week, take them off and announce that I was better because I had meditated and people had prayed. This was still an amazingly quick time frame to have healed, and my professors thought it was remarkable, but at least it was within the realm of acceptability, even if barely so. They could accept that instead of 6 weeks the healing took a week, but they would never have believed a day and a half. It would have been outside their realm of possibility, and I imagine I would have been kicked out of school.

I have hesitated to talk publicly about some of my more unusual experiences because I suspect it may interfere with acceptance of my research among certain more religiously conservative audiences, but what the heck? I am trying to be more authentic, so here goes.

I had another experience when I was a graduate student in Galveston. Back when I was 20, I had spent some time during the summer at an ashram and began meditating and doing yoga. I soon let it all slide and regressed back into a normal bachelor's life. By the time I was in graduate school, several years later, I was content just living at the beach, drinking beer, and eating chicken-fried steak. One night I went to see a movie at the mall. It was *Back to the Future*. I was driving home from the theater in my pickup truck on a back road near the wharf when all of a sudden the inside of my truck started glowing violet. Honest. I thought there was a fire somewhere, so I rolled down my window and looked out. But there was no fire. So I thought, "Cool, I'm having one of those experiences I've read about."

I didn't freak out and crash the truck or think I was going mad or anything like that. I knew that violet was the color of the highest chakra and I was thinking, "Okay, I'm having the thing where the air goes violet." It was very exciting. I tried to wave it away, and it didn't go. Windshield wipers? Nope. Blinking my eyes real fast? Uh-uh. So I pulled the truck over and turned it off and just sat there. Eventually, I restarted the truck and drove on and the color began to fade out, but right before I was supposed to make the turn to go home, a thought came into my mind to turn right and go to this other mall. So I did. I ended up in the bookstore and went over to the section labeled Eastern Philosophy or whatever they used to call it. Of all things, a Ruth Montgomery book fell off the shelf at my feet. It was one of her books that talked about walk-ins and aliens and things like that. I thought, "Oh my God." But I read it and ended up reading all of her books and then every book I could find on Kabbalah and whatever other metaphysical topics were on the shelves of bookstores in Galveston, Houston, and Dallas. I started meditating again and, through various synchronicities, ended up back in synagogue after an absence of many years. All of this happened when I was 26 years old, which is interesting because the number 26 in *gematria,* or Cabbalistic numerology, represents the numeric value of the name of God. A very auspicious age for "initiation," I suppose.

Another experience with altered consciousness: I lived in Virginia Beach for 8 years and had a friend who owned a flotation tank business. I floated nearly every week and had just about every type of experience you could have. Once, I believe I bilocated.

It happened while I was on a dry flotation table. Music was piped up through the table adjacent to each chakra, and I was simultaneously hooked up to one of the Edgar Cayce radial appliances. I slowly shifted consciousness and found myself, I swear, in Tiger Stadium in Detroit in line to get tickets for popcorn. The Tigers were playing the Yankees that day.

This was the same day, same time. It wasn't a normal dream because I didn't fall asleep. I was in my body, and then I felt a little "poof." But it wasn't a typical out-of-body experience either, because I was in line there, and people were interacting with me. I had a corporeal form; I wasn't just some astral body floating around going through the walls. I remember looking out on the field; the players were warming up, and there was a clock, and it read 1:15 PM. After a moment or so, poof, I was back in my body on the table. I thought, "Well, that was weird." When I checked the clock, it was 1:20 PM. At the time, I lived in Virginia and didn't follow the Detroit Tigers. I couldn't have cared less about them and didn't even know whether they were playing that day or not. But after I went home I found out that they did indeed have a game that day against the Yankees and that the first pitch was scheduled for 1:30 PM.

I think these experiences are just part of human life and part of what it means to be a human.

I don't try to analyze or interpret them as a scientist, in terms of mechanisms because I'm not sure how valuable it would be to do that. I once published a paper documenting the national prevalence of psi experiences in people's lives, without much explanation. I did so because I think that simply documenting them and showing that they are part of what it means to be human is enough. The sense that something isn't real until we have broken it down into pieces to "understand" it is bizarre. To me, being a scientist is a sacred calling. It is a calling to try to examine reality, document what is going on, and, if possible, try to understand it. If we can't understand it, then we should just encounter it, document it, and see it for what it is.

Next Steps

I would like to begin investigating physiological and psychophysiological correlates of love and actually find some way to assess love as it happens, so to speak, perhaps by studying people who are in the midst of loving, feeling love, or having loving experiences. I'm not talking about measuring brain chemistry, necessarily, but examining whether there may be effects on various physiological systems and on outcomes like overall health, physical functioning, and emotional well-being.

Neurochemistry, *per se,* is not my primary interest. Moreover, the idea that the mind is something that exists or happens solely inside the brain is a strange notion. As for what and where the mind is, the theosophical view is that there are interpenetrating, overlapping subtle bodies. We have an etheric template, an astral or emotional body, and a mental body. The mental body is the part of us that vibrationally contains our thoughts and thought forms.

In that sense, what we see with our eyes when we look at a human being is only the densest precipitation of matter. The body is what we manifest as in the third density or dimension. But there are other parts of us energetically that go all over. The third-dimensional manifestation is simply where our physical sensations are "contained," if we can use that term. Our emotions are contained in another part, as are our thoughts. So when we try to remember something or are gauging thoughts, it does not occur "in here" in the brain. It does not occur "out there" either but in some different kind of place.

CHAPTER 17

DAVID LUKOFF, PhD

The Importance of Spirituality in Mental Health

David Lukoff, PhD, is a licensed psychologist in California, and professor of psychology at Saybrook Graduate School and Research Center in San Francisco. The author of more than 50 articles and chapters on spiritual issues and mental health, he is also co-author of the *(Diagnostic and Statistical Manual)* DSM-IV category "Religious or Spiritual Problem."

Dr. Lukoff trained in psychology and anthropology at the University of Chicago, Harvard, and Loyola University of Chicago, and has been a member of the faculties of Harvard, the University of California-Los Angeles (UCLA), the UCLA Neuropsychiatric Clinical Research Center for Schizophrenia, Oxnard College, California Institute of Integral Studies, and the Institute of Transpersonal Psychology.

An avid fan of the Internet, Dr. Lukoff is also the webmaster of the Online Guide to the Transpersonal Internet and the Spiritual Emergency Resource Center, both of which offer self-help and professional resources for spiritual problems. He recently founded Internet Guided Learning to promote the use of online learning in the area of spirituality and mental health.

In keeping with Dr. Lukoff's interest in the Internet, in the Fall of 2000, I interviewed him via e-mail and the World Wide Web.

For the past 30 years, transpersonal psychology has explored experiences in which the sense of identity extends beyond (hence, *trans*) the individual or personal to encompass wider aspects of humankind, the natural world, or the cosmos. Such states are notoriously difficult to study, as William James pointed out in his classic book *Exceptional Human States*. But James's philosophy of radical empiricism argued that a true science must be based on the study of all human experiences, not just those that can be manipulated in a laboratory. The discipline of transpersonal psychology attempts to study reports of transpersonal experiences and behaviors scientifically, using both quantitative and qualitative methods.

Transpersonal psychologists have been particularly interested in the experiences and practices of the great religious traditions. Other important topics have been altered states of consciousness and spiritual issues in mental health. Transpersonal psychologists have avoided judging the reported phenomena exclusively by the standards of normal science and consider whether certain unusual states point to human possibilities that are alternatives to or even superior to ordinary functioning.

These are topics that have been assiduously avoided by mainstream psychology for the past 80 years since behaviorism took a stranglehold on academic psychology. But there has been a significant shift in the field of psychology toward openness to transpersonal phenomena and clinical approaches within the positive psychology movement. Martin Seligman, PhD, former president of the prestigious American Psychological Association (APA) and well known for his work on helplessness and depression, recently stated that spirituality and religion have a "major role" to play in addressing the epidemic of depression that swept across the United States and other countries in the 20th century.

One way spirituality can significantly affect depression is by fostering positive beliefs and behaviors while ameliorating the effect of negative ones, thereby remaining consistent with positive psychology's focus on improving life quality and meaning. Maslow, a founder of the transpersonal psychology movement, and Carl Rogers, one of the founders of the humanistic psychology movement, argued for the investigation of the positive aspects of mental health some 30 years ago, but Seligman has taken a very empirical approach that speaks to the powers that be in the scientific and research worlds.

Of course, there have been hundreds of studies demonstrating the health benefits of religion, and there are also several spiritual well-being scales already in wide use that have demonstrated validity. I am all for quantitative approaches to transpersonal topics, though I consider such methods to be limited in their capacity to deepen understanding of the phenomenon. Stan Krippner has described how similar the therapeutic objectives are of the Brazilian healers he studied, who perform exorcisms, to therapists who do cognitive modification to alter negative thinking patterns. I think we have much to learn from indigenous and religious traditions about healing—and most spiritual practices have something profound to contribute about how to be happy.

That is another virtue of transpersonal psychology—its focus on the need for personal experience with the transpersonal dimension and the importance of having a spiritual discipline. My experience over the past 12 years has been the mind-body-spirit practice of aikido. I think it would be quite difficult to use transpersonal therapeutic approaches without some grounding in a spiritual practice. This also sets transpersonal psychology apart from the mainstream. Some transpersonal psychology graduate schools—such as the Institute for Transpersonal Psychology, Saybrook, and the Naropa Institute—actually require that students follow a spiritual practice in some programs. I am sure that none of the graduate schools approved by the American Psychology Association have such a requirement.

Spiritual Emergencies

Spiritual emergencies are crises during which the process of growth and change becomes chaotic and overwhelming. Individuals in such episodes often suddenly and dramatically enter into new realms of mystical and spiritual experience. However, they may also become fearful and confused and have difficulty coping with their daily lives, jobs, and relationships.

Sometimes such experiences result from intensive involvement with spiritual practices such as meditation or yoga. In the West, the connection between spiritual practices and psychological problems was first noted 50 years ago by an Italian psychiatrist, Roberto Assagioli, known primarily as the founder of psychosynthesis. He described how people may feel especially inflated and grandiose as a result of intense spiritual experiences. But teachers of Asian spiritual practices have known and written about this for hundreds of years. One term used in the Zen tradition to refer to this type of pitfall on the spiritual path is "the stink of enlightenment."

Stanislav Grof, a psychiatrist and previous scholar in residence at Esalen, and his wife, Christina, coined the term "spiritual emergency" and founded the Spiritual Emergency Network in 1980 to identify and make referrals to therapists of individuals who were experiencing psychological difficulties associated with spiritual practices and spontaneous spiritual experiences.

Basically, spiritual awakening is often a tumultuous process, but it is not a sign of mental illness. A recent survey showed that the vast majority of therapists today do not consider mystical experiences to be psychopathological, but this is a change from the past views of Freud, Albert Ellis, and other leading psychological theorists who viewed religious experiences as psychopathological. Mystical experiences can be overwhelming and disruptive but once integrated, often lead to positive transformation of the person's health, spiritual well-being, and relationships. Allen Bergin, PhD, a psychologist and author of several books on spirituality in therapy, described the power of such spiritual emergencies as the mental equivalent of nuclear energy. They have tremendous healing power for the individual—and even for society—but can also be destructive if not channeled properly.

I have written several case studies of individuals who had such overwhelming spiritual experiences and were hospitalized and medicated for months ("Myths in Mental Illness" in the *Journal of Transpersonal Psychology*). Later, it became clear that these were positively transformative experiences. We can do much better for such people by creating a safe therapeutic environment for them to be able to go safely through the experience. Russell Shorto's book *Saints and Madmen* describes how I have worked with spiritual emergency patients over the past 20 years by providing confirmation, radical respect, and witness to the significance of the changes.

To set a context for my work, it is useful to know that I went through such an experience myself, back in 1971. Triggered by my first LSD (lysergic acid diethylamide) experience, I spent 2 months convinced that I was a reincarnation of Buddha and Christ, and wrote a 47-page holy book to unite the world around a new universal religion that I would create. Seemed like a good idea at the time.

Fortunately, I was not hospitalized or medicated. My friends provided food and shelter and spent time just talking to me. I really feel quite grateful that I was allowed to go through the full experience. It is a touchstone experience in my life and set me on a spiritual journey.

I needed to understand what happened to me. How could this Jewish boy (I was 23 at the time) have believed himself to be Buddha and Christ, about whom I really knew very little? I entered Jungian analysis, read, and listened to Joseph Campbell tapes and went to many of his workshops to enable me to understand the experience. I also worked with shamans and Native American medicine chiefs who helped me to integrate this experience and taught me how to control entry and exit from such ecstatic states.

I also became a psychologist, but that didn't help me to understand my experience. The language in psychology is a discourse about psychopathology. When I started graduate school in psychology in 1974, I learned that my experience would have been diagnosed as schizophrenia in the *Diagnostic and Statistical Manual*, 2nd edition (*DSM-II*). In the *DSM-IV*, it meets the criteria for a hallucinogen-induced psychotic disorder. But I consider it my spiritual awakening. And obviously those two rather different interpretations would lead to different treatment approaches.

Kundalini

Kundalini awakening is probably the most common type of spiritual emergency seen in clinical practice. The *Spiritual Emergence Network Newsletter* reported that 24% of their hotline calls concerned kundalini awakening experiences. In the Hindu tradition, kundalini is spiritual energy presumed to reside at the base of the spine. When it is awakened, it rises like a serpent up the spine and opens the chakra psychic centers situated along the spine from the tailbone to the top of the head. The opening of the chakras is accompanied by consciousness expansion.

However, individuals not prepared for the sudden onset of these experiences can become confused and disoriented by the many physical symptoms. Sensations of heat, tremors, involuntary laughing or crying, talking in tongues, gastrointestinal distress, and animal-like movements and sounds can all be part of this syndrome. Kundalini awakening can resemble many disorders, medical as well as psychiatric. But here, too, the outcome is likely to be positive if the person's experience is validated and guided.

Spiritual teachers know how to do this. Jack Kornfield described a person who underwent a kundalini awakening at an intensive meditation retreat. Jack is both a psychologist and a seasoned meditation teacher, but I think it was his training in meditation practice that led him to know how to help the person through the experience. When the participant in the silent retreat charged into the dining room and began yelling that he saw everyone's past lives and demonstrating karate maneuvers at triple speed, Kornfield recognized that the symptoms were related to the meditation practice rather than signs of a manic episode (for which they also meet all the diagnostic criteria except duration). Under Jack's supervision, the meditation community handled the situation by stopping the man's meditation practice and starting him jogging 10 miles in the morning and afternoon. His diet was changed to include red meat, which is thought to have a grounding effect. They got him to take frequent hot baths and showers and to dig in the garden. One person was with him all the time. After three days, he was able to sleep again and was allowed to start meditating again, slowly and carefully.

This type of spiritual emergency most commonly occurs as an unintentional side effect of yoga, meditation, qigong, or other intensive spiritual practice. Some theorists include psychotherapy, giving birth, unrequited love, sorrow, high fever, and drug experiences as other triggers, and some believe kundalini awakening can occur spontaneously without apparent cause. I agree with Bonnie Greenwell, PhD—a transpersonal therapist whose research and clinical work focuses on kundalini awakening problems—that the term *kundalini* is most applicable to problems specifically associated with meditative practices. Appendix I of the *DSM-IV* includes "qigong psychotic reaction," which is similar to kundalini awakening.

Cross-Cultural Perspectives

Possession is actually a common experience in many cultures, but in Western industrialized cultures such experiences are not normative and may lead to inappropriate diagnoses of dissociative or psychotic disorders. One of the difficulties in this clinical area is that some forms of possession are linked to mental disorders, so training in differential diagnosis is a necessity for therapists to be able to make treatment decisions.

Mircea Eliade, the great scholar of comparative religion, described how psychotic-like episodes often serve as the initiatory illness that calls a person into shamanism. In his classic book on shamanic cultures, *Shamanism*, that brought this vital therapeutic modality to the attention of the West, he states: "The future shaman sometimes takes the risk of being mistaken for a 'madman'. . .but his 'madness' fulfills a mystic function."[1] Anthropological accounts show that babbling confused words, displaying curious eating habits, singing continuously, dancing wildly, and being "tormented by spirits" are common elements in shamanic initiatory crises. In shamanic cultures, such crises are interpreted as an indication of an individual's destiny to become a shaman, rather than a sign of mental illness. Other experiences seem more universal, such as near-death experiences and visionary experiences.

Some people who have such experiences are future poets, visionaries, and even social leaders. John Perry, MD, the Jungian analyst who, in the 1970s, founded an innovative treatment called Diabysis for first-episode psychotic patients, treated such people as visionaries in the making. He tried to facilitate the movement and expression of their psychotic experiences to a personally meaningful resolution. Some visions occur at a very personal level. I think my utopian vision was this type and applied only to me. But others currently in our mental institutions are

---

[1]Eliade M: *Shamanism: archaic techniques of ecstasy* (W. Trask, transl.). New York, 1963, Harper & Row.

visionaries. Some are clearly highly creative individuals. Kay Redfield Jamison, PhD, a professor of psychiatry at Johns Hopkins University, conducted research showing the genetic connections between high creativity, such as that found among distinguished award-winning poets, playwrights, visual artists, and bipolar disorder. As a bioethics committee member of the Human Genome Project, she has warned against the long-term effect of trying to eradicate bipolar disorder because of its demonstrated association with creativity and leadership.

The DSM-IV

I began working with the Spiritual Emergency Network in 1980, and the proposal grew out of our work to increase the competence of mental health professionals in working with spiritual issues. In 1990, Francis Lu, a clinical professor of psychiatry at University of California-San Francisco; Robert Turner, a psychiatrist in private practice; and I took on the task of getting a new diagnostic category for spiritual emergence problems into the upcoming fourth edition of the *Diagnostic and Statistical Manual,* the book that everyone half-jokingly calls the Bible of mental illness. It has a profound effect on treatment and training of health professionals, and so we set out knowing there would be a few years of work involved and that it could end up going nowhere.

As many have documented, creating or eliminating diagnostic categories is, at least to some degree, a political decision. Remember that the *DSM-IV* is really the American Psychiatric Association's own document. They appoint all the committees with only minimal cross-disciplinary representation, and the APA Press publishes the book. Really, the *DSM* is a little industry in itself, with casebooks, treatment manuals, pocket guides, and so on. Given the dominance of the APA in the creation of the *DSM,* we knew that getting support of committees inside the APA was critical.

To build support for adding a new diagnostic category, we expanded the range of clinical problems to include religious problems. We got the support of the APA's Religion and Psychiatry Committee and also the Task Force on Subcultural Issues. Our proposal for the category was submitted in 1992. It was based on an extensive literature review documenting case studies on and surveys about the frequent occurrence of religious and spiritual issues in clinical practice. To add to the political dynamics of the process, another key event was when the *Journal of Nervous and Mental Disease* published our entire proposal. It was their lead article, and this helped the proposal's credibility. We made sure the entire *DSM-IV* Task Force received copies of the article, which appeared a few weeks before they would be meeting to make a decision about this new diagnostic category.

Articles on this new category appeared in *The New York Times,* the *San Francisco Chronicle, Psychiatric News,* and the *APA Monitor,* where it was described as indicating an important shift in the mental health profession's stance toward religion and spirituality.

As we had proposed, the category is listed not in the section on "Mental Disorders" but in the section reserved for "Other Conditions That are the Focus of Clinical Attention." Bereavement is listed in the same section, because it, too, is disruptive to a person's functioning but is a normal reaction to an extreme loss. Spiritual emergencies are also disruptive, but they are normal reactions to certain kinds of intense spiritual experiences. Elisabeth Targ, MD, a psychiatrist on staff at California Pacific Medical Center, mentioned in a talk at a conference on spirituality and mental health that a patient admitted to their inpatient psychiatric unit had been discharged with "Religious or Spiritual Problem" as the diagnosis. That's the first use of the diagnostic category in an inpatient setting of which I'm aware.

But the category actually is much broader. It covers religious problems such as loss of faith, changing denominations, and leaving a cult. It also covers religious and spiritual issues that arise in treating mental disorders. The *DSM-IV* specifically allows for problems to be diagnosed even when they are related to a mental disorder. Thus a person in a manic episode who has religious delusions would receive this diagnosis if the treatment addressed his or her religious beliefs. I have used this diagnosis in my work at the San Francisco Veterans Affairs Medical Center with patients in substance abuse treatment when their relationship with a higher power is a focus of therapy. Therapists working with health issues are dealing with these issues routinely. I have led a number of pain management and chronic illness groups in which I used religious and spiritual beliefs and practices as potential coping resources, such as meditation and prayer. When patients' beliefs and past experiences make it difficult to access these resources, such as when they believe their illness is a punishment, then this diagnostic category is also appropriate.

However, the category is not that widely used. Economics is another driving force in diagnostic usage, and insurance companies do not generally reimburse for nonmental disorders. But it has had a major effect on training. Psychiatric residency programs now must demonstrate that their training addresses religious and spiritual issues. The APA has published three major books on this topic in the past two years, though it has not mandated training on this type of cultural competence. Interestingly, nursing has had an ongoing recognition of this component of treatment. In the several literature reviews we published, the nursing journals had many more articles on spirituality than did the psychiatry and psychology journals. And "Spiritual Distress" was first recognized as a nursing diagnosis back in 1983, a decade before it was recognized in psychiatry.

I think the *DSM-IV* category does reflect a major paradigm shift with spirituality being recognized as a part of mental health. Of course, it starts with the problems, but increasingly the benefits are also being recognized. It is amazing to me how widespread the use of meditation in healthcare settings has become. Thirty years ago just a few transpersonal psychologists were exploring its applications in healthcare.

How Mental Health Affects Physical Health

In the clinical sciences and healthcare, there has been an acceptance over the past 20 years of the significant role that mental health plays in physical well-being. This journal [*Alternative Therapies in Health and Medicine*] has certainly played a role in raising awareness of the health benefits of mental activities such as visualization and meditation. The danger is that there is a tendency to reduce these practices to brief interventions and to leave out the spiritual dimension.

Mind-body techniques can be prescribed like a medication, done mechanically, and have minimal effect even though a regimen is followed. I believe there must be a soul connection to the mind-body therapies, a belief in their potency, in the value of the technique, respect for the teacher of the technique—all the same factors that go into creating an effective therapeutic alliance. The National Center for Complementary and Alternative Medicine considers religion and spirituality to be a type of mind-body medicine, but it seems it needs a category of its own.

Meditation is the first spiritual intervention to break through into mainstream healthcare. Meditation is now widely taught at mainstream clinics such as Kaiser Permanente in the Bay Area as a technique for relaxing the body and calming the mind. Thirty years ago, articles on the beneficial effects of meditation appeared only in the *Journal of Transpersonal Psychology*. It was still considered a religious practice, not appropriate for healthcare settings. I think the shift was initiated by the pioneering work of Herbert Benson at Harvard Medical School. He demonstrated the benefits of meditation for several medical conditions. He argues that medicine must incorporate self-care methods like prayer and meditation because God is good for us, and it doesn't matter from a health point of view whether God exists or not—there are clear health benefits to believing. And if God happens to exist, all the better, he says.

That's the mind-body practitioner still holding on to the intellectually unassailable agnostic stance. I am more of a transpersonal therapist. In most clinical situations, I want to promote a spiritual connection. However, not on any one particular path. I support patients who are Jehovah's Witnesses or any other tradition in their faith. But techniques such as meditation inherently are something more. They create the opportunity for the meditator to experience a connection with something larger. Mind-body techniques all have parallels, if not in their origins, in ancient spiritual practices. I think for the mind-body technique to be effective, the therapist must be sensitive to its spiritual origins and dimensions.

In other words, over time, engaging in practices like meditation, yoga, t'ai chi, and their offshoots into aerobics, dance, and other such activities will lead to spiritual experiences (and occasional spiritual emergencies). How much of the benefit for the hypertensive meditator is derived from the physiological training to lower arousal, and how much comes from the deepening satisfaction that comes from meditation-related spiritual well-being, which is also known to be associated with lower hypertension?

Surveys show that people want spiritual interventions from their health professionals. Yet the therapeutic potential of spirituality has been neglected. Spiritual interventions are not a standard part of the curriculum in mental health training programs (with the exception of a few programs affiliated with a religious institution). I think professional programs are not sure how to integrate spiritual competence into the curriculum. Many conferences on exactly this topic, as well as books, are now appearing, so this field is clearly evolving. The Templeton Foundation has funded the development of dozens of programs on religion and spirituality in medical schools. I think over time this will have an impact on the healthcare system.

One of the keys to acceptance of spiritual interventions will be finding appropriate practices and language that can be widely shared in secular healthcare settings. Even spiritual teachers aren't sure how to approach this. I share the Dalai Lama's view that we must find—all of us together—a new spirituality. This new concept ought to be elaborated alongside the religions in such a way that all people of good will could adhere to it.

Moments of silence are one of the most universally accepted ways to create a sacredness to a period of time or event. Invoking Christ or any other denominational religious figure in a secular healthcare setting is not appropriate. I have struggled with this issue in my work at Camarillo State Hospital, University of California-Los Angeles Neuropsychiatric Institute, and the San Francisco VA for more than 25 years. Working with serious conditions such as schizophrenia, depression, posttraumatic stress disorder, and chronic pain, I have taught meditation as a mind-calming technique to patients. It is still rare to see mind-body techniques taught on psychiatric inpatient units, but there is growing support for outpatient interventions that are not only sensitive to religious and spiritual issues but actively use patients' religious and spiritual beliefs and values. This can range from using religious or spiritual practices in the treatment sessions (e.g., conducting a loving kindness meditation from Buddhist practice) to adoption of Christian imagery in cognitive-behavioral interventions.

Spirituality

Except for moments of unitive experience, we experience reality through many culturally defined filters. I think of spirituality as one of those filters. Humans are meaning-seeking, meaning-creating beings, and spirituality is one way of engaging meaningfully with the world.

It's so pervasive that it's like health. One is always dealing with one's health. One may have bad health to deal with, and one can also have a spiritual connection that is poor. I heard a panel presentation at the APA about a new diagnostic category for lack of religious connection. The panel debated about whether the multiple benefits associated with religious belief and participation—lower rates of depression, hypertension, faster recovery from surgery—made lack of religious connection a mental health problem!

Like physical health, our spiritual life is largely affected by the choices we make and the practices we follow. I came across a chapter titled "Behavioral Approaches to Enhance Spirituality" in *Integrating Spirituality Into Treatment,* edited by William Miller (APA Press). At first I was put off. It seemed like a mechanistic approach to a metaphysical issue. But as I read it I could see the validity of focusing on—or managing, as behaviorists would say—the everyday decisions that affect our spiritual life. With substance-abuse patients at the San Francisco VA Medical Center, my work has often involved behavioral interventions, such as helping them connect to their higher power through participating in Alcoholics Anonymous, meditation, and attending religious services.

Health professionals are often involved with spiritual issues. My wife is a social worker at the Petaluma Hospice. Part of her work involves helping patients and their families face death, find some meaning, accept suffering, let go, be grateful, say goodbye. These have been elements of religion for thousands of years, and now health professionals are often in that role as well. We need to learn new methods and techniques that aren't taught in graduate school. Christel has become a storyteller. In our workshops at the UC-Berkeley program on Grief and Loss, and in her clinical work, especially with children, she uses traditional folktales that speak to death and grief issues. In my therapy groups with pain and chronic illness patients, I include meditation and affirmations, which I consider a form of prayer. We cultivate an attitude of hope and gratitude through exercises. I explore with patients how their religious life does or does not support them. All of the preparation for this clinical work comes from my own personal life, not from my psychology training. These are techniques I practice in my own life to help cope with my chronic physical condition, Crohn's disease.

Part Five

Conversations About the Art and Science of Healing

"As integrative medicine emerges, it will come through not only science but also contemplation, self-reflection, and working with the force of health as well as treating disease."

—DAVID RILEY

CHAPTER 18

DAVID RILEY, MD

Integrating the Science and Art of Medicine

David Riley, MD, graduated from the University of Utah School of Medicine in 1983. He is currently a clinical associate professor at the University of New Mexico Medical School, is board-certified in internal medicine, and is a certified yoga instructor. In 1993, he completed a three-year training program in homeopathy at the Hahnemann College of Homeopathy in Albany, California, and most recently has been studying osteopathy with Jim Jealous, DO.

Dr. Riley serves as editor-in-chief of *Alternative Therapies in Health and Medicine* and is the founder of the Integrative Medicine Institute, an organization that conducts practice-based outcomes research on effectiveness, safety, patient satisfaction, and costs when complementary and alternative medicine (CAM) therapies are integrated with conventional medicine. He has conducted many clinical trials and is currently involved in a variety of clinical research projects. He was the principal investigator on the first International Integrative Primary Care Outcome Study, a multicenter outcomes study that evaluated patient outcomes when CAM therapies were integrated into primary care.

A board member of the Homeopathic Pharmacopoeia of the United States, Dr. Riley is also a technical adviser to the Food and Drug Administration for regulatory issues concerning homeopathy. Dr. Riley's primary interest in medicine is improving patient care through the evidence-based integration of conventional and CAM therapies.

I have worked with Dr. Riley for many years. My admiration of him is two-fold: he has an amazing depth and breath of knowledge and he is committed to his personal spiritual path. I interviewed him at his home in Santa Fe, New Mexico, in the summer of 2001.

At first blush, research may appear fairly cut-and-dried, even to the extent that some would say the term *medical literature* is an oxymoron. That has not been my experience. I've found research to be a powerful tool for communication of valuable information. At the same time, it has some of the characteristics of a coded message that is used in private societies or tribal rituals. The main point is that research is not only about objective data; it is a much richer intersection of personal and cultural beliefs with what we know and how we establish what we know and believe and why.

Of course, it is the "currency" of information exchange in the scientific community. If you want to communicate with the scientific community about complementary and alternative therapies, you will be much more effective if you use their language.

I used to believe that the results of research would give me definitive answers that would be forever memorialized. This has not been my experience; in fact, I usually have more questions when I finish a clinical trial than when I began. The answers you get out of clinical research are largely the result of the questions that you ask and the way you ask them, your hypotheses, and your methods. Those questions and answers pass through our visible and invisible cultural filters, which sometimes accept as true answers that may later be shown to be false and dismiss answers that cannot be explained or that are incongruent with the cultural tradition.

So, for example, medicine is attached to finding material explanations for physiological changes and illness that occur in the body. It seems to follow from the reasoning that since we can see the body and the body is a physical entity, there must be a physical or material explanation for illness. We seem to have difficulty believing that mind-body forces, spirituality, and other nonmaterial energies that we all accept as real in everyday life can cause illnesses or stimulate health. I don't want to deny the physical and material causes of disease, but they seem to exist on the surface of a much richer reality.

The essence of science is curiosity, and these phenomena that cannot be easily explained with our current models need to be accommodated. This touches on the question of what constitutes evidence. There's a tendency in scientific circles to ignore evidence that challenges the conventional model—the very evidence that should pique one's curiosity is dismissed! I think we have to look at all of the evidence, not just the evidence we like. All of these anomalous data that are dismissed comprise an extensive body of uncontrolled clinical observations that make up the raw material of science, from which one can develop a testable hypothesis. For me, this is the essence of science and the reason I get excited about science and the scientific method.

We need to recognize that some CAM modalities do not easily fit into the biomedical model. Most of these treatments can be researched and studied scientifically; however, it will be challenging to do so, and we may need to expand our view of the scientific method. We will almost certainly need to look at a broader base of evidence than that which is derived solely from randomized controlled trials. We do that already in surgery, for example. Many commonly accepted conventional medical therapies have limited evidence for their effectiveness. Just today I saw someone who, in the 1950s, was treated with radium radiation for birthmarks and is suffering the consequences. It is a myth that most of what we do in conventional medicine is research-based. One of the common hallmarks of CAM therapies is that they are individualized to the patient and often used in combination with other therapies and lifestyle recommendations. It will be challenging to study these therapies, and it probably cannot be done using the cookie-cutter approach so common in contemporary medical research.

In conventional pharmacology, for example, the general plan for some time has been to isolate biologically active plant components, patent a synthetic analog, and bring a drug to market. These drugs often have one very powerful action that overwhelms the body's ability to respond. Botanical preparations are different. First of all, most of them are not patentable and therefore cannot economically justify a $200 million drug development cost. Second, in most botanical preparations, the whole plant is used. It is full of compounds that may have paradoxical effects that stimulate different actions in different patients.

When you offer the body a choice of responses, multiple outcomes may occur. How does one test this? Are the group characteristics that are evaluated in a typical, randomized, controlled trial the best way to go? Perhaps not. A less reductionistic model that can handle multiple variables with a variety of possible outcomes might be necessary. This is one of the reasons I am interested in overall outcomes rather than specific effects.

There are many ways to conduct an investigation. Imagine a mural on the side of a large building. If we step back far enough from the mural to see it in its entirety, we will miss many of the details, but hopefully we will have an overview. If, however, we stand close and use a telescope to look at the mural, we will get a very precise, in-depth view of a very small portion, but we could not begin to offer a description of the whole mural.

I am interested in the overall mural. One of the areas of research I'm most interested in is health services research—in particular, observational or outcomes research. I enjoy looking at what happens in a practice-based setting. Even though I may not be able to control for variables in the same way I can in a randomized controlled trial, the data sets and information that emerge are very rich. In the process of controlling for all the variables in a randomized controlled trial, you set up another set of artificial circumstances that differ from the real world of medicine. I want to evaluate how a medical therapy works in a practice-based setting, use that information to educate providers and patients, and help design better clinical trials.

I think it is interesting that the research that has had the most impact in the field of alternative medicine to date are the surveys by David Eisenberg at Harvard. And these were not randomized, placebo-controlled, clinical trials.

I think the effectiveness of any medical therapy has a nonspecific component. This means that how I relate to my patients and how they relate to me, the effect of coming into my office, and all sorts of other things have an impact on the outcome of the treatment. This is in addition to the medication I may give or the therapies I use. I don't believe these nonspecific responses are linear or trivial. The study of placebos by Ted Kaptchuk and the exploration of the therapeutic encounter by David Reilly raise important questions about what it means to treat patients.

Problems in Research

Here is a commonplace scenario. There are three arms to the study: one arm gets nothing; one arm gets treatment X; and one arm gets treatment Y. Thirty get better even though nothing is done; only 20 get better with treatment X; and 50 get better with treatment Y. The typical conclusion is that treatment Y is good.

But there are some difficulties with this reasoning. You are assuming a stable placebo response across time and across groups, and I am not aware that the placebo response has been shown to be stable or linear. When calculating results in conventional clinical research, we generally assume that the total response of the treatment has two components: one is the effect of the medication or treatment, and the other is a placebo response. If you add those up, you get the total response. But we assume there is a linearity across patients, across time, and across treatments that has not been demonstrated.

It may be that for those who are highly suggestible, the placebo response is 80%, and for those who are not suggestible, it is 20%. It may be that in a clinical trial, those patients who are compliant with therapies get a better response than do those who are not, regardless of whether they receive the real medication or a placebo. Because we don't know what the placebo response rates actually are, we can't control for them even though we try. It may be that the people enrolled in any given clinical trial have, for any number of reasons, a very high placebo response.

When you reproduce exactly the same time trial with exactly the same cohort of patients somewhere else in another part of the world, the nonspecific or placebo response may be totally different. I would not assume that because you get a 30% response in the first group, you will have a 30% response in the second group. Yet that is an unspoken assumption that is common in interpreting the results of medical research. It may be that the use of placebo in medical research has more to do with limiting observer bias than measuring effectiveness or efficacy.

I am currently working on health services research that involves collecting practice-based data. We are collecting outcomes data from patients and providers, offering practitioners a useful and simple way to collect information and offering this data to the scientific and academic medical community, as well as the providers who participate in the clinical trials. I believe this type of research effort is creating the balance and momentum necessary to advance integrative medicine and impact the delivery of healthcare without CAM becoming just another therapy for a specific disease or condition.

Patient involvement is critical, and patients' perceptions of outcome and satisfaction are a key ingredient. And these outcomes should be independent of the practitioner to get a clear sense of the patient's response. Practitioner involvement, particularly from those in a "real-world" medical setting, is necessary for understanding what is happening outside the rarified setting of academic medicine. In a real-world practice setting, this information can become part of the patients' charts, and the forms take less than 4 minutes to fill out. Then, of course, there is a scientific structure around the project provided by those with experience in health services research. The structure of this project respects the three stakeholders in integrative medicine: patients, providers, and science.

My Practice

My practice evolved over the years, and I am continuing to explore alternative therapies, how they influence the therapeutic environment, and how they affect me. Mostly I try to maintain a position of "not knowing"—not knowing what I am going to do when somebody comes in the door. The further I go in this exploration, the less of an agenda I try to have concerning what I think the patient will need before he or she arrives and before we've had the chance to be together. An encounter with a patient should be therapeutic for both of us. The patient may be coming with certain expectations; nevertheless, I try to stay in a space where I don't know until I do know, then move in that direction. There is always a delicate balance between intellectual knowledge, intuition, and what the patient wants. I try to use whatever knowledge I have to challenge my intuition, using my intuition to keep me in the state of not knowing, but trusting that I will. It is not easy; I often recognize the state of balance by noticing that I am not there.

I am board-certified in internal medicine, so I use the biomedical model of conventional medicine as a grounding and springboard into other therapies. I use homeopathy, therapeutic yoga, counseling, and, less commonly, herbs and dietary supplements. I have a particular interest in manual medicine, probably beginning with yoga, and I am currently studying biodynamic osteopathy as developed and taught by Dr. Jim Jealous and his colleagues.

The practice of homeopathy is superficially similar to conventional medicine. You have a presenting set of symptoms; some are important; some are not. You do a physical exam, and based on an integration of this information, you select a medication. In some cases, on the surface at least, you might not be able to tell the difference between a conventional medical encounter and a homeopathic one. One big difference with homeopathy is that I am maintaining an awareness of and integrating symptoms experienced by a patient on different levels, from emotional to mental to spiritual, in addition to the physical manifestations of illness. The art of homeopathy is matching the symptom picture of the patient with symptoms associated with the remedy. It is also not uncommon for me to see patients on conventional medications that must be continued. I often will prescribe a single homeopathic remedy—one dose of a medicine.

It is actually even stranger than that. It is often one dose of a medicine that, from a pharmacological point of view, has no material substance. And then I wait and see what happens.

I would say that 20% to 30% of the time, I can have a significant effect on a patient's problem, and between 60% and 70% of the time, I have some effect on their condition. About 20% of the time, homeopathy has no effect at all on my patients. I used to believe that whatever therapy I was passionate about was going to cure the world and that when enough practitioners and patients learned about it, everyone would begin to use that therapy. I am coming around to the belief that the therapy chooses the provider and the patient as much as or more than the other way around.

I began to realize that there are patients for whom homeopathy—or any therapy, for that matter—is just not going to work. I've had to learn to keep an open mind and to recognize what I can and cannot treat or whom I can or cannot treat. On another level, I believe that my job as a provider is to find the therapy that I can most effectively use as a fulcrum for healing and to recognize that, at some very important level, all healing is self-healing. I have to learn to get out of the way.

I would say that most patients come to me expecting to get some sort of complementary therapy in addition to a conventional medical evaluation. My commitment is to try and develop a plan with my patients that will work for them. Interestingly, my most difficult patients are often those who I believe need conventional medical treatment and are afraid to go that route.

A large component of success with any therapy is the practitioner doing the therapy and his or her belief and experience with that therapy. The practitioner must find the therapies through which he can provide the most benefit to his patients. Some of it is not related to the therapy but to the nonspecific healing effects that go on in a therapeutic encounter.

One of the dilemmas in alternative medicine is that patients have such high expectations and hopes, yet we also have a culture in which patients are desperately searching for the right pill or the ultimate cure. People have come to me sometimes with shopping bags of stuff that they were taking—literally a shopping bag full. When a person is on 10 nutritional supplements, two or three Chinese herbal medical formulas, two or three Western botanical formulas, maybe some conventional medications, and a combination of homeopathic remedies, I don't know where to start except to tell him or her to stop and listen to what his or her body is saying. What I want to create is a partnership—a relationship that works both ways. I believe this is one of the things that makes the encounter therapeutic. Finding a balance, though, is challenging.

Yoga and meditation have been two gifts for me personally—they have taught me to be more patient. I continually practice being more patient and learning to watch and wait. The answer will come at some point. It may already have come, in which case I have to go back and take a look at it in terms of my previous encounters with the patient, or it may come at the end of a patient visit. I have to fight the tendency to interject or jump right in and "get to the bottom of things." The most valuable information is usually somewhere around the edges or in the nuances of a patient encounter. Maybe it's in the way the patients are dressed or what they say in the first 5 minutes. More often than not, particularly with chronic medical problems, these subtle things, which are directly related to why the patient was in my office, are important.

Yoga

Yoga was actually my introduction into alternative medicine, though I didn't realize it at the time. When I was newly married and a medical student in Salt Lake City, Utah, my wife and I took a yoga class. We both went on to become certified as yoga teachers, traveling to India to study and taking many yoga intensives. I can still remember going to my first extended yoga working in Austin, Texas, and doing yoga for 6 to 8 hours a day for at least 2 weeks. I came out of that workshop with a different body than I went in with—my understanding of it, the way I moved, my knowledge of what the possibilities were; it was a transformative experience.

After that, we started teaching yoga classes and created a wonderful community of friends in Salt Lake City around our classes. I gradually became aware that the experiences I was having while teaching yoga were what I wanted to have while I was practicing medicine. Over time

I incorporated therapeutic yoga and what you would call restorative yoga into the therapeutic encounters with my patients. Getting people in touch with their breath, teaching them some simple postures, working with them to develop flexibility and strength—all seemed to be useful and helpful for my patients

The breath is a doorway between the body and other levels of consciousness and can be a fulcrum for the process of integration. When I'm doing yoga—and for some time afterward, particularly if I go to a meditation retreat where I am focusing on the breath—I become much clearer on what is going on inside of me and around me. It's as though I'm accumulating reserves of energy and insight. The more I can strengthen a person's internal reserves, the more likely she is to activate her own self-healing process.

Yoga is one of the philosophical systems that evolved in India. One of the classic yoga texts was written by Patanjali 1000 to 2000 years ago. Interestingly enough, Patanjali hardly discussed the postures, but over the years, they seem to have evolved into a preparation for meditation practice and a physical discipline in their own right. Patanjali focused on yoga as a path to self-realization. There is a well-described eight-fold path in yoga that begins with right living, a sort of "golden rule" and evolves through the postures, breathing, and meditation to *samadhi,* a state in which the person can become unified with *Paramatma,* or the collective universal mind. In this respect, yoga overlaps with other Eastern philosophical and religious traditions such as Buddhism, which also originated in India.

One of my favorite stories is about the Buddha and an encounter he had after he became "enlightened." As he was passing through a village, people looked at him because they recognized him as a prince but knew that something was different. So they asked him a number of questions: "Are you this; are you that; are you a god?" And he would say no. They finally gave up trying to figure it out and asked, "What are you?" The Buddha's response was, "I am awake."

That is a nice place to be—to be awake. It is a continuous state that is available all the time. One of the most profound realizations I ever had was the idea that at the moment you realize you are not awake, you are awake. The very act of realizing that you are not awake can only come from a state of being awake. I find it comforting to realize that each moment holds the potential to awaken once again.

Oriental Herbs versus Western Herbs

Some of the herbs are the same, whether they are Chinese or American. The biggest difference is that in Oriental medicine the herbs are commonly used in combination formulas prescribed according to Oriental medical diagnostic criteria. Western herbal medicine more easily fits into the biomedical model, with the caveat that each herb may have a variety of active ingredients, each influencing and balancing the activity of the other.

All of which raises a good point: from the outside, it is easy to look at the various categories of alternative therapies and assume that each one is a unified field with a consistent set of principles. Nothing could be further from the truth. In homeopathy, there are at least a half dozen different schools of thought. Some people use single remedies, some use combinations, and some practitioners use machines to select remedies for their patients. In China, the practice of traditional medicine is about 80% herbs, and most practitioners specialize in either herbal medicine or acupuncture, not both. In addition, the practice of traditional medicine changed and became much more Western during the cultural revolution, when many of the spiritual aspects of traditional Chinese medicine were persecuted. These aspects do seem to live on in the five Elements and the six Energetic Phase traditions.

Has Medicine Lost its Way?

Even though individual practitioners may be an exception, it feels to me that conventional medicine has in many ways lost its connection with the patients it serves. It has become so enamored with the business of medicine, from high technology to patent-protected pharmaceutical drugs, that it has gotten off track. I wouldn't want to abandon the marvelous diagnostic and treatment technology that we have—I would just want to maintain the connections with our patients and ourselves. When we lose these connections, we are limiting our effectiveness.

Consider the World Health Organization statistics for the top 30 developed nations. On virtually every marker of societal health, the United States is not in the top 10. It would be one thing if we were spending twice as much as everybody else and were at the top. Then you might say, "You get what you pay for." But we are paying the most and ranking below most of the developed world on the major indices of health.

Many patients' desire for alternative medicine is a desire for meaning and connection with their doctors. One of my fears is that conventional medicine will simply adopt alternative therapies in the same way it has adopted its technological advances. Western medicine has backed itself into a corner. In the 1930s, we started seeing surgical advances, sulfa drugs, and antibiotics on the horizon, and we had the illusion that we could cure everything quickly and efficiently without side effects. Things started unraveling in the late 1950s and 1960s, until we got to where we are today. One of the key events in this change was the thalidomide disaster.

For the first time, it caused people to question the safety of the drugs they were taking. The successes of conventional medicine are phenomenal and should not be underemphasized. When you think about what you can do, particularly in surgery and the intensive care unit, it's amazing. But somehow, this is not where most medical care takes place—it is much more mundane. Most medical care is in the nuts and bolts of a mother taking care of her child or someone with an ache or pain, perhaps worried if this or that symptom means they have some terrible disease. Do you really want to give therapies that have powerful side effects and may suppress the self-healing capacity of the body just because you can, when there may be other avenues available?

Look at conventional cancer therapy. There are specific examples where it is clear that it changes life expectancy. In the treatment of childhood leukemia, for example, very few new drugs have been introduced in the last 20 years, yet the survival rate has increased dramatically.

What's changed is that cancer specialists have individualized the chemotherapy regimens. They are using combinations of chemotherapy drugs in lower doses, resulting in less toxicity. Doctors have begun taking into account how the individual patient's tumor cells may respond to a given drug, developing individual life strategies for treating the patient. The emphasis of individualization is a cornerstone of most alternative medicine, and here we find it in conventional medicine as well.

To me, the real question is: does disease serve a positive purpose?

Is it a realistic goal to think that we can eradicate disease and still be in a state of natural balance? What is our relationship to nature and the world around us? Does the appearance of an illness in a child actually strengthen and educate the immune system in a way that a vaccination cannot? We know that immunity rates are much stronger when you are exposed to a natural disease than when you are exposed to an artificial disease through an immunization. And is it a realistic goal to try to wipe out all disease? It raises another question about our whole relationship to nature and the world around us. Is nature something to be dominated and controlled or something to be worked with? Our insistence on dominion rather than cooperation is, in my opinion, a fatal flaw in our view of the world.

Why Alternative Medicine?

For almost all people involved in alternative medicine, there is something that happened early on in their careers where they saw a response that was so dramatic they couldn't dismiss it. For me, other than the personal transformation I underwent with yoga, it was one of my first experiences using homeopathy. A patient came to see me with a frozen left shoulder. He was left-handed and a talented but poor pen-and-ink artist. His frozen shoulder had gotten so bad that his hand was in his pocket all the time. He couldn't take his hand out without using his other arm to pull it out of his pocket. Then his arm would just hang down. He was also a diabetic.

I referred him to an orthopedic surgeon who did a radiographic study with a dye injection that documented the frozen shoulder and underlying capsular adhesion. But he didn't think the patient would respond well to manipulation under anesthesia, because he was afraid he might rupture his rotator cuff. The patient was then seen by a variety of specialists with no real improvement. When he came back to see me, I had a homeopathic remedy that was supposed to be good for inflammation and injury, so I said, "Let's try this. What have we got to lose?" I injected about 1 mL of this sterile solution into his shoulder capsule the same way you would inject steroids and told him I wanted to see him in 2 days. He returned the next day, and as he came up to me he started grinning. He raised his arm up over his head and fully extended it toward the ceiling, swinging the arm around. He had a totally normal range of motion—in less than 24 hours. I was amazed. I thought, "this is really interesting, and I am going to have to learn a lot more about it."

Why Homeopathy Works

We don't know scientifically why homeopathy works. I was involved in an interesting project with Arthur Zajonc that was supported by the Fetzer Institute to bring together scientists involved in cutting-edge basic science research. We made the assumption that since testing and measuring devices have gotten more sophisticated, perhaps we could find a tool to explore possible mechanism of action theories for homeopathy. So far we have concluded that for homeopathic remedies in which there is a molecular substance present, we can postulate a theory for how they might work based on existing information, whether it be clathrate formation or some other process. But for homeopathic remedies in which there is no substance present—where you pass Avogadro's number and it is unlikely there is even a single molecule of the substance—we don't have a good model that can be tested for postulating how it could be effective. We can only say that it appears to be effective empirically, without knowing why.

One of the more interesting metaanalyses on homeopathy was done by Klaus Linde and Wayne Jonas and published in *The Lancet* in 1997. It evaluated 89 randomized, controlled trials and asked the question "is the response in these trials compatible with the hypothesis that homeopathy is a placebo response?" They found that homeopathy was 2.45 times more likely to be effective than was the placebo response, with a 95% confidence interval.

We seem to be attached in medicine to measuring a material dose of something, and homeopathic remedies with "nothing there" strains credulity. An explanation of how homeopathy might work has many attributes of a Zen koan. It is very hard to wrap your rational mind around homeopathy. It could be that informational patterns can be imprinted on some types of solutions and then transmitted to the body. We don't know for sure and we don't even know for sure how to test the mechanism of action theory for homeopathy.

It may be that one of the main contributions of homeopathy in particular—and alternative therapies as a whole—will be a reevaluation of what we consider an acceptable risk-benefit ratio in medicine. We may look back in the not-too-distant future and say, "Wow, those interventions were pretty toxic." Hopefully by then we will be using medicines that are less damaging.

Advice

If I were giving advice, I would first recommend that practitioners be happy doing what they are doing. If you're not happy doing what you're doing, you should be doing something else, particularly when you are taking care of patients. To be happy, you must find the therapy that works for you.

Second, keep an open mind about things that you don't understand, without abandoning your skepticism. And, finally, listen to your patients and take time for self-reflection.

For patients, I would say, "focus on prevention." Then I'd advise them to trust their instincts about what they think might be going on. And, finally, they should find a provider or providers they trust and create a partnership.

When people have medical problems it's easy, from the patient's perspective, to say, "I can't be happy until I fix this problem." One of my challenges is to help somebody yet not have them get hooked into my being the answer to their problems, even if I may be able to help that specific problem. Happiness is not dependent on your medical state. That, for me, has been a huge realization, and it has made treating patients more enjoyable. I also believe that you can change your genetic and physiological structure through self-observation and that there is potential for healing to occur under almost any circumstances.

When you are meditating, the general instruction if you have a pain is to just look at it and watch what happens; invariably it changes. Sometimes the pain will go away; sometimes it will change. All of a sudden you will notice that, in fact, this pain you're having over here may be connected to something going on over there. It may be connected to a specific thought process, or you may only get this pain when you think about a certain subject or sit in a certain position. All sorts of insights and subtleties exist in the web of connections.

In an interview I read in *Yoga Journal* several years ago, Chogyam Trumpa Rinpoche said that we are all perfect the way we are and there is always room for improvement. I like this as a foundation because if you think you are perfect the way you are and there is nothing to do, it's easy to become lazy. It's also true that if you think you always have to improve yourself, then you might not experience satisfaction with where you are now. As integrative medicine emerges, it will come through not only science but also contemplation, self-reflection, and working with the force of health as well as treating disease. Science cannot find the answers to everything, but it can help keep us from getting too far off track.

CHAPTER 19

WAYNE JONAS, MD
The Science Behind Healing

Wayne Jonas, MD, is the director of the Samueli Institute. From 1995 to 1999, he served as the director of the Office of Alternative Medicine (now the National Center for Complementary and Alternative Medicine) at the National Institutes of Health (NIH). A former Lieutenant Colonel in the U.S. Army, he previously served as director of the medical research fellowship at Walter Reed Army Institute of Research, Washington, DC, where he taught research methodology and conducted laboratory research in immunology and toxicology. Dr. Jonas is also an Associate Professor in the faculty of the Department of Family Practice and the Department of Pathology at the Uniformed Services University of the Health Sciences in Bethesda, Maryland.

Dr. Jonas received his medical degree from Bowman Gray School of Medicine in Winston-Salem, North Carolina, and completed his residency training in Family Medicine at DeWitt Army Community Hospital. In addition to his conventional medical training, he has studied homeopathy—in which he is currently licensed—bioenergy therapy, diet and nutritional therapy, mind/body methods, spiritual healing, electroacupuncture diagnostics, and clinical pastoral education.

I originally interviewed Dr. Jonas in 1996 when he was the new director of the Office of Alternative Medicine (OAM). However, because that interview focused on the OAM and because Dr. Jonas is one of the leaders in this field, I asked if I could reinterview him for this book and talk more generally about his views on the subject of healing. He agreed, and in the spring of 2002, we met at the Samueli Institute in Newport Beach, California.

Healing Research and the Samueli Institute

The Samueli Institute (which I now direct) is a private, nonprofit, nonaffiliated research institute. It was founded by Henry and Susan Samueli, both of whom have a great interest in healing, in science, and in bringing the two together. I have an interest in bridging science to healing practices, ancient and modern, inner and outer, Eastern and Western, so the Institute is a great match for us all.

Our mission at the Samueli Institute is to investigate the underlying science of healing. Healing is the process of recovery and repair whereby individuals, communities, and the environment get better, feel better, and become more whole. Our belief is that there are fundamental concepts in healing that cut across medical modalities from different cultures around the world and also unify terms such as *complementary* or *conventional*. We think that all healthcare systems and practitioners are interested in healing and the process of healing.

Yet there is little research that is focused on the science of healing. What happens in healing? How can it be facilitated? What are the mechanisms whereby we become healthy, and how can we bring those consistently into our medical care? These questions are our focus.

The institute is especially interested in the interaction between healer and healee. We are interested in optimal healing environments, in the therapeutic relationship, in how thoughts and consciousness influence healing, in how energy comes off and through the body and influences healing, and in other types of nonchemical and nonmolecular interactions in biology. Homeopathy, energy medicine, therapeutic relationships, placebo effects, and mind-body therapies that deal with consciousness fall into these categories. Again, we are interested in understanding scientifically what are the fundamental mechanisms underlying these processes and developing methods for reliably measuring their therapeutic effects so we can use them more effectively in practice.

There are five main domains on which we intend to focus. One is homeopathy because both the founders and I have an interest in that, and I have completed research in this area. Another domain is consciousness. How does intention and attention influence healing and the healing process? How does consciousness interact with living systems? Another area is energy medicine—is there energy that flows off of and through the body? What controls it? Can we measure it? A fourth domain is bioelectromagnetics—how do frequencies such as laser, millimeter waves, and ultrasound facilitate healing processes? Finally, we have a program on digital biology that asks whether informational or electromagnetic signals can be digitized and delivered via information technology to stimulate healing and induce biological systems to recover.

These are our five domains of research focus and grant support. We have put most of our initial efforts in the area of homeopathy and consciousness and are now developing programs in energy and energy measurement.

Homeopathy

In the area of homeopathy, we have a number of projects that look at neuroprotection. Our primary question in this program is whether one can use homeopathic preparations of neurotoxins such as glutamate or more traditional remedies such as *Arnica* to reduce damage from stroke or brain trauma? We are also looking at remedies that may influence cancer, both in terms of quality-of-life and at the molecular level. For example, we are exploring the use of very low-dose carcinogens that are also homeopathic remedies in cell and animal models and looking at the mechanisms whereby these induce recovery or repair processes. We are also investigating clinics that treat cancer patients with homeopathy, such as those in India where there is extensive use of homeopathy for treating cancer and other serious illnesses. We want to see if their work can be documented through NCI-NIH–type best-case series and prospective evaluations to determine if there is an effect, what kind it is and whether it can be quantified and measured.

Preliminary data indicate that low-dose effects do have therapeutic value. When I was at the National Institutes of Health (NIH), we did a best-case series on a clinic in India that treated cancer, often fairly advanced cancer, exclusively with homeopathy. The National Cancer Institute (NCI) evaluated that series of cases and felt that some benefit was there. NCI is now in the process of following up with this clinic. We are on a parallel track with similar types of clinics. Whether these will uncover useful cancer therapies or not, I have no idea, but it appears well worth investigating.

I don't think we are any closer to answering how or why homeopathy works. There are a lot of hypotheses, including one that invokes the placebo effect. We held a meeting in Freiburg, Germany in January 2002 that brought together some of the best researchers in homeopathy from Europe and Great Britain. They reviewed and discussed the state of the science in homeopathy.

Their conclusion was that the state of the science in homeopathy is dismal. There are no decent laboratory models to explore or explain what is observed clinically. And the clinical observations are not always consistent. In addition, there are no accepted and testable theoretical models for homeopathic action. Also, practically no funding entity supports research in homeopathy. Moving forward scientifically requires high-quality research methods and sufficient research support and infrastructure to do state-of-the-art science. That doesn't exist in this field. There are a few individuals doing research and very few groups supporting it. It is a small field and to do high-quality research is going to take considerably more effort.

While there are inadequate results to say that we know how to apply homeopathy consistently, or where we should apply it, or when it works, or when it doesn't work, there clearly are enough intriguing results to say that we ought to investigate this area. It may turn out that homeopathy is just an extremely good way of applying the therapeutic relationship. The classical homeopathic interview, for example, involves a detailed interaction and interview with the patient. It involves looking for changes over a long period of time and setting up expectations and beliefs for change and working with those. These are all things that we know have a therapeutic effect. So it may be that with homeopathy, we've developed a good way of applying the therapeutic relationship. If so, we need to understand that too. And we need to begin to explore how to maximize that in all medicine.

Consciousness

I use the term *information biology* to get at the idea that biological systems respond to information and not just to energy, not just to molecules, and not just to matter. Specific configurations of information are important, and living systems are attuned and sensitive to those types of information. Information may have an independent effect from the carriers of that information, such as the energy or the molecules that store it. So we are interested in exploring these mechanisms.

Consciousness is a good example. We have been looking at the research on mental and spiritual healing, practices that are part of all healing systems in all cultures. Is there any science in it? We now have done a systematic summary of the quantity and quality of research in the area of mind-matter interaction, mental interaction with living systems, prayer, distant healing, and energy medicine. These things aren't energy in the classical sense. Consciousness is not like a light beam that travels at a certain speed and attenuates at a distance. Consciousness has an instant effect. Consciousness involves some other kind of connectivity than energy in which the information exchange or interaction is always occurring. We are interested in exploring how that works. If consciousness does have an influence on healing directly through connectivity, this could be a fundamental mechanism whereby all healing works across all systems. Investigating that will be useful and could also help us understand something fundamentally different about the world that hasn't been explored before.

Consciousness involves the detection of our interconnectedness. But it doesn't appear to act like a physical phenomenon in that you send it; it travels through time and space; and then somebody receives it. There are lots of ways of communicating information. For example, we currently think that communication in biology acts like the mail system. I put a molecule in the bloodstream; it gets transferred through the bloodstream and arrives at a cell; it hits the receptor; and then the cell opens up the "letter" and finds the message. That's like the Pony Express. Another way to transfer information in the body is like the telephone system. The brain functions this way. It is not a chemical that is transferred through the nerves; it is an electrical impulse. The chemical is delivered at the end, and then the message gets delivered.

But there are other ways of communicating. For example, look at wireless communication. Perhaps this is the way in which bioenergy, as in qi in Chinese medicine, is transferred. Another possibility is that there is a level at which biological systems are already connected that doesn't fall into normal, three-dimensional space and time transmission. This is what Larry Dossey calls *nonlocality*. In quantum mechanics they also call this nonlocality, but whether these concepts are the same thing or not is unknown. Both of these concepts express the idea that there's already a connectivity on some level through different dimensions than the ones handled by the five senses. Accessing that connectivity and utilizing it is another way of communication. The idea is this type of information can be accessed through consciousness, through our minds, and through our awareness.

We have supported several projects investigating consciousness. We just finished a summary of the science of consciousness and healing using standard critical evaluation methods. We have had two meetings on this topic and have published two Proceedings. Laurence Rockefeller has been cosupporting this project with us. Currently, our German office is exploring whether electroencephalograms (EEGs) correlate on some kind of nonlocal level. Two individuals are placed in separate electromagnetically shielded, sound-proof booths and their EEGs measured simultaneously. In one individual, there is an EEG evoked potential produced when a flash appears on a little checkerboard screen in front of the person's eyes. Then they simultaneously look for any correlated changes in the EEG of the other person who is not having the evoked potential. We want to see if there is any direct interconnectivity between the EEGs under those circumstances. The preliminary evidence indicates that there is, but much more research is needed before such an observation is confirmed and understood.

The mythology in this field is that if individuals are bonded, let's say they're in love or twins, then there will be a greater connection in their EEGs. But Harold Walach and his colleagues in Germany looked both at individuals who knew each other, as well as individuals who had not met. The phenomenon of connectivity seems to occur in both sets of people whether they were bonded or not. So, the connectivity may or may not have something to do with bonding. This is something worth exploring, and we're trying to develop tools to do that.

Can Healing Be Measured?

One of the challenges in healing research is that we don't have a way of measuring when someone is healing or not. We need some objective and reliable neurological or physiological measures that turn on or turn off when in the healing mode. If you had such measures, you could know when healing was occurring or not occurring. Until this happens, we only have very crude methods for studying healing. We can determine if a 'healer' has gone through a certification program. But what does that mean, since there are no standards and such programs are extremely variable? Currently, if you don't see any effects from healing, you don't know if it has to do with the competence and skills of the healer or the treatment just doesn't work.

There are increasingly sophisticated ways of measuring neurological states that allow us to catch the real-time functional phenomena of consciousness. I'm talking about new neuroimaging technologies like multichannel EEG, magnetic encephalography, monitors for heart rate variability, and autonomic function. These are tools that may be fruitfully applied to these areas. Prior work on meditation has given us clues as to what might be the most useful measures. We know EEG changes occur, that heart rate varies, and other physiological and cellular changes happen during meditation. So we're exploring some of these measurements to see if we can come up with a way of fingerprinting or characterizing when someone is turned on during a healing state.

Scientific Rigor and the Samueli Institute

I would like to say more about how we go about establishing scientific rigor at the Samueli Institute. Quality science is essential if we are to avoid erroneous claims and concepts. The Institute is nonprofit and nonaffiliated. We are not connected with any specific university or research institute, but we make connections and partnerships and develop projects with research institutes around the world. My background and the background of the deputy director of the institute, Ronald A. Chez, MD, is one of full-time academic medicine and high-quality, rigorous, scientific peer review. So we follow that pattern.

We solicit grant proposals from individuals who have an interest in and the ability to conduct high-quality research in healing, and we work directly with them to develop their research applications. Then we convene an independent body of prominent scientists to peer review the grant applications. The committee members write formal reviews and then convene for a couple of days to score all of the applications. If an application meets quality scientific standards, we'll take it to our board of directors, who have the final say over which projects are funded. The process we follow is modeled after ones that exist at the NIH, but ours allows more flexibility to work with investigators who are delving into innovative and multidisciplinary areas.

I should mention that all of our investigators are asked to look at both positive and negative effects of their treatments. Of course, we always hope that we can find effects that will be clinically useful, but in the process, it is essential to explore whether the effect could be adverse. Adverse effects can occur with even apparently harmless therapies. Larry Dossey wrote a book called *Be Careful What You Pray For* in which he documents cases from many cultures around the world in which prayer and intention are used for bad as well as good. So if there are positive effects, then there is always the risk of adverse effects as well.

For information dissemination, we follow the standard scientific process also. Once research has been done, it needs to be looked at and discussed by the larger scientific community and that's where the peer-review publication process comes in. We always ask individuals who apply to us for grants where they intend to publish the results of their research and when. We expect all results, positive or negative, to be written up and submitted for publication in peer-reviewed journals. So we look for individuals with a track record of publishing and who have the ability and willingness to do that.

Some Current Projects Investigating Consciousness

One of the most intriguing areas that we are currently involved in is the exploration of consciousness. Our investigators are investigating questions about the nature of consciousness and how it interacts with biological systems. The EEG studies mentioned earlier are an example of this.

We're also interested in looking at whether the attention that someone pays to another individual alters the autonomic nervous system. There's been preliminary work showing that if I am paying attention to you, if I'm staring at you or I am trying to calm you or excite you, and even if you are not aware that I am doing this, you're autonomic nervous system reacts, and your heart rate changes. In other words, you "know" and respond on some level what my consciousness is doing. This is intriguing because we all know that when you walk into a doctor's office and you're worried, the attitude and the focus of the physician may have a profound effect. But it may be that the doctor's intention has a profound effect even *before* you walk into the office. The internal state of the physician or healer may be continuously influencing the patient. If so, we need to attend to that in the therapeutic relationship.

Related to this is another pilot project looking at whether the nervous system is able to detect an event before it occurs. For example, one of our investigators has done pilot work on monitoring the autonomic reactivity before a stimulus is applied. The subject is exposed to high-decibel white noise—not painful but very irritating—that causes a marked jump in the autonomic sympathetic discharge that's reflected in the electrodermal activity of the hand. In a series of pilot experiments, the investigator has shown that a rise occurs in autonomic activity several seconds before the noise is actually played. So there is a precognitive response in which we detect a stimulus before it happens. This is called a *prestimulus response* (PSR). If this can be quantified and amplified, this could be valuable tool.

I spent 24 years in the military and still have a great interest in investigating areas that may have value for the military and military medicine. If people could be signaled by their own nervous system 3 or 4 seconds before something is going to happen, they would have an advantage in responding. This might be very valuable on the battlefield or in situations such as car accidents. These are our early and rudimentary ways of exploring the idea of interconnectivity across space and time that accompanies consciousness.

Energy Medicine

There is controversy over the concepts of energy versus consciousness. The question is not whether they exist but how they are related. I think the difficulty revolves largely around how the word *energy* is used in reference to healing and the different meanings we have about that word. In standard Western science, *energy* has a very specific meaning and definition that generally has to do with electromagnetic forces or other types of forces such as gravitation. It is a very precise definition, and these energies are measurable with instruments. That's how we define energy in the West.

Traditional healing systems also talk about energy, such as Chinese medicine or Ayurvedic medicine. Those concepts are not the same as the energy of physics. Take the Chinese term for life energy, *qi*, for example. We translate qi as energy, but actually if you look at how the term is used in Chinese medicine and science, it does not have the same characteristics as the term energy in the West. It has some characteristics that are similar, such as the transmission of force, but it also has characteristics of consciousness, such as nonlocality. One's mind can control it, direct it, and accumulate it. And that is not the case with energy in the Western sense. These are different concepts, and yet we use the same term.

We don't currently have a good, single term for this concept in Western medicine, but there are a number of terms that have been used. They're not part of mainstream science, but there are, for example, concepts of vital force, L-fields, bions, orgone, and the like. But those are also not the same as standard energy used in Western science.

So definitions become crucial. If you're going to talk about energy in a scientific way, you need to mean the standard Western scientific definition. And if you're going to talk about qi or *mana* or *prana,* you need to use a different term, perhaps *biofield* or *bioenergy.*

To address this, the Samueli Institute is going to have a conference the goal of which is to obtain operational definitions for the various terms in the area of energy medicine and healing. We also will be creating guidelines for standards of research in these areas. I found the same need when I was at the NIH in reference to complementary and alternative medicine. There are scientists who want to do research in this area, but like any new area, there's a lot of confusion about definitions and standards, misunderstandings across disciplines, quality issues in research, and ignorance about prior data and historical background as people begin to learn about these new areas. One needs to have both good science and a good understanding of the concepts being investigated: what are the underlying assumptions and background data and what are the tools best used to explore healing. Finally, the Institute is interested in determining how this can pragmatically be applied to developing healing environments in medicine.

Healing Environments

Another one of our main goals is to explore the components and application of an optimal healing environment. This is being done in conjunction with the Metronic Foundation. If you were to set up the optimal circumstances of intention, energy, physical environment, and therapeutic interactions, all focused on facilitating healing processes as opposed to simply eliminating disease, what would these be?

Obviously, one needs to eliminate disease if you have disease, and that's where conventional Western medicine has its great strengths. At the same time, especially with chronic illnesses, supporting and stimulating the inherent healing capacities of the body is crucial. So, how do we optimize that? How can we create an environment that supports and stimulates healing? We are beginning by defining the components of an optimal healing environment and how we go about evaluating and applying these in our healthcare system.

Even in the conventional literature, a fair amount of this has been looked at in this area already, for example, belief, expectation, and what maximizes placebo effects. These tend to be things that also maximize healing in general. Dan Moore and I published an article in the *Annals of Internal Medicine* called "Placebo Effect: Reformulating It as the Meaning Response." The placebo effect is usually studied by looking at how the context and meaning of a therapy are altered which leads to the positive effects that we then call the placebo effect.

For example, a warm type of interaction frequently will enhance the therapeutic effect as can the color of a pill or the context in which it is delivered. In a society that believes that injections are a powerful way of delivering a therapy, injections of a placebo work better than a pill of placebo. Different cultures will respond differently because of the meaning. Blue pills tend to be sedative; orange pills tend to be stimulate. This works in most European cultures except for Italy, where blue pills are calming for women and exciting for men. Why? For women in Italy blue is most often associated with the Virgin Mary, a very soothing image. And for Italian men, blue is most often associated with the national soccer team, a stimulating image. The meaning and the context of how therapy is delivered is crucial in all societies and all cultures and can lead to healing.

Inner Work

In my opinion, it's important to balance the inner and the outer life. The outer, intellectual, workaday world is an essential component of our lives, but there is also the inner, subjective aspect. Cultivation of all those skills helps to keep us fully human.

We have a meditation room here at the Institute, and we encourage people to use it. It's a place where individuals can go to intentionally engage in their own inner work. We put a copper wall on one side of the room because copper is an electromagnetic reflector and when you get close to the copper wall, you can feel the electromagnetic waves that come off your body and reflect back. Sitting in front of the copper wall and meditating seems to enhance the inner process.

We borrowed the idea from Elmer Green who measured the electrical and magnetic activities that were coming off the bodies of meditators and healers. Green had a copper room with electrodes on all the walls. He, in turn, got the idea from an ancient Tibetan practice of meditating in front of a copper wall. The Tibetans claimed that it enhanced lucidity and the meditative process by reflecting back the components of electromagnetic energy involved with the meditative process. Now, if we are able to study those components, we might understand how to capture and use the power of mindfulness more effectively. So studying the electromagnetic aspects of healing becomes an aspect of our work.

Electromagnetics

It may be that electromagnetic interactions with biological systems will be useful in healing. This idea is a popular one. The effect of electromagnetic energies at low frequencies has been explored in standard science for a long time. NASA, for example, has been investigating if there are ways to enhance wound healing with electromagnetic frequencies because in space, wound healing slows down. The gravitational field seems to be an important context in maintaining proper wound healing.

There are a number of instruments for delivering electromagnetic energy that are of interest. For example, our coinvestigators have explored low-level lasers. They are looking at low-level light, which, at certain frequencies, seems to stimulate cytochrome-C and enhance adenosine triphosphate (ATP) production leading to accelerated wound healing. Again, the use of magnets is popular although hardly any clinical research has been done on the effectiveness of magnets for healing.

Digital Biology

Many of your readers know that almost 20 years ago a scientist by the name of Jacques Benveniste published an article in *Nature* in which he claimed to show that ultra-high dilutions of IgE produced specific biological effects. He also claimed that the mechanism whereby this occurs has to do with electromagnetic frequencies that can be delivered electronically. In other words, chemical signals can be digitized, stored on a disc, and transmitted, even over the Internet. Obviously, if this were true it would be revolutionary.

Professor Benveniste had reported that he could digitize a thrombin inhibitor signal that would slow the coagulation rate between thrombin and fibrinogen, just like the chemical thrombin inhibitor can. He set up several experiments in which a thrombin inhibitor was digitized, placed on a disc, and then played back to a thrombin-fibrin mixture. Because of the profound implications such a discovery would have, we decided to independently examine this idea and attempt to replicate, verify, or disprove his claims and to do it in a rigorous way with randomized, double-blind methods and with experts, including skeptics, involved in the process.

First, we had Professor Benveniste and his team come to our lab and do the initial experiments. Our team included a hematologist who is familiar with the coagulation process, several expert consultants, including an engineer looking at the frequency and electronic issues, a statistician looking at the statistical and redesign issues, a sociologist to observe the overall replication process and make sure that we are managing communications between participants correctly, and also a skeptic who observed all aspects of the work.

Many people think it strange that we have a sociologist on our team. However, when I was at the Office of Alternative Medicine at the NIH, I found that many times, it was not lack of scientific methodology that prevented us from investigating complementary and alternative medicine. One can develop a good scientific methodology. But in highly controversial areas, it was the social process that interfered with being able to do the science. Scientists are human and do not check their biases and opinions at the laboratory door. So we have incorporated into our replication a management method for dealing with the social aspects of research to ensure that we can execute high-quality science properly.

Conclusion

At the Samueli Institute we are investigating the underlying aspects of healing. Mr. and Mrs. Samueli have been very generous in setting up and supporting the infrastructure of the institute, and we have been able to fund innovative and cutting-edge projects. Our ultimate goal is to catalyze interest in the area of the science of healing and the biology of healing in the scientific and medical communities and get others to get involved.

It will be fundamentally important to bridge many concepts and disciplines that have been separated for too long: the ancient and modern, the East and West, the clinic and science, the alternative and the conventional. We are not identified with any of those, we simply hope to stimulate a new synthesis of the best of healing and the best of science. And we seek to bring the concept and practice of healing to the public in a credible and scientific way.

CHAPTER 20

Ted Kaptchuk, OMD

Subjectivity and the Placebo Effect in Medicine

Ted Kaptchuk, OMD, received his undergraduate degree from Columbia College in New York and his doctorate in Oriental medicine from the Macau Institute of Chinese Medicine in Macau, China. Dr. Kaptchuk is currently associate director of the Center for Alternative Medicine Research at Beth Israel Deaconess Medical Center and an assistant professor of medicine at Harvard Medical School.

Besides writing numerous articles in medical journals, books, and monographs, Dr. Kaptchuk is the author of *The Web That Has No Weaver: Understanding Chinese Medicine.*

In 2000, when the meaning of the placebo effect was being broadly debated in the medical literature, the editors of *Alternative Therapies in Health and Medicine* asked me to talk to Dr. Kaptchuk and record his perspective on this controversial phenomenon. This interview took place in Dr. Kaptchuk's home in Cambridge, Massachusetts, in the spring of 2001.

I'm a product of the 1960s. When I finished my regular academic education at the university, I wanted to do something that would affirm the values, practices, and perspectives of other cultures—especially what we used to call the Third World. I also wanted to do something beyond rioting and causing mayhem; healing seemed sensible. Chinese medicine was mostly unknown in the West at the time; it was not so much China that attracted me as it was a medical system that was radically "other" and not part of the dominant medical system. So I spent five years studying Chinese medicine, mostly in a town called Macau, near Hong Kong.

Intellectually, attending medical school in China provided an entirely different vision of human beings and the cosmos. Thinking in yin-yang terms, continually seeing phenomena shift in context or relationships—that required a radical realignment. Actually, seeing yin and yang or wind or dampness as simply as I can see the color of my shirt was mind-boggling. Also, I was adopted by an old-style Chinese family, and Chinese behaviors such as concern with face, being hyperpolite, and veneration for the elderly became second nature. I expressed myself in Chinese metaphors and dreamed in Chinese languages. I could barely remember pizza and kosher pickles.

When I returned to the United States, I started teaching. Teaching was important because I needed to reflect on what I had learned, and I felt I had a debt to China to transmit in the West the knowledge I received. I also started a private practice. There was a place in Cambridge called Quack Row, where a whole bunch of "weirdos" were, so I opened my practice there.

At this same time, other forms of healing had an attraction. Maybe I wanted more mind-boggling experiences and intellectual vision. Maybe I wanted to go beyond Chinese chauvinism. Maybe it was that I thought patients should have the benefit of all insights and practices available. For all these reasons, I went to India on my way back from China. But I realized I didn't have the internal stamina to remain overseas to learn Sanskrit and Hindi after learning

Chinese languages. Later, I worked at the British Broadcasting Corporation for 4 years as a television series writer. During that time I wrote a series on the healing arts and visited healers of every kind around the world. I became excited by the structure of various kinds of healing—what is shared, what is distinct, what is commensurate, what is necessarily absolutely "other." I became interested in what I call *metamedicine*.

For me, the best learning seems to take place in the context of disagreement more than agreement; contrasting conceptual models help to prevent complacency, self-serving avoidance, and dishonesty. The challenge of an "alien" environment (such as Harvard) seemed attractive—like wanting to see what it'd be like to be a dinosaur in an environment dominated by mammals. When money became available, I was invited to participate in some research efforts, primarily because of my scholarly background in Oriental medicine and alternative medicine. But much of my focus rapidly turned to studying the a priori epistemological assumptions of the people around me, of modern medicine and modern science.

I feel like a participant-observer. I always try to do what you're supposed to: scientific research, academic teaching, and peer-review publication. But I also remain an outside observer who tries to make sense of the fundamental gestalt of the biomedical culture. Also, I have used the opportunities at Harvard to study statistics, epidemiology, medical history, and anthropology. (By the way, statistics also can be mind-boggling.) I didn't expect this Harvard appointment to last more than 6 months. Now it's been 12 years. I seem to be part of the community and people have been generous in overlooking my strangeness and have encouraged me to be critical and even heretical. I've become a hybrid—a committed scientist and, at the same time, maybe a prehistoric and prescientific outsider trying to look at science.

The Placebo Response

To begin simply, the placebo effect is an inherent capacity within a person to evoke renewed senses of well-being, intactness, and authenticity. This endowment is especially elicited by the symbolic and behavioral activities of the patient-healer encounter. The mediums through which such placebo effects seems to work include the power of belief, expectation, hope, imagination, will, intention, preference, and commitment, as well as the ability human beings have to change their relationship to disease and its meaning.

The placebo effect is one of the contradictions in modern medicine's conceptual structure. It is an oxymoron-like enigma having to do with an effect produced by something that is inert—that is, the effect of something that has no effect. Any discussion about placebo reveals as much about modern medicine's metaphysics as it does about any mind-body effects. The placebo effect is an important challenge to the biomedical belief that healing is primarily a stimulus-response nexus, a cause-and-effect relationship of a specific physical intervention with a circumscribed outcome.

Often people do not notice that there is no such thing as a placebo effect in Chinese medicine, Greek medicine, shamanism, or any other system. Only modern medicine speaks about a placebo and a placebo effect. I think this is related to the fact that there is no such thing as an inert substance outside Newtonian physics.

Since the scientific revolution, we've known that an outside physical impulse is always necessary to bring anything (including human life) into new movement or to alter or end previous movement. The central image of change is the impact of billiard balls with predefined mass and velocity. Humoral medical systems (e.g., East Asian, Ayurvedic, Greek) are grounded in a physics that sees transformation as primarily having to do with the development of tendencies inherent within a particular configuration of life—an unfolding of preexisting potentials.

Of course, humoral systems also understand that external forces, such as purgatives or diuretics, have dramatic impact and power. But external physical treatment is not thought to be the main cause of transformation; external stimulus is meant to resonate and evoke what is already inherent.

Other systems, such as shamanic medicine, which is centered on belief, imagination, and will, sees change as having to do with the intentionality of the spirit realm and sees causality as primarily nonphysical. In opposition, biomedicine privileges external physical forces (in the form of drugs, surgery, and so on) changing a relatively inert human being.

The placebo effect is one way to see that a Newtonian healthcare model is too simple when it comes to human life. Any health outcome that does not fit biomedicine's primary explanatory model of physical cause-effect reasoning can operationally be dumped into the wastebasket of placebo effects. This disposal system is actually a policing system that eliminates subversive and threatening phenomena. The placebo effect is a prime culprit.

A different way to conceptualize the placebo effect is to call it the outcome produced by the dummy control arm of a randomized controlled trial (RCT). Besides being a measure of the psychological component of the experimental ritual, this placebo arm also—importantly—includes the self-healing aspect of the natural history of disease and the statistical concept of regression to the mean (which has to do with the fact that a variable extreme on its first measurement will tend to be closer to the center of distribution at a later measurement).

The Asbjørn Hrøbjartsson and Peter Gøtzsche metaanalysis published in the *New England Journal of Medicine* argues that the placebo effect is primarily natural history and regression to the mean. One of the historical problems in placebo discussions is that the placebo arm of trials is only designed to help understand the verum active treatment. The placebo arm actually does not give information that allows one to distinguish between what giving the dummy pill does compared with what "natural history" or "no treatment" would do on its own. The article explores this question by examining trials that happened to include both a placebo arm and a "no-treatment" arm. I thought it was a creative article, and I admire what they did. But I have several responses.

First, this study only challenges the narrow concept of a placebo effect that has to do with the outcomes of dummy controls in RCTs. The authors do not challenge the broader notion that the placebo effect is composed of a package of "nonspecific" interactions that may include communication of concern, intensive monitoring and diagnostic procedures, labeling of the complaint, explanation of the disease process, or any of the expectations and behaviors that can be manipulated in the patient-healer relationship. The authors explicitly state that their study did not deal with this arena. (The mass media entirely overlooked this caveat.) Why the authors avoided any challenge here is undoubtedly because they are aware that many RCTs exist that compare different kinds of physician behaviors or patients provided with different expectations. For example, I'm sure the authors were aware of Di Blasi's *Lancet* systematic review of one type of these trials. Di Blasi found consistent evidence that physicians who adopt a warm, friendly, or reassuring manner are more effective than those who keep consultations formal or do not offer reassurance.

My second response to the article is that the outcome of the placebo arm in RCTs has always had a polemical and rhetorical dimension. In fact, I published an entire discussion on this in *The Lancet*. The placebo effect that Beecher found in 1955 was very shaky, but the medical profession adopted it uncritically because it helped justify the adoption of the placebo-controlled RCT. If you have a fierce bogeyman placebo effect that clouds clinical judgment, you supposedly need placebo controls to test for efficacy. But, in fact, when compared with natural history in RCTs that just happened to have a no-treatment group, the placebo effect has not consistently been robust. Beecher intentionally hid this. Sometimes it is not present; sometimes it is. Sometimes it is very dramatic. It should not have been unexpected that a metaanalysis across many conditions with extremely heterogeneous outcomes will not demonstrate a stable effect.

Nevertheless, there have been two domains in which the placebo effect has been uniformly robust: physiological experiments on subjects given sugar pills under laboratory experiments and prospective clinical experiments designed to study placebo effects. These experiments began with Wolf's early experiments in the 1950s giving pregnant women ipecac (which makes you vomit) and having it relieve nausea when accompanied by an appropriate suggestion. The placebo effect in this kind of experimentation has consistently been robust up to the present. Beecher deliberately confounded this effect with the dummy arm of an RCT.

My third response to the article is that you don't overturn a concept because of one metaanalysis, especially if there is other evidence that argues in a different direction. And there is much of this kind of data. *The New England Journal of Medicine* paper argues for the absence of a strong placebo effect by comparing the placebo arm with "no-treatment" arms in RCTs designed for altogether different purposes. But another way of studying placebo effects in RCTs is controlling for them with another type of placebo—for example, saline solution versus sugar pill. This type of experiment is usually prospective with a hypothesis about placebo effects and is better blinded than a no-treatment arm.

Believe it or not, there have been many such experiments. For example, Grenfell and colleagues randomized 70 hypertensive patients into treatment with saline injection versus sugar pill. Patients were followed for up to 143 weeks. The injected placebo worked significantly better than did the oral placebo. I've written a technical review of such experiments in the *Journal of Clinical Epidemiology*. If a placebo has no effect beyond natural history, changing the type of placebo in an RCT should make no difference, but it does. One could also extend this perspective and examine the enormous literature on expectation manipulation. A good example is the entire series of experiments performed at different sites between 1970 and 1985 in which identical saline inhalators given to asthmatic patients could either start or stop asthma attacks depending on the instruction. Again, we're not dealing with natural history here.

My fourth response to this study is that any decision on placebo effects should look at the meticulous mechanistic studies of the placebo effect. I'm thinking especially of the recent work of Fabrizio Benedetti, Donald Price, and Irving Kirsch on humans or Robert Ader and Robert Herrnstein's Pavlovian conditioning research on animal models. It is hard to argue that the placebo effect does not exist after reading these kinds of experiments in which the effect of symbolic representation can clearly be traced in neurochemical pathways.

So to summarize my response: I think the Hrøbjartsson and Gøtzsche paper is important and will stimulate research and debate. But other research avenues suggest that it's too early to abandon the powerful placebo.

Questions About Placebo

If you give a drug with a needle and you give water with a needle, the assumption is that there is an equal placebo effect in both arms, but this needs to be demonstrated. For example, it may be that the placebo effect is bigger or smaller in one arm depending on its interaction with the drug. Or maybe the active arm outcome is the result only of the verum. Maybe the placebo effect is as big as the drug but does not happen as often. Maybe doubting you're receiving a real treatment affects the verum and placebo differently. For me, it raises a related question: Can you separate a verum effect from a placebo effect? Isn't this a lot like separating the body from the soul? What does this separation mean? For the earthly realm, at least, do any of these components have an independent existence? Is their separation the consequence of an inadequate medical metaphysics or the requirements of an awkward research method that must be further refined? Does separating them destroy what it is you're searching to understand?

In one study, the placebo effect of the needle was greater than the effect of the pill. Personally, I think it's because in our culture, the needle is perceived to be more powerful, so there's a stronger belief system in play. There's reasonable evidence here. But obviously, more research would be helpful.

So, presumably, coming into the trial, a person's belief system will affect how he or she reacts to the healing being given. In experiments, modern medicine controls for belief by removing knowledge of the intervention. When a person's knowledge is removed, he or she doesn't know whether the treatment is real, so presumably the placebo effect is evenly distributed. But one of the questions I am pursuing is this: how do we know this method of intentional ignorance produces accurate information? Maybe removing knowledge has consequences that we don't understand. For example, when I studied in China I was taught that, in most situations, patients should know what's going on because that will produce the most powerful results.

For me, it is an epistemological assumption that the act of removing knowledge does not interact, in some way, with the drug or sugar pill. Maybe the interaction is unequal; maybe the drug or placebo has a better effect or worse effect with knowledge. A lot of my work is related to how we know that the clinical research methods adopted after World War II—such as blinding, random assignment, and probabilistic inference—has ecological validity and is generalizable to the real world. How do we know that it doesn't produce artifacts like the Hawthorne effect or Heisenberg principle, where if you measure something it may change the reality of it? Does the removal of human knowledge—creating artificial states of ignorance—make a more accurate portrayal of what an intervention really does? In what exact way is it more accurate? What does this accuracy mean in terms of patient care?

From what I've uncovered so far—and it's still a work in progress—it seems that the modern placebo-controlled trial apparatus is not necessarily neutral; it actually interacts with what you're studying. It can produce complex phenomena. The effects of the real drugs and the placebo are often significantly different in real clinical situations compared with the hermetically sealed enclosure of the masked RCT. Human subjectivity can undermine objectivity even under double-blind conditions.

For example, in 1990, just before informed consent became mandatory in France, researchers took 49 consecutive hospitalized patients with cancer pain (not requiring opiates) and secretly randomized them to be informed—or not informed—of their participation in a double-blind RCT crossover experiment. Completely unaware of the experiment, 25 control patients received naproxen and a placebo pill in random order (they thought they were receiving routine care for pain), and the other informed patients were asked to join a double-blind RCT testing a pain medication. The trial compared the effect of a drug and placebo in an RCT with their effect when given when patients thought they were receiving routine care.

The outcome of both the drug and the placebo in the two different arms were significantly different. In some situations, knowing you're in a trial seems to be able to significantly change the effects of both drug and placebo. Such experiments suggest that more needs to be understood concerning the ecological validity of research methods. I could give other examples but, perhaps not surprisingly, I've written an extensive review of similar kinds of experiments elsewhere.

The Body's Natural Healing Abilities as Different from Placebo

Supposedly, the body's innate healing ability is different from placebo, but the recent article in *The New England Journal of Medicine* says that's not true. If you group together more than 100 trials and you crunch the numbers, the data appear to say it isn't true. But I think there is sufficient evidence to believe that there is something called the *placebo effect* beyond natural history. I've already given some examples, but maybe you'd like to hear more.

There are two recent metaanalyses by Tom deCraen and colleagues showing that giving four sham pills is better than giving two sham pills in peptic ulcer disease and that sham injections are better than placebo pills in acute migraine. Again, if it is only natural history, there should be no difference. Another wonderful experiment is by Dick Gracely and colleagues, who told dental patients that they could receive either placebo, narcotic analgesic, or narcotic antagonist. Then the patients were randomized unknowingly into two arms: in one trial arm the dental patients randomly received either placebo, narcotic analgesic, or narcotic antagonists, whereas the other arm provided only a placebo or narcotic antagonist. Treating dentists knew the possibilities of intervention in both trial arms, but the medication administration remained blind. The placebo response was significantly worse in the second group (without narcotic possibility) compared to the first group. The large placebo effect detected was dependent on practitioner expectation and clearly more than just natural history.

Pathology versus Experience

The placebo effect is an important critique of any narrow reductionist perspective in biomedicine and any equally narrow approach within alternative medicine. The bottom line is that the placebo effect demonstrates that an exclusively billiard-ball model impoverishes any understanding of health and illness.

The existence of a placebo effect means that imagination, expectation, anticipation, hope, belief, adherence, and intentionality have an effect on treatment both in terms of active or ritual components. As fully conscious and interacting beings, the healer and the patient are an integral part of the healing process. Any conventional or alternative medicine that exclusively privileges the appearance of objectivity is full of its own hubris.

The dynamic of symbols, meaning, and the human imagination is critical for healing. An understanding of inward tendencies cannot be neglected. Any science (even an alternative medicine type science) that neglects art is insufficient for understanding healthcare.

One of our tasks as healers is to say what's wrong with the patient. It has the appearance of an objective assessment process. This applies not only to modern medicine but also across the board to chiropractic, East Asian medicine, Ayurveda, or homeopathy. We label patients. We tell them what's the problem. Your kapha is too strong; your wind is going in the wrong direction; you've urinated in the wrong direction and now the god of the north is angry; your electrolytes are out of balance; or this or that. But one of the absolute truths of medicine that is avoided across the board in all medical systems is that there is no one-to-one correspondence between what the healer says is wrong and the state of the patient.

Now, what do I mean by that? I mean, many kids get strep throat growing on their throats, but most never get strep throat. More people have objective diabetes than have the symptoms of diabetes. Cancer lives in people for years before we detect it. People walk around with tuberculosis all the time. Everybody's yin and yang is out of order, and who doesn't have a spinal subluxation? With all of this, some people feel good, and some people don't feel good. The so-called pathology—the objective-like diagnosis—doesn't predict the human experience.

The so-called intervention is aiming at only a piece of the puzzle. Relying on objectivity in medicine is putting a veneer over an ocean of subjective perception.

Let me illustrate this with a story. In the Jewish *Midrash*, God creates the world in 6 days and rests on the seventh day. So one question is: When did he create old age? The *Midrash* says that God created old age when Abraham was walking with Isaac to the sacrifice and Abraham complained that he didn't look older than Isaac. So God made old age at that point. And then the next question is: When did disability arise? It turns out that the patriarch Isaac was blind and couldn't distinguish Esau from Jacob. So the *Midrash* says that disability came into the world at that point. So the next question is: when does illness come in? No one was sick in the very early stories of the Bible. The *Midrash* says that sickness came into the world when the patriarch Jacob didn't feel good. Before this time, sometimes feeling bad was routine. Jacob, however, was the first person to turn his head toward heaven and say, "God, please take away this pain." At that moment, illness came in. The *Midrash* says illness does not exist until the moment people, as self-conscious human beings, want things to be different.

When we get cancer, we obviously want to get rid of that cancer. But on some level the *Midrash* is saying that it is not only an objective reality; it's also the inner world of the person that makes this an illness. So the questions of where people sit in their inner world and who they are in relation to themselves and the entire creation are important. These are absolutely human questions—subjective questions of evaluation and meaning. I think this interpretive realm has a close relationship to the placebo effect.

Penicillin is a great drug, and it really does get rid of infections. Surgery does its job; needling with acupuncture does its job; spinal manipulation does its job. In some situations these interventions get a person beyond what self-healing would do. In some situations, these interventions are part of a process of shifting our self-relationship to the complaint, shifting our self-relationship to our own identity. Yes, even the most physical surgery, successful or otherwise, can involve a shift in identity.

What Is Healing?

Ultimately, medicine's job is not to relieve suffering or eliminate it. Medicine's job is to relieve *unnecessary* suffering and to help shift our relationship to necessary suffering.

Both active intervention and rituals alone probably help small discomforts and illnesses. Sometimes even big discomforts are relieved. But there is some level at which all medical systems blank out and pretend to be looking elsewhere. In fact, there are always some things we can't fix. But we can change self-relationship, and that's very powerful. Let's pretend shamans don't have drugs that work in the form of pharmacologically active herbs. Let's pretend that acupuncture doesn't work, and let's pretend that we have an infection that can't be treated with an antibiotic. Ultimately, we are confronted by suffering that cannot be relieved. This is at least one of the dimensions of healing that the placebo effect points toward.

Maybe this is where I should try to be explicit about what I mean by healing in the context of our discussion: I would say that healing is providing relief in the face of unnecessary suffering; in the face of necessary suffering, healing evokes a depth of humanity deeper than the tragedy of any illness. Both active and ritual interventions have these capacities. Depending on particular situations, one can be more powerful than the other.

One of the things I learned as a practitioner of Chinese medicine was that there is always room for transformation. That's one of the beautiful aspects of Chinese medicine's metaphysics. We probably all know that as healers. But there's a way that's not spoken about enough. In any situation, there's always a possibility for people to have a different relationship with themselves.

This absolute subjectivity—this ultimate self-reflection—is so much more profound than the simple placebo effect of giving a pill. The simplistic placebo effect just points a finger at an ocean of healing that resides in self-relationship and utter subjectivity.

If the placebo is going to remain a scientific concept, the following question must be answered; it's the mechanism question. If you give a person a drug and it causes a chemical reaction in the body that causes an effect and if you give a person a placebo and get the same effect, has the same chemical reaction been caused, or is the effect from the placebo happening via a different mechanism?

There is much evidence showing that the placebo analgesia is related to endorphins and other endogenous opioids. Opiate antagonists such as naloxone and opiate agonists such as buprenorphine predictably alter placebo effects under laboratory conditions. That's one mechanism. Other researchers are now scrambling to get objective evidence of other mechanisms using magnetic resonance imaging or various methods from psychoneuroimmunological science. More objective and hard reductionist research would be great here.

Mind and Will in Chinese Thought

But the bifurcation of the world into objective and subjective is less rigid in Chinese medicine, and any boundary is fluid; the two realms merge. Traditionally, the Chinese have no need for accurately measuring things and making things independently verifiable by an outside observer. In traditional culture, no one would consider "blinding" or "randomizing" patients as an enhancement to improve knowledge detection. Qualitative relationships were more critical than quantitative considerations. Dynamics of flux are primary; stability was secondary. Ancient texts always understood that a person was able to transform himself, at least on some level of being and self-awareness, by an exertion of will. Physical and nonphysical realms interacted and merged. Will and mind are important in all situations.

I recently rewrote my first book, *The Web That Has No Weaver,* to deal with such issues. They got neglected in the first edition because I was under the influence of modernist interpretations of Chinese medicine. Since at least the Republic period, China has sought to modernize itself, and for Chinese medicine this has meant attempting to appear more objective and a lot more materialistic than its original formulations. After many years of studying ancient texts, I reread the first edition and realized that much of the ancient perspective—which included an in-depth understanding of psychospiritual issues—hadn't been fully transmitted to me in Chinese medical school. So I wrote the second edition hoping to make up for this serious deficiency.

Mind and will are seen in the context of what the Chinese call spirit. For the Chinese, spirit is the dimension of human life that is not restricted to ordinary time and space. Mind is that aspect of spirit that describes the consciousness of possibilities. It's about transformation, creativity, and understanding the value of things moving from one state of being to another. Will is deeper and has two dimensions: a yang dynamic dimension of arduous effort of volition and a yin dimension of profound receptivity and recognition of the inexorable and the entire process of destiny, or what can be called the "will that has no will"—the will that goes through us that we only notice when we turn around. Will is related to the unknown, as are wisdom and fear. Fear is the visceral-emotional feeling of the unknown; wisdom is consciousness embracing the unknown.

Questions of how one establishes a sense of wisdom, how one abides in the world that changes all the time, and how one makes connections in time and space that are appropriate all are critical to traditional healthcare. Being able to do meaningful activities even though one is sick: how do you get that strength? How do you find will? How do you get the intelligence and awareness of possibilities to be able to know when to hold on and let go? How can meaningful activity and good deeds still be performed when one is sick? Forgiveness. When and how should one forgive others or oneself? These are central problems. And it goes on and on.

Forgiveness and Good Deeds

For the Chinese, forgiveness is connected to the human sensitivity to boundaries, both in terms of bodily activity and the boundary between self and others. This sensitivity is regulated by the psychospiritual dimension of what the Chinese call the noncorporeal soul. This spiritual capacity has to do with creating the specific virtue of "human kindness." (There are many other virtues, such as wisdom and faithfulness.) When the boundary capacity of people is unbalanced—for example, when it's grandiose—there can be excessive anger or pushiness, or when it's too small, there's insufficient self-esteem or lack of assertion.

Forgiveness is transforming the energy of disturbed boundaries into the virtue of "human kindness." People have the psychospiritual potential to forgive others or themselves. Taking anger and moving this emotional energy toward forgiving other people is self-transformation. In regard to self-esteem, saying "I didn't take enough space in the world" is also a self-transforming process. For the Chinese, this energetic of human-kindness, forgiveness, anger, and self-esteem extends into physical problems such as body rigidity or insufficient bodily mass, migraine headaches, or certain types of menstrual problems. It also extends into particular herbs or acupuncture points. For the Chinese, these herbs can resonate or evoke disturbed boundaries into becoming more balanced borders.

But any evoking of forgiveness with physical interventions also must have the subjective participation of a certain style of patient-doctor relationship and the subjective commitment of both partners. The herbs and acupuncture can only help to bring out the potential. To summarize: forgiveness is understood in the context of an energetic of the noncorporeal soul, human-kindness, anger, self-esteem, migraine, chronic menstrual problems, and such herbs as chrysanthemum and peony and liver meridian acupuncture points. All being is on one gradient or another in a great chain of resonating being. All phenomena interpenetrate and interact. Going back to the original questions on subjectivity—for the Chinese, objectivity and subjectivity mutually create one another.

The most important thing is what you pay attention to when a human being comes into a patient-healer relationship. What things are central? Mainstream doctors might use lab reports or imaging techniques. A homeopathic doctor might notice if the baby especially likes being hugged. For a shaman, it's what kind of rituals did you break? Chinese doctors feel the pulse. Systems access different components of who we are.

One of the important things that I've learned is that we practitioners need to acknowledge that what we're seeing is only a piece of reality. One of the important lessons of looking at multiple medical systems is that any single system does not touch all of reality. Even putting all systems together might not be enough—and maybe it only creates clutter. Holism is an elusive goal.

Ultimately, medicine, at its best, can never enumerate or know everything about a person. At best, medicine is an art that resonates with the elusive truth. Ultimately, we are dealing with poetic resonance, evoking the possible. The artistry of any system needs to transcend its own conceptual limitations. This applies both to mainstream and alternative medicine.

I work in the conventional medical world. I do research, and I have patients who have specific entry criteria, a predetermined outcome, and are randomized, blinded, and studied as the mean outcome of a cohort using probabilistic logic. I also worked in a world where blinding a person was bizarre and randomizing was incomprehensible—where objective outcome was so much less important than process and one could not consider a person as anything but a nonreplicable event.

I've worked in and enjoyed both situations. My inner world struggles with how to reconcile objectivity and subjectivity. For me—and I guess this is a projection of my inner struggle—the debate between alternative medicine and conventional medicine and this new amalgamation some people are calling *integrated medicine* is about how one reconciles solid objectivity arrived at independent of belief and culture with the absolute uncontestable importance and meaningfulness of subjectivity. How can these two different approaches be reconciled without destroying the internal validity of either? Any synthesis won't be easy. Maybe it shouldn't be resolved. Putting everything into a box and calling it *integrative* may be an unreflective way to short-circuit an important process that may require generations and multiple avenues of exploration.

Psychospiritual Issues in Chinese Medicine

I'd like to make just one further point to finish an earlier discussion: I raised the question of psychospiritual issues in Chinese medicine. It may be helpful to say that it is critical that we practitioners remember that our job is to heal body and soul (and I emphasize *heal*) and not save the soul (and I emphasize *save*). Sometimes this boundary between healthcare and spiritual/religious ministry gets lost. Being healthy is different from being spiritual or religious. Any blurring here can be dangerous.

Healers have power, and patients are necessarily vulnerable. It is important not to abuse this power. Healthcare should be open to helping patients explore the transcendent dimensions in their life. Any deep healing should offer people, if they want, the option and positive support of examining authenticity, freedom, morality, self-identity, and self-relationship. Issues of being moral, having commitment to values, and engaging in religious or spiritual practices are important. But healers need to be careful not to impose their own forms of spirituality onto patients. At times, healers may need to be aware of how their patients are struggling with such issues and support these efforts, but we must be careful not to explicitly—or even subtly—impose, even by simple example, any of the practices or commitments of our own spiritual values. This has the potential of subverting patients' freedom. In practice, making this distinction is difficult and deserves an extensive discussion. I just want to raise it for a moment.

But mostly, I'd like to thank you for an opportunity to talk about some of the things I've been mulling over.

CHAPTER 21

DAVID REILLY, FRCP, MRCGP, FFHOM

The Therapeutic Consultation

Most people know of Dr. David Reilly as the "Scottish physician who published the home-opathy paper in *The Lancet.*" Although true, this notoriety hardly speaks to the depth of Reilly's formal medical education or his varied accomplishments as a researcher. Nor does it speak of his interest and inquiry into the nature of the human spirit.

Reilly comes from a traditional medical background. He graduated with commendation from Glasgow Medical University in 1973 and is a member of both the Royal College of Physicians and the Royal College of General Practitioners. In 1987, he was awarded the first RCCM/MRC Research Fellowship. In 1992, he was elected as a Fellow to the Royal College of Physicians and Surgeons, one of Britain's highest medical honors. Currently, he is Honorary Senior Lecturer at the Royal Infirmary in Glasgow and the lead Consultant Physician at the Glasgow Homeopathic Hospital

His interest in culture, in the process of manifestation, in human feelings, in the mind-body relationship, and in man's inherent healing abilities led Dr. David Reilly to explore other realms of knowledge. Integrating information and wisdom from these areas with what he knew as a physician, Reilly has come to believe that the "therapeutic relationship" is one of the most important aspects of medical care. I interviewed Dr. Reilly in 1995 in Santa Fe, New Mexico, while he was visiting some American friends.

Before I went to medical school I read a lot around human beings—about experience and illness and health—and was intrigued by hypnosis and inner mind work. I had to put it on the back burner, but eventually I reached a crisis point. I remember the particular moment. I'd been reading around the relationship of nutrition and illness in Crohn's disease and inflammatory bowel disease. There was a doctor from Cambridge whose published work showed that if you withdraw some allergens, sometimes it helps. Not that it's curative, but it's supportive. At that point I was a registrar (resident) in a busy teaching hospital. We were standing around the bed of a lady who'd had surgery so many times for her inflammatory bowel disease that there was not much gut left. And each time they removed the gut, the biopsy showed eosinophils, which are cells of allergy invading through the gut wall and going into the lumen. As we stood around the bed, the patient told us that whenever she took milk, her pain became much worse. I looked the consultant in the eye and said, "In view of these facts, how about a trial of a dairy-free diet?" He completely rejected the suggestion with that time-honored phrase I've heard so many times since, "There is no scientific evidence for that whatsoever."

Something in me said, "I've got to get out. This is now the moment."

The practice of medicine is often truly unscientific. So often there is information lying in one corner that isn't applied in another corner. Throughout my journey I've been trying to learn about the human elements of that: the fear, the prejudice, the attitude, the movement of knowledge. What traps people within particular perceptions? What moves people from one place to another? That sort of awareness is part of what I've tried to bring to the examination of complementary medicines.

My first water in the desert was the British Society of Medical and Dental Hypnosis. I did some of their postgraduate courses. It was the first chance I had to bring together more systematically some of the strands I'd been studying and thinking of and spontaneously developing with my patients. Then came the moment I mentioned earlier. Right after that, there was an advert in the *British Medical Journal* for a registrar at the homeopathic hospital in Glasgow. I had never been there and knew nothing about homeopathy. But the advert said, "An interest in nutrition may be of value."

When I crossed through the door, I thought, "I like it." The people I met had a more flexible, open attitude and feeling. I joined the unit and watched and listened. I had no confidence whatsoever in homeopathy in terms of the dilutions, but I was very intrigued by the system of care.

Homeopathy

Many physicians think that homeopathy, as a science, exists only in the little vials of dilutions, but the funny thing is the dilutions are often the least part of it. The biggest part is human engagement and a system for approaching illness and disease that is not based on judgment or theory. Homeopaths had an interesting dilemma 200 years ago that, in a way, persists. They didn't know how the medicine worked, so they did not marry their observations to any transient theory of what human illness is or what recovery is. This led them to do something fairly radical—they listened to their patients. If a patient says, "I have a pain and it's on the right side of my face, and it tends to appear at 3 PM," the homeopath will write this fact down.

Conventional training made me think I was an expert. Now, what an expert does is this: In comes the patient, and he has this one-sided headache. You cross-correlate one or two points and say, "This is migraine." Having made your diagnosis, the fact that it comes on at 3 PM is no longer of interest to you.

But homeopaths try to match up the physiological and emotional disturbances of the person at this time with a pattern of disturbance recognized with different drugs. So if the headache comes on in the evening or the morning, suddenly or gradually, if it's helped by heat or by cold or if it changes with barometric pressure, it's recorded. What's the mental content during this headache? Is the person withdrawn or sad? Do they want to be cuddled or cared for? Are they weeping? All of these things are taken on an as-is basis and documented. So patients suddenly realize this practitioner is interested in what they are saying. That's powerful medicine. There's no doubt that that, in itself, is deeply therapeutic.

The other thing is that homeopathic medicine never perceived the mind and body as separate, so it never went down the tracks of conventional medicine and many of the dead ends of conventional medicine in that regard.

Thurston Brewin, a radiooncologist in Glasgow, published papers that observed that in malignancy, people's food cravings often subtly change. The way a dog may seek out grass when it's sick, certain people will go off certain foods and they'll begin to crave others during significant illness. He claimed that on successful resection of the tumor, these cravings may normalize. But a subtle signal of reappearance of the tumor created a disturbance in taste sensation again.

That information was completely ignored by conventional medicine because it didn't fit into how people viewed things. But if you open the homeopathic books, there's 180 years of unbroken development of observation, of a correlation of food cravings and reactions and illnesses, and—more importantly—of mental content, such as the shift in the response pattern that emerges from the person in trauma and how that relates to the onset of physical illness and its expression.

People who do our introductory homeopathic course tell us that even if they don't use homeopathic medicines, their perception of the patient has become enriched. And their consultation has become more effective and more therapeutic in its own right.

The Basic Homeopathic Course

In our course, we first try to respect the good intentions and desires of these people who have gone into healing professions, who are genuinely doing what they conceive to be the very best for their patients, who are afraid—and so they should be—of unscientific and exploitive forms of care. I take the group and start from where they are and what their fears and needs are, and I show them a patient. I root the course in patients—not in theory or philosophy.

We start with a video of a man who has severe headaches. Participants have a sheet of paper on which they take down whatever they think is of interest in this man's case. Most people might write one or two words. "Possible migraine or cluster headache," or something. Then we pause the video and say, "Okay, what do we think is wrong with this man?" We discuss diagnosis, perception, and it turns out he has cluster headaches. Some of the group may not be aware of that diagnosis, so they suddenly realize we're dealing with human beings and medicine and that we have something to share conventionally. So we talk a little about cluster headaches. What's known about it and how it presents and so forth.

The group is asked how they might treat the case, and they make various suggestions. Then I reveal that this man has had all of the drugs mentioned. I put up an acetate overhead that lists his previous medication. It contains all of the medicines they suggested. "That's why you're all here," I say, "because all of us are seeking whether there are other meaningful, valid, therapeutic approaches that might work when our conventional medicines don't work or that might be better."

So then we roll the video, and the man describes his reaction to the homeopathic medicine he received. This man was referred to me back in 1984 on an open-admission policy to the neurological institute because of a high suicide risk. He was chronically invalided with the cluster headaches. I gave him counseling and emotional support, and he wept a great deal. I used auricular acupuncture, which very interestingly swapped the sites of the attack but did not heal him. I admitted him to the (Glasgow) homeopathic hospital for observation and did something that I do very, very rarely: to judge the impact of the circumstance and of the ritual, the first medicine I gave him was placebo. He was enthusiastic about it, but it didn't work. Then I swapped to the active medicine, and it worked in seconds.

On the tape, he describes how, from a few doses, the remission emerges and then continues for months. This is intriguing for the audience, and they begin to wonder: how could that happen?

At the end, I say to the group, "Okay, we're here to study this and wonder together. What does this mean? Is this placebo? It could be. The literature shows that sometimes a second placebo will work when a first won't. And if so, why did it work, what did I do, and what can we gain from it? Or is it the homeopathic medicines? That's the dilemma that homeopathic physicians have presented for two centuries. Patients all around the world and clinicians all around the world continue to say it works. So let's have an adventure together. Let's clear our minds and see what the claims are, what the sciences are, what the clinical experiences are, and then you will have a chance to try a few medicines for yourself."

By the end of the first day, they've learned a little about five simple applications of homeo-pathy. Then they watch the video a second time and I say, "Take a note of anything you find of interest." And the pens hit the paper. They're noting that it's on the right and that it came on suddenly and that he's agitated and angry during it, and it came on after grief. They have had this private, inner experience of a shift in perception.

They go away and try the kits. Six weeks later, we ask how many people have tried homeopathy. Maybe 90% of the hands will go up. Then I ask how many people consider that it's been working, and we have lots of statistics on this, but it will always be over 80%. I challenge them. "Well, what does 'worked' mean? What is 'worked' in medicine? Is what you've experienced science or not?"

Changing the Culture

Getting my paper on homeopathic research published in *The Lancet* was extremely difficult on one level. But they have a saying in Britain: "If you can't stand the heat, get out of the kitchen."

I have thought a lot about what research is, and the best thing I can say is that it is an act of communication. This could be communication with yourself, privately, or with people close to you who share your views or with others who are distant from you and don't share your views. As an act of communication, therefore, it behooves you to resonate with the people with whom you would like to communicate. I understood that. In 1983, when I first went to the homeopathic hospital, I stood in the library. It was a remarkable experience because of these books, published in continuity for 200 years. I thought, "Is this crazy? Imagine if 10% of it is accurate. Think of the implications for healthcare."

So I began to construct in my intent. I began to think, what moves a culture? What shifts attitudes? I reckoned that human beings are the same everywhere, and they're locked into the same constraints, which includes culture, peer pressure, belief, and exposure. Medicine's belief system has its own religious roots, the ritualistic or symbolic, and the catalysts that move it— such as articles in *The Lancet*. So I took that on board and set it as a goal for the inquiry. I picked models of research that were easily communicable and understood, which is why I chose pollen and hay fever.

Most people have been exposed to the idea that you can give pollen shots for hay fever. Therefore, the only new concept was the homeopathic dilution. I used standard methodology and off-the-shelf, validated outcome measures. I visited multiple university departments. I presented the idea for the research to skeptical colleagues because I think it's important to go to people who are your worst enemies rather than your best friends and try to understand where they're coming from.

So, every step along the way was very carefully constructed. And when the pilot study worked, I must confess, I was very shocked.

Let me put my cards on the table. My preconception was that homeopathic dilutions—not the system of homeopathy but homeopathic dilutions—were definitely a placebo. But I wanted to put flesh on the bones of my prejudice. I wanted to test my hypothesis, which is what science is. So the title of the project was, "Is Homeopathy a Placebo Response?," and the pollen and hay fever were just a model to address the specific question. When it came out positive, my gut level said, "This is a mistake."

I wrote to all the departments that had given me the advice to start with and said, "What do you think? What could be the flaw here? What's the mistake? What does it mean?" I took certain ridicule in quite a few environments and was accused of being unscientific for looking at something that was not plausible. I sent the pilot study to *The Lancet*. They refused it. So we took on board all the criticisms from every forum that we could gather; we incorporated them and reran the study a second time the next year, five times bigger.

We built into it solid protection against the possibility of fraud. We had one of the senior lecturers from the Glasgow University department of medicine personally look at every diary and check the results off the visual analog scales in the diary against the computer printout. This was a duplicate of the printout that the statistician had already received, which was independently correlated. And the statistician was not a homeopath and not interested, so he was neutral. It came out positive: clinically and statistically significant. So I was able to write back to the editor of *The Lancet* and say, "You recall the pilot paper? Your referee's comments? Well, here's the second piece of work, taking on board the ideas." And they took it.

After it was accepted, I spoke to the editor for the first time and thanked him for having the courage to take the paper. He thanked me for recognizing that it took courage. He said that they had gone over this paper with a fine-toothed comb and couldn't fault it and therefore felt it was science and it was data and it should be published. And I suppose, privately, that was one of the nicest moments for the team.

Then the feedback, the criticisms, and the arguments rolled in to the second paper. Things like, "Who cares about hay fever?"—which misses the point. It has nothing to do with hay fever. Also, I was now tainted and called a *homeopathic researcher*.

I was then awarded, with my co-worker Morag Taylor, the RCCM/MRC Research Fellowship at Glasgow University. So I went to the department of respiratory medicine at the University and said to Robin Stephenson, the head of the department, "How would you like to be the man that proves homeopathy doesn't work? I have the grant."

We set up a new trial that was still allergy, treated with the allergen, but it was with asthmatic patients, principally with house-dust-mite allergy. But this time we didn't do it with homeopathic researchers; we did it with conventional researchers. We didn't do it with homeopathic patients but with conventional patients already attending the department. We had them rediagnosed by the respiratory people, including laboratory tests and histamine provocation. We had the drugs made independently in France, sent straight to the pharmacists, double-blinded, who recoded them and administered them to the patients. The respiratory doctor monitored them throughout, and the homeopathic doctor, Neal Beattie, chose the allergen.

Within 7 days of receiving the randomized active medicine, those patients receiving the homeopathic remedy showed a clinically statistically significant greater drop in symptoms. We sent the results back to *The Lancet* after we took over 2 years in the analysis of it, and they accepted it.

By now there was a cultural debate growing as to whether the clinical trial evidence was proving sufficient to validate an unconventional therapy. A review was published after 100 trials of homeopathy, with 77% showing results in favor of the therapy. So I began to wonder, would 200 trials be evidence? Would three hundred trials be evidence? What is evidence? So I sat down in the last month before sending the paper to *The Lancet* and thought, "What do three positives in a row mean?" And a very simple answer came back. It's one of two things: either we have shown homeopathy works and that it works more than placebo, or we've shown the clinical trial doesn't work. We've shown the clinical trial, with predictability, reproducibility, clinical and statistical significance, can produce three false positives in a row.

I put that in the paper and the editor, much to my surprise, ran an editorial called "Reilly's Challenge."

I would say the first paper, in particular, did change the culture. What I learned is that medicine and religion have the same roots. The high altar is *The Lancet*, and a sacrifice has to be laid upon the altar with certain validating rituals occurring prior to the moment that it's placed there. And there must be magical symbols within the paper. There's a small one, and it's the letter *p*, for example.

I don't know whether the magic has affected the American culture or not, but certainly I've seen it shift the British culture. I've seen people take homeopathy with much more seriousness than before. I've seen the articles contribute to the general shift in attitude. That's why I search my heart very deeply, and why Morag, my partner, and I had to have the highest possible standard of science. Because think of the responsibility if this was sloppy science, if this was bad results, if this was distorted data? The cultural implications for me would be unthinkable.

I know now that homeopathy works clinically. I accept that. I know good consulting often works even better, which is my big interest in medicine. And I know the results of these trials are accurate. What it all adds up to, I wait to see. Maybe the small clinical trial is not a valid tool. Maybe you need a thousand in a group for any clinical trial to be meaningful. If this is the case, the implications are far more important for conventional medicine than for homeopathic medicine.

The Therapeutic Relationship

I've learned that things like relaxation techniques and acupuncture and homeopathy can be very useful tools in your toolbox. And what I'm about to say is not meant to invalidate that. But what I'd like to add is that, sometimes, oddly enough, therapies are the least of the issues. It's in the intention and integrity, the quality of the meeting, the trust, the relationship, the shared walk together of the person and the carer, where the magic really happens, where things really move and people experience radical changes in how they're coping or not coping, and in the quality of their life, and where transformations occur.

So having gone to some depth in formal techniques, what I've been exploring is what simply happens when you're with someone and you talk and you listen, allowing an effective consultation to unfold, feelings to be expressed, and trust to be established—and to bring to that situation some simple, positive intention.

I see changes occurring that are very radical sometimes. About 50% of my patients are in chronic pain. They've seen surgeons and had injections and x-rays and drugs, and they've also seen psychiatrists, yet often, no one has ever really let them tell their stories. No one has let them just speak and tell the story about the stresses that have come to their life, where things went off the rails, and how they responded to that and how it touched their inner world and the fears that developed and the inner fragmentations and conflicts that grew up. Being with the person to help place that back together somehow, to me, is the heart of medicine. It's the heart of care, and I think people are missing it.

People should be aware that there are many practitioners within the field of alternative medicine who are every bit as mechanistic, power-oriented, interventionist, and invested in "the therapy" as elsewhere. One of the things that moved me 15 years ago was that people were going to the psychiatrist and the cardiologist and the general practitioner. Now they're going to the aromatherapist, the homeopath, and whatever. Sometimes that's good. But for the group of patients I see, there's a missing ingredient—some sort of ancient, simple, human faculty and method of interaction.

Something struck me very powerfully about 18 months ago. For the first time I spent some time with a shaman. His name was Emaho, and I suddenly realized that what I was doing was simply operating in an ancient, traditional way—the ancient, traditional relationship of a person who's unwell seeking the counsel and presence and wisdom of someone who can help him on that path. I was doing something similar to the work of this man—but within my cultural metaphors, within its structures, within its ideas—and that was important. There are many people who are so rooted into where they're born and their family and the culture that they will not connect, perhaps never connect, with these wisdoms from other cultures. But there is something simple and basic about the relationship of people's inner world to the body, to their health, to their outer world, and to the forces that shape this inner world and produce fragmentation or cohesion with it and to the symbols that activate and move it.

It's actually okay to reconnect with some of the feelings that took you into medical school. The fact is the first patient you saw was a dead one and you cut him up, and you began a process of brutalization and loss of sanctity. When medical students are around the body on the first day of dissection, they are there as human beings. They stand in silence. They stand in awe. By the end of 9 months, they have been systematically broken down. I actually believe that has much more of an impact than people realize. Practitioners have lost a feeling of awe or a feeling that it's okay to be a human being. It's a big, big part of what it is to be sitting with this patient right now, sitting together as friends, as fellow travelers whose paths are crossing on a journey.

I've been trying to demonstrate to the homeopathic community, and I think they're uncomfortable with it, that all the phenomenology of homeopathy—very powerful and rich as it is—can be elicited without the use of the remedies on many occasions. Often when I have therapeutic consultations with people, something's happened; something's been touched. I'll ask them at the end if they would like a homeopathic medicine or not, and about 40% will say, "No, I don't want one." That's perhaps my most satisfying moment, because people know that something's been touched and moved, and they would like to go away and see what the product of that is.

In the asthma study, we began with people receiving a single placebo, which they didn't know was placebo, but we did. One month later, they received either a placebo or the homeopathic medicine. And this time, no one knew. Totally double-blind. We had certain people who had no reaction to the first medicine and a dramatic reaction to the second or a positive reaction to the first and a negative reaction to the second. We charted these reactions for each patient, and some displayed the phenomenon that homeopaths call *direction of cure*. I've put up these acetates in front of homeopathically trained colleagues and asked them, "Who received homeopathy at the second prescription, based on the phenomenology that's exhibited?" Most people get it wrong.

What we found is that many people respond to the second placebo and not the first or respond in opposite ways to the two placebos. The magic seems to be in the clinicians and the people partaking in the ritual, because that's what care is, when they change inwardly as to what they feel about the therapy. So when we knew there was a chance of an active medicine, something was transmitted to those patients. Is it demeanor? Is it tone of voice? Is it something more subtle? To my mind, that's what all of us should be examining, without being overattached to the particular tools in a toolbox.

I saw a lady last week—chronic abdominal pain, 9 years, thought originally to be coming from her pancreas. She had surgery on three occasions, multiple drugs, computed tomography (CT) scans, the works. She comes into the unit. After the end of the experience, that woman describes a dramatic change in herself: a reduction in her pain, a falling into place of how this pain may have developed, and the stresses in her life. And what I now know is not to sit too comfortably in saying why this occurred.

The receptionist who greeted her, the atmosphere of the building, sitting down with the nurse and being touched, the crying she did, the sense of receiving love and attention, the intense homeopathic interview, the experience with myself of a sudden release of memories, seeing a thread through the experience, and the homeopathic remedy which, interestingly, she elected to take. The product of all that was a transformation and a change.

I've studied it my whole life. At head level, I'll never understand it. But at the heart level, there is a healing capacity in people. It's natural. It's not anything esoteric. It's not spiritual in the sense of otherworldly; it's part of being a spirited person. There is a reality of a healing relationship, and no matter how much it might be abused or professionalized, or dehumanized, there is a reality in it, and useful things do occur when a focus is brought in that way.

Inquiry is as rich and varied as life. Scientific methods are just tools to help you in your inquiry. Why do we need to rip everything down into categories? You know, so-called "art," so-called "science," so-called "therapeutics" as opposed to inquiry? Why limit ourselves? You can't chop down a tree with a scalpel. If you want to know if a swallowed substance or an administered substance seems to have therapeutic potential in and of itself as opposed to the richness of medicine, then a placebo-controlled trial is a wonderful tool to do that. But it only applies sometimes, in a limited way. We've been doing outcome studies, writing to people 2 years after we saw them, phoning them, sending inquiries, making sure that we get at least an 80% capture of those populations. We make sure we start on one day and move sequentially forward until we have the 200 patients, so there isn't a personal bias in the selection. We make sure the person that approaches them is not the doctor originally consulted, so the person is free to give an honest opinion. To me, that's science. To me, science is a web that you weave to catch a prejudice.

The Future of Medical Care

We're going to build a new Glasgow Homeopathic Hospital within 2 years. We want it to reclaim healing as a part of everyone, not owned by people who call themselves healers. It's all from within us. There's nothing more amazing than life and the fact that life tries to heal and can also destroy. In this building, I would like to see a blending of the sciences and the arts, of high technology being available in a human atmosphere, with kindness, with fun, with confrontation if it's needed, against a background of trust, with a range of therapeutic options.

I think it's important to introduce the concept of specialists and generalists when we discuss holism. Some people think that because homeopathy takes a whole-person history—mental, physical, and environmental—that that's holistic medicine. That's nonsense. Holism involves looking at or accepting the multifaceted nature of one person and of that person's care.

Hospital specialists can be trapped in the ivory tower, immersed in the in-depth knowledge they have of a specific territory and being dismissive of the general practitioner's superficial knowledge of that territory and not understanding that the generalist—the whole strength of the generalist—is to have an overview of a situation. This applies in complementary medicine as well. Complementary specialists should recognize that they're specialists and should begin to talk about the bounds and limits of their own competence and their own perception. They should know that their strength is their specialization, and it's their weakness as well, because of the narrowness of view.

So how is the healthcare system to put that together? And how is the single patient to put that together? What if one person's care would benefit from the perspective of a number of people, or a number of viewpoints?

The hospital is experimenting with how those ingredients will mix together. It is a center struggling toward more balanced or integrated care management for particular patients. We hope this small place will be a quiet point of inspiration about a therapeutic atmosphere and an approach to care that might offer something to the community around it, and receive something from that community.

When does the acupuncturist refer to a physician? When does the physician refer to an acupuncturist? That's exactly the dilemma we were talking about between the different specialties of orthodox medicine. That's why I'm still very impressed by the possible role of an informed generalist. In Britain, the primary care team plays a critical role in that. That's why the homeopathic course, at its foundation level, is not about turning people into homeopathic specialists. It's about making them able to talk to their patients in an informed way about whether the approach might or might not help.

The system of primary and secondary care did not evolve without reason. Why did orthodox medicine grow up as a generalist/specialist split? I think there's wisdom in it. So make the primary care physician and the rest of the primary care team have amongst them a rich awareness of the potentials of these therapies and specialists. That's how I'd see it. We're in a strong position to do that in Scotland, because we've built up the credibility through the education. For instance, 20% of Scotland's general practitioners have completed our basic training in homeopathy.

So these ingredients are coming together. And I say to the folks reading this that there are places in the world where the prejudices are beginning to break down and the contact is beginning to happen, and better care is resulting from it. It's inspiring.

Earlier, I mentioned the shaman. Emaho talks about such radically simple things as kindness. The thing that struck me when I first saw him work was that he came into the room quietly and simply and began his workshop by meeting every person in the room, saying "hello" by engaging his eyes with that person's eyes for a few seconds until there was a natural nod of the head or smile. Something about the uncomplicated humanness of that, I understood. I understood that was something I was also striving for, stripping away the mystery.

He has evolved a dance called the *fire dance*, which some people think is an ancient tradition. In fact, it evolved spontaneously in Edinburgh on one of these visits. There's music and movement and a ritual, and a center and a couple of candles, and flowers, and a lot of focus. One by one in the dance, people will go into that center to be held or touched, or have some sort of experience. But again, what personally fascinates me is this commonality in all human beings and all human culture and across time, of the things that touch our hearts, that make us feel loved, that make us become more aware of ourselves. I so enjoyed the apparent difference of it, a shaman of another tradition, and yet it was exactly the same as a nurse sitting with someone before an operation, with a few words of kindness, holding the patient's hand.

I guess my thing is trying to just watch and feel and see the links and acknowledge that I, like everyone else, am caught in my way. I'm called a doctor. I've had this training. I do homeopathy. But that doesn't matter very much. The religion, the medicine, the bits and the bobs. In the end, we've got these feelings and experiences and we're alive, and we have certain needs. We are just human beings.

Part Six

Conversations About Consciousness and Intentionality

"The power of consciousness to act nonlocally in health is the elephant in the living room of medicine."

—LARRY DOSSEY

CHAPTER 22

LARRY DOSSEY, MD

Healing and the Nonlocal Mind

Best known for his books on prayer and his thought-provoking, entertaining editorials in *Alternative Therapies in Health and Medicine,* Larry Dossey, MD, is an international advocate for the powerful roles consciousness and spirituality play in health and healing.

Dr. Dossey graduated with honors from the University of Texas at Austin and earned his medical degree in 1967 from Southwestern Medical School in Dallas. Before completing his residency in internal medicine, he served as a battalion surgeon in Vietnam, where he was decorated for valor. He is a diplomate of the American Board of Internal Medicine.

Dr. Dossey served as consultant to Hillary Rodham Clinton's Task Force on Health Care Reform in 1993 and as consultant to the Section on Alternative Medicine of the British Parliament in 1993. He lectures nationally and internationally at medical schools, hospitals, and scientific conferences. His concept of *nonlocal mind,* which he introduced in 1989 in his book *Recovering the Soul,* has helped define the current emerging scientific image of consciousness.

Dr. Dossey is the author of nine books, including *Reinventing Medicine; Be Careful What You Pray For. . .You Just Might Get It; Prayer Is Good Medicine; Healing Words; Meaning & Medicine; Recovering the Soul; Beyond Illness; Space, Time & Medicine;* and *Healing Beyond the Body.* Dr. Dossey has served as executive editor of *Alternative Therapies in Health and Medicine* since its inception.

High on my list of heroes, Dr. Dossey has been a great teacher for me not only because of his brilliant mind, but also through the gentle way he lives his life. This monologue is from the conversation we had at his enchanting home in the hills of Santa Fe in the summer of 1999.

The Era approach to medicine is a shorthand way of looking at the changes through which we are all living in the evolution of medical care and of trying to make sense of these transitions. Era I began in the mid-1800s with the advent of science into medicine. Era I can be called "mechanical medicine" because it views the organism as a mindless machine. Era II began in the 1950s, about a century later. When I was in medical school it was called *psychosomatic disease*, and now the favored term is *mind-body medicine*. Era II acknowledges that consciousness exists and affects the body, but it is limited because it essentially equates the mind with the brain. In the Era II view, consciousness is a refined machine—a sophisticated expression of the brain's chemistry and anatomy.

Era III is a radical departure from both Era I and II. It views consciousness as something fundamental in its own right—something that isn't produced by the brain or body and that has the ability to affect not only one's own body but the body of other individuals as well, even at a distance. For me, the operative term that captures the essence of Era III is *nonlocal*. *Nonlocal* implies that you cannot localize consciousness to specific points in space such as the brain or body or even to specific points in time such as the present. Consciousness is simply indifferent to spatial and temporal limitations. It can act remotely, instantaneously, powerfully. There is a ton of evidence supporting this idea, and any medicine of the future that deserves to be called scientific is going to have to honor these facts.

Eras I, II, and III aren't rigid categories. They overlap, and therapies based on them can be used simultaneously.

Questions like these run through *Reinventing Medicine:* If we honor the nonlocal aspect of the mind, what would medicine look like? What difference would it make in how we practice medicine? And what scientific evidence supports a nonlocal, Era-III approach to healing?

I'm convinced that the impact of a nonlocal view of consciousness would be profound. The evidence is overwhelming that intentions do make a difference at a distance and that they can have life-and-death consequences. For instance, Mitchell Krucoff, MD, and Suzanne Crater, RN, at the Durham Veterans Affiars (VA) Hospital at Duke University Medical Center, are putting nonlocal intentionality to the test. Early results are remarkable—a 50% to 100% reduction in side effects from invasive cardiac procedures, such as catheterization and angioplasty. Elisabeth Targ, MD, and Fred Sicher have tested distant healing intentions on patients with advanced AIDS at California Pacific Medical Center in San Francisco and have demonstrated an impact on mortality and morbidity. I could mention other studies as well. These experiments conform to good science—they're double-blind, controlled, and prospective in design.

These studies didn't just drop out of the blue. They rest on a foundation of solid work showing the ability of human intentions to affect the metabolic activities of simple organisms—growth rates of bacteria, yeast, and fungi; the healing of wounds and the rate of tumor growth in animals; and growth rates in plants. These studies have been done quietly over the past 30 years and have been reviewed by Daniel Benor, MD, in his book *Spiritual Healing* and in my 1993 book *Healing Words*. They rest, in turn, on even more fundamental data—the capacity of human intentions to affect the nonbiological, nonliving microworld, as Dean Radin has recently reviewed in his book *The Conscious Universe*. These nonhuman studies are usually overlooked, but they are vastly important. They make up the "bench science" or the basic science that is vital to any field.

So there aren't just one or two tantalizing studies out there demonstrating the nonlocal impact of the mind, as cynics claim. There are hundreds. They span distant domains in nature, from the subatomic to the human. They show consistent findings. They've been replicated in laboratories around the world.

Let me put it this way. The power of consciousness to act nonlocally in health is the elephant in the living room of medicine. During our mechanically obsessed twentieth century, nobody has wanted to acknowledge the presence of consciousness. But there it sits, for all to see. In fact, the evidence favoring this view is so strong that to fail to deal with it involves ethical and moral issues, like holding out against a new antibiotic or lifesaving surgical procedure. The data, in my judgment, are that strong.

So what's the problem? Why don't we get on with things? Currently we are in the awkward process of overcoming our emotional and intellectual indigestion about these phenomena. A doctor actually told me recently, "Don't bother me with Era III. I'm still getting used to that mind-body stuff of Era II." I understand his reluctance. When I first encountered the nonlocal behaviors of my own mind, I, too, ran in the other direction. So a lot of my work has been aimed at helping my profession take the first baby steps in developing a comfort level with nonlocal therapies. The question is: How do we give birth to this? How do we midwife this process and help it find a home in healing?

My Personal Experience

I experienced a series of precognitive dreams the first year I was in medical practice. Three different times, I dreamed of medically related events before they actually happened. One of these was so detailed and elaborate I was utterly stunned. Then the precognitive dreams stopped, and I haven't had one since. It was as if the universe had delivered the message and hung up the phone. Now it was up to me to make sense of the experiences. I realized in a heartbeat that my conventional worldview was in deep trouble. If I could dream of events that had clinical significance before they happened, then space, time, and consciousness didn't function the way I was taught.

Now, I'm no psychic. I started out as a typically trained Western physician who wanted absolutely nothing to do with this stuff. I had seen people put on medication for taking these sorts of experiences seriously, and I equivocated in dealing with them. So I responded like a cowardly, spineless weenie; I denied them. But they were always in the background, festering in my unconscious mind.

Through the years, I found enough empirical evidence supporting this side of reality that I was finally able to make a place for my experiences. I eventually honored and embraced them, let them become real for me, and allowed them to make a difference in my life.

Interestingly, one of the experiences that helped me make peace with nonlocal reality came in the wake of my time in Vietnam. I was assigned as a battalion surgeon to a group of airborne paratroopers. I spent a year with them, frequently in combat situations. Sometimes one of them would be in danger, and I would put my life on the line to help him. When I came back to the States I was severely troubled by what I'd done because I had violated every vow I made before going. I tried to figure out why I renounced all of my common sense and behaved so irrationally. I found insight in an essay by the German philosopher Schopenhauer in which he asked the same question: why is it that when one individual sees another in danger, this individual is willing to give his life to save that person? His answer was because at that moment there are not two people, there is only one. Although there are two bodies, there is only one consciousness. So the rescuing person is not trying to save someone else; he is trying to save himself.

I've seldom read anything that seemed to validate my own experience so totally. I knew Schopenhauer was right! So this gave me a way of honoring what had happened to me and helped me pay attention to other experiences pointing in the same direction. It helped legitimize the idea that my consciousness was not totally an individual, personal affair and that it might function outside my body in the world.

Early on I also stumbled onto the philosophical writings of the Nobel physicist Erwin Schrödinger on the unitary nature of consciousness. For Schrödinger, there is only a single mind, a universal consciousness. I was tremendously inspired by his vision. Here you have one of the greatest scientists who ever lived, whose wave equations lie at the heart of quantum physics, boldly asserting the nonlocal, unitary nature of the mind. I still recall how, after seeing patients all morning, I'd close my office door during the noon hour and devour Schrödinger's writings. He helped me see that one could be a good scientist and also honor the side of consciousness that had revealed itself to me. So, on my short list of heroes in science, Schrödinger is close to the top.

The Spectrum of Consciousness

Sometimes there is a focused kernel that I call *I*, a localized little nugget of awareness that's experienced as the ego. At other moments that totally evaporates, and I feel I am a part of everything there is. The movement is fluid; one state informs and empowers the other.

There is a profound concept in Buddhism called the *mutual coarising of opposites*, in which opposites are defined in terms of each other. I see the sense of *I* and the universal sense of oneness and unity in this way. One state makes the experience of the other possible. As the Buddhist aphorism says, "After ecstasy, the laundry." The point is, we would not be talking about oneness if we did not have some corresponding experience of the particular. So this "codependence of opposites" is a very precious idea to me. It helps me relate my sense of "I-ness" to my experience of the universal.

I am deeply skeptical of generalizations about how to get healed. Often healers cite a case in which an individual takes an aggressive *I*-oriented stance against the illness and the illness goes away, and they proceed to proclaim that this is the secret to healing, the one way to do it. But this is nuts, because there are other cases in which the exact opposite approach works, in which the *I* is surrendered. In healing, there is no room for dogmatism. We need to honor the mystery of healing, admit our ignorance, and keep all our options open.

One of the most introverted people I have ever met—so introverted she spoke in a whisper—told me after a lecture, "Twenty years ago I had metastatic breast cancer, and do you know what I did to get rid of it? Nothing." She continued: "I didn't fight the cancer. I just quietly went inside and the cancer went away."

Then she started crying and said, "But nobody wants to hear my story. Do you think anybody who was healed by doing nothing would ever be interviewed on *Oprah*?" Of course, this woman's "doing nothing" was not really "nothing." Surrendering the I is hard work!

Prayer

A major question is whether prayer works because of some specific, direct impact of consciousness or because of some metaphysical or transempirical factor, to borrow Jeff Levin's term. In other words, does your intention—whether we call that a prayer, a wish, or something else—tweak the universe? Or does the Absolute, however named, intervene and create the effect? Since we don't have any god meters, I don't know how we can decide scientifically between these two possibilities. I can't conceive of an experiment that would settle this debate.

For me, either possibility is pretty wonderful. I am struck by the fact that these effects suggest a benevolent side to the universe. After all, there is no obvious reason why prayer should work. Why should your empathic, compassionate prayers, wishes, or intentions make a difference? The universe would be a lot simpler if it went on its merry way without bothering with what you thought. But it does take our consciousness into consideration—and this suggests a charitable, caring, wonderful side to the world. What we call this is up for grabs. God? Goddess? Allah? Brahman? The Tao? Universe? It's up to you.

As the evidence for the nonlocal effects of the mind are becoming better known, scientists are agonizing about how to respond. What's the best way to model the mind to account for the evidence? I enjoy trying to stay abreast of these theories, which are popping up like weeds. One of my favorite theoreticians is David Chalmers, a cognitive scientist and mathematician at the University of California-Santa Cruz. Chalmers suggests that, based on the evidence, it's time to bite the bullet and declare consciousness fundamental in the world, perhaps on a par with matter and energy. In other words, consciousness can't be reduced to anything more elemental. The brain doesn't make it; the body doesn't produce it. It exists on its own, and it is everywhere.

But this sort of talk is deceptive because it really doesn't answer anything. What does it mean to say that consciousness is fundamental? That it's nonlocal? This is really recycled stuff; spiritual masters have said the same thing for millennia. So these "explanations" are basically illusions. They make us feel better when scientists proclaim them, and they help legitimize the data surrounding consciousness. But let's not kid ourselves; they just substitute one mystery for another.

I agree with you that intentionality and prayer should not be equated. We dishonor the richness of prayer to call it a mere wish, thought, or intention. I keep a little formula in my mind: intention + love = prayer. Most folks would expand this equation even further by adding a term for the Absolute.

But let's not be too hard on intentionality. One of the reasons researchers favor this term is that scientific journals are highly allergic to the term *prayer*. So many researchers say, "I'm going to call this stuff something that will help me get my paper published." But this creates confusion. If you look at most of the studies, you don't have a clue about the particular mental strategy used by the healer. Is he or she using prayer? If so, what kind and in what way? Or is a robust desire or a casual wish being employed?

Lawrence LeShan tried to sort out these questions back in the 1960s and 1970s by interviewing healers about the strategies they used. He found a few who themselves tried to function as the source of power that made the change happen, which he called *Type II healing*. But by far, most of the healers identified with something greater and more powerful than themselves and attempted to serve as a conduit for this healing power. LeShan called this *Type I healing*. The great majority of healers seem to use this approach. They relax their sense of *I* and allow themselves to be absorbed into a power that is greater and wiser than themselves. This is basically what healers do in "centering" themselves before they invoke healing.

To call this strategy *intentionality* may overemphasize the *I*, which takes a back seat in this process. But certainly there is some relation between prayer and intentionality. After all, one intends to pray in the first place. One day we'll lose our squeamishness about the term *prayer* and call it what it is—an invocation of the power of the Absolute, however the individual terms that.

Time

The healthiest place to start is to admit that we don't know what the heck we're talking about where time is concerned. We're in good company. Richard Feynman, the Nobel physicist, was once asked what time is. He responded that he didn't know; it's "too difficult," he said. St. Augustine said he knew what time was—until somebody asked. Yet we all think we're experts on time. What a laugh!

Most of us carry around the idea that time flows and is divisible into a past, present, and future. But with all due respect, there has never been an experiment in the entire history of science that shows that time flows. And there are moments when our experience of a one-way time is violated, as in my own precognitive dreams, during which I saw the future before it happened.

I'm convinced that the nature of time is crucial to healing. William Braud, director of research at the Institute of Transpersonal Psychology in California, has reviewed more than a score of experiments that strongly suggest that consciousness can reach back into the past and influence events that presumably have already happened but which have not yet been actually observed. It appears that the past, to some extent, is not fixed. Braud has introduced an enchanting term—*seed moments*—for past events that may still be manipulatable by consciousness.

The idea that we can affect the past may be shocking, but it isn't fantasy. The studies are real, and they won't go away. They are related to what is called the *observer problem* or the *measurement problem* in quantum physics. The basic idea is that if an event at the quantum level has not actually been observed, it may perhaps be changeable at a later time, even though it lies in the past. According to Helmut Schmidt, the physicist who has laid the experimental foundation of this field, unobserved quantum events are those in which "nature has not yet made up its mind," as he puts it. Schmidt says that one doesn't really change the unobserved past because it is not yet fixed. Following observation, though, the event does become fixed, incapable of being influenced further.

But we shouldn't get carried away with a quantum-physical explanation for these events. Physicists are groping in the dark just like everybody else in trying to understand them. There's no consensus among physicists about what's going on here, including what is meant by "observation" and "measurement." Some physicists call this area not quantum physics but quantum metaphysics, in ridicule. Quantum theory may eventually prove bankrupt as an explanation for these happenings. Some novel, future model we can't foresee may be needed, which will leave current concepts in physics in the dust. But we shouldn't wait around for a perfect explanation before we come to terms with them.

I began to play with the implications of these phenomena for healthcare in my book *Healing Words*, with what I call *time-displaced healing*. If you go to your doctor for a routine physical examination, you have all sorts of tests—radiographs, blood tests, and so on. Before anybody actually observes the results of your tests and "fixes" them, might it make sense to sit down and try mentally to steer the test results in a positive direction? Before a radiologist reads your mammogram, should you image, intend, or pray that it be normal?

A mammogram or blood test is of course not a quantum event, but it reflects quantum events in the body.

Perhaps all diseases are reflected at the subatomic, quantum level, so that these "observer" or "measurement" effects apply to disease in general and indirectly to the tests that reflect them. If someone's disease hasn't been fixed through identification or diagnosis, measurement or observation, could it be changed to a more benign state or even eradicated? Of course, most of us think that our "medical past" is unchangeable. But if we take the experimental evidence seriously, there's no reason we should not try to manipulate the critical "seed moments" in our past in which illness originates.

But to do this we must be willing to flirt with new ideas of time, in which it ceases to be the irreversible, one-way, monolithic entity we assume. Funny thing is, most esoteric spiritual traditions and perhaps all native cultures have no trouble with a nonlinear view of time—what Eliade called *the myth of the eternal return*. I can't tell you how fascinated I am by the possible relevance of this to health.

The most precise studies employ a random event generator, which is a computer-like gadget that spits out, over time, equal numbers of zeros and ones or pluses and minuses. So you let the machine run and you record its output on a magnetic tape that nobody looks at. Then you sit down and try to influence the machine to produce more ones than zeros, or vice versa, though it has already run. Afterward, somebody examines the record of the magnetic tape—and they shockingly discover that the machine's output wasn't random after all, as it should have been, but actually corresponds to your intention. Apparently you have been able to reach back into the past and influence a quantum-based event—the function of a random event computer. These studies are simple, elegant, and precise. They've been independently replicated by a great many researchers at several different laboratories, and meta-analyses of these studies have been published in prestigious physics journals.

I've found that this stuff horrifies a lot of people. They have their hands full with the present; to tack on responsibility for what has already taken place is going too far. But if the ability to nudge the past presents us with awesome responsibility, it gives us a stunning opportunity as well. Ah, we'll get over it! This is going to be one of the most exciting, cutting-edge issues we'll be dealing with in the coming millennium.

We really must be adventuresome here. It's irrational to suppose that the nonabsoluteness of time is relevant only to the microworld of quantum physics and not to human bodies, which are composed of quantum-sized events. Sooner or later we'll have to face the importance of this area to health and wellness. Actually, I've started applying these ideas on my own.

When I go in for a physical, I know I'm going to get poked, probed, and x-rayed and that my doctor will draw blood. I take a multitemporal approach to influencing the results of all these observations and measurements. Before my appointment I image the outcome of each test and try to push it in a positive direction. After the test—but before it's been read, analyzed, or observed—I do the same thing. I would challenge anyone to do this. I can't think of any harm in doing so. So I say go for it. Try to invoke the nonabsoluteness of time on your behalf. There's nothing to lose, so have fun with it.

White Crows—A Symbol for Anomalies

A flock of white crows—Willam James's term for events that don't fit in—is fluttering around in the form of telesomatic events. These are incidents in which one individual who is empathically or lovingly connected with a distant individual experiences a change in his or her body at the same time the distant individual is experiencing a change. For instance, in one case a mother is writing a letter to her daughter who has gone off to college and whom she misses desperately. Suddenly the mother experiences such severe pain in her hand she has to stop writing—at the same time her daughter, it turns out, burned her hand in a botched experiment in chemistry lab. Telesomatic events are exceedingly common; hundreds have been reported. Scores of them have been investigated in fanatical detail by Ian Stevenson of the University of Virginia. Telesomatic events point toward a nonlocal quality of consciousness and the role of love and empathy in uniting us across distance. This body of evidence alone could revolutionize our basic understanding of consciousness.

White crows are always fluttering around dreams, as I found out with my own precognitive dream experiences. In one nifty case, a woman dreamed that a nurse was holding a light to the dreamer's lower leg as if to show her something. This happened every night for a year. Then a focus of osteomyelitis erupted at the spot, requiring surgery. In another instance, a man dreamed he was back in the army in combat. He was being shot at and took refuge in the hollow of a huge tree. The bullets penetrated the tree, however, as well as his lower lung—where a lung cancer was found later.

Do we dream *of* the future or do we dream the future into being? Well, Philosopher Stephen Braude of the University of Maryland believes that precognition actually causes things to happen in the future. If you dream of a plane crash and it happens, have you caused it? This is pretty sobering stuff. Of course not everybody agrees with Braude. But even if he is correct and we influence the future through our dreams, we don't have to accept the "bad" dream. We can always go back to the drawing board and redream or reintend a more optimal future. This is commonly done in native cultures.

I'll let the ethicists handle the "should we?" in this. But even if we consciously decided not to probe the past and the future with our minds, we would wind up doing so anyway, because most of these phenomena take place unconsciously. So we can't opt out of transtemporal tampering.

There are probably several reasons why this human capacity has been driven into the unconscious. For one thing, to admit that we can shape the future and influence the past is a burden many people are unwilling to accept. Better to assign the past to history and the future to fate. It gets us off the hook. For another reason, we humans have a way of dealing harshly with seers, prophets, shamans, mystics, and diviners who snub time. These people make us uncomfortable—so uncomfortable we've often killed them as witches, warlocks, blasphemers, and heretics. Little wonder that people don't want to own their transtemporal abilities and use them publicly!

But these abilities won't go away, probably because they've become internalized in the course of our long evolutionary history. These capacities have obvious survival value and therefore would tend to be genetically transmitted in succeeding generations. They're in our genes, we're stuck with them, and we can't get rid of them—nor should we want to.

As an example of how transtemporal awareness favors survival, consider what happened one March evening in 1950 in Beatrice, Nebraska, when all 15 members of the church choir turned up late for practice. One woman hadn't finished her housework; two guys were listening to the tail end of a sports broadcast; one girl was doing homework; another was taking a nap; and so on. Normally, choir practice started promptly at 7:20 p.m. At 7:25 p.m., however, the gas boiler exploded and demolished the little church. But nobody was there, and nobody got hurt.

Biologist Lyall Watson, one of our greatest observers of white crows, chased down this story in his book, *The Dreams of Dragons*. He states that the odds against chance for all 15 choir members being late on the same evening are more than 1 billion to 1. My proposal is that a bit of unconscious nonlocal knowing was occurring, permitting the choir members to scan the future, identify a threatening situation, and take proper action.

Here's another one from Watson that makes the same point: William Cox, a researcher in North Carolina, looked at the number of riders on trains that had accidents such as derailments and collisions. He studied many trains over many years, in all kinds of weather. Cox found that there were always fewer riders on the wrecks than would have been predicted by chance.

Another example is from research on SIDS—sudden infant death syndrome. Researchers from the Southwest SIDS Center near Houston asked parents whose child died from SIDS whether they had ever had a premonition that their child would die. A total of 21% said yes. In comparison, only 2.1% of control parents expressed such a fear. The SIDS parents were apparently able to intuit the "health future" of their child. Yet when the SIDS parents expressed their concerns to their physicians, they were placated or ridiculed. In no case were they taken seriously, and in no instances did the doctors recommend taking extra precautions.

How should we in healthcare respond to the ability of ourselves and our patients to intuit things nonlocally? We can respond like the SIDS physicians—dig in our heels and ridicule these experiences. But in view of the laboratory evidence favoring the ability of consciousness to function outside of space and time, we'd better knuckle down and ask some tough questions.

Does Being Ethical Make a Difference?

The good guys don't have a monopoly on nonlocal mind. A 1994 Gallup poll found that 5% of Americans actually pray for harm for other people—and that's just the 1 in 20 who will admit it. The key question is whether these negative prayers, wishes, and intentions have any effect. I wrote a book, *Be Careful What You Pray For,* exploring this troubling area. Personally, I'm convinced that there are compelling data that prayers and intentions can harm—so convinced that if I knew my doctor or nurse was having a bad day and was emanating negative thoughts I wouldn't want either one taking care of me.

It's amazing how squeamish we are about this. People want to say that intentions and prayers either work positively or not at all. If this is true, then intentionality is the only known "therapy" that is totally free of side effects, which I consider implausible.

If negative thoughts can harm nonlocally, we ought to be talking about "preventive medicine" for them. It's no accident that every culture that has entertained nonlocal mind has devised ways of dealing with its dark side.

Perhaps the best way to prevent harm from other people's thoughts, intentions, and prayers is to live a life of compassion and integrity, so as not to evoke their malevolent intentions in the first place. We can also counter negative intentions and prayers with positive ones. In the *Oxford Book of Prayer,* for example, there is an entire section on prayers of protection drawn from all major religious traditions, East and West.

But we ought not to become paranoid about being done in by the malevolent intentions of millions of nasty people out there. Research by Dr. Loudell Snow of Michigan State University shows that most hexes and curses in the United States come from people you know well, people who are your intimates—spouses, children, siblings, lovers, in-laws. So, again, if you behave impeccably toward others, you are not likely to provoke their negative, nonlocal intentions. Be nice. Not too complicated.

The Negative Side of Prayer

After I'd written two books on the positive side of prayer—*Healing Words* and *Prayer Is Good Medicine*—I began to get nasty letters. People said things like, "I know you meant well, but you have turned prayer upside down. You completely misunderstand it. So I'm going to pray for you and help you." Some of the letters virtually dripped with venom and were unsigned. Some people said I was possessed by the devil and bound for hell. They enclosed religious tracts describing my destination in lurid detail. For a long time I wrote back to these people saying, "I am grateful you are willing to pray for me. Thank you for your prayers." Then one day, as these letters kept coming, I realized that these people weren't doing this out of love and concern for me. They wanted to manipulate and control me and force me through prayer to come over to their side. I was really thickheaded about this. It took me a long time to see the light.

I felt attacked by these people. Then I came across the 1994 Gallup poll I mentioned, showing that 5% of Americans—over 10 million folks—actually pray for harm for others. It became increasingly obvious to me that the shadow side of prayer is real, and I decided to write about it.

I didn't rush into this decision. I discussed it with friends. Some were horrified. They said I would popularize hexes and curses and set off an epidemic of negative prayer. I would set back research in positive prayer. Then I talked with my friend Sandra Ingerman, who also lives in Santa Fe. Sandra is a scholar of shamanism and author of *Soul Retrieval*. Should I dabble with the dark side and write a book about it? After shamanically journeying in search of the answer, Sandra said, "Yes, it is the right thing to do. You are protected, but be careful."

I do feel protected by the good wishes, intentions, and prayers of thousands of people. I also have my own rituals and prayers that are very fulfilling and strengthening. I feel this far outweighs the negative stuff that's directed to me. So I decided to take an in-depth look at the negative side of prayer, and that's how the book was born.

I have legions of allies. I support them, and they support me. Plus I have the abiding certainty that I'm immortal anyway. This can make you reckless, but it can also make you fearless and more courageous in doing your work.

I can't see any other conclusion than immortality for all of us. If you reason through the implications of a mind that is authentically and genuinely nonlocal, you realize that nonlocality is not a halfway sort of deal. Nonlocality implies infinitude in space and time. If you are spatially nonlocal you are omnipresent; if you are temporally nonlocal you are immortal. These are divine qualities—what many great spiritual traditions call "the Divine within."

This changes the way you approach life. For one thing, a nonlocal view of life can enhance your sense of humor. All of a sudden you realize we are not talking about progress, salvation, or becoming something that you are not but about waking up to an extant fact. This is why many of the great wisdom traditions use the term *enlightenment* to describe the process of realization.

Enlightenment implies turning on a light and seeing what was there already. So the task is one of realization and waking up, not of moving from A to Z in an agonizing, tortured process of growth and transformation. This scenario has been phrased a million ways in a thousand traditions, but it invariably involves the idea of indwelling perfection waiting to be realized—again, the Divine within. When we realize there's nothing to do and, moreover, no *I* that could become enlightened, we feel lighter, freer, happier. Contrast this with the effort, time, and money we expend on personal transformation, and all of a sudden the situation seems uproariously funny. The answers were there all along, nothing had to be done, and it was all free.

The question many people ask is: If we are immortal, then why bother with all this healing business? But why not bother with it? I can't think of anything better than trying to bring healing to someone else. When love and compassion flower in our lives, the natural response is to help others. Helping others is simply what awakened humans do. Many of the great spiritual masters in history have been healers. The miracles they performed often involved healing. Jesus was called the Great Physician.

If we can hold immortality in our minds while we try to help others in the healing arts, then we can have fun. We know the patient will eventually die—the statistics are convincing—but so what? The nonlocal aspect of his or her consciousness couldn't sign off even if it tried. If we can hold onto this paradox, we might be able to introduce something into medicine that has recently been missing—a light heart and a sense of humor. That would be a change!

The Question of God

I believe in the Absolute—the uncharacterizable, unanalyzable, indescribable, ineffable Absolute. This term is too sterile for lots of folks, but for me any other name is idolatrous and shamelessly anthropomorphic. I will bend over backward not to assign any human qualities to the Absolute.

But I receive them with gratitude. Another paradox, right? The most impersonal view of the Absolute becomes the most personal, the most immediate, fulfilling, real.

Let me tell you a story. When *Healing Words* came out in 1993, one of the major television networks did a primetime story on the role of prayer in healing. They sent one of their best interviewers to Santa Fe to talk with me. They wanted to film the interview at the nearby Santuario Chimayo, an old rustic Catholic church known as the Lourdes of the Southwest because of the reputed healings that take place there. The dirt there is said to have healing power, like the water at Lourdes. People come from all around to take some of this blessed dirt from a little hole in the floor of one of the church's anterooms, which they rub on the afflicted part of the body. One wall is hung with crutches the lame have left there.

We were there late in the day and there was a huge problem. The interviewer was recovering from a cold and sore throat, and when he would get halfway through his monologue he'd start coughing. This happened time after time. The camera crew was frantic because the daylight was fading, and the project appeared to be headed for disaster. So I asked the interviewer to hold on for a moment. I went into the church, got a handful of the enchanted dirt, and massaged it into the interviewer's throat, from his chin to below his Adam's apple. He probably thought I had lost my mind. Then I asked him to try it again. His voice was clear and powerful. He was so shocked he recorded his monologue three times to make sure his "healing" wasn't a fluke.

Here's another story. When I was finishing my training in internal medicine at the VA and Parkland Hospitals in Dallas, I had a patient who was an elderly black man who had disseminated lung cancer. He was terminal and refused all treatment, and there was nothing medically we could do for him. The congregation from his church circled his bed during visiting hours and prayed nonstop. I was a good mechanistic doctor in those days and didn't think this would make any difference. He wanted to go home to die, so I discharged him. I was certain he would expire in a few days, and I eventually forgot about him. A year later I got a request from one of my colleagues at the hospital to come by and see this man again. He had been admitted for a bad case of the flu. The first thing I did was to go down to the radiology department and put his old chest radiograph and the current one side by side. The earlier one showed cancer everywhere, but the new one was clean as a whistle. It was as if the man had been raised from the dead, with prayer as his only treatment. If there are miracles, this was one of them.

The Personal versus the Collective

If we take seriously the experimental evidence supporting the nonlocal effects of consciousness, the idea of a strictly personal universe is in trouble. The intercessory prayer studies, for example, clearly show that I can influence your reality at a distance, even when you're unaware that I'm doing so. And you can do the same for me. So we have to put "personal universe" in quotes. Our world may seem strictly personal, but the personal is more permeable than we imagine.

I once asked Pir Vilayat Inayat Khan, perhaps the greatest living Sufi master, the same question. What is the relationship between the universal and the particular or personal? He said with a laugh, "Oh, Larry, don't worry about it! It isn't one or the other. It takes both." For me there is a delicate interplay between the global and the particular, the universal and the personal—the mutual coarising of opposites we mentioned earlier. It's like a magnet. You can't have a magnet with just a positive or negative pole; you have to have both.

As philosopher Alan Watts once put it, "The greatest metaphysical principle in the universe is that every inside has an outside and every outside has an inside." It's that simple yet that profound. So we wouldn't be talking about the universal without a corresponding experience of the particular.

I thought we might get into this discussion, so I brought along a passage from author Edward Abbey that makes the point. Abbey, who died a decade ago, was a brilliant writer and passionate defender of the environment of the American Southwest. Like Alan Watts, he was an unregenerate rogue, raconteur, and trickster. He hated piety, and he excoriated "spiritual" people who were always searching for "reality." Here's a dose of Abbey:[1]

> When I write paradise, I mean not apple trees and only golden women but also scorpions and tarantulas and flies, rattlesnakes and gila monsters, sandstone, volcanos, and earthquakes, bacteria, bear, cactus, yucca, bladderweed, ocotillo and mesquite, flash floods and quicksand, and, yes, disease and death and the rotting of flesh. Paradise is the here and now, the actual, tangible dogmatically real Earth on which we stand. Yes, God bless America, the Earth upon which we stand. . .For my own part, I am pleased enough with surfaces. In fact, they alone seem to be of much importance. Such things, for example,

---

[1] From Abbey E: Quoted in Williams TT: A eulogy for Edward Abbey. In An *Unspoken Hunger*, New York, 1994, Vintage Books.

as the grasp of a child's hand in your own, the flavor of an apple, the embrace of a friend or lover, the silk of a girl's thigh, the sunlight on rock and leaves, the feel of music, the bark of a tree, the abrasion of granite and sand, the plunge of clear water into a pool, the face of the wind, what else is there, what else do we need?

There you have it—as Blake put it, a world in a grain of sand, heaven in a wildflower, infinity in the palm of your hand, eternity in an hour. The opposites are in cahoots, playacting as if they're not. And an insight into this interdependency can come through the nonlocal manifestations of consciousness, which just explode the absoluteness of personal isolation and particularity, space and time, and so on. That's one reason I believe nonlocality is such a fertile area: it's loaded with scientific and spiritual dynamite.

In Closing

I'm fascinated these days by how modern neuroscience seems to be playing into the hands of ancient spiritual ideas. The brain scientists incessantly assure us that we are deceiving ourselves to believe in the reality of anything that could be called an *I* or a self. The neurotransmitters are really in charge. At the end of the day it's all brain chemistry.

In an absolutely crazy way, this is a profound teaching. Many of the great spiritual traditions have maintained for millennia that the ego, the self, the *I*, is an illusion. It's as if the brain scientists are in league with the mystics and don't have a clue about this situation. The scientists, of course, would be scandalized if they realized this and would deny any such connection to high heaven. I really do think this is a hoot.

One more thing. We've skated on some pretty heady ideas during our conversation. But we can be too cerebral, too rational, in trying to understand healing and consciousness. If we stay too much in our heads, we become ungrounded and we lose our power.

A tale from Greek mythology makes the point. Antaeus, the son of Poseidon, was a giant wrestler who was invincible as long as he was touching his mother, the earth. He had won all his battles until he met Hercules. All Hercules had to do to win was simply lift Antaeus in the air and hold him there, while he writhed and lost all his strength.

Most academic explorers of consciousness have become modern Antaeuses, writhing in the rarefied, detached atmosphere of the intellect. That's why the fundamental breakthroughs in consciousness and healing are not likely to emerge from computer labs or think tanks. Those of us who get our hands dirty as healers have a magnificent advantage. The earthy, gritty world of bedsides and bodies, excreta and blood, pain and suffering, are a magnificent way to stay grounded. Moreover, sick rooms and hospitals are fabulous breeding grounds for the nonlocal behaviors of consciousness. Visions, premonitions, nonlocal communications between doctors and nurses and patients, intuitions, and the distant healing effects of intentions and prayer—these are everyday fare in our lives. This gives us a rich source of data the "experts" on consciousness never see, and whose existence they deny.

Staying grounded is a challenge for me. My first impulse on waking up in the morning is to grab coffee and something to read. My wife's is to go outside, sit on a rock and talk to birds, flowers, and the leaves on trees. I swear they talk back. Fortunately, I draw strength from her, because part of her grounding is mine as well. Nonlocal mind is like that.

CHAPTER 23

MARILYN SCHLITZ, PhD

Consciousness, Causation, and Evolution

The editors of the journal *Alternative Therapies in Health and Medicine* are very interested in consciousness and intentionality and their effects on health. Consequently, I was introduced to and asked to interview Marilyn Schlitz, one of the leading proponents in this field. Dr. Schlitz is an anthropologist and vice president of science and education for the Institute of Noetic Sciences (IONS) in Petaluma, California, where she develops and oversees programs in three areas: emerging worldviews, inner mechanisms of the healing response, and extended human abilities. Author of numerous papers and book chapters on the topic of consciousness studies, she is currently involved with numerous research projects that explore the relationship between subjectivity and the physical world.

Dr. Schlitz has taught at many universities and colleges, including work as a lecturer in the Department of Psychology at Stanford and as an instructor in the Department of Sociology and Anthropology at Trinity University. In 1994 she received the Thomas Welton Stanford Psychical Research Fellowship. She received her doctoral degree in anthropology from the University of Texas–Austin in 1992 and her master's degree in behavioral and social sciences in 1986 from the University of Texas–San Antonio.

It was my pleasure to interview Dr. Schlitz in La Jolla, California, in the summer of 1998 while she was in town to give a keynote address.

While on the Apollo 14 space mission, astronaut Edgar Mitchell saw the earth suspended in the vast void. As he gazed at our planet, he had an epiphany during which he experienced a profound sense of connectedness for which none of his scientific education had prepared him. The sense that we are something larger than the material part of our being occurred to him, yet his epistemology wasn't adequate to explain this sense. So he came back to the earth with the idea of starting an institute that could investigate aspects of experience that didn't fit within the materialist model. But he also wanted to bring scientific rigor and critical thinking to that domain of experience.

The notion was that we have harnessed our collective cultural power to map the external physical world, but what happens if we bring that same level of commitment to understanding the inner world—in particular, to understanding the relationship between inner and outer? That way of thinking led Mitchell to choose consciousness as the central organizing premise of the Institute of Noetic Sciences (IONS); in turn, the idea launched a series of research projects investigating the mysteries of the mind.

We are trying to create an umbrella term big enough to hold all the different definitions of consciousness. The dominant scientific definition is that mind and brain are one, that in order to understand consciousness you must understand the brain, and that consciousness is reducible to brain activity. Buddhism, however, talks about the six levels of consciousness, with sublevels of consciousness in each level, and uses different words to describe the different states of consciousness. There are also religious and spiritual views that involve consciousness as the ground of all being—the essence of life and reality and our place in it. Social scientists see it in our cultural interactions and belief systems. So to come up with one definition isn't easy. We have marginalized subjectivity in our culture, so we lack the language to describe these qualitative aspects of experience.

My own definition involves an integral model in which consciousness is all of those things: the brain as well as what is beyond the brain. It is rooted in terms of ourselves as unique human beings as well as in relation to all sentient beings and potentially the whole system of life in the cosmos. There is something very intelligent about the way the universe operates and, to me, that is a manifestation of consciousness.

Until recently, the idea of spirituality wasn't an acceptable topic because we're supposed to keep science and religion separate. But we now know that these realms aren't as isolated from one another as we previously thought. Consciousness is a label we have used to describe the ineffable, and today, *spirituality* is a term we use as much as "consciousness." In both cases, we're talking about something that is not easily measured or quantified—something that transcends our individual egos. They are probably different things, but once again we lack a linguistic framework and tend to lump them together.

Consciousness requires, at this point in our understanding, an integral definition. It requires that consciousness be the first person—it's about my own subjectivity, my inner experience, my sense of who I am. It also requires a second person—engaged consciousness is somewhere in the medium between us. It is about culture, language, and the way we create concepts through our interaction with each other—concepts that provide us with cognitive categories for organizing our experience. So the first person is mediated through this second-person relationship.

But consciousness is also about the third person. According to the conventional scientific definition, it's about the brain, about something that can be measured in an "it" form. So if you want to understand consciousness, it's about all of these, and I would add that it's also about the *we*, the transpersonal *we*, which is the larger sense of consciousness from the spiritual dimension. It's about connection to the most holy of whole—that sense of life, earth, the universe. There's something about the intentionality of nature and life that is pure consciousness.

Prayer and Intentionality

Traditionally, prayer presupposes an engagement with "an other," which is different from experiences just involving the self, such as positive thinking and intentionality. But from the current scientific perspective, I don't think we can distinguish between intentionality and prayer.

We recently held a scientific meeting on clinical studies of prayer and healing at Harvard. This meeting was geared toward introducing people who are engaged in this research, thinking clearly about methodology and talking about the challenges and opportunities of doing this type of research, and encouraging collaborations. There's limited funding for this research, so if four or five laboratories collaborate on a clinical study, the sample size and statistical power increase. And, happily, all these things happened at our initial meeting. We put together a group of researchers who were interested in looking at the effects of intentionality or prayer—of some kind of transpersonal interaction between two people—within the context of clinical studies.

We're now in the process of planning our next meeting, where we want to talk about the phenomenology of prayer and healing. What are the inner aspects of how one does this type of thing? Can we begin to understand what's going on in people's subjectivity even though we must rely on verbal reporting?

A lot of people are interested in doing this type of work. When people commit themselves to service, they have a sense that they want to do something good for humanity. I also think it's about camaraderie: they know they're going to be working in a group, and there's something powerful about knowing you are no longer isolated, that you are not the only person doing this kind of frontier science.

Our work has been about establishing proof of principle that one person's intention may affect another person at a distance in ways that are measurable. For 10 years, William Braud and I conducted a series of experiments in which we worked with psychics, experimenters, and unselected people from the street. And we did not find significant differences between any of these groups. Still, it remains an important research question.

Healers across cultures and throughout history have made claims that healing can occur at a distance. Anthropologists have documented these claims anecdotally, but so far there have been few attempts to try and validate these claims. So Braud and I brought these claims into the laboratory and set up experiments that would allow us to examine these reported abilities under conditions that ruled out conventional sensory interactions. We conducted 13 experiments involving a biofeedback-type design; instead of trying to regulate one's own physiology, a healer from a distance tries to regulate the physiology of another. Today, people in this field have conducted many experiments in a variety of laboratories throughout the world. In addition, a handful of clinical studies have been conducted, suggesting that distant healing is a useful treatment for heart disease and AIDS. Overall, we found highly significant evidence for a nonlocal healing interaction.

But even though the results suggest that people can do this, we still have the problem of plausibility. People don't frequently have the experience of this, so they can't relate to it. However, people commonly report being able to detect someone staring at them at a distance. This concept has "street validity." So the question is this: Can we begin to understand what's happening in these situations? Is it due to peripheral vision (i.e., they are able to perceive motion changes), or is it something transpersonal? Is there some kind of subtle information or energy exchange? We set up an experiment to test this and found that there were significant differences in the average amount of autonomic nervous system activity in the distant staree when the starer was projecting his or her attention toward the distant person. I conducted two experiments using this paradigm, both of which produced significant changes in physiology during the staring periods.

However, a colleague in England, a card-carrying member of the skeptical community, has tried similar experiments and experienced chance results. He invited me to come to his lab in England and we set up a collaborative project working in the same lab, with the same equipment, the same randomization procedures, and the same subject population. Everything was identical, except that I worked with half the people and he worked with the other half. We found that we both replicated our original findings. I got a significant effect, and he didn't. We have now replicated the effect in a second time in my lab and have engaged in a third study to look more closely at what is going on. Not only does there appear to be some kind of transpersonal communication that occurs between two people, but the intentionality of the researcher may be a vital factor in influencing the outcome of the studies.

The Rainforests

The rainforest project focuses on the dream-sharing practices of two indigenous tribes who live in the Amazon—the *Achuar* and *Huaorani* Indians. They wake up every morning before dawn and share their dreams, with the idea that people don't dream for themselves. Instead, they dream for the collective. They believe that every dream is precognitive, that dreams portend what will happen in waking life. They also believe that the dream state is more real than what Westerners would consider real and that in some sense the waking state is an illusion. They believe they connect to their ancestors or to a larger cosmology through their dream states.

Our research concerns the ways in which these tribes move from the *I* state of consciousness, the subjectivity of inner experience and the dream state, to the shared experience of collective action. For example, if somebody has a dream that portends a good hunt, how do they interpret the dream in such a way that they reach consensus and act upon it?

We're working in collaboration with five students from the tribes. Right now, they are keeping journals about who comes, who shows up. Is it equally male-female? How do they go about doing the interpretation? I'm more interested in how they reach consensus than in the dream interpretations *per se*. That will be a piece of it, but that's not really what the project is about. Rather, it is about collective consciousness and how we can move from subjective experience to collective action.

The metamessage of the project is about helping to create a more sustainable dream for our own culture. Again, we have ignored subjectivity, and in the process we have paid a big price. When you look at the problems of the rainforest and deforestation and oil exploration—it isn't about their dream. There's nothing wrong with their dream. Those things are really about the dream of the north. So the question becomes: is there a way that chronicling these people can help them to better value their own process? With acculturation, they may lose that. Also, is there a way to translate this process back to our own culture? Perhaps the indigenous peoples can teach us about something we either never had or lost in the process of becoming "civilized."

How they do things is quite thoughtful. I was invited there by the tribal leaders of the Achuar Federation to present the project at their congress, and it was both the most exhilarating and challenging talk I have ever given. They wanted to know what "noetic" meant. I defined it as *direct knowing* and used the analogy of how they are able to get information about medicinal plants through dreams. If a person is sick, he or she reads the dream to find out which plant to pick in the forest. After this explanation, Santiago, the president of the Achuar Federation, said, "Excuse me, but my understanding was that 'noetic' meant 'multiple ways of knowing.' Which is it? Direct knowing or multiple ways of knowing?"

In my whole history of working in this area I had never had anybody from our culture ask me a question like that. They've asked me what "noetic" meant, but we rarely make distinctions between direct knowing and multiple ways of knowing. We just know rational knowing and "other" kinds of knowing. But here in this ostensibly "primitive" culture they are extremely sophisticated about intricate levels of consciousness and inner experience.

For about 3½ hours they challenged me: "Why isn't it 10 scholarships instead of 5? Why isn't it 4 years instead of 2?" At the end, they called for a vote. We missed approval of the project by one vote. I was floored.

But what happened was that a significant minority, the traditionals, wanted to dream on it. They didn't want to be forced to make a vote right away. So they went to bed that night and dreamed. Before dawn, everybody was busy talking. You could hear them all over the village. They came back at 9 o'clock and unanimously approved the project.

The Remission Project

The remission work started under Brendan O'Regan's leadership. He was interested in the healing system. We know there is an immune system and an endocrine system and a nervous system, but what about a healing system? Or can you simply reduce healing to immune responses? What role does the mind-body-spirit relationship play in this healing system? Brendan thought the best place to look for something like a healing system would be cases of exceptional healings among people who had had spontaneous remissions or experienced some type of miracle cure.

Although he tried to study this, there was tremendous prejudice against it. Disease was (and still is) the model. Survival was not a topic for research. It was too idiosyncratic, too rare. So he did a massive search of the literature and found thousands of case reports of people who had had remissions.

Armed with the evidence that remission does occur, he went to the Northern California tumor registry and obtained the names of people in a limited geographical area who were still alive 10 years after a stage-IV metastatic diagnosis. There were 117 people on the list. He was able to get medical records for most of them. These were sent to an independent pathologist who, in 100% of the cases, confirmed the initial diagnosis. So the recoveries weren't due to a misdiagnosis. They really were due to a healing response that we don't currently understand.

Unfortunately, Brendan was sick and died before he completed the project. So when I came to the institute, I thought, "This is interesting. It's now 20 years later. What if we go back to the registry and look again? How many of those people are still alive?" We found more than 100 people who were still alive 20 years after a stage-IV diagnosis. The large number was due to better search capacities and increased population in the study area.

We conducted interviews with these people, looking for ways the cancer experience has played a role in their life history. Was it a transformational experience? Many people report that the experience was a positive thing because it forced them to reframe their lives. Many report some sense of gratitude to their doctors, their families, themselves, or God, for helping them. We recently published our findings on this. We feel that this focus on survival rather than on death is an important perspective.

Also, we don't always have to be normative in our research. Most of science is done on the bell curve. We focus on the majority. But what about those people who are on either end of the probability distribution? Are they just random, or are they a meaningful cohort that will allow us to understand something about the healing system and about the process of survival—something that can be turned into treatment modalities or options for others who are facing a terminal diagnosis?

There is a tremendous amount of individual difference—more difference than similarity, in fact. That's one of the challenges for us: how much can we be normative about our conclusions, finding generalizable patterns, and how much can we really articulate the differences in people's life experiences and how they react?

The fundamental thing we should do now, in this time of tremendous change, is question—question everything. Of course, it's disconcerting to question everything. We want to believe in things. And one thing we can believe in is that the answers we get are based on the questions we ask, so we'd better be careful about the questions we ask.

On Evolution

We are evolving moment by moment. Whether we see the evolution in our lifetime is a separate issue. But the nature of evolution is a critical question for the twenty-first century. What is unique for humans is our consciousness, our ability to self-reflect and understand our own mortality. Our challenge as a species is to own our role in the process. We are evolutionary agents in a way that no other species ever has been, which is both an opportunity and a challenge. How do we bring full consciousness to the process?

Take genetic engineering, for example. We are now able to create new life forms in the course of an afternoon, when it previously took millions of years. That's never happened before in all of history. It's never happened on this planet to any other species.

Nature creates new life forms all the time. And nature is self-correcting. But now we have the capacity to get out of right relationship, out of harmony, with nature. So how do we bring wisdom to bear on our great knowledge system? Values are fundamental. Instead of going about genetic engineering and waiting for the values conversation to catch up, we need to engage the values question first and understand the long-term implications of our present actions.

It seems that nature instinctively knows how to keep things in balance, while we do not. My guess is that we have an ability to judge good and bad, and nature doesn't judge good and bad. The idea of intrinsic goodness or badness is a human construction. Nature has the ability to function as a system and maintain integration of the system, but it doesn't have any kind of judgment. It has an intrinsic functional capacity; life forms either succeed or fail because they work within the system. It isn't because one organism is good and the other is bad.

But we have the capacity to bring judgment in. The challenge is in becoming conscious participants about our judgments and our assumptions in that process. How do we bring our highest self to our unique capacity, to be the sense organs for the planet in a way that has never been done before?

One way is to start asking the deeper questions about what it means to be conscious, sentient beings on this planet. I would argue that our culture's emphasis on objectivity has gotten us out of a right relationship with nature. Something about our sense of a world "out there" that we are detached from may contribute to the variety of environmental and social problems we face today—overpopulation, environmental degradation, inner-city violence. If we can gain a better sense of the whole and our place in it, rather than apart from it, I think we may reengage in the world and help steward it more responsibly.

Inner versus Outer Reality

I believe that if a person can change something in his or her own consciousness, that it will then produce changes here in shared reality. If enough people change their thoughts and their actions, the world will change. At least our perception of the world will change.

One of the things I love to think about is ontology. What is reality? And how do we know it? Throughout history the definition of reality has changed profoundly from culture to culture, from time to time, and we are equally committed to a worldview. As we become more aware of the arbitrary nature of these constructions, I think we can become more active participants in creating a new vision. Rather than just deconstructing our worldview, which is the postmodern perspective, it's about reconstructing. Once we realize it's arbitrary, that our consciousness does play a role in shaping experience, then I think we can bring full awareness to that process and visualize what we want to happen in the twenty-first century. And then, as a significant constituency, we can put our collective dreaming together to manifest it.

Having said all that, we are not omnipotent. There are subtle ways consciousness interacts with reality, but there are physical manifestations in reality that don't easily succumb to our intentionality. Part of the process of bringing consciousness into it involves becoming more humble, more willing to give up ownership and ego, and recognizing that we do have a unique role to play, but that it is one of coparticipation with nature—not *over* nature, but *with* nature. So I think our consciousness shapes reality, but reality also shapes consciousness. It's a two-way street.

We have assumed that causation is due to physical processes. But it may be that consciousness is causal as well. It may be that it is a two-way street. Our subjectivity may be as important as the objective aspects of the brain, for example, and our feelings and inner experience may have their own causal possibilities.

Take intentionality, for example, and our staring experiments. If consciousness is able to influence another physical being at a distance, then causation isn't simply about our brain influencing our motor system but about transcending the physical. This suggests a different kind of causality that isn't as easily reduced to strictly a materialistic model. Also, within the notion of causality, we assume, from a Newtonian point of view, that there are causes and an effects. But with the notion of systems theory, it is increasingly clear that there are multiple causes—multiple dimensions—especially in complex systems such as human biology, society, or nature.

So causation isn't a simple, linear process anymore. It is a multidimensional, participatory, collaborative process between multiple points of causation. If you consider quantum mechanics and some of the models that have been built on backward and forward movement, you see that the space-time matrix in which we are grounded isn't the only model of reality. We have structured our space-time continuum in a linear fashion because that works much of the time. A tree grows, a baby matures into an adult, and so forth. We see a linear progression. But it may also be that in certain domains of experience, any kind of linear cause and effect relationship is just one aspect of what is possible.

The Big Bang Theory

The complex thing about the big bang theory is that we assume that there is only one universe. But there may be many universes coexisting simultaneously. We talk about a big bang because it's a plausible model within our own cultural framework for understanding something we don't otherwise understand. But even that is being questioned now, and I don't know where it's going to go.

To me, it's about relationship. There is this sense that all of life and all of experience are about some relationship between parts. In the past we looked for the elementary particle, and once we looked further at the elementary particle we found that it was made up of other elementary particles, and so on. What we finally determined was that this thing we call *matter*, the sense of a table, really isn't about anything absolute called *matter*. It's about the relationship between a set of subatomic particles that make it up and give it the appearance of stability. But when it's in dynamic form, it is a very nebulous and continuous process.

Of course it's changing. It's evolving. So why should the notion of nonlocality in healing be considered far out, when in fact the universe is so mysterious we have only clues as to how it came to be or where it's going? We want continuity because that helps us on a psychological level, but it is much more complex than that. The challenge is to hold the mystery, to be in awe of the mystery and fully engaged in it, and then to recognize that it is part of human nature to seek answers. The discovery process has been fertile for us as a species.

That's my main line of inquiry: how do we learn to live with the questions, and how can we hold open the possibility that we'll never have the answers and have that be all right? Then again, if you're living with the questions, what does the purpose become? One of the things that drives people is the desire to know. But if you don't have that drive, if you aren't operating off that stimulus, then what?

Living in the question is about wanting to know. It's about trying to formulate the right questions so that the answers we find are more appropriate to the fullness of lived experience than the answers we get when we live in a box. The box tells us, "These are the kinds of questions you are able to ask," and they fit within a certain causality model. If you break out of that box, you have to formulate new questions to get a new set of answers. So part of the discovery process is discovering the questions that lead to a better set of answers.

I believe in the Buddhist precept of reducing suffering, whether it's for humans or animals or plants or "any sentient being." For the universe as a whole, the quest is to create a more life-affirming, sustainable vision for future generations.

Various studies have been published showing change in brain physiology when people enter contemplative states. So if you have a meditative experience, there is a change in brain activity. But you don't get enlightenment through changes in brain states.

It's about correlation, not causation. You're finding a correlation between a certain state of consciousness and brain chemistry, but that doesn't imply that either one of those things is necessary for the state of consciousness to occur. It's like stages in a research program. Eventually, you can get at causation. I love reductionism as long as people remember that it's only one step in the process. For example, right now in the epidemiology data on spirituality and health or religion and health, there are strong correlations between religious participation and health outcomes. Those who participate live longer, have fewer visits to doctors, and so on. But that doesn't give us a clue as to causation.

So in terms of causation, you begin to ask, "What are the different possible mechanisms of action that would lead to that kind of outcome? Is it social support? Is it belief? Is it diet? Is it altruistic love?" There are a variety of different explanations. Then you ask a more specific, focused question, and you try to manipulate the question in such a way that A causes B. But that's further down the road, and right now we have no answers to the causal questions about consciousness.

Work at the Institute

At the Institute of Noetic Sciences, we worked with Jeff Levin, one of the people who pioneered the work on religiosity and health from a social-epidemiology perspective. He's been looking at the idea of altruistic love as a possible mechanism for positive health outcomes associated with religious and spiritual participation. The study is based on Sorokin's work on altruism, and the notion that if you give love to other people, it may improve your own health and well-being. Again, the study is correlational, but he found significant correlations between health and the degree to which people report altruistic behavior.

Another project we've gotten into involves the health impacts of transformational practices. We look at those "Eureka!" moments people have that are, again, very idiosyncratic and might involve something as mundane as washing dishes or as profound as going to the moon and back. There's a whole continuum of possible triggers for transformation. The question involves the role that practice plays in moving a person from an exceptional experience to a "transforming" experience?

It is our hypothesis that people live in a box, but if they are able to transcend the box through whatever this "Eureka!" moment is, they can change the way they behave in their lives. We're looking for how these moments lead to profound transformation that causes them to live differently and that will potentially change the way they manifest reality.

We've approached this from a number of different perspectives. We collected transformational stories and conducted a qualitative content analysis. Rhea White, a transpersonal psychologist, coded a series of narratives that people have written about the difference between the exceptional experiences and transformational experiences so we could better understand that distinction. We interviewed people who had advanced cancer and people who traveled to foreign lands and who, through the process of meeting people from other countries, have found that their lives change. We brought together teachers of transformation in the Northern California area to look at common elements of their program and have begun to interview masters from the world's spiritual traditions. Eventually, we plan to conduct a longitudinal study that will explore specific outcomes such as quality of life and altruism and emotional intelligence, based on participation in transformational practices. The question is this: Do any of these transformational experiences actually have long-term consequences?

Another big program area for us is integral medicine. Through a series of grants over the last couple of years, we've studied what's been happening as the area of CAM emerges. Medicine is changing so fast that there's virtually no keeping up with it. Allopathic medicine is changing, and alternative medicines are changing. I hope we can hold the best of both to create something new that honors the integrity and wisdom inherent in both. We have focused on a deep examination of the values underlying alternative, complementary, and allopathic medicine. What are the common core attitudes and beliefs people bring to these practices, whether it is a medical student starting allopathic training or an alternative practitioner at the end of his or her career?

Subtle energies or biofields are another area. We have a number of projects examining their possible role in healing. Qigong practitioners, for example, claim they are able to activate our qi energy, that there's something innate in our healing system that is manifested through martial arts practices. But they also claim they can do intentionality at a distance, that they can project their qi so it has measurable outcomes in the physical world. We're working with a molecular geneticist named Garrett Yount at the California Pacific Medical Center on a study of the impact of qi on cell cultures—in particular, cells that have been cloned from brain tumors. Garrett is interested in whether it's possible for qigong masters to cause changes in gene expression.

Our research program functions in a couple of roles. As a research organization, we do in-house research and sponsor an extramural program. We always try to provide small amounts of funding for renegade ideas that can't seem to get support from conventional funding agencies but which hold great promise for breakthrough.

The second part is perhaps our most important function: we serve as an information clearing-house. People come to us for information on remission or distant healing or contemplation practices, for example. We have access to the current research, and we know the key people doing the work. So we've been very helpful to people at a time when they are in serious crisis. In this way, IONS offers discernment in areas in which there is so much information that it's hard to know how reliable it is. We have published a meditation bibliography with Michael Murphy and Steve Donovan that is a definitive source book for research on meditation; we have put it online so that it is available to the international community.

But going back to the question about evolution, there are two change models: one is adaptive change and the other is generative change. Adaptive change is the Stephen Hawking model—how we synthesize ourselves into a form that can deal with and adapt to the particular problems we are creating in the world. And that's good. One of the functions IONS can play is to help people cope as change happens faster and faster. But it's also important that we work toward generative change—figuring out what model we think is most useful to the future and how to get there, how we can create specific markers for ourselves as a culture to begin to achieve a sustainable future.

In my view, our work is about creating a story that recognizes that various models of reality coexist and that they change over time. We have a role to play in that change. It's about recognizing that there are different kinds of epistemologies to consider. Science is a very powerful and important one; wisdom traditions are among some of the others. We need to learn from all of them so we have a larger frame in which to hold the whole. Our ultimate goal is to help nurture the emergence of a more life-affirming and sustainable worldview for future generations—a worldview that honors all dimensions of our human experience, both physical and metaphysical. Ultimately, we serve as hospice workers for the old paradigm and midwives for the new. This is both our challenge and our opportunity.

CHAPTER 24

ANDREW WEIL, MD

On Integrative Medicine and the Nature of Reality

Perhaps alternative medicine's best known advocate, Andrew Weil, MD, is director of the Program in Integrative Medicine of the College of Medicine, University of Arizona—the first effort to change medical education to include information on alternative therapies, mind-body interactions, healing, and other subjects not currently emphasized in the training of physicians. He also holds appointments as clinical professor of medicine and clinical assistant professor of family and community medicine at the University of Arizona. He has a general practice in Tucson that focuses on natural and preventive medicine and diagnosis.

Dr. Weil received an AB degree in biology (botany) from Harvard in 1964 and an MD from Harvard Medical School in 1968. From 1971 to 1975, as a fellow of the Institute of Current World Affairs, Dr. Weil traveled widely in North and South America and Africa, collecting information on drug use in other cultures, medicinal plants, and alternative methods of treating disease. From 1971 to 1984 he was on the research staff of the Harvard Botanical Museum and conducted investigations of medicinal and psychoactive plants.

Dr. Weil is the author of nine books: *The Natural Mind; The Marriage of the Sun and Moon; From Chocolate to Morphine* (with Winifred Rosen); *Health and Healing; Natural Health, Natural Medicine;* and the international best-sellers *Spontaneous Healing, Eight Weeks to Optimum Health,* and *Eating Well for Optimum Health.* His newest is *The Healthy Kitchen* (with Rosie Daly). He publishes a monthly newsletter, *Dr. Andrew Weil's Self Healing;* maintains a popular Web site—http://www.drweil.com; and appears in three videos featured on PBS: *Spontaneous Healing, Eight Weeks to Optimum Health,* and *Eating Well for Optimum Health.* A frequent lecturer and guest on talk shows, Dr. Weil is an internationally recognized expert on drugs and addiction, medicinal plants, alternative medicine, and the reform of medical education.

I interviewed Dr. Weil on his ranch near Tucson, Arizona, in the spring of 2001. His ranch, which is in the middle of the Arizona desert, has an unexpected and beautiful stream flowing through it.

I think the whole alternative medicine movement is in a good place. It is still a consumer-led movement, but it's gaining a real response from academic medicine. At this point, I believe it's unstoppable and that it will result in a transformed system, including the system of medical education. By "transformed system," I mean a total transformation of the healthcare system with a strong emphasis on prevention and lifestyle medicine. I mean a totally different system of reimbursement and different kinds of institutions and facilities. Much needs to happen before all that comes to pass, but I clearly see us moving in that direction.

I've long had a vision of a healing center, which I see as a hybrid between a spa and a clinic. If you were well, it would be the kind of place you would go for a preventive lifestyle analysis or, if you were sick, a place you would go, not for critical or terminal situations but for routine complaints. It would be under the direction of generalist physicians with an integrative perspective and would offer many modalities of care. But the emphasis would be on learning how to live—how to eat, how to exercise, how to grow food, how to eat in restaurants, how to shop, how to use natural remedies—all of that.

But it will take a lot of work. For instance, I don't see us making much progress with people's eating habits until we engage the corporations that produce the food. For instance, our Program in Integrative Medicine at the University of Arizona has been completely unsuccessful at changing the food served in the hospital cafeteria. It should be easy, because nobody's happy with what's served there. We even talked to the food providers about just having one dish a day that was approved by the Program in Integrated Medicine or at least having basic labeling of nutritional information. But they've stonewalled on everything. It's not the registered dietitians who are the problem; it's the food contractors.

Marriott and a few other corporations have a lock-hold on all the food service in this country's institutions, including hospitals, and they only look at bottom-line profit. So they have to be convinced they can make as much or more money serving healthy food. But much of this comes back to the fact that our health professionals are so uneducated about nutrition. There's a glaring defect in the training of doctors and nurses that must change. If we had an informed, enlightened medical profession, it could be a powerful voice on issues like this.

Changing Medical Education

We've created a Consortium of Academic Health Centers for Integrative Medicine, and at the moment we have 12 member schools: Columbia, Duke, Harvard, Georgetown, Albert Einstein-Yeshiva, University of Maryland, University of Massachusetts, University of Michigan, University of Minnesota, University of Arizona, University of California–San Francisco, and Jefferson. And I think we'll shortly admit Cornell. We are currently funded by an outside group of philanthropists. Our goal is to have 25 member schools so we speak for one fifth of the nation's medical schools. At that point, we could begin to exert an influence on the American Association of Medical Colleges and the National Board of Medical Examiners. As you know, we're looking for radical change, which includes building self-care into the training of doctors. Medical education can't work at cross-purposes to the attainment of a healthy lifestyle.

Ralph Snyderman and I just wrote an editorial called *Integrated Medicine: Bringing Medicine Back to Its Roots,* which argues that the whole healthcare system needs radical restructuring and that integrated medicine should be the cornerstone. This editorial was the first official announcement of the consortium and we submitted it to the *New England Journal of Medicine.* Ralph just e-mailed me that it was summarily rejected with the comment that it contained nothing new. (NOTE: This essay has since been published in the 02/25/02 issue of *Archives of Internal Medicine.*)

Transforming medical education has always been my vision. Learning about alternative systems of healing, the natural healing mechanisms of the body, mind-body medicine, lifestyle medicine including nutrition, and self-care must be mandatory.

The Program in Integrated Medicine

The focus of our program here at the University of Arizona is just that—changing medical education and creating new models for training physicians. The program is training its fourth group of fellows this year, and there's been a lot of change since the beginning. We're still in the midst of thinking about how to do it best. For instance, we're still not sure how to structure the second year of the fellowship. One possibility is to have separate tracks for research, administration, and clinical care. Also, there has been talk about adding an optional third year. But I think we're producing the beginnings of a new generation of doctors who will begin to change the culture of medicine. And in my view that's what's needed most—more so than evidence for or against alternative therapies.

However, what's given the program the most vitality is the development of distance learning via the associate fellowship because that's forced us to organize the curriculum into a form that will eventually be publishable. For example, we're working on a nutrition module that could be the basis of a nutrition course for undergraduate medical education. Distance learning also gives us the ability to reach more doctors.

There's a big gap between what consumers expect and want from their doctors and how medical schools train them. It's out of frustration that most consumers go into the world of alternative medicine. I think their first choice would be to go to a medically trained person who is open-minded and able to make recommendations and referrals and give advice on how to live well and shop in health food stores and things like that. We are trying to close the gap by developing new educational models for healthcare professionals.

We chose the term *Integrative Medicine* for our program for a specific reason. When I travel around the country speaking, much of what I do is try to get people to distinguish between complementary and alternative medicine (CAM) and integrative medicine. I see CAM as only one piece of integrative medicine. Two other pieces that I think are important are the recognition of the innate healing mechanisms of the body and the reconnection of medicine with nature.

Another is whole-person medicine—treating patients as mental, emotional, and spiritual beings and community members as well as physical bodies. Other important aspects of integrative medicine are lifestyle medicine and the centrality of the doctor/patient relationship in healing. Yet another is shifting the emphasis of public health away from a narrow focus on water purification and prevention of infectious disease to the much broader issues of how kids eat, the epidemic of obesity, stress, healthy aging, and all that. All of this—more than just CAM—is what integrative medicine is about. If all we achieve is getting doctors to prescribe herbs some of the time in place of or in addition to pharmaceutical drugs, that would be a very limited achievement.

The Innate Healing Mechanisms of the Body

At every level you look at, the body has the capacity for self-diagnosis, self-organization, and repair and regeneration. That's the most wonderful thing about the human organism. It's such a shame when that is not emphasized in the training of doctors and is not a focus of research or practice. It's actually easier to talk with kids about the concept of the body's healing system than it is to talk with colleagues. When a kid gets a cut, you say, "Watch what happens," and the child immediately gets the concept that the body has the capacity to heal itself. But when you talk with physicians about it, they dismiss it as New Age fluff. But it's not New Age fluff. It's biology.

When I approach a patient, I'm always conscious that Nature's there and waiting to move things in the right direction. I just have to figure out how to help. It's very comforting as a physician to be aware that you've got Nature as your ally. Good treatment is about facilitating healing. It attempts to identify obstacles to healing and remove them. Even if you're dealing with overwhelming illness or illness that's not curable, it's still possible to move people in the direction of healing.

Over the years, many patients have told me that the most important thing I did was convince them that it was possible to get better. Even though I couldn't tell them exactly what to do—I may have told them to experiment or given them suggestions or sent them here or there—many people have said that no other medical authority ever told them that it was possible to get better, and that started them on the road to improvement.

My general thought is that healing comes from within and that all the external methods we use simply activate the healing process or unblock it in some way. But when you see these people who call themselves healers, they seem to do something to another person. So my question is, "What's happening? Are they actually causing it? Or are they somehow working on the belief?" I don't know for sure, but I suspect that when somebody touches another person and that person gets better, the healer has somehow activated an internal mechanism.

I have seen healers work, and I've also experienced it myself. About a year and a half ago, Rosalyn Bruyere was here working with the fellows, and I had a viral infection that was just hanging on and on. My throat was sore, and I could not shake it. So I asked her if she could do something. She told me to lie on a table, and she put her hands on my throat. Immediately, I felt strong vibrations from her hands. After a few minutes, I could feel the vibrations going down to my toes. What was especially interesting was that when she took her hands off, the vibrations continued for 10 minutes. I could feel them running through my body. The next day, I was completely better. Now, I don't know if that would have happened anyway, but if I get sick again I would certainly go back to her. And, again, what I felt was not subtle.

I've also written about some of my experiences with cranial osteopathy from Dr. Robert Fulford. I saw very dramatic results in the patients I sent him. Within hours of his doing gentle manipulation, chronic problems disappeared. It was very impressive.

Homeopathy and acupuncture might operate in that same realm as well—they both may be forms of energy medicine. I think energy medicine is a field that's going to come into its own in the 21st century. In the near future, we'll have a better understanding of subtle energies and the human biofield and how these various therapies interact with it.

A Patient Story

There was one woman I worked with who was the wife of a faculty member at the University of Arizona. She had widely metastatic breast cancer, but she actively experimented with alternative treatments, lifestyle changes, and spirituality. She lived for a good long time after the cancer had spread though her bones. I would not have thought it possible. I had never seen anybody with that much cancer throughout the body keep it in check. The experience reinforced my sense of what the body is capable of. Even if people have overwhelming disease, there is a lot one can do. She finally died, as we all will, but she certainly outlived the predictions of the medical experts who saw her.

I get a lot of feedback from people who tell me that they've read suggestions in my books and have followed them and now they're completely rid of some chronic problem that other doctors told them they couldn't get rid of. I love getting letters like that.

The Nature of Reality

The real question is "What is the relationship between internal reality and external reality?"

I don't know what's out there, but I have a feeling that whatever it is, we only perceive a narrow slice of it. Just as we only see a portion of the electromagnetic spectrum as light, I think there's a lot out there that we can't perceive. Other forms of life may perceive things we don't, just as dogs' noses can smell odors we can't. So I'm sure that what we perceive as reality is only one part of it.

Second, I have a feeling that there is subtle and complex interaction between what's in here and what's out there. Buddhists teach that sense perceptions are the result of the interaction between sense organs and objective things, which is not to say that there is nothing out there or that it's all projection. What they are saying is that we are active participants in the way we perceive reality. This certainly is true when we assign positive or negative qualities to things. For instance, there is no such thing as a bad odor in objective reality. There are just molecules. "Badness" of an odor results from an interaction of a molecule with a receptor in the olfactory organ. So it's a combination of objective and subjective that leads to our experience.

The most interesting thing I took away from all my work with psychoactive drugs and altered states of consciousness was the conviction that objective reality can be modified by modifying internal reality. An example is fire-walking: the result is totally dependent on your state of consciousness.

This is relevant to healing because when you are sick you want to change your reality. And there are ways you can do it. The recent *60 Minutes* program on my work made fun of my saying I had lost a cat allergy during an LSD (lysergic acid diethylamide) experience. But it's true. I had a lifelong allergy to cats, and in one instant it was gone. Another experience I've not mentioned before was that as a youth I was never able to get tanned. I grew up being told I had "fair skin." My experience of the sun was always that my skin got bright red and then peeled off. I accepted it—that was just how I was.

One day during this same period (I was about 28 years old) I tried lying in the sun without any clothes on in an altered state. I had decided that I was going to change my response, and I did. I got a tan that day and have ever since.

I love this kind of stuff. It seems to me that maybe whatever is out there is a collective— that "out there" is simply a collective molding of the raw stuff of reality. And if there is a collective consciousness that molds reality into the way we see it, maybe it could all be changed if there were a change in collective perception.

The main point of *The Natural Mind* (1972), the first book I wrote, was that drug experiences don't come in the drugs; they're in the nervous system. The drugs simply act as releasers of these experiences. What the drug does is something neutral and ambivalent, but then it is shaped in a positive or negative direction by the person. My book *Health and Healing* is an expansion of the idea that healing is something internal that can be released or triggered by things you do externally. Belief plays a great role in this.

A colleague recently told me that if we had a dramatic experiment showing the reality of energy healing, it would change everything. I said to him, "I used to believe that we lived in a rational culture where people's minds were changed by evidence, but I've learned that's not the case. No matter what you show some people, they'll say, 'That's not evidence.'" What we have to do is change the culture of medicine.

We need a new generation of people who see and think differently. That's really what we're trying to work at with the program—to build a critical mass of people in medicine who think and act in a different way so the whole system can change.

Personal experience is the key. The therapies that I can present most convincingly to my patients are those I have experienced myself. I know they work because they worked for me. If I know something by my own experience, there is no way anybody is going to argue me out of it.

Again, look at fire-walking. What the skeptics were originally saying was that people could do it because of an insulation effect. If you put a drop of water in a hot skillet, it will dance around and not evaporate because there is a microlayer of air that evaporates and insulates it. Then when that didn't hold up, they came back with the idea that the hot coals appear to be hot but really don't conduct heat very well. The analogy was being able to stick your arm in a 500° oven briefly and not get burned because air is a poor conductor of heat.

However, the second fire-walk I did was a shorter, cooler walk than the first—you could get across in three steps—but the group energy was horrendous. In retrospect, I should never have done it. I definitely got burned on that occasion—the coals conducted heat just fine. Subsequently I did a 40-foot walk on much hotter coals. But I was in the right state of mind so I didn't feel heat and didn't get burned in the slightest. The crucial variables were my state of consciousness and the group energy that I experienced.

Again, this is very relevant to medicine, because there are some patients with whom you're not going to have a good encounter and you can sense that immediately. So I think you should head them off at the door and send them elsewhere. Conversely, you know right away with some patients that you can engage them and help them, or you might know which practitioner a patient will respond to. You need to pay attention to those intuitions.

In the 1970s I spent a lot of time with South American Indians and shamans. The shamans I visited were a mixed bag, running the gamut from alcoholics to people who were masters. The best ones were very skilled, highly intuitive therapists who knew how to sense the structure of a client's belief system and to take the belief projected onto them and reflect it back on the person in a way that increased the possibility of healing. There's a lot that medical doctors can learn from shamans. It's all in the realm of the art of medicine, especially how to take projected belief and use it.

This is the stuff we don't teach that we need to teach. Any time a patient walks into the presence of a doctor, this magic is going on. A doctor is a power figure and will elicit projection. But there's a way of working with projection creatively to increase the possibility of healing.

Intuitive Knowing

I think intuition is unconscious material that bubbles up into consciousness. It may be based on or triggered by subtle perception. All of us have intuitions, but we're not trained to listen to, trust, or act on them. But I think that all good diagnosis is based on intuition, and all the great clinicians and diagnosticians I've met have been highly intuitive, even though they might not admit it to themselves.

There is a trend I see in medicine of not only not honoring this but actually discouraging students from using intuition and telling them to pay attention only to objective data. We need to change that.

Personal Practices

I have a meditation practice, and my early work with altered states was all moving in the direction of opening channels between the unconscious and conscious mind. I think anything you do that opens you to intuitive knowledge is good. But then there is the work of training yourself to pay attention to the intuitions, to trust them and act on them. That's a separate process.

Initially I practiced Zen, which I learned mostly from reading. Then I received formal instruction in Vipassana meditation. Now I try to do some daily sitting meditation, where I focus on my breathing and on body sensations. My relationship with my practice changes over the years—there are periods when it's easy and periods when it's very hard. But it's been useful. I think it's improved my concentration and evened out my moods in a good way. I'm committed to the practice and try to use it throughout the day, not just in the period of sitting. I constantly work at it.

The only religion with which I feel any kind of affinity is Buddhism, and the institutional aspects of Buddhism leave me as cold as do the institutional aspects of other religions. But as a philosophy, Buddhism works for me. I believe there is a mystery out there. There's something greater, but I have no conception of what it is. And I think that any attempt to describe or think about it is futile—you just can't do that. Our minds weren't designed for the task.

But I certainly have a sense of it and a sense of destiny. I like the feeling that I'm doing what I'm meant to do here. That sense is comforting. Sometimes I get annoyed with my life and wish that I could have been a chef or a gardener, but I know that isn't what I was sent here to do. I'm doing what I am supposed to do and using my talents and abilities in the way that I am supposed to.

Cooking

I've always been a generalist; I've always had too many interests. The dean of students at Harvard Medical School used to call me in every few months and berate me for not taking medical school seriously and for having too many outside interests. He always told me I was a dilettante and managed to make me feel really bad. One day I looked up *dilettante* in the dictionary. It comes from the Italian verb "to enjoy," and as soon as I knew that, he could never make me feel bad again.

I do a lot of things—like cooking and gardening and writing and hiking. I could imagine at one point doing something totally different from medicine, but right now I feel an obligation to work with this movement until our program has become financially stable, and the whole movement is solid and going in the right direction. I want to use my position to help all that happen.

I was always fascinated by it, but as a kid, if I was in the kitchen, I would be told that it wasn't where I should be. So I didn't really get a chance to cook until I was in medical school. I would get into such awful moods when I had to work in the hospital for 72 hours—it was more brutal back then—but I found that coming home and cooking, making order and beauty, detoxified me. So that's when I first got serious about cooking. It's something I really like to do. I like making food with other people and I like serving people good food.

I have written a new cookbook with Rosie Daley. Most people who write about food and health don't get how pleasurable food is. I think that a disservice has been done in sabotaging that aspect of food. For me, food is one of the major sources of pleasure in life. It should be enjoyed. So I want to give people the sense that you can have all that enjoyment and be good to your body as well.

Healthy Aging

My next major project is a book on aging. It's about healthy aging and what, realistically, we can do to increase our chances of arriving at old age the way we'd like it to be.

The big question is how much of it is genetically determined and how much is environmentally determined. There's pretty good evidence that a lot of how you age is influenced by environment and lifestyle. The first thing we should do is not deny aging. There's a huge amount of that in our culture. I want to take a hard look at cosmetics and plastic surgery and what all that really represents. What happens when you tell people, "You're looking younger"? I see that as very unhealthy. I want to look at the rise of this whole antiaging medicine trend as well.

The other thing I want to talk about is the Buddhist idea that aging begins at the moment of conception. It's not something that suddenly happens to you at age 60. Conventional medicine has the view that you suddenly age, but aging begins at the start of life; it's a lifelong process. The other Buddhist idea that I want to introduce is that awareness of aging can be part of spiritual awakening. The four heavenly messengers who were sent to awaken Buddha from his sleep as the prince were an old man, a sick man, a corpse, and a renunciate. So his enlightenment began with the sight of an old man, when the future Buddha realized that his beautiful young body wasn't going to last.

I'm interested in the areas of our experience in which we value aging. I want to consider old trees, cheese, wine, whiskey, and steak. What are the qualities that we appreciate in aged things? I think they include roundedness and smoothness as opposed to angularity and a kind of deep strength combined with mellowness.

I also want to look at the appeal of antiaging fantasies. There is the fountain of youth, the magic potion that you take, the place where you go where aging slows down. These are very powerful fantasies. And I want to look at the MacArthur Foundation's study on aging. The two outstanding characteristics it found in populations of healthy old people were maintenance of physical activity throughout life and maintenance of social and intellectual connectedness.

Probably the worst thing that happens in our culture to old people is isolation. Increasingly, we segregate old people with other old people. This is not true in cultures where people live in extended families.

I'm 60, and my daughter is 10. So a good place to start is to be physically active and connected—to be interested, connected, and engaged with the world and with other people. Nutrition is certainly part of it. Even though you can find very healthy old people who have eaten horrible food all their lives, maintaining a good intake of antioxidants, eating lots of vegetables, avoiding the bad fats—all of that is very sensible.

I think it's the resistance to aging that wears the body down. It's the tendency to defend yourself against what you don't like that creates the problem. It's better to accept it and flow with it.

The Environment

I am also highly concerned about the environment. You watch a place like this, the Tucson Valley, which was probably one of the most beautiful valleys in America not long ago, and it's being completely filled in by city. We're doing in the water and the land and the air.

My all-time favorite bumper sticker is the one that says "Nature bats last." If you take the stance of fighting a battle against nature, you're doomed. I don't think we'll do in the planet or do in all life, but I certainly think we could do in ourselves and end civilization as we know it.

I think medicine has a big responsibility in this area. Michael Lerner and Commonweal gave our program a grant to survey the world's medical literature for systems of detoxification. Iris Bell, our research director, and I are working on it. Specifically, we are looking at what's been proposed as ways of ridding the body of chemical toxins and what validity these methods might have. In the case of nutrition, it seems to me if the medical doctors were educated, they could stand up as one powerful voice and fight the fast food providers and the soft drink companies in the schools. And if doctors were really educated about the relationship between the environment and disease, they could be a very powerful force to stand up to industry and government on many of these issues.

But at the moment, the profession has abdicated its responsibility in this area.

It's a huge issue. It's easy to feel completely powerless, but there are steps you can take in your own immediate life that can help. The one I've been most directly involved with is organic agriculture. I've never used pesticides or exterminators. Most people who live here have the exterminator come once a month and spray the house. They spray for scorpions and black widow spiders, for example. I don't spray, and I don't have problems with those creatures.

I would bet money that diseases such as Parkinson's disease and ALS (amyotrophic lateral sclerosis) are going to turn out to be due to toxic injury to very sensitive parts of the brain.

What Is Medicine?

Having spent a lot of time with Native Americans, especially in the 1970s when I was investigating shamanism, I was always struck by the fact that when they used the word *medicine*, it had a much larger meaning than our word *medicine*. When they talked about *medicine men, medicine women, medicine places, medicine people*, it was a much bigger concept that embraced magic and religion, as well as what we mean by *medicine*. I call it *Medicine with a capital "M,"* and I think our culture desperately needs it.

Our medicine and our culture have disowned magic, which we tend to think of as antiscientific and antirational. But to me, magic is what we were talking about earlier. It's about the relationship between internal reality and external reality and how you can change or modify external reality with internal operations.

And anybody can do it. It's part of the wonder and mystery of existence, and I deplore the fact that science has become a kind of religion for many people—one that aims to make wonder and mystery go away. There is a saying that the bigger you build the fire, the more you become aware of the extent of the darkness. I like that because there is this idea that science will ultimately roll back all that we think is unknown and mysterious and that we'll know everything. I don't believe it. It is legitimate for science to try to figure out mechanisms and cause-and-effect relationships, but it doesn't have to make the wonder go away.

The relationship between what's in here and what's out there is built right into Native American medicine. We need that. I want to see that perspective come back into our medicine. Being able to instill or awaken in patients a sense that they can get better is an example of practical magic. We should help them understand that change on the level of consciousness can translate into physiological reality.

Part Seven

Conversations About New Views of Health and Healing

"Curing is about solving a physical problem on a physical level, which is very important, but healing is about using whatever adversity you're trying to heal to learn the truth of who you are."

—MITCH GAYNOR

CHAPTER 25

DEAN ORNISH, MD

Healing the Heart, Reversing the Disease

Ten years ago, neither the medical establishment nor the American public accepted the fact that heart disease could be reversed through changes in diet and lifestyle. But thanks to the work of Dean Ornish, MD, patients with cardiac disease now have proven options to invasive surgery. His extensive research has shown that the progression of heart disease can not only be stopped, it can be completely reversed through diet and stress reduction, and his cardiac programs are now being used in hospitals and clinics throughout the United States.

Dr. Ornish received his medical degree from Baylor College of Medicine in Houston and completed his internship and residency in internal medicine at Massachusetts General Hospital and Harvard Medical School in Boston. He is the author of *Stress, Diet & Your Heart: Dr. Dean Ornish's Program for Reversing Heart Disease; Eat More, Weigh Less;* and *Make It Easy: Everyday Cooking,* all bestsellers. In addition to his work as president and director of the nonprofit Preventive Medicine Research Institute, Dr. Ornish is a clinical professor of medicine at the University of California–San Francisco School of Medicine. He served on the White House Commission on Complementary and Alternative Medicine Policy and as a consultant to former President Clinton and his chefs.

In the summer of 1995, I interviewed Dr. Ornish at his offices at the Preventive Medicine Research Institute in Sausalito, California.

I began doing this work in 1977 when I was a second-year medical student at Baylor College of Medicine in Houston. At first, bypass surgery was exciting. There's an Aztec-priest quality to cutting someone's chest open and exposing his beating heart. But after a while, it became disheartening, literally and figuratively. We would operate on people, and their chest pain from heart disease would go away, but then, in most cases, they would go home and eat the same diet, not manage stress well, not exercise, and continue smoking. And their bypasses would often clog up.

So for me, bypass surgery became a metaphor for an incomplete approach. It was literally "bypassing the problem," rather than addressing the underlying cause. It's like mopping up the floor from a sink that's overflowing without also turning off the faucet. If we don't address the underlying cause of virtually any problem, then more often than not the same problem tends to come back again, or we find a new set of problems. For example, studies show that if people don't change their lifestyles within 4 to 6 months of an angioplasty, 40% of the angioplastied arteries will have clogged up.

If we can address the more fundamental causes, then we find that, in many cases, and especially with heart disease, the body has a much greater capacity to begin healing itself and often more quickly than we once thought. Our research has shown that for patients who have severe heart disease, within a few days to a few weeks, chest pain tends to diminish, often dramatically.

Within a month we've measured that the blood flow to the heart often improves, and the ability of the heart to pump blood often improves. Within a year, we've found that even severely blocked coronary arteries may become measurably less blocked. Our newest findings indicate that there was even more reversal overall after 4 years than after 1 year. So instead of getting worse and worse over time—the so-called "natural history" of heart disease—we're finding that patients often may get better and better.

These findings are giving many people new hope and new choices that they didn't have before. When I first began doing this work, I thought that the younger patients with milder disease would be more likely to experience reversal, but I was wrong. The major determinant of how much or how little people improved wasn't how old they were or how sick they were. It was primarily how much they changed their lifestyles, both after 1 year and after 4 years. We found that there was a direct correlation between adherence and outcome.

That's very hopeful news for many people because it's saying that as long as you're stable, it's never too late to begin making these changes, and, for that matter, it's never too early either.

In the beginning, it was very difficult to get funding for this work. When I went to the major government agencies like the National Institutes of Health or private agencies like the American Heart Association, they'd say, "Why should we waste our money funding research that isn't likely to show anything?" My approach was to say, "It may be impossible, but let's find out. Even if we show that heart disease can't be reversed, that will be as interesting as if we showed that it can be, as long as it's done with proper scientific design, proper scientific technology, and proper scientific rigor."

Ironically, we're using the very latest in high-tech, state-of-the-art medical technologies to prove the power of these very ancient, low-cost, and low-tech interventions. But we were caught in this catch-22. Without the funding, we couldn't demonstrate that it might be feasible, and without the demonstration that it was feasible, nobody wanted to fund it. Besides the fact that they thought heart disease couldn't be reversed, most people said, "You have an untestable theory. Even if it were possible to reverse heart disease by making the kind of comprehensive changes in diet and lifestyle that you recommend—a low-fat vegetarian diet with less than 10% of calories from fat and virtually no cholesterol; an hour a day of stress-management techniques including yoga-based stretching, breathing, meditation, imagery and progressive relaxation techniques; moderate exercise; stopping smoking; and psychosocial support—this is too hard a program to follow. People can't do it." Doctors would say, "I can't even get my patients to eat less red meat. You expect them to give it up completely and do meditation and exercise and quit smoking and come to these regular meetings and talk about their feelings in a group? Forget it. No way. It's too hard."

The Life-Style Heart Trial

We enrolled our first patient in the Life-Style Heart Trial in January of 1986. The specific aims were: Number one, how can patients be motivated to make and maintain these changes in a real-world setting? Number two: What are the longer-term effects on their risk factors, like blood cholesterol levels? And number three: What happens to the blockages in their coronary arteries?

We found that these patients, by and large, were able to follow the program, and that, on average, they did get better. Within a year, the patients in the experimental group who followed the program showed some overall reversal of their coronary artery blockages, whereas the patients in the comparison group, who followed conventional diet and lifestyle changes, on average, got worse. They were following the guidelines recommended by the National

Cholesterol Education Program, the American Heart Association, and others, meaning, a 30%-fat diet, with 200 to 300 milligrams of dietary cholesterol. And on average, the patients who followed their physicians' instructions got worse.

We reported these findings in *The Lancet* and later in the *American Journal of Cardiology, Circulation,* and the *Journal of the American Medical Association.* Those findings formed the basis of my second book, *Dr. Dean Ornish's Program for Reversing Heart Disease.* The first book—*Stress, Diet and Your Heart*—was published after my first two studies.

Based on the results after 1 year, we received funding from the NIH to extend the study for 3 additional years. And what we found is that there was even more reversal overall after 4 years than after 1 year in the experimental group who followed the program, whereas the patients in the comparison, or control, group got worse on average after 4 years than after 1 year.

When I began doing this research, the idea that heart disease could begin to reverse was considered radical. Now it's become fairly mainstream. Most cardiologists believe that heart disease can be stopped or even begin to reverse, not only because of our work, but also the work of others who have shown that a variety of interventions may reverse the progression of heart disease. The skepticism that remains is "how practical is this?"

Nova did a 1-hour documentary on our patients in the Life-Style Heart Trial, and they followed the first four patients all the way through their first year. At the end of the broadcast, the producers asked Dr. Eugene Braunwald, who at the time was chief of medicine at Harvard and wrote the standard textbook on cardiology, "Do you think this is real?" And he said, "Yes, this is scientifically valid, but it'll never play in Peoria."

So the next level of our research was to say, "How practical is this? Can we train other health professionals in our program to teach it? Can they, in turn, motivate their patients in other parts of the country to make and maintain lifestyle changes to this degree in a real-world setting? And what are not only the medical outcomes but also the cost outcomes?"

We're now trying to find out if other people, in other places, can do it. We've set up a demonstration network of eight hospitals that's coordinated through our nonprofit Preventive Medicine Research Institute. We went to individual hospitals and asked them if they would pay a *pro rata* portion of what the research and training would cost. We began with Immanuel Hospital in Omaha, then Mercy Hospital and the Iowa Heart Center in Des Moines. So we're not in Peoria, but we're close. The other hospitals in the study are Beth Israel Hospital in New York City; Richland Memorial Hospital in Columbia, South Carolina; Broward General Hospital and Medical Center in Fort Lauderdale; Beth Israel Hospital at Harvard Medical School; Mt. Diablo Hospital in Concord, just outside of San Francisco; and the Scripps Clinic and Hospitals in La Jolla, California.

Mutual of Omaha was the first insurance company to pay for the program. In the past, insurance companies were reluctant to pay for programs like this, because they viewed them as preventive, and they would say, "Why should we spend today's dollars for some future benefit that may or may not occur? And even if it does occur, we know that up to 25% of the patients change companies within a year, so chances are that patient will be with some other insurance company who will get the benefit." We suggested to the insurance companies that, rather than viewing this as a preventive approach, they view it as an alternative therapy for selected patients who are (a) motivated to do it; and (b) clinically stable. Bypass surgery and angioplasty clearly have their place in someone who is unstable or who has critically severe disease. If someone comes into the emergency room and they're having crushing chest pain in the middle of a heart attack, that's not the time to feed him vegetables and teach him to meditate. That's the time when drugs and surgery can be lifesaving. But most patients who get bypass surgery and angioplasty don't fall into that category.

So we proposed that the insurance companies view this as an alternative treatment for patients who might otherwise have gotten a bypass or an angioplasty. For every patient who goes through our program and doesn't need the surgery, somebody saves approximately $50,000 immediately. In addition to the short-term savings, there may be long-term savings. Many of the bypasses and angioplasties clog up and have to be done multiple times, whereas we have evidence that the patients who stay on this program tend to get better and better over time.

The insurance companies said, "That sounds great, but we don't think people can do it. It's too hard." So the missing links, really, are the data to show that people will do it and that most don't need the operations that they otherwise would have had. So we began our study.

Our preliminary data are very encouraging. Mutual of Omaha is collecting our cost data and providing matched controls concurrently, based on their age, gender, disease severity, and left ventricular function. Our preliminary data are that about 90% of people who were eligible for bypass surgery or angioplasty have been able to go on my program instead of having those operations. Mutual of Omaha has calculated that for every dollar they've spent, they've had over $5.55 in immediate savings and much more when you factor in the savings in medications, the redos of the angioplasties or bypasses, and so on. Right now, there are 12 insurance companies paying for our program, but if we continue to show them that for every dollar that they are spending, they are saving $5.55, then clearly, we hope that in the near future many more insurance companies will cover this program.

This, in turn, becomes a flying wedge, if you will, for other kinds of approaches that may be less well documented. If we can show in this area where the science is so advanced, that a less-expensive therapy is not only medically effective but also cost-effective, then I hope this will encourage NIH and other agencies to fund studies of other alternative therapies, to see what works, for whom, under what circumstances, and to what degree—because clearly, not everything in traditional medicine works in all circumstances, and not everything in alternative medicine works. The goal is to find what works best under what circumstances, for whom, at the lowest cost and the highest quality.

I think there are a lot of health-policy implications to this. We have 41 million Americans who don't have access to healthcare—more precisely, disease care—in this country. If we simply take those 41 million Americans and put them into the medical system and do what we've been doing—for example, bypass surgery and angioplasty—healthcare costs go up exponentially. So then what do we do? We have painful choices. Do we raise the deficit? Do we raise taxes? Do we just not treat entire categories of people? Do we ration healthcare like is done in England, where they don't treat people after a certain age for certain illnesses? None of these choices are very good.

We're trying to show that there's a new model for healthcare that's not only more cost-effective but also more compassionate. There's a lot of anxiety and fear and loathing among many physicians—and, understandably, because they are getting squeezed. They are being forced to see more and more patients in less and less time, at less and less reimbursement. The irony is that at a time when the scientific evidence of the psychosocial factors and their role in health is increasing, physicians have less and less time to spend with their patients. We're trying to create a new model for medicine that's both more cost-effective and confident and compassionate—a model where it actually saves money to spend more time with patients addressing these fundamental questions of health and illness.

A primary determinant of how medicine is practiced in this country is not only science—science is important—but also what insurance pays for. If insurance doesn't cover it, it's very difficult for doctors to do it, even if they want to do it. So if we can change how medicine is reimbursed, then we may change how it's practiced. This even goes back to influencing medical education—because, in the final analysis, we physicians do what we get paid to do. And we get trained to do what we get paid to do.

Adherence Factors

I never try to get people to do anything. I don't tell my patients what to do. As soon as I try to get people to change, even in the name of helping them, I am now engaged in a manipulative relationship with them. Medicine uses words like "compliance," which has a horrible connotation to it. It's like one person bending his will to another. I don't do that. I used to. When I first began doing this work 19 years ago and saw how much better people were getting, I would say, "Why don't you do this? Why would you do that?" But I realized that once I was in that kind of a manipulative relationship with them, I was doing more harm than good. If they weren't able to change, they'd blame themselves and feel guilty or ashamed, which only made them want to eat more fat or smoke more. And they would be less likely to tell me, because they didn't want to feel embarrassed or didn't want to make me feel bad or didn't want me to get angry with them. So I wouldn't really know what they were doing. I'd think they were doing everything right, but they wouldn't get better, and I'd think maybe something was wrong with the program, when the real problem was that they just weren't doing it.

So I don't do that. If you had heart disease, I'd say, "My goal is to give you the latest scientific information from my work and the work of others, so that you can make informed and intelligent decisions. Whatever you decide to do is fine because you're the one who has to take the consequences. If you decide you want to have a bypass, I'll find you the best surgeon. If you want to have an angioplasty, I'll find you the best invasive cardiologist. If you want to go on drug therapy, I can prescribe that for you. If you want to change your lifestyle, we've developed this program."

Then we'll go through the risks, the benefits, the costs, the side effects—and whatever they choose is fine. I'm free, and they're free, and they know that they can be honest with me if they're having a problem with it. I have seen what a powerful difference these choices can make in people's lives. But whether or not they want to make those choices is really up to them.

The adherence to medication is less than 50% after a year, and that's just taking a pill. But we've been showing that 90% of the people who choose to be in our programs have been able to stay with it now, and not just in California but in Omaha and Des Moines and South Carolina. Why is that? Because we get away from the idea of "risk-factor modification," which is how cardiologists often talk about the reason for changing behavior. Most people don't really believe that anything bad is ever going to happen to them. Intellectually, we know that we're all going to die, but we don't think about it most of the time. If someone's had a scare, if they've had a heart attack or they've gotten hospitalized for chest pain, their denial has broken down. They'll do just about anything that their doctor asks them to do, for about 2 or 3 weeks, maybe a month, maybe 6 weeks. Then they tend to go back to their old patterns—but that's because doctors are asking them to change behaviors out of fear. "If you don't do these things, something bad may happen to you." Most people can't relate to that.

Instead of asking people to change out of fear of dying, we're asking them to change to increase their joy of living. You feel better. You have more energy. You think more clearly. If you have chest pain, the chest pain tends to diminish. For people with severe heart disease who can't work without getting pain, can't have sex without getting pain, can't even take a shower or shave without getting pain and within a few weeks they can do virtually all of those things, they often say, "I know what my choices are now. I like eating meat—but not that much. I like doing these other things even more. These are choices that are worth making because I feel so much better now." People are not afraid to make big choices if they think it's worth it.

The paradox is that I think it's actually easier to make big changes all at once than to make small, gradual changes, or moderate changes. Because if you make moderate changes, you get very little benefit. If you only go on a 30%-fat diet, you have the worst of both worlds. You have the sense of deprivation from not being able to eat everything that you enjoy, but you're not making changes big enough to get much benefit. Your cholesterol, your weight, your blood pressure don't come down very much. If you have heart disease, you tend to get worse.

However, when you make comprehensive changes, you usually feel so much better so quickly that choices become clearer and, for many people, they're worth making—not to keep something bad from happening, not to live longer (although you probably will), but to live better.

The Training Program

When we teach the staff of the hospital programs—which include a cardiologist, an exercise physiologist, a cardiac nurse, a registered dietitian, a psychotherapist, a stress-management instructor who is really a yoga teacher, a chef, a program director, and a medical director—the way we train them is that we bring them out here to one of our week-long retreats. We've learned that the best way for them to teach it is to experience the program. And the rationale for the week-long retreats—not only for them but for everyone—is that within a week, if the changes are intensive enough, you really do feel the benefit. It's not just being convinced of it intellectually. Whether you have heart disease or not, you'll feel much differently by the end of that week than you did before, and then you get it.

The health professionals come a day early and stay a day later, but during most of that week, we ask them to go through the program just like everyone else. They're not set apart. They are going through it to experience it, for the very reasons that you're asking about. The best way we have found for them to teach it is to understand it experientially.

The Role of the Physician

The physician became the priest approximately 300 years ago when the Catholic Church lost its position as the holder of the cosmology. They used to say that the earth was the center of the universe and everything revolved around it. Then in the 16th century, an Italian scientist, Giordano Bruno, came along and said, "No, I think that the earth revolves around the sun." The Church responded the way that people often do when their paradigms are threatened, and burned him at the stake. A hundred years later, Galileo said the same thing, but he provided the telescope so people could see for themselves that the earth wasn't the center of the universe. Under the threat of the Spanish Inquisition, he was forced to recant, but by then it was too late. People could see for themselves. And from that time on, the scientists, and ultimately the physicians, became the modern-day priests. They say, "This is how the world is."

I think it's appropriate for the physician to not just be a technician but also to deal with what Sir William Osler called "the art of medicine." There is the science, which is clearly important, and we shouldn't lose sight of that, but the art of medicine—whether you call it "spiritual" or "psychosocial" or "mind-body" or whatever—falls into what I would call "the art of medicine," and that's been an important part of medical tradition for centuries.

You ask me if the mind affects the body, or if the body affects the mind. It's like the story of the blind men and the elephant. One has the leg, and he thinks the elephant's like a tree; one has the tail, and he thinks it's like a snake; and one has the ear, and he thinks it's like a bat.

But we all have different pieces of the elephant. In his classic book, *The Structure of Scientific Revolutions,* Thomas Kuhn talked about how reality is infinitely complex and infinitely vast. Our minds can't really grasp things that are infinite, so we reduce them to more manageable proportions by coming up with models or paradigms or worldviews that say, "This is how it is." We can handle that.

One model of the universe, the Cartesian model, says that the mind and the body are separate. And science has tended to evolve in that direction. But it's wrong to say that it's all mind or it's all body. Some would say that the mind and the body are just different manifestations of the same thing, or that there's the physical body and an astral body, that there are all different levels of body, some of which can be seen and some of which are more difficult to see. The point I'm trying to make is that, as part of my training as a physician and my education, the more different systems that I can understand, the more pieces of the elephant that I have, the more clearly I can see the emerging whole. No one system has all the answers. They're all models. Some are more useful than others, and some are more useful under certain circumstances than others. But the goal is to try to see things from as many different perspectives as possible, without losing the rigor within that individual perspective.

I find it useful to be grounded in western science. It gives me a base that I can then explore other perspectives from, much as Wynton Marsalis has said that being trained in classical music helped him when he learned jazz, or how training in classical ballet is helpful in exploring modern dance. The goal is to not get caught in believing that the model is the reality. The model is a very useful perspective of that reality, but it is only one of many perspectives.

I went to India with Sri Swami Satchidananda in 1979 to study Ayurveda and naturopathic medicine and look at their different health systems, and I got a bad case of amoebic dysentery. It was the middle of August, 100°, and I had unrelenting diarrhea. I was getting more and more dehydrated and lost 20 pounds. I tried all the local remedies, the Ayurvedic treatments, the nature cures, the homeopathic medicines. Whatever system we were studying, I would try that. But I just kept getting sicker and sicker. Finally I said, "The hell with it!" I took some antibiotics and was well the next day. So I came back from India with this very healthy respect for what Western medicine does well.

Then in medical school, I learned what it doesn't do so well. So the goal, the key, is to really find what each system does well and what it doesn't do well and not to try to force everything into one approach or system.

Meditation

Being in the moment, being aware in the moment, is a goal of meditation. The moment is really all there is. So much of stress is about worrying about the past or the future: "I should have done it this way" and beating yourself up. Or "Oh, my God, this might happen or that might happen." But meditation, in whatever form, brings you into the present moment. There are a lot of practical implications from that. The first is that although people often tend to view meditation as withdrawing from the world, it's really about embracing it more fully. When you meditate, in whatever tradition, you become more aware of what you are doing in that moment, and, in general, you can focus and concentrate better, so you can perform better. Whether it's in the business world, school, or the academic arena, when you concentrate and focus better, you perform better.

People think about meditation as being in a cave in the Himalayas. Sometimes people think of me or my program in this way, which is quite the opposite of the way that I like to experience life. Whether it's food, sex, music, art, massage, or anything that involves your senses, when you really focus on it and when you really pay attention to it, it's a lot more enjoyable. I used to eat while reading or watching TV or talking to somebody, and I would look down and my food was gone. I'd say, "Who ate this food?" because I was focusing on the news, rather than on what I was eating. If you really focus on what you're eating, it makes things much more sensual, much more joyful.

A third aspect of meditation is that your mind begins to quiet down and you begin to experience more of an inner sense of peace and joy and well-being and to realize that that feeling came not because you got something that you thought you needed in order to be happy or you didn't get something that you were afraid of getting but rather you simply quieted down your mind and body enough to experience what we have all the time if we don't allow it to be disturbed. It's an empowering realization, even if it's only a glimpse of that, because it redefines for people where their sense of peace and joy and well-being comes from. Once they realize that they have it already unless they allow it to be disturbed, then the question shifts from "How can I get this in order to be happy and peaceful?" to "What am I doing that's allowing my inner peace to be disturbed?"

So often, patients who have heart disease believe that their happiness comes from outside themselves. "If only I could get (blank), then I'd be happy." Until they get it, whatever it is, they feel stress. If somebody else gets it and they don't get it, then they feel really stressed and hostile, and that hostility has been linked very strongly with heart disease. Even if they get it, there's this moment of feeling, "Great, I got it," which is what makes it so seductive because it seems like the good feeling came from outside oneself. But the feeling doesn't last. It's soon followed by, "Well, now what?" It's never enough.

So being in the moment—using the stretching and breathing and meditation and visualization techniques—can be powerful tools toward providing people with that direct experience of what it means to feel at peace and to realize that it came not because they got something they thought they needed but rather that they quieted down their minds and bodies enough to experience what they have already—if they don't disturb it.

The more work you do on yourself, the more you have to offer other people. For instance, I practice yoga every day. I couldn't do what I do otherwise.

I got interested in yoga when I became profoundly depressed. Suffering can be a catalyst for transforming one's life. The word *healing* comes from the root, to make whole. The word *yoga* comes from the Sanskrit, meaning to yoke, to unite, union. So these are very old ideas. The ancient swamis and rabbis and priests and monks and nuns who developed these techniques didn't develop them to unclog their arteries or lower their cholesterol and blood pressure. They developed them because they helped to quiet their minds and bodies to give them the direct experience that on one level we're all separate—you are you, and I'm me—and on another level we're part of something larger that connects us all.

By the way, when we work with people, we work within their own religious or secular framework. We don't ever try to get people to chant in Sanskrit if they don't want to do that. For example, they can meditate on a prayer or something secular. If they're Catholic, they can use the Hail Mary prayer or rosary beads. They can use the word *amen* or the word *om* or *shalom* or the word *one*. It doesn't really matter as much what they meditate on as that they do it in a way that's comfortable and consistent with their own belief systems.

Ultimately, these practices are not just about managing stress or coping with stress or dealing with stress. They're really about transcending that isolation that I think really is a root cause of so many of the self-destructive behaviors and emotional stresses which, in turn, are such major contributors to so many of the illnesses that people suffer from.

CHAPTER 26

MITCHELL W. KRUCOFF, MD

The Mantra Project

Dr. Krucoff currently serves as director of the Ischemia Monitoring Laboratory and director of interventional clinical trials for the Duke Clinical Research Institute (DCRI), as senior staff in the Interventional Cardiac Catheterization Laboratories at Duke Medical Center, and as director of the Cardiovascular Laboratories at the Durham Veterans Administration (VA) Medical Center. Dr. Krucoff received his bachelor's degree from Yale University in 1976 and his MD from George Washington University in 1980. He completed his residency in internal medicine at George Washington University in 1983 and his fellowship in cardiology at Georgetown University in 1985.

Since 1990, Dr. Krucoff has served as a member of the board of directors of the Sri Satya Sai Institute of Higher Medical Sciences in Puttaparthi, India. He has published more than 50 articles in refereed medical journals and has written numerous book chapters on various aspects of cardiology and coronary care. He is the principal investigator of the Monitoring and Actualization of Noetic Trainings (MANTRA) Study Project at the DCRI.

In 1999, I interviewed Dr. Krucoff with his partner, MANTRA co-principal investigator Suzanne Crater, at their offices in the VA Medical Center at Duke University in Durham, North Carolina.

A number of threads have come together in this particular tapestry (the MANTRA project) over the past 10 years. In 1989, Suzanne and I began working together with patients with very advanced heart disease. At that time there was nothing being offered to these patients other than ongoing chest pain, prolonged hospitalizations, and, ultimately, death. Unblocking coronary arteries through catheter-based "interventional" methods on such high-risk patients was new territory.

In this context our interactions with patients and families were focused not on the general complications that can occur with these procedures—bleeding, infection, stroke—but on death and issues around dying. At the time we believed that in such very sick patients one in three would not make it through these new procedures, and we obtained informed consent from patients with these figures. We were very consistent about our communication patterns with patients: speaking with them directly, giving them time to reflect, meeting with the whole family present. At the end of a year's work, instead of a 33% procedural death rate, the data showed a 3% death rate.

Although we didn't understand it at the time, looking back, our work with patients and their families frequently involved spiritual issues. Duke University is in the middle of the Bible Belt, and our patients were typically spiritually grounded people. They did not always have a formal education, but many were farmers who understood life cycles and had religious faith. Families, and often the local pastor, were almost always present and frequently prayed with and for the patient during our discussions, as they went to the cath lab, or both. Looking back, the atmosphere was unique. Clearly, new technical innovations partially explained why these people did better than expected, but there was also something else that we now believe has more to do with something that began with the preprocedural interactions.

What happened next was that through a series of "coincidences" we were put in contact with the creation of a very unique hospital in Puttaparthi, India. This hospital is a 300-bed, two digital catheterization laboratory, five operating theater, state-of-the-art, free-care facility that was built by Sri Satya Sai Baba in a rural area of India where, until recently, there was no electricity and most people had never seen a toilet, much less a cath lab. We were involved in its original design. At the end of the first year of operation, the hospital hosted a symposium to review its activities. The day before the symposium we rounded in the hospital and found ourselves immersed in something we had never seen before.

In U.S. hospitals, everyone basically fights off depression. Patients don't want to be in the hospital, and their families are worried about them. Cardiovascular disease is almost always shrouded in a life-and-death atmosphere, and in the western world death is taken as a bad thing. But the patients at the institute in Puttaparthi—people who could barely breathe and were waiting for a catheterization or surgery or who had just had surgery—were beaming. As we went from bedside to bedside, they just beamed. It was a different kind of atmosphere than we had ever walked through in a hospital setting. And the reason everyone was beaming was very clear—this was God's hospital. These folks believe that Sri Satya Sai Baba is an avatar, meaning they believe he is a reincarnation of Rama in human form. So, very literally, God came on rounds and physically touched them.

As Suzanne and I flew home over the Pacific we talked about how such a powerful atmosphere had to have an effect on the immune system, the healing characteristics of tissue, on pain thresholds. Likewise, we talked about how western healthcare had drifted toward a depersonalized, packaged, high-efficiency, high-technology, time-driven system. We discussed how we might systematically go about reconsidering and studying the notion of what, exactly, constitutes a "healing space," and the MANTRA Study Project began to take form.

Over this same period a small group of cardiology doctors, nurses, and statisticians with common research interests at Duke evolved into what is now the 700-person Duke Clinical Research Institute. This group developed models for clinical outcomes research, mostly examining the safety and efficacy of new pharmacological therapies and new device therapies. This progressively formalized think tank operates at Duke and also organizes and conducts clinical trials in multiple centers across the country, the continent, and the globe. With outcomes research models we developed tools that are useful to examine any new medical therapy. Through global experience we gained an appreciation of how different cultures can influence clinical outcomes differently, within their particular physical surroundings and practices, even when they use the same high-tech drugs and devices.

When Suzanne and I returned from India, we did an informal poll of two dozen prominent academic cardiologists as well as an equal number of nurses and technicians in our medical center. We asked them the same question, stressing that they should take the question seriously and give us a serious answer. The question was: If you went back to the year 1 on the Christian calendar, to a community of Christians who not only believed in Jesus but who physically lived with him, and you did balloon dilatations of their coronary blockages, would you get the same results as we do in the 1990s?

Seventeen of 24 cardiologists and all 24 nurses and technicians responded, "No, they would do better." If nothing else, that poll highlighted beliefs about faith that are held in the academic community in healthcare.

Another important "thread" during this same period involved Suzi completing her master's degree as she became a nurse practitioner. In that process she encountered and trained in some alternative practices such as Reiki and touch therapy. Over the course of her training we had some defining experiences with very sick patients. This was an experiential turning point that further promoted our interest in posing clinical research questions. The first time you see a nontraditional practitioner take away chest pain or put a patient in agony to rest or interrupt a heart attack without adding another drug or device at the bedside, you say, "Nice coincidence." The second time you see it you say, "This is interesting." By the third time you say, "We need to study this."

Two additional threads fell into place just around that time. The first question we had about studying things was "How do you study it?" If we examined a spiritual phenomenon, a relaxation technique, or a prayer environment, for instance, by sticking a patient with a needle to draw blood every hour to measure catecholamine levels, we would likely change the atmosphere just by virtue of how we performed the study. The Lotus Sutra, which is very dear to us, is like a 3000-year-old version of the Heisenberg Uncertainty Principle. It says that you have to be aware of the tools you use to study a phenomenon, lest you alter the phenomenon with the tools you use.

About 15 years ago I started an electronics laboratory in Washington, DC, focusing on physiologic monitoring in patients with active coronary disease. I moved the lab to Duke in 1989, which was how Suzi and I met: we worked together doing revascularization research for the Ischemia Monitoring Laboratory. Over the years we had been talking to electronics manufacturers about "seamless" noninvasive monitoring. The dilemma of what happens to patients with chest pain who call an ambulance, go to a community hospital, and are ultimately put in a helicopter and flown to Duke (where they go from the cath lab to the coronary care unit [CCU] to the ward) is that pieces of their record—like their electrocardiograms, their heart rhythms, and so on—become fragmented and frequently get lost along the way. For general clinical use, we had been after the industry to build a capability that would keep all these pieces together.

In the mid-1990s Marquette Electronics in Milwaukee, Wisconsin, supported our interest by creating such a "Unity" monitoring system for the MANTRA study patients. This technical capability allowed us to noninvasively and continuously look at heart rate, blood pressure, ischemia, and heart rate variability, which are physiologic reflections of autonomic nervous system tone and vascular tone. These data were all recorded digitally and sent to the core laboratory offsite, where they could be analyzed by someone who was blinded to both clinical details and patient treatment assignments. From a research point of view this gave us noninvasive, objective, blinded measurements with which to measure therapeutic effects. In fact, the whole front end of this monitoring system is identical to what CCU patients have on them anyway: press-on electrodes, blood pressure cuff, that sort of thing. So Marquette gave us a tool at a time we just happened to need it most.

We used this monitoring capability in the MANTRA pilot in a "stress test" paradigm. In a stress test, a patient is hooked up to the monitoring system, examined at rest, and then put on a treadmill that forces him or her to exercise—a predictable period of stress. Following this period of stress, the patient is monitored and examined while he or she recovers. This "rest-stress-recovery" model was the basis of the MANTRA pilot, except instead of being stable outpatients, the MANTRA patients were flat on their backs in a hospital CCU. The stress for these patients was not a treadmill, but an invasive heart catheterization and balloon angioplasty, after which they recovered in the CCU. With the Marquette Unity tool, we were able to seamlessly monitor these patients even though they moved from the CCU to the cath lab and back again.

The last thread that fell into place was the awareness of hospital administrators that integrative medical therapies might be good marketing and even cost-effective, because compared with new drugs and devices, noetic therapies are cheap. In the 1990s, cost-effectiveness was an inescapable currency. Fortunately, beyond this administrative perspective, our medical center chancellor has a genuine interest and wants to see good research to create data sets in this area. A radiology group at Duke started working with imagery and tracked its cost effectiveness compared with giving patients valium and then having a nurse make sure the patient was breathing for the next 4 hours. They used imagery during invasive radiologic procedures to see whether it helped manage anxiety and pain. So that kind of awareness began to develop at Duke Medical Center as the MANTRA Study Project took form.

The Feasibility Study

When we conceived the feasibility pilot study about four years ago, it was *feasibility* with a capital F. There were many practical questions, such as whether patients would allow themselves to be enrolled into such a protocol or whether they would be too uncomfortable to be touched or to relax. Another question was whether the Duke and VA staff would think it was outrageous and ridiculous or whether they would be willing to allow a study of these therapies to happen. As it turned out, the Duke mind-body community is both fascinating and deep. There are many thinking people spread across many disciplines who are not only open to these kinds of thoughts but also practice or develop some of these thoughts. The staff enthusiasm for this project has been overwhelming.

Another feasibility question concerned whether we could demonstrate a therapeutic benefit in this population, and if there was a difference, was it substantial enough for us to design a definitive trial to prove it? Finally, the feasibility of the monitoring system—would it work, would it give us the endpoints we needed for the study—was an unknown when we first designed the pilot.

So as all this came together, the final version of the feasibility pilot protocol centered around the rest-stress-recovery paradigm but in a relatively acute patient population who came in with either unstable angina or acute heart attacks. "Stress" in this setting is a pretty predictable "snowball." When people are physiologically uncomfortable—they feel chest pain, can't get their breath, or break out in a cold sweat—and they are told in an ambulance or an emergency department that they are having a heart attack, emotional and spiritual issues around their own mortality and death are superimposed on the physical misery. From a mechanistic point of view you can see how such an experience quickly amplifies all the wrong kinds of things. A stress reaction pours adrenaline into the body, which accelerates the heart rate, constricts blood vessels, and stimulates clotting. These are all wonderful if you have to run away from a gorilla, but they are all bad for you if you are having a heart attack. Then, to top it all off, we send a diligent young cardiology fellow in to tell you that we're going to stick a hole in your leg with a needle and run a plastic tube up into your heart, squirting dye and blowing up balloons in the coronary arteries, with procedural risks that could cause a stroke, kill you, or worsen your heart attack in our attempt to fix it. No matter how mellow or spiritually inclined the patient is, this is pretty tough turf for a human being.

In the midst of all this, our final feasibility issue was whether it was feasible for trained noetic practitioners to make contact with a patient for 30 minutes without disrupting the flow of care but with enough interaction to affect something physiologically and spiritually. Also, it was not clear whether different therapies might work with different patients—for example, touch therapy: would these patients want to be touched, or would they be too uncomfortable to be touched?

When we began this work, these were all unknowns. This is what the pilot study was all about. The pilot was not trying to prove anything definitively. It was meant to generate a preliminary data set and experience to determine whether, statistically and logistically, it would be feasible to do a definitive trial.

Suzanne and some of our steering committee members pulled together several baseline assessment instruments that we hoped would add some insight into who our patients were and how they responded. These were acquired in addition to collecting the descriptors that we routinely do in studies of patients with heart disease, such as age, gender, and smoking history. There were three instruments: the Koenig Spiritual Activity assessment, the Spielberger anxiety score, and a visual analog scale. Harold Koenig at Duke developed the spirituality survey. With remarkable simplicity, it characterizes three elements: the patient's involvement in community-based spiritual activities, the patient's personal daily prayer or meditative rituals, and the patient's sense of his or her own spirituality. The Spielberger instrument is widely known. The visual analog scale was developed for our pilot by Jon Seskevich and Jim Lane at Duke. It measures nine subjective self-assessments—happy, worried, fearful, satisfied, short of breath, and so on—before and after the noetic intervention, all before going to the cath lab.

So the routine was that a patient would appear and informed consent would be obtained. Then the patient was randomized to one of the five treatment arms. If he or she was randomized to touch, stress relaxation, or imagery, one of our volunteer noetic practitioners was called in. So three of five patients would have a trained person come to their bedside and do something with them, so they knew and the staff knew which therapy had been assigned. But for two of every five patients, the standard therapy and the prayer group assignments, no one would appear. They knew through the informed consent process that if no one appeared then that meant there was a 50-50 chance they were being prayed for in addition to whatever else their pastors, hospital chaplains, or families were doing.

As we use the term *noetic* in the MANTRA acronym, we refer to interventions that have physiologic or spiritual effects without using a drug, device, or surgical procedure. Within the pilot's prospective, randomized study design we did our best to stay away from "brand names" associated with any of these noetic methods—we didn't want to get caught up in the politics or become an advertisement for anybody's particular technique. Suzanne and Jon Seskevich created generic scripts for the imagery, touch, and stress relaxation techniques. They collected a fabulous group of 22 volunteers, all of whom had completed some type of noetic practitioner training. These folks were so motivated that they were willing, on a volunteer basis, to staff a call system 24 hours a day, 7 days a week for this study for a year.

Very aware of the prayer study reported by Randolph Byrd, we also included double-blinded, off-site, intercessory prayer as a fourth noetic arm. Unlike the Byrd study, however, we wanted to get past the perception of advocating any particular religion, so we created our "Mother Theresa Model." When we formulated our study, Mother Theresa was still alive, but was ill off and on. Our image of what happened every time the newspapers announced that she was ill was that millions of prayers of all shapes and sizes were said on her behalf. So for our pilot study we compiled a diverse group of prayer groups, including the Carmelite nuns in a monastery outside Baltimore; the Unity Church's prayer center in Missouri; the Abundant Life Christian Center, a fundamentalist group in North Carolina; a Baptist prayer group and a Moravian church group, both from North Carolina; two Buddhist monasteries, one in Nepal and a smaller one outside Paris, France; and the family who runs the Virtual Jerusalem Web site, who will take a prayer we type in, print it out on paper, and put it into the cracks in the Western Wall in the Jewish tradition. Every patient who was randomized to the prayer arm was prayed for by all these groups at the same time.

Examining the methodologies of how each of these groups pray, what images and words they use, who is involved in the praying, how often they pray, and what time it is on their end is really wonderful. In the spectrum of prayer models our groups include everything from the prayer warrior who literally slings prayers like arrows against evil on the face of the earth to the virtually transcendent type of prayer that is part of the imaging in the Buddhist tantras.

Our fifth arm was standard therapy. We instantly had to weather questions from our own staff, such as "Does the standard arm mean that if I routinely pray for my patient that I can't pray for them? What if I routinely touch my patient?" So we had to make it very clear that if a patient was assigned to standard care it did not imply that the staff should go in and be cold or mean to the patient.

But the patients receiving touch therapy were not also getting prayer. In fact, one of the shortcomings in the pilot was that we had no way to look at potential synergy between these therapies. That has been corrected in the more definitive phase-II study design.

The Intricacies of Prayer Research

There are lots of truly fascinating questions. For instance, if the patient presents at 10 o'clock and will be in the cath lab by 11 o'clock, and she randomizes to prayer but the prayer group doesn't actually assemble for Vespers until 5:00 PM, is that too late? Or is the intention enough? Or is time even linear with regard to prayer effects? Is there a dose response to prayer? Is it more effective to pray for 10 minutes than for 2 minutes? If 10 people pray, is that more powerful than 1 person praying? And how does prayer work on health matters, anyway?

All of these mechanistic questions are interesting but very difficult to answer with current knowledge. We have approached the efficacy of prayer from the perspective of clinical outcomes models, which are more phenomenological than mechanistic. Clinical outcomes research asks a question such as "If you systematically add prayers from all over the world to people undergoing angioplasty for heart attacks, is there a measurable incremental therapeutic benefit?" The clinical outcomes model then establishes the level of statistical certainty that the therapy, rather than chance, is causally related to the improved outcome. It begs the mechanism question.

Clinical outcomes is the hallmark of new therapies evaluation and data-driven medicine. It is what we do at Duke Clinical Research Institute. If we were a basic lab studying cell growth, we might concentrate more directly on questions of mechanism. But what we study is what we do at the bedside and how the patient does as a result of what we do.

Clinical bedside application is a key part of our whole project focus, right down to our acronym. The "tra" in MANTRA stands for "trainings." It was clear to us as we returned from India that if we had to have an embodied god or saint to make rounds to enhance healthcare, we would never be able to touch most American healthcare institutions. But if we could define some of the elements that constitute a true healing space through reproducible methods, methods in which practitioners could be systematically trained, we could train doctors in medical school or nurses in nursing school the same way we teach them to start intravenous lines or to take a blood pressure. What we are studying is not what a master or an avatar can do, but what an ordinary human being in healthcare, if well trained, can accomplish at the bedside.

Results

Our conclusion from the pilot data was that a study of these methods in these patients was feasible. Staff acceptance was overwhelmingly positive. Our scientific peers have been very interested in our study design and in the results. Our first submitted abstract of the data was accepted and presented to the scientific sessions of the American Heart Association, the largest cardiology meeting in the world. Of the 170 candidates who fit the protocol criteria of unstable angina or acute infarction who were heading for the cath lab, 150 (88%) enrolled in the study, so it was clear that patient acceptance was very high. Patients were equally randomized across five therapeutic "noetic" arms—including standard therapy, healing touch, stress relaxation, imagery, and off-site intercessory prayer. With all therapies, working with patients proved to be very well received.

One of the things we realized soonest was that we would never be in a position to address that question of whether prayer works or not. Duke is in the middle of the Bible Belt. Almost everybody is being prayed for all the time, and we are not aware of anyone who has designed a prayer-proof room for clinical studies. So the question "Does prayer work?" cannot be answered scientifically as we understand science. What we can ask is this: if, above and beyond what is routinely part of our healthcare environment, one systematically adds prayers from prayer groups all over the world, will there be an incremental, measurable benefit—yes or no? That is a question that we can study with a scientific investigation. And that is how we styled the pilot.

When all noetic therapies together were compared with the standard therapy group, there was around a 30% reduction consistently over every adverse outcome we measured. Although these changes are not statistically certain or "significant," they are very intriguing. The best results were from the prayer arm, in which adverse outcomes were reduced 50% to 100% relative to the standard therapy group. Again, definitive statistical proof was not the goal of the pilot, and these are not statistically definitive results. But if these changes are indeed the result of the noetic therapies, proving their validity can be done in a very feasible population size in a phase II study.

Analysis of these data with regard to our baseline assessment instrument descriptors was also very intriguing. Visual analog data, for instance, were analyzed with regard to the degree of change in the measured variable—that is, was there an increase, decrease, or no change in levels of hope, satisfaction, and so on before and after the noetic intervention? Interestingly, not only were there consistent and marked changes across the patients who were treated with bedside therapies, but there were equally large and positive changes in the patients treated with double-blinded off-site prayer.

Our results were interesting along these lines. Patients strongly rooted in a spiritual community did well, regardless of whether they were assigned standard or noetic therapies. Among patients who were not rooted in their communities, those receiving noetic interventions seemed to have better outcomes than did those receiving standard therapy. On the personal spiritual activity scale, patients who prayed on their own at least once a day or who felt strongly that their spirituality was important to their daily life seemed to do better when assigned a noetic intervention than did those assigned to standard therapy. So it seems noetic therapy is like "water in the desert" for patients who are alienated from their community and seems to connect to an "open channel" in patients whose personal spiritual activity is strong.

On the anxiety scale, people who are anxious relative to people who would characterize themselves on a questionnaire as not so anxious don't seem to have different clinical outcomes *per se*. Independently, then, the anxiety score does not seem to drive outcome. However, people on the high end of the anxiety scale who got noetic therapy seemed to do better than did high-anxiety folks who got standard therapy. Again, from this perspective the noetic therapies look like clinical "water in the desert."

We hope to expand on all of these data in the phase II study.

Phase II

In phase II we have designed a multicenter, multiregional trial. The power calculations from the pilot study data suggest that to have an 80% certainty of proving a real effect (i.e., an alpha of 0.05 and a beta of 0.8), a population of 700 patients would be required. In phase II we are asking two independent questions and looking at synergy, so we have a 1500-patient study planned. Patients will be randomized to double-blinded prayer or not, then subrandomized to a bedside, hands-on noetic therapy using a combination of music, imagery, and touch, or no such therapy. With this design we will also be able to examine whether the use of prayer and hands-on therapy have synergistic effects.

Because the best results in the pilot were from the prayer arm, we could have eliminated the bedside therapies and gone forward to study where the biggest effect appeared to be, but our own staff wouldn't let us. They wanted us to continue to study the bedside intervention. Because the bedside therapies were relatively equivalent, Suzi and Jon created a consensus methodology with the collaboration of the noetic practitioners from all of our phase II sites, which we call the "music-imagery-touch" or MIT intervention.

One thing we did not do in the pilot study but will do in the larger trial is ask the people in the double-blinded prayer setting to which group they believe they were assigned. We will use a predischarge question such as "Do you think you got assigned to prayer, yes or no?" I want to ask not only what they suspect but whether they think they really know. We are bouncing this around the steering committee right now.

How the Study Changed our Practice

It is very clear that by putting these data into the cardiology mainstream—even putting the examination of these questions into the mainstream—we are at some level acknowledging practices that are going on all around us all the time. We discovered during the pilot that many of our bedside nurses were touch practitioners or prayer warriors but never told anyone about what they were doing. Our work has allowed open discussion of things like prayer and relaxation and music, and just this dialogue has changed the quality of the healing space in our little cardiology corner. It has been like its own water in the desert phenomenon. It is not just Suzi or me who has changed but our whole environment through allowing what was already there to surface and blossom in the light of open, serious examination of safety and efficacy.

Working with our practitioners and this area in general, we have also been touched by another application of prayer or a meditative moment: the centering moment of the practitioner. Many practitioners, before they begin a healing session, say a prayer within themselves to clear their own hearts before approaching the patient. Unlike intercessory prayer, this centering prayer is more a prayer of supplication that may benefit the patient by making the healer more calm, more focused, more aware of the patient.

Some years ago we started using Thich Nhat Hanh's book *Peace Is Every Step* for our cath lab fellows in training. This book is about recognizing the noxious stimuli in the world, such as the alarm in the morning or a pile of dirty dishes in the sink, and training yourself to use them as stimuli to stop, consciously take one mindful breath in and out, and smile. And the smile is very important.

When a young physician first enters a cath lab, it is a terrifying experience. Suddenly you are responsible for this human being on the table who is surrounded by all kinds of gadgets and catheters and things that you have never touched before. Your heart thumps; you are dripping with sweat; and you lose your ability to think. We call the first weeks of cath lab training "plunging into the sea of adrenaline." It is a very profound experience. Just as the trainee begins to get a feel for the environment, a case comes along in which every time the fellow touches the catheter it goes in the wrong direction, and as she tries to compensate, the misdirection gets worse instead of better. When this happens, the world feels like it is spinning. That is a predictable reality for every trainee in the first weeks of cath lab training. If we can train our cardiology fellows at a time like this to take one conscious, mindful breath and smile—to recenter and clear their minds and hearts—it becomes a profound learning experience not only for their future as practitioners in cardiology but also in their lives as human beings. So we now keep a stock of these books in the office and distribute them as a routine part of our training.

On a very personal basis, I used to say a prayer every time we deflated an angioplasty balloon. Now we make it a point to say a prayer before we go into the cath lab—before we enter the patient's space.

There are many prayers, but there is one that came to us from Mother Theresa's healing village in Calcutta that we use most often. It goes:

Dear Lord and Great Healer,

I kneel before you since every great gift must come from you. I pray, give skill to my hands, clear vision to my mind, kindness and meekness to my heart. Give me singleness of purpose, strength to lift up a part of the burden of my suffering fellow men, and a true realization of the privilege that is mine. Take from my heart all guile and loathing, that with the simple faith of a child, I may find You.

Before MANTRA, on a good day we were probably good healthcare practitioners. On a bad, rushing day, when the grant had fallen through and kids were sick and everything was coming apart at the seams, we were probably not as good. If we were lucky, one of us was having a good day while the other was having a bad day, and maybe we could pull each other through. What MANTRA has done is help us think systematically about where these moments are as well as where the clear spaces are and how to create them in key moments. So I think the biggest change has been that now we don't just pray randomly, but we concentrate on taking the moment to say a prayer before every angioplasty, before entering the cath lab, before entering a patient's room. We see the whole process of clearing your heart before going to the bedside as important to learn as the mechanical techniques of the catheterization itself.

Why Prayer Works

I tend to conceive truth, meaning, growth, healing, and what I would characterize as the more divine elements of life as centered around the notion of harmony, balance, flow, and equilibrium. Using these types of terms, disease states can be seen as disequilibrium, whether of mind, body, spirit, or combinations of the three. What brings tears to your eyes, what lifts your spirits, what brings joy—these are basically the same process to me. They represent a reequilibration, a harmonization, a restoration of flow and balance. Some of the photos on my office wall are of patients whose mortal flesh has passed on. In several of them, even death presented itself as a release from a less harmonious existence to a higher one. In some ways this simple vision lends a certain clarity to the direction of this work, to the defining of a healing space as one which supports the transformation of suffering.

In Closing

One thing we haven't talked about that is a very real part of this is not the effectiveness of noetic therapies but their safety. We feel it is important to respect the fact that any one of these noetic strategies may potentially cause harm in the wrong population at the wrong time, even prayer. For instance, in a patient having a heart attack who is on the edge of shock, tightly constricted blood vessels is a key component to maintaining blood pressure. If you relax those blood vessels suddenly or too much, the patient will die. So relaxation may actually have some potential to exacerbate disequilibrium.

Intuitively, enthusiasts often assume that there are no toxic side effects with healing prayer or assume that if we mix Catholic prayer with Buddhist prayer with Jewish prayer they don't counteract each other or cause some kind of spiritual toxic inflammatory reaction. Similarly, with imagery and relaxation techniques it is generally assumed among enthusiasts that these therapies all build equilibrium and contribute to healing. In fact, this is a very bold assumption. Few things in medicine that are effective are completely free of risk or side effects. For our phase II study, we will form—as we would with any serious investigation of a new therapeutic agent—an independent group called a *data safety monitoring board*. The role of this board is to confidentially peek at the data along the way and to make sure, for ethical reasons, that no one is being obviously harmed by participating in the study.

This can occur from either of two settings. If the theoretically therapeutic treatment is actually harmful, the data safety monitoring board will be in a position to detect this early. At the other extreme, if the therapy is far more effective than anticipated, it may be unethical to withhold it through the end of the study. Again, the data safety monitoring board is positioned to detect such a difference early through a process that preserves and actually enhances the integrity of the study along the way. It is a way of questioning what's going on, a patient advocacy kind of questioning that does not expose the data prematurely.

We think our strongest sense of where human perception can discern real truth comes not from the conviction of seeing and knowing that something is true but from questioning—from being able to ask the most challenging questions of our most precious observations. One characteristic of truth is that it is not obscured but is clarified when questioned. Questioning whether prayer works, questioning whether prayer can be dangerous under certain circumstances, questioning the safety and efficacy of noetic therapies, questioning our bias and intuition in these areas—these are the most definitive ways to make sure that what we come to believe and practice bears some relationship to the truth.

CHAPTER 27

KENNY AUSUBEL

Ecological Medicine

Kenny Ausubel, an award-winning journalist, filmmaker, and environmental entrepreneur, is founder and president of Bioneers, an organization that "unites nature, culture, and spirit in service of the restoration of Earth and our relationship to the web of life." Ausubel also founded the nonprofit Collective Heritage Institute and cofounded Seeds of Change, a biodiversity organic seed company.

Ausubel is the author of three books: *Seeds of Change: The Living Treasure; The BIONEERS: Visionary Solutions for Restoring the Earth,* a book profiling the Bioneers culture; and *When Healing Becomes a Crime: The Amazing Story of the Hoxsey Cancer Clinics and the Return of Alternative Therapies.* His feature nonfiction film, *Hoxsey: How Healing Becomes a Crime,* was chosen for the Best Censored Stories award in 1990.

I met Kenny Ausubel when, in 2002, we began a collaboration with the Bioneers to produce our seventh annual Alternative Therapies Symposium—Medicine and the Planet: The Coming Age of Ecological Medicine—which was held in March, 2003, in Seattle, Washington. This interview took place at Ausubel's home in the mountains outside of Santa Fe, New Mexico, in June of 2002.

When I was about 19, I experienced some fairly serious health problems that were not able to be addressed by allopathic doctors. As a consequence, I fell through the rabbit hole into the world of alternative medicine, not because of any philosophical inclination, but out of desperation. I realized I had to get out of New York City and landed on a small farm in northern New Mexico where I began to learn about alternative therapies, nutrition, and growing organic food.

In the midst of my own drama, I got a very chilling phone call one night from my mom, who told me that my father had cancer. Six months later, he was dead at the age of 55. It was a very traumatic experience for me. Then, 2 weeks later, I got a newsletter in the mail claiming cures for terminal cancer patients using a metabolic and nutritional regimen. Like most people at that time, I believed what the doctors told me—that cancer was largely incurable and the only effective methods were surgery, radiation, and chemotherapy. But with my father freshly buried, I decided if there were anything to the alternative claims at all, I needed to know about them.

So I embarked on a journey of discovery. I was also a working journalist, and in the course of this process, I came across the story of the Hoxsey cancer treatment. In its time, from the 1920s through the 1950s, the main Hoxsey Cancer Clinic in Dallas was the largest private cancer center in the world, and it had gained tremendous support. The treatment primarily employed herbs, which today are all well documented as strong anticancer plants. But during Harry Hoxsey's era, the medical establishment vilified and suppressed the treatment, along with many other "unorthodox" approaches. I realized that, like everything else, medicine is political and, to some degree, a fashion victim embedded in the temper of the times. The real story of the Hoxsey treatment was that it had been politically railroaded instead of medically tested. In fact, a 2001 federal report found "noteworthy cases of survival" using the Hoxsey treatment among terminal cancer patients and says that it merits further investigation. The Hoxsey treatment is certainly not a panacea, magic bullet, or cure-all, nor was it ever claimed to be. But clearly, it is a valuable therapy that many people have benefited from.

I made a feature documentary film about the story, which was released in 1987 and played on national TV and in movie theaters. It also had a special showing for members of Congress just at the moment when these kinds of policies were poised to change.

Seeds of Change

Because Hoxsey is an herbal treatment, part of the research involved botanical medicine. Through the research, I met Christopher Bird, author of *The Secret Life of Plants*. Several months later he called me at my home in Santa Fe, and he asked if I would make a film about a very unusual garden on an Indian pueblo north of Santa Fe.

As you drive up the Rio Grande Valley, the pueblos, which are mainly set on the Rio, have a long tradition of agriculture. It is really a culture of farming, where food and farming the land are the center of the celebration of human culture. San Juan Pueblo had hired Gabriel Howearth to create the garden. Gabriel had been all over Mexico and Latin America learning about indigenous agriculture, and as people began to trust him, they shared with him what for them was the most precious of gifts—the gift of seeds. Native peoples often believe that through the seeds speak the voices of the ancestors. In turn, we become the ancestors for the generations to come in this sacred transmission. Consequently, Gabriel had amassed an extraordinary seed collection of rare traditional and heirloom varieties, mostly foods and herbs, which he then stuck in the ground at San Juan Pueblo.

I had been a gardener and farmer for a few years, but this was my introduction to biodiversity in the garden. I had never seen anything like it. It was the first time I'd seen quinoa and amaranth, the sacred grains of the Incas and Aztecs, along with entire societies of tomatoes—every shape, size, and color imaginable. The scents were intoxicating, the tastes astounding. It was nothing like the dead produce you find at most grocery stores.

In any case, I then learned that all these seeds were under threat because of patents in the seed industry and that most of the seed companies were now being acquired by the chemical and pharmaceutical companies that also produce the pesticides and synthetic fertilizers. It was ironic to me because these were the same drug companies that had opposed the Hoxsey remedy.

The experience was a wake-up call for me about the danger to the agricultural biodiversity of the planet. I came to understand that biodiversity is the very fabric of life from which life is made. It's the reservoir of all the adaptations that life has made over 4 billion years, and when there is a crisis or a challenge you go to that reservoir because it is the source of resilience for evolution itself. Yet here it was under escalating threat. We're in the midst of the Earth's sixth great spasm of extinctions, but the first bearing the fingerprint of the human hand. The Earth will regenerate, but it takes 10 million years to reach the kind of level we have now—not a human time frame.

Gabriel approached me a couple of years after I had finished the movie and asked if I would help him raise money to start a health center and an organic farming project. As an independent filmmaker, you're not independent at all; you're totally dependent on funding, so I had become a fundraiser by necessity. As I talked with him, the thing that struck me was that the important aspect of the work was the preservation of these seeds. We ended up putting our heads together and starting a company called Seeds of Change, whose strategy was to start a market partnership with backyard gardeners, who prize and cherish diversity.

Gardeners are always leaning over the fence and saying to their neighbors, "What's that you've got there? Could I trade you some of this?" We thought it might be a valuable strategy to help actually bring diversity back into the food system and, in turn, preserve these varieties in a very practical way.

Seeds of Change continues today. I left in 1994, shortly before the company's acquisition by M & M Mars.

The Bioneers

During this period, I'd become concerned about environmental issues and started making a focused effort to find out what other solutions might be out there. Clearly, Hoxsey represented part of a solution toward treating cancer. Saving seeds seemed part of a solution to restoring biodiversity. I figured there must be other solutions out there and other people doing interesting things. Sure enough, one by one by one, I began to meet some extraordinary people.

The common thread was that they had peered deep into the heart of ecological systems to understand how nature does it, to learn what nature's operating instructions are, and to glean from that how we can live better in this world. One of the most striking people I met, who remains an elder in the Bioneers movement, was a fellow named John Todd.

John is a limnologist, a pond man. He lives on Cape Cod and founded the New Alchemy Institute, which did a lot with solar energy in the late 1960s and with food production and fish farming in large, solar greenhouses. John was disturbed because Cape Cod is basically a sand spit—anything that goes into the land there goes right into the water table and comes right back to us. He was witnessing the deaths of a number of his friends at very young ages, 30 to 40 years old, and recognized that these deaths were probably tied to environmental contamination and pollution. So he started to look at how we could remedy that and what that would take.

He looked at natural ecosystems, particularly what's called the pond-marsh-meadow ecology, to understand how nature purifies water. He then designed solar greenhouses and mimicked these ecologies within these structures. He would run dirty water, usually sewage water, through a whole sequence of translucent tubes and tanks holding microbes and plants and animals, like snails and fish. Sure enough, when the water came out the other end, it was virtually pure enough to drink.

He found out how to do this through an inadvertent discovery. He had encountered a tremendous problem with the tanks for his fish farming. The tanks would collect poop and eventually suffocate the fish. One night before going home, he mindlessly took a piece of Styrofoam from one of his planters, punched a hole in it, stuck some watercress in it, and tossed this little raft into the fish tank. When he came back after the weekend, the water was clear. This revelation led him on his journey to create "living machines" because he discovered that in nature there is no waste.

This waste that we call poop is nutrients out of place. Everything in nature is somebody's lunch or source of energy. Waste equals food. This principle became John's guiding light. Similarly, biodiversity is a fundamental principle in the natural world as the source of resilience.

John Todd sees his work as farming because when you create greenhouses to treat toxic waste water, you can also grow things. For instance, you can produce cut flowers as a business. Not something people would eat, but certainly something ornamental. You can take what was previously viewed as a cost and turn it into a benefit and a revenue stream. The economics are one of abundance.

I fell upon more and more folks creating innovative approaches founded in basic principles of biology. One afternoon I was with a friend of mine, who is an investor and philanthropist, raving about all these amazing projects and how no one knew anything about them and how the people involved didn't even know each other. My friend said, "Why don't you have a conference?"

I said, "That's an interesting idea."

And he said, "I'll fund it."

So that's the genesis. In 1990, about a year after Gabriel and I started Seeds of Change, I began the Bioneers.

The idea behind the Bioneers was to look into the heart of nature and to understand what nature's solutions are and how we can learn from that to live more lightly on the planet.

The work of the Bioneers that we highlight has always been highly practical. While philosophy and vision are interesting and compelling, at the end of the day, we are interested in what we can actually do. We knew in 1990 that the natural world was already well on its way toward an environmental crisis, and certainly things have only intensified since then. The real issue for me was that I don't want to sit around being depressed—I would like to know what we can do to make progressive change and improve the state of the environment. What we did was bring together the visionaries who have both feet on the ground and who can put their ideas into practice and to look at models that can be replicated widely and spread around the world.

Our initial focus was on biodiversity and food and farming issues as well as bioremediation and natural treatment systems for decontaminating the environment. Since then it's expanded. These days the conference has more than 100 speakers who are involved in a diverse spectrum of projects uniting nature, culture, and spirit. You would weep over what ends up on the cutting room floor because we can't fit it in. The growth and expansion of this work is very inspiring.

Some of it is grass-roots activity, which is very important work, but some of it is starting to operate on a large scale today. One example is an architect and designer named William McDonough, who just wrote the book *Cradle to Cradle*.

Bill was contacted by an upholstery and furniture company in Switzerland that had massive problems with its production process. In Switzerland, of course, industrial-quality water is actually drinking quality. They have some of the most rigorous standards in the world, yet there were heavy metals and nasty chemicals and toxins coming out in the factory water. It was a real problem. After Bill designed the new system, the inspectors came back and thought that their measuring equipment was broken because the wastewater coming out of the plant was cleaner than the water going into it.

He is currently designing a $2 billion dollar facility for the Ford Motor Company at their Rouge River plant [in Michigan], which is where Henry Ford started the assembly line. Bill calls it a disassembly line. He will literally deconstruct the harm that has been done by these industrial processes and create a facility that produces more energy than it uses—purely renewable energy—and simplify the entire production process into a closed loop that will emit no poisons whatsoever. In fact, he aims to actually restore the vast wetlands ecosystem there over the next seven generations.

Green Technologies

Paul Hawken and Amory and Hunter Lovins, who wrote the book *Natural Capitalism*, have looked at a whole range of industrial applications of green technologies. Oftentimes, green technologies are rejected because capital costs are too expensive. But they found that green practice actually cuts costs in half, quadruples profits, and creates jobs. It's worth remembering that the industrial system at large is 94% waste. That represents a huge business opportunity.

A few years ago, Massachusetts created a Toxics Reduction Act, and 800 out of 1000 companies signed on for it. They found that it improved their production and cut their costs. Insurance analysts have said that climate change alone will bankrupt the economy by 2065. Not dealing with these issues is a sure route to bankruptcy and environmental destruction and all sorts of other painful experiences. In fact, going green in these very intelligent ways is good for the economy, creates jobs, and is helping to restore the planet.

I like to call these the *true* biotechnologies. When you look at what some people are doing in the name of biotechnology, it is more like biocide. Genetic engineering is a misnomer: it is genetic roulette. It is unpredictable, and it is the equivalent of splitting the atom on the molecular level, and we all know what harm nuclear technologies have wrought.

A good example of a true biotechnology is the work of Paul Stamets, a mycologist from Washington state. Paul is a brilliant fellow who has written several classic texts in this field. He is not only a mushroom collector but also a first-rate scientist.

The medicinal and nutritional properties of many of these fungi are well known already, particularly in Asia. There's a maitake fraction moving through the FDA now that has strong anticancer properties. The antiviral remedies from fungi that are going to come out in the [next few] years are also remarkable. But Paul is also an ecologist and spends a lot of time in the rainforest in the Pacific Northwest saving these species, cloning them in his laboratory, and keeping an extraordinary gene bank. He asked the question: if these fungi are medicines for people, then might they not also be medicines for the earth? What are they actually doing in the ecological balance?

Paul is now convinced that the mycelial mass that underlies most land masses in the world is a vast communications network. There's one mycelium that is as large as half the landmass of the state of Michigan.

Mycelium is all the little filamentary threads. What you see above the surface is the fruit of the mushroom. The actual roots and threads are a whole network that grows as much as an inch a day depending on what area it is in. Paul has made a strong case that it is actually the earth's original Internet. This is where the concept came from, this huge moving grid.

What he found, however, was that these fingialso have bioremediation properties. After a diesel fuel spill near his farm in Washington, the state set up a project to try to remediate it. They set it up as a competition, and five companies participated. Each one was given a large cell of contaminated soil to try to cleanse. Paul managed to get involved in this task, and he inoculated his cell with oyster mushroom spores. Well, everybody came back about a month later. The cells were covered with tarps, and one by one, they started removing the tarps. In all the other companies' cells, there was no visible change. The stench of hydrocarbons was overwhelming. But when they got to Paul's cell and ripped the tarp off, it was blanketed with oyster mushrooms, some of them 12 inches in diameter. When they tested the fungi and the soil, it was more than 99% remediated. There were virtually no hydrocarbon residues.

The message here is, again, waste equals food. These mushrooms treated these hydrocarbons as food. If we're lucky, mushrooms will turn out to be like people and they will like junk food, because there are plenty of hydrocarbons to go around.

Paul has gone even further and applied this theory to farmland where *E. coli* H:0157 is a tremendous problem. He's discovered a species of fungi that will actually defeat and then digest *E. coli*. The implications of this are gigantic.

When some of this work got out of the bag, Paul got a call from the Department of Defense. Forget Saddam Hussein—the United States government has the biggest stockpiles of chemical and biological weapons components in the world, and these are arguably some of the most deadly items around. What do you do? How do you get rid of it? This is a major problem.

Paul ended up sending the Department of Defense 28 samples of fungi to try in a blinded experiment, not telling them what these things were, and about 6 or 8 months later he received a very excited call back from the Pentagon. Two of the mushrooms worked. They actually were able to digest these heavy-duty poisons, no residue, no nothing. One of them did it in four months.

When you are looking at a planet that is so seriously contaminated, what are you going to do? Take the former Soviet Union, where there was a centralized authoritarian party, no checks and balances, no accountability, and often no documentation. They don't even know where they have dumped the stuff. Or Eastern Europe. They were having a party, unmitigated and unregulated pollution on a huge scale. Are you going to declare these places sacrifice zones for generations to come? The methods of cleanup for the Environmental Protection Agency's (EPA) Superfund sites are ineffective and wildly expensive. It's in the trillions of dollars to even approach remediating these sites. But using fungi is a highly practical strategy that could be decentralized. You don't need a high-tech engineer; you need a gardener.

Again, the importance here is to look beneath the surface at the guiding principles. The restoration of diversity is one of the keys not only to our survival but also to our prosperity in the future. Nature does not favor centralization or monocultures, yet this is exactly what we have designed. It's a giant bullseye for extinction. If we really understand the fact that waste equals food, there are no byproducts, only products. You look at every system through these kinds of lenses.

Kinship and the Principle of Interdependence

There are several other basic Bioneers principles. One is kinship. From the microbes to the mammals, we share far more in common at the molecular level than we have differences. It's about a half percent of DNA that separates the human being from the chimpanzee. We share about 30% of our DNA with fungi, much more than we do with plants. There is a literal kinship to all life. This is not a metaphor or an abstraction. The overriding message is interdependence, that life is connected and you cannot throw things away. As my grandmother used to say, it's all relatives.

Mycelial mats answer the ancient Zen question "Is there a sound when a tree falls in the forest and no one is there to hear it?" You can bet that the fungi are the first to hear it, and they send messages almost instantaneously through these mycelial networks: food! The idea of connectivity is really a guiding principle for how we need to live in this world.

Dr. Lynn Margulis, who developed the Gaia hypothesis with James Lovelock and who is probably the premier biologist in the world, came up with the endosymbiotic theory of evolution. She said that the bacteria originally were warring. They were cannibals trying to eat one another. When neither side could conquer the other, they decided to cooperate. That was when cellular evolution and multicellular organisms originated. It was out of rejecting cannibalism in favor of cooperation.

By the way, Dr. Margulis also says that bacteria rule. Bacteria are 80% of the biomass of the world. It is much more their world than ours. We're latecomers. We're the tiny new tip on a branch of the tree of life.

Similarly, she says that the predator that extinguishes its prey will also perish. The wolf puts the lightning in the step of the deer, and this is coevolution. It's not a dominator model. So what you find in nature—and nature is not all warm and fuzzy—is that while there's plenty of competition, the overriding principle is cooperation, or mutual aid in human cultural terms. It is an entirely different way of looking at life.

This is very different from Darwin's "survival of the fittest." The idea of Darwinism—survival of the fittest—has been greatly distorted. What Darwin actually said was survival of those most fit for their specific environment, not survival of the meanest or the strongest. That philosophy has led us to the abyss, and it doesn't work biologically or culturally. In fact, it was a deliberate distortion by the nineteenth-century robber barons to justify their brand of predatory monopoly capitalism.

But I think we are going to enter a new era of cooperation. It is clear that things like climate change cannot be solved unilaterally. It is going to take global cooperation. Ecology doesn't respect national borders; they are totally irrelevant to the issue.

I have an ecological fable. Overgrazing is a tremendous problem, and cows have become the poster child of environmental destruction, particularly here in the western United States. In New Mexico there have literally been bullets flying between environmentalists and ranchers. Dan Dagget stepped into the breach with a group of citizen diplomats and put the ranchers and the environmentalists in the same room and started to ask questions. They said, "Put your opinions aside for a bit, and let's talk about values. What do you care about?"

Well, it turned out that everybody cared about the land, including the ranchers. And, of course, if ranchers go bust, they are followed by condos and development, and nobody wanted that. People realized, "Okay, we all want the same thing." So Dan said, "Let's talk about management practices." Then they started to look at how they were managing the animals.

It turns out that the prairie ecology actually coevolved with large ungulates—hooved animals—and these animals are essential to the prairie ecosystem. Their hooves tear up the soil in such a way as to allow seeds to take hold, and the animals' poop fertilizes the land. There is a coevolution that's healthy and productive. The whole is greater than the sum of the parts, a standard that we find consistently as a measure of genuine synergy.

What the management issue turned out to be is called "move 'em and mob 'em." What you don't want is for the animals to be in one area for too long, and you don't want them there when the grass is too young, because if the grass gets eaten down to the stub, it never recovers and regenerates. By moving the animals about every 10 days and timing their presence in tune with the cycles of the plants, you cultivate a sound ecosystem.

The basic premise behind the system that the two groups developed was that ecology is not about things; it is about *relationships*. When you restore the relationships, you restore the ecological health.

This group took abandoned mining sites here in the Southwest—which look like the moon, a crust like talcum powder, not even dirt, much less soil—and they spread grass seed out on the land. Then they spread hay on it and then alfalfa on the higher parts of the slopes so that the animals had to traverse up and down the slopes in a zigzag pattern to eat. When you see the photographs 6 months later, there is grass that is chest high.

Other folks have tried throwing the grass seed out and mulching and watering it, but nothing ever grows. It was the animals that made it happen. But the real point of the story is that ecology is not about counting things so much as it is about mapping relationships. Ecology is really the superb art of relationships and understanding the interdependence and interplay among all the organisms.

Community is another keystone of biology. Like an orchestra, while the soloist may be especially important or striking, in the end, it's about the symphony.

Restoring our Environment

Michael Lerner (Commonweal) was among the first to recognize that environmental health is destined to become the central human rights issue of this new century, and that this issue has tremendous political traction if all the people working in the field of environment and health can come together. Michael works very closely with a lot of health-affected communities through the Commonweal Institute he founded. He has also been seminal in the group Health Care Without Harm, which is working to reduce and eliminate toxins from the medical waste stream, which ironically is one of the worst.

They have launched a global effort to get rid of mercury thermometers—a single one can kill a 20-acre lake—as well as dioxins. Medical incineration is the single greatest source of airborne dioxin, and of course IV bags contain dioxins that leach out, creating great harm, especially to infants, the elderly, and people with compromised immune systems. This kind of work has evolved now into a much broader ecological medicine movement keyed less to an individual's health than to understanding that personal health depends on healthy ecosystems. The practitioners' first commitment is to create ecological conditions conducive to life.

One of the beauties of biology is that its facts are also our metaphors. Perhaps the single most troubling human health indicator today is that mother's milk is arguably the single most toxic human food, so toxic that it could not be legally sold on store shelves in developed countries. The milk of human kindness is poisoned. What more do you need to know?

But restoration is not just about technological fixes. Bizarre as it may sound, for most of the environmental problems that we face today, we know what to do. We actually have the solutions, or certainly know what directions to head in. So why aren't they being implemented? What you find is that it is largely either political or economic roadblocks of one sort or another.

To restore the environment, we need to look not just at technological solutions but also at the social strategies that are going to achieve conditions whereby we can implement these solutions.

Let me give you an example. One of my very favorite people in the ecological medicine movement is Diane Wilson, who is a fourth-generation shrimper on the Texas Gulf Coast. The Texas Gulf Coast has one of the richest, most diverse ecosystems in the world. Diane was in her shrimp house one day sorting shrimp when another shrimper came in clutching the *Houston Chronicle*. The paper had an article saying that her little county—Calhoun County, population 15,000—was the most toxic county in the United States. It blew her mind.

Diane, who only had a high-school education, had five young children and was the head of the PTA. She knew she had to do something. She started holding meetings and talking to people and doing research. She found out that a company called Formosa Plastics was so bad and its ecological practices so egregious that it was kicked out of Taiwan. That was when it came to Texas, and Texas gave it $200 million to relocate. It had been convicted of various felonies and was notorious for kickbacks to the Oval Office, and on and on.

Almost single-handedly, Diane has gone up against Formosa for the past 15 years. She ultimately turned to direct action and held several hunger strikes. After she had gone through the whole process with the courts, and there was no question that the company was making an illegal discharge into Lavaca Bay, the issue went to the federal level with the EPA.

One day she decided to call the EPA and check on how the case was going. Well, the EPA official mistook Diane as the lawyer for Formosa Plastics—named Diana—and started saying, "Even if you're convicted, we're not obligated to take enforcement action." Diane couldn't believe her ears. She had done everything by the letter of the law, but the system was corrupt from top to bottom.

So Diane removed the engine from her shrimp boat and in the middle of a northern storm, got another shrimper to tow her out to the discharge. She planned to sink her boat on this illegal discharge as a permanent monument to the company's lies and chicanery. Somebody betrayed her, and she was busted by the Coast Guard, which charged her with terrorism on the high seas. But the Associated Press wire service was there, and 60 *Minutes* showed up, and all the other shrimpers—Vietnamese, Anglos, Hispanic, everybody—all these people who had never talked before—came out in a big armada to defend Diane.

What ultimately happened was that Formosa agreed to a zero emissions policy. Thirty days later, when DuPont and Alcoa heard that Diane was coming after them next, they, too, agreed. They have yet to fully implement it, but the irony here is that zero emissions technology has been used for years and years, particularly in the Middle East, because it also conserves water. It costs a little bit more in initial capital costs, but after that, it is cheaper and, of course, it eliminates environmental harm and all social costs of illness and pollution.

It is one thing to know about zero emissions and promote the technology, but how do you get the system to change? Sometimes it takes standing in your integrity in the way that Diane has done and being outrageous, as she puts it. She likes to quote Thoreau's remark on his deathbed that his only regret was that he had been too "well-behaved."

This is like the tobacco settlements. Years ago I suggested that, in effect, fast food represents manslaughter. I was delighted when some lawyers said they were going to sue some of the fast food companies on the principle that they are deliberately and knowingly causing damage to people's health with a product that is proven to be harmful.

Medicine gets very complicated because medicine itself is a highly toxic enterprise. One of the most disturbing aspects is pharmaceutical pollution. We all know about antibiotic resistance and the tremendous danger that this represents to medicine right now, but what people don't realize is that these antibiotics don't biodegrade. They go through your body into the land and particularly into the water. So we are breeding resistance everywhere, and in addition, pharmaceutical drugs also pass through your body and are turning up in the water supplies. We are getting subclinical doses on tap from a plethora of drugs. In effect, we are all becoming involuntary subjects in a mass medical experiment, and there's no control group.

It turns out that the industry has known about this for 10 years, but they haven't known what to do about it. For instance, researchers are finding intersex fish in the Great Lakes—fish that have both genders—most likely from the hormones in birth control pills and other kinds of estrogenic drugs. Of course, these fish will no longer be able to spawn, so it could lead to extinctions as well as other health effects. Researchers are also finding massive amounts of caffeine, antidepressants, and anticholesterol drugs in the water, not to mention Viagra.

Here's an interesting conundrum for medicine. Pharmaceutical drug prices are the biggest single driver of exploding healthcare costs. So whenever I hear about making prescription drugs cheaper, I have to question if that is really the ticket. They do have a place, but overuse and overmedication are being driven by a profit motive, not by real human need nor by a prudent approach. What are we going to do about the ecological harm that they are causing? Who is responsible, or more accurately, who is liable? This is a serious problem that medicine is going to have to confront.

Then there is nuclear medicine. Every day, we witness on TV the terrorists and dirty bombs, and where is the easiest place to get these nuclear materials? It's out of the hospitals. Not to mention the fact that they are indisposable—we have no way to get rid of the so-called waste. Do we really need this kind of medicine?

So from top to bottom, the greening of medicine has a very important agenda. The kind of work the Bioneers do is to help find the opportunities in these crises. For example, the Vienna Hospital Association contracts with a large network of organic farms around Vienna to supply organic food to hospital patients. When you have people in hospitals, supplying good nutrition should be near the top of the priority list. At the same time, you can clean up the environment. Munich now pays farmers to farm organically in the local watershed to avoid chemical poisoning of the water. This is ecological medicine. It's so huge in its implications that we are just beginning to crack it open. It's up to the power of the imagination from here on.

The impending context is that we are about to face the biggest public health crisis we've ever known. Infectious disease, already the world's top killer, is being dramatically increased by ecological disruption, from climate change to habitat destruction. Levels of toxicity are unparalleled, with all the consequences that brings. The great healthcare advances of the nineteenth century were principally public health measures such as cleaning up water supplies and diminishing overcrowding. Prevention is the key—creating the conditions for health and wholeness. We need to focus once again on creating the public health infrastructure and priorities, and making sure those get funded adequately. In many places in the world, those systems are functionally nonexistent, and in most places woefully inadequate.

Resources

My life has had so many left turns and unexpected developments that I never pretend to give anybody advice. But I think it's clear that there is no question that we are entering an ongoing environmental crisis—serial crises—and that all of us are going to be increasingly affected. The environment is going to move to the center of the stage and be the single most important issue in all of our lives.

It's going to take a tremendous amount of imagination and a great deal of passion and the involvement of millions and millions of people. The first step is just recognizing this reality and committing that you're going to do something. I also think it is important for people to follow their hearts. You are going to know what's right for you to do. You will know where you have particular skills or gifts or where you are moved by something. Oftentimes you get involved in a small way, but one thing leads to another, and who knows where you'll end up in that regard?

I would certainly recommend in practical terms that people look at the Bioneers web site. We have lots of resources and are very collaborative, so we work with many other groups that we respect and feel are effective. In the medical field, in particular, I'm sure people know about Healthcare Without Harm, Pesticide Action Network, and other such organizations. In fact, we're helping build a national network of people in this field, so if people want to get connected, these organizations are all on the web site.

One important point that is often ignored is that the worst toxic dumping takes place in low-income communities comprised of people of color. It's not happening in their backyard; it's in their front yard. I've been reading about the computers that are shipped to China for disassembling. The Chinese people are taking apart these supertoxic tubes. The water is completely polluted in all of these villages, and the people are having horrible sores on their bodies. They are dropping dead. So we've just exported the problem to other places. We haven't solved it at all; we've just sent it out of this country because companies couldn't get away with it here.

The other reality is climate change. Ninety-five percent of the population growth—another 3 billion people—is going to occur in less-developed countries where there is no public health infrastructure. What will happen? There are 25 million ecological refugees in the world today and in 10 years that could be 250 million refugees. What will the Mexican border look like? Is it going to be an armed camp? But you can't stop the diseases from migrating. Two billion people in the world, a third of the world's population, live on a dollar or two a day, literally. This is just not viable.

We are never going to solve environmental problems without also solving social justice problems. People need to realize that when we say it is all connected, it means there is no escape. The wealth gap is perhaps greater than it's been since the time of the pharaohs. But it's in nobody's interest to have that kind of a disparity and to have that many people living in squalid conditions. The health implications alone should be enough to wake people up. That's another issue we deal with at Bioneers because the problem of the ecological health of the planet will never be solved without also solving social justice.

CHAPTER 28

MITCHELL GAYNOR, MD

The Capacity to Heal

Mitchell Gaynor, MD, the director of medical oncology at the Strang Cancer Prevention Center in New York, received his medical degree at the University of Texas—Southwestern Medical School in Dallas. He is currently an assistant clinical professor of medicine at the Cornell Medical Center in New York and the medical director at the Weill-Cornell Center for Integrative Medicine.

Dr. Gaynor writes and speaks on cancer treatment and prevention. A lifelong interest in religion and spirituality prompted his research of the healing effects of meditation and sound. He is the author of *Healing Essence: A Cancer Doctor's Practical Program for Hope and Recovery* and *The Healing Power of Sound*.

I interviewed Dr. Gaynor in the fall of 1997 at his offices at the Weill-Cornell Center for Integrative Medicine in New York City and had the pleasure to hear Dr. Gaynor demonstrate the sounds of his Tibetan bowls.

Healing Essence was created at the request of my patients and came out of my efforts to help them deal with their anguish and pain. For most of my life, I've been interested in meditation and the transforming effects of music and sound. I've studied many different philosophies and religions—from Sufism to Judaism to Buddhism—and I found a commonality in each different path. The commonality is that everything leads one toward a perspective of "essence." There are other words for it—"soul," "higher self," "inner being"—but it's the part in each of us we're here to discover.

Let me tell you a story. I work with singing bowls, which are similar to Tibetan bowls, and last week during a session, a patient asked me about silence. I said, "Let your mind become very silent." Then I took her through the guided imagery process. After the meditation she told me, "I kept hearing things. Even in the silence, there was still sound."

That's a very important observation. This patient was saying that she was having trouble creating silence. Silence is a capacity; it's like a cup or a container. Really, there's no such thing as "silence." Silence is simply the capacity to contain sound. And this is a great analogy for everything we do in life. No matter what adversity you're trying to overcome in life, one of the key things is that you will never overcome the adversity with force. The only way to overcome any adversity or negativity in your life is to turn it into a capacity. So if what you're dealing with in life is anger, you're never going to deal with it by trying not to be angry. The way to deal with it successfully is to turn the anger into a capacity for the infinite part of yourself, so the anger becomes the capacity for experiencing infinite forgiveness.

If you are dealing with sadness, you're not going to heal just by trying to be happy. You'll do it by turning the sadness into a capacity for experiencing infinite happiness and infinite joy.

Because of the Healing Essence program, every day of my life, several times a day, I see people transcending their problems and fears. I see them turning a fear into a capacity to experience faith and trust. It's a very beautiful transformation. So the key in life is not to see these things as fixed obstacles that you are trying to overcome but rather to turn them into a capacity for experiencing the infinite traits of your essence.

Early Influences

The death of my mother from cancer was one of the things that propelled me, but it wasn't the only thing. The qualities she manifested when she had the illness and was dealing with it did give me an understanding of what was possible for people. Looking at her courage and the love she had for her children gave me an idea of what the resilience of the human spirit can do.

But there was another influence. My father employed a Pueblo Indian by the name of Fernando Dominguez as a yard worker. It was from him that I first heard the word "essence." My father had told Dominguez to cut down a certain tree, but when Dominguez touched the tree, he realized it was still alive. Rather than cut it down, Dominguez nurtured it back to life. Then, at one point, Dominguez was placed in a mental institution against his will. He was one of the most spiritual people I had ever met, but for practicing his own customs and traditions he was thrown in a psychiatric hospital. My father arranged for Dominguez to be released and explained to the doctors that there was nothing wrong with him. But the whole situation made a lasting impression on me.

Dominguez was able to "introduce the sacred into the profane." We live so much of the time in competition with one another—countries against each other, religions against each other. It's easy to go into a monastery or up to a mountaintop or into a church, synagogue, or mosque and feel the sacredness of life. But it's very different—though critically important—to be able to feel that sacredness of your essence and that sacredness of life in the presence of the real world, in the presence of people who are dealing with cancer, in the presence of politics and wars. And that's the real goal in life.

The Healing Essence Program

Healing Essence is a book and a program about people taking charge of their own healing. Each of us has a natural life force, a natural energy inside us that we can tap; when we do this, we change our perspective. If you are afraid of losing your hair during chemotherapy, your perspective can shift. You can see that you are a lot more than just your body, that your beauty comes out through your heart. People need a much broader sense of who they are. The guided imagery technique I use is a seven-step process. These steps are simply ways of reaching your core, your essence, that part of you that can't feel afraid, sad, or hopeless.

In brief, here is the process:

Experience

Experience where in your body you feel the judgments you have about your illness. Feel their exact location, size, shape, color, and temperature. Visualize them as energy.

See

Visualize the light of your essence located above the top of your head. Visualize it as a white, comforting, luminous light that emanates from your essence or higher self.

Surrender

Surrender your judgments to the higher power of your essence by visualizing their energy being released upward into the light of your essence.

Empower

Empower and strengthen this healing by visualizing the white light of your essence flowing from above your head down to the area where you most experience negative judgment.

Nurture

Nurture the idea of a life free from negative judgments. Visualize these judgments as clouds and imagine them dispersed by the white light of your essence, leaving a clear, bright blue sky.

Create

Create a space for your higher power to continue to guide you by visualizing a channel through which the light of your essence can continue to flow in and the negativity you are working with can flow out.

Embody

Embody and externalize this healing by visualizing the light of your essence flowing into each cell of your body.

The Strang Cancer Center

At Strang, we believe that illness is a manifestation of many things. For the most part, Western medicine has just looked at the illness. In other words, if you're dealing with a tumor, Western medicine has looked solely at the manifestation and said "you must cut the tumor out" or "you must radiate the tumor." It does not look at all the things that transpire behind the manifestation. We believe it's important to look at the manifestation, so we do bone-marrow transplants, chemotherapy, radiation, surgery—all the things that any academic medical center would do. But that's only a part of our program. We also try to identify the causes behind the manifestation and deal with as many of those causes as possible.

Now, what do I mean by "causes behind the manifestation"? For one thing, I'm talking about genetic factors. Certain people are at higher risk of cancer and other illness because of their genes. We look at nutritional factors—what a person's diet has been, what he's putting in his body that he shouldn't be putting in, and what his body needs that it's not getting. There is a tremendous amount of data about the nutritional factors involved. We have done work on cruciferous vegetables and have isolated a substance called *indol-3-carbinol,* which is the only substance ever identified that can shift the estrogen in a woman's body from the type that predisposes to breast cancer to the type that actually prevents breast cancer.

Indol-3-carbinol is found in broccoli, brussel sprouts, cauliflower, and cabbages. A study was published a couple of years ago about an area of China where people had a lot of esophageal cancer. The researchers found that people who drank at least 2 cups of green tea every day, which contains a lot of phenols and polyphenols, had about a 40% decreased incidence of esophageal cancer. Recent studies also show that people who eat garlic have lower incidence of stomach and colon cancers.

We have something called *phase II enzymes*. In every organ in our body, phase II en-zymes break down carcinogens that we ingest through eating and breathing. These phase II enzymes can be enhanced by a number of factors. There are substances in algae, grass juices, and antioxidants that can enhance them. For instance, a study came out showing that people who eat 10 or more servings of tomato-based products per week have a significantly lower incidence of prostate cancer. That's very likely because of the lycopenes that are in tomatoes.

But it isn't just diet. We also look at emotional factors. For example: What traumas have people been carrying around their whole life? In Chinese medicine, physicians look at the flow of qi, or life force. They believe that there are blocks in a body—whether it's from an injury, emotional trauma, whatever—that interrupt the flow of qi. To a degree, I believe that they are correct, that we do carry these negative emotions, these traumas that we've experienced, in our body. And while I don't think that it is the only factor that leads to illness, I think it's a contributing cause.

So we approach everything in an integrative manner, by looking at people's dreams, at their diet, and at what traumas they are carrying in their bodies and in their unconscious.

We look for certain recurrences in dreams. A very common dream with cancer patients involves being on a road or a freeway—there are always all these different roads—and trying to get back to where they were supposed to be going. That dream is about people wanting to find their center again, people wanting to find their core, their direction in life, because cancer is so disruptive. Dreams are a window to a person's essence and to the unconscious. It's important for people to find their way back to their essence and to look at what fears, traumas, resentment, and anger they have been holding onto so they can let go of them and look at life from a different perspective.

I was once treating a young woman for Hodgkin's disease. When she came in for her first cycle of chemotherapy, she told me that her greatest fear was that there wouldn't be any tomorrow. Then she did the Essence Guided Imagery program and started on the 28-day healing path. A month later she came in and said, "The most wonderful things have happened." Her perspective had changed, and she was living each day as if there were no such thing as tomorrow. So she was able to take her worst fear and transform it into her greatest comfort. She was able to transform her fear into a capacity and realize that the concept of tomorrow was just that—a concept. Having done that, she was able to live in the moment.

These are the types of transformations that people have. So many of my patients have told me that having cancer was the best thing that ever happened to them. You may find that difficult to believe, but when you hear their reasons for it, it is always that they learned how to look at life from the viewpoint of who they really are, and that nothing could get to them anymore. They were able to go through life with a totally different perspective.

Guided Imagery and Sound

Guided imagery and meditations with sound can change patients' perspectives by helping them view themselves as much greater than the people they thought they were. Most of us think we're in these bodies and that there's this huge world around us with all these forces that are totally beyond our control. We think things happen to us because of bad luck, bad fate, or bad karma, and we see ourselves as limited and victimized. If that's your perspective, you'll create that in your life. What the imagery techniques and sound meditations do is help you go deep inside, where you literally can begin to experience yourself as your essence—as being vast rather than limited—and begin to experience infinite qualities such as love and peace and joy.

I start all of the guided imagery meditations by having people do deep breathing. As they breathe, they picture their in-breath as a waterfall flowing into a clear blue mountain lake located in the upper part of their abdomen or solar plexus.

Then I have them breathe in positive traits with the word "infinite" before. So I'll go through "infinite love," "infinite peace," "infinite harmony," "infinite wisdom," "infinite joy," "infinite healing." As they say these words, people begin to get a sense of the part of themselves that can experience these things, and their perspective of themselves broadens dramatically. When you look at your problems, fears, and doubts from the space and perspective of your essence with those infinite traits, they look totally different. It's not that you're trying to look at them differently—it's that you cannot help but look at them differently.

The Shadow Principle

Jung said that if you do not confront your shadow, it will come back to you in the form of your fate. That's a chilling commentary, but I think there's a great teaching in the statement. From the time you're a child, you begin forming your perspective. We all start out as children who consider themselves very vulnerable and weak. Many people have a lot of traumas during that time. For instance, I've seen people who were abused as children—physically, emotionally, sometimes sexually. I see people carry all this armor that they put around their heart to protect their vulnerability. That armor comes across as a shadow, in the sense that people want to believe that they're strong, but behind that wall of armor lies a very weak, vulnerable child. People may be very angry to protect themselves against trauma, and some people may even become quite selfless to protect the part of themselves that they see as guilty.

When people who have deep-seated feelings of worthlessness or powerlessness are able to let them go and understand how the feelings have been manifesting as armor—as a shield around their heart that never lets them experience love and vulnerability and peace—it can be very painful. But if you are carrying these types of things in your body, it's absolutely critical to confront them if healing is going to occur.

Most of us exist on a very superficial level. We deal with the conscious thoughts, with our work, with our families, with various other people. And most of us get along pretty well just dealing on the surface. But the problem is that there is a whole depth beneath the surface that most people live their entire lives unconscious of. It's the whole depth of your being, your innermost longings, your innermost dreams, your innermost truth about why you're here in this life. Most of us stay unconscious of all those things. They are there, but we are too busy living on the surface.

So what does this have to do with cancer? Many people live their lives stressed out, frustrated about their jobs, or unhappy with their relationships. Life is not fulfilling for them, but they are still dealing on that surface level. Then, boom, they get an illness such as cancer, and their perspective is completely shattered. Suddenly, all these unconscious things come up like a tidal wave. It usually manifests as a tidal wave of fear—fear of losing their hair, fear of dying, fear of who is going to take care of their families. All the surface stuff becomes totally unimportant. The person who was a very strong, successful businessman, the person who was the perfect mother or teacher—all these masks that people wear don't serve them when they are confronted with an adversity like cancer. So the key is not to let the unconscious surge of fear overwhelm you. And there is only one way to keep it from overwhelming you: you have to get to your essence.

Healing Process

When somebody comes to Strang, we first take a careful history. We do a physical exam, look at the pathology reports, and talk to the doctors who have been working with the patient. Then we talk to the patient about what we need to do medically—what the problems are, what the prognosis is—and we answer all those questions. Then we move into how the patient is feeling about the illness. We look at what traumas she's had in her life. What does this current illness remind her of? What's been going on for the last 5 years? Has she been through a divorce? Has she been through a job loss? Has she been dealing with a sick child?

The first time a patient's in with me, I identify his or her core fears and issues. Then I make recommendations. First I'll make my medical recommendations—whether it's for chemotherapy or radiation or bone marrow transplant. Then I'll make recommendations in terms of psychologists, acupuncturists, massage—that type of thing. Sometimes I'll recommend healers who work with cancer patients. Then we talk about diet. We have the Anne Fisher Nutrition Center at Strang, which is a nutritional oncology program. We do a lot of work analyzing a person's food records. As you can see, we approach our care from a multidisciplinary standpoint.

It usually takes me a minimum of $1\frac{1}{2}$ hours for new patients, sometimes 2 hours. Then I see them every time they come in for the chemotherapy or routine office visits. The nice thing about having an integrative program is that every time a patient comes in for medical reasons, we can deal with other issues. Also, I have support groups every other week in which I teach people meditation using sound, voice, and tone in conjunction with imagery.

I believe that all healing is fundamentally self-healing because the shift is happening within the person. The people I refer to are mostly psychiatric social workers, psychologists, and nurse practitioners who are doing things like therapeutic touch or healing imagery work. But I believe that people who are in the healing profession should look at themselves as healers. What that means is that there's a distinction between curing and healing. Curing is about solving a physical problem on a physical level, which is very important, but healing is about using whatever adversity you're trying to heal to learn the truth of who you are. It's transforming whatever the adversity is into a capacity to experience whatever it is you need to experience, which only your essence can provide you.

But it's a big mistake for people to give their power away. If they're working with a healer or a meditation teacher or a yoga instructor, it's a mistake for people to give that person the credit for what they're experiencing. That person is merely a facilitator. If you go on a trip and want to climb a mountain but you don't know the way, you get a guide to show you the best paths to take and the location of the pitfalls. But he can't climb the mountain for you. So it's important for people who are in healing professions to stay focused on the fact that they are just the guide, that the patient is the one who must make the journey. And it's very important to acknowledge people who have made that journey, because they are the ones who did it.

Let me tell you a story. I once took care of a young man who had a relapsed lymphoma and was admitted at New York Hospital for a bone marrow transplant. He was 29 at the time. When I first met him, I said, "What's the thing that's bothering you most now?"

He said, "I haven't slept a single night in 3 months."

His doctors had given him valium and sleeping pills, but nothing was working. So I said, "What do you think about before you try to fall asleep at night?"

He said, "I'm afraid I won't wake up."

Right then, I took him through one of the guided imagery techniques for releasing fear, and he fell asleep during the process. He was able to sleep through each night of the entire hospitalization. We all know how important sleep is for recovering from any illness, much less a bone marrow transplant, and he got through it. He was out of the hospital in less than 3 weeks' time, and now, 3 years later, he's still doing very well.

So it's not that these techniques were able to release him from all his fear. But by using the techniques, he was able to connect with a part of himself that could allow him not to be afraid—at first just for a few seconds, then for a few minutes, and so on.

Surrender

It's important that the concept of surrender be correctly understood. Surrender, to many people, means giving up or quitting. That's not what I'm talking about. I'm talking about the surrendering of judgments and doubts, about letting go of your judgments and doubts concerning what's happening to you or somebody you love and getting to a place where you can eventually let go of all suffering.

The only way you can let go of suffering is to let go of judgment. You see, all of us are going to have pain in our lives. We're all born with bodies. We're all born with minds. So all of us are going to have pain in life. It's an inherent aspect of the human condition. But that pain is very easily transcended, unlike suffering.

Suffering is when you look at an unwanted condition like an illness, divorce, or job loss, and you start asking, "Why is this happening to me?" So many people tell me, "Doctor, the whole world is in chaos."

I tell them, "Go out tonight and watch the sunset and wait for the stars to come out. And just listen. You'll see and hear that the world is not in chaos—nature and the world are in absolute perfect order. It's our minds that are in chaos. Our minds create the chaos through judgment and doubt." Once people are able to see that it's not the world that's chaotic—it's their thinking that's chaotic—then they have the power to transform their thinking. I find sound to be one of the most powerful ways of doing that.

The Tibetan Bowls

About 5 years ago, I took care of a Tibetan monk who introduced me to Tibetan bells and bowls. Tibetan bowls came from the Bon people of Tibet. They were very interested in sound. Most of the bowls are made of seven different metals, including silver, gold, tin, mercury, and lead. To make a sound, you can either strike the bowl or turn a stick around it. There's little written about the Tibetan bowls, but they are a very sacred part of Tibetan culture. When the Chinese invaded the country and started looting the monasteries, these bowls made their way to Europe and America. The bowls emit this beautiful sound with many overtones. So you'll hear a fundamental sound, then you'll hear the harmonics from all the different metals vibrating at different levels.

I'm not the only doctor involved with this. Jeffrey Thompson, MD, in California, has shown how the sounds from the singing bowls can induce relaxation responses; Mark Ryder, a PhD at Southern Methodist University, has worked with sounds and chants, showing how they can positively affect our immune system; and Con Potanin, MD, in Tennessee, has successfully used the singing bowls with patients who are dealing with heart disease.

I think using the bowls is a profound and rapid way of going very deep. I am fascinated by the fact that the overtones induce this profound relaxation response in people. A lot of the mantras that are used in yoga, for instance, can be done with your voice in resonance with the bowl, which can bring out overtones in your own voice. The Tuvan singers are the masters of overtones, or what is called "throat singing." Many Tibetan monks use overtones in their healing rituals and prayers. I have also studied with David Hykes, who is a master of what is known as the "harmonic chant."

I'm amazed that modern western medicine has neglected the breath so much. All of yoga is about the breath. And, really, voice is nothing more than audible breath. It's so important to be able to teach people how to use their voice—how to use their breath—for healing. If you look at the fundamental force in life, it's the breath. When I try to make people conscious of their breath, I try to make them conscious of the force of their breath. In other words, instead of being conscious of the air moving through your mouth and nostrils, be conscious of the force behind that. What's the force that is causing the air to move in and out of your lungs? Because that's life.

Health and the Environment

I believe our society is undergoing a major shift. When I say "our society," though, I'm talking about the world, not just western society. People around the world are beginning to recognize that the way we've been living has not served us or our planet.

I am very alarmed about the increasing incidence of certain cancers, for instance, and the fact that there are so many damaging things that we've done to our planet over the last 50 years—like the number of pesticides, polychlorinated biphenyls (PCBs), and other types of pollutants that we release into the environment. No wonder there's been an explosive rise in melanoma. A study in the *New England Journal of Medicine* exonerated dichlorodiphenyl-trichlorethan (DDT) and PCBs as potential agents in the etiology of breast cancer. But I think the study was flawed. In 1996, a different study in *Science* showed how you could look at an individual pesticide in a laboratory model and show some degree of estrogenicity, but when several different pesticides were combined, they acted synergistically, becoming far more estrogenic than if you totaled the estrogenicity of each one. But the *New England Journal* study didn't take that factor into account.

Also, PCB and DDT exposure *in utero* or in adolescence may affect developing breast tissue, resulting in cancer decades later. Blood tests would not help define this risk. The study did not look at blood levels of these toxins over the course of a woman's lifetime, nor did it measure tissue levels of these toxins.

There must be reasons that Japanese women have one seventh the incidence of breast cancer that American women do. There must be reasons that Asian men have one thirtieth the incidence of fatal prostate cancer compared with American men. It's really important to start looking at what we're doing to our planet in terms of global warming, the destruction of the rain forests, and the pollution of our rivers and streams—all of those things that have come about because of unconsciousness and lack of caring for other people. But people are waking up to that, and I think one of the reasons is that people are starting to look inward at who they really are and why they are here.

I think there are a number of factors contributing to the increase in cancer, many of which we probably still don't understand. Probably the most disturbing statistic about cancer is the rising incidence. Every day, I see younger and younger women coming in with breast cancer. Bailar and Gornik published a paper in the 1997 *New England Journal of Medicine* that demonstrated that mortality due to cancer in 1994 was 6% higher than the rate in 1970. The paper also revealed that cancer mortality increased by 15% to 20% between 1970 and 1994 in persons older than 55, with a recent decline in older men. I think it's absolutely key that we start looking at nutritional modalities for cancer prevention, that we give credence to the idea that we can't live our lives with a lot of negative emotions like stress and depression and pessimism and think that they are not going to affect our health. We must be proactive in demanding that our water, air, and food be clean.

Because of our integrated approach, because we are looking at the causes behind the manifestations, I believe that Strang is making truly revolutionary advances in understanding how cancer develops and how to deal with it once it's already developed, as well as the steps that people can take to prevent cancer in the first place.

We believe that every person interested in cancer prevention should eat eight servings of a variety of fruits, herbs, and vegetables daily. These should include cruciferous, yellow, and sea vegetables as well as soy, green tea, garlic, rosemary, and curcumin. I also believe that organic produce is best. We still do not know the long-term effects of pesticide exposure at times of organ development such as *in utero* or during adolescence.

However, I must emphasize that the benefits of eating nonorganic fruits and vegetables appear to far outweigh the risk of not getting these foods because you are worried about pesticides.

We have all been through challenges or problems that, at the time, have left us feeling that we would never experience happiness or peace again. Then, at some point, you realize that precisely because of the situation, you can experience a clarity and vision you have never known. It's my experience that this is true of all "adversity" in life.

CHAPTER 29

Alan Abromovitz, MD

Integrated Patient Care: One Physician's Story

Increasingly throughout the United States, physicians and other healthcare providers are using and integrating alternative, complementary, and cross-cultural medicine in their practices. One of the "pioneers" of the integrated practice is Alan Abromovitz, MD, who has been using alternative medicine to help patients at his medical practice in Phoenix for more than 30 years.

Abromovitz received his bachelor of science degree in zoology from the University of Arizona in Tucson; his medical degree from the University of Tennessee College of Medicine in Memphis; and his licentiate, bachelor's, and master's of acupuncture from the College of Chinese Acupuncture in Oxford, England. In addition to these disciplines, he has studied homeopathy, mind-body integration, folk medicine, parapsychology, biofeedback, chiropractic, and osteopathy. Dr. Abromovitz is currently a clinical assistant professor in the department of osteopathic manipulative medicine at Michigan State University College of Osteopathic Medicine and was a founding member of the Arizona board of Homeopathic Medical Examiners.

In the spring of 2000, I interviewed Dr. Abromovitz at his offices in Phoenix, Arizona.

The practice I have now primarily revolves around the treatment of chronic disorders and pain. I see people with cancer, migraines, injuries, and trauma, or people who have had multiple surgeries and grown worse. Most of the time these patients are fairly desperate. Occasionally we get people who want to deal with their mental and emotional aspects, with their personal lives and their spiritual growth, but most of the practice is focused on people of all ages who are traumatized, hurt, or in pain. They are suffering; they are not sleeping; and they are taking a lot of drugs and medications.

Our job is to restore the system to balance, to reduce or to eliminate the need for drugs and to stimulate the body to heal itself.

The first thing I do is take an extensive history because in the traditional acupuncture system—the Five Element system—all physical illnesses are believed to be a manifestation of an imbalance of energy within the body, mind, or spirit, or somewhere in all three. The key, however, is to start taking care of people at a place they are willing to accept. If some patients think that pills or surgery are the only way, then it is important to let them know you understand and relate to where they are and to make them feel accepted.

Sometimes you talk about the things they've been through in childhood. You can tell from observing how they react and respond to questions whether they still carry the things that cause illness—resentment, jealousy, anger, fear, hurt—all these types of mental emotional blockages. The surface "personality" is the part that runs the show and makes decisions for most people. Most decisions don't come from a god-centered self. They come from the surface ego-personality identity, which is there to interface with the physical world. You have to relate to that part of them so they can begin to develop an understanding that you are here to help them and that you are not going to judge them as being good, bad, right, or wrong.

So the first thing is to establish the nature of the person's life experiences and the physical symptoms that accompany this. For many people it is something that happened 20, 30, 40 years ago—a triple rollover car accident, falling off of a horse, and so on. Chronic problems are multidimensional problems and, if they have been there for a long time, the body has adapted to the limitations and restrictions that are present and has consequently developed more problems. If you have pain in your foot and can't walk, you end up with hip and knee pain and then lower back and neck pain. So we have to find out where in the body the system is manifesting the disease, illness, or disorder. But we also find out how the person feels about the care he or she has had because if the patient has had poor care or the kind of care in which practitioners haven't taken an interest in that patient, then he or she loses faith. But you have to have faith. As long as you give it a little help, the body really does have the ability to heal itself virtually regardless of what is wrong with it. It is a miracle.

People react to the world in a defensive way because they see it as competitive. The truth is that nature is totally cooperative. Competitiveness creates separation; cooperation creates harmony. So the idea is to try to cooperate with people, relate to them where they are, and help them move along by expanding their awareness of the possible problems, as well as how their lifestyles, mental attitudes, and experiences are continuing to guide their decisions and choices. Then talk to them about the fact that there is a presence in all things, which we can call *energy* or *qi* or *God*. It is that part that we ultimately want to help the person connect with and touch because that is where all the wisdom, healing, and love emerge.

You generally don't begin with this because people are concerned with their pain and the fact that they can't sleep at night. But you can gradually introduce reading material, audio- and videotapes, and other things that will help them expand their awareness to realize that they are part of an unbelievable energy that manifests as physical things in the world. And this energy is directed by their own desire, their own imagination, and what they expect to happen. It ultimately comes down to their belief structure. The story I tell people is that if they believe the world is a scary place, they are going to react and respond to everything around them in a semiparanoid manner. They are going to be frightened and untrusting of the world, and the world is going to respond to them in that way. They are going to see the scariness that they feel inside reflected back in their lives.

If you can help people change their attitudes by changing their beliefs to that of the world as a friendly place, then suddenly their expression of friendliness draws out that same caring energy in the world. The world is the same, but their experience of it is totally different.

I start with most patients by talking about religious beliefs in the context of their upbringing. If you set up a mass of ideas and laws for people to follow, it makes them trust the system rather than themselves. That is the key: if you trust yourself and are able to listen to your own insight and your own inspiration and take action on it, then you are healthy. But if you believe that the things inside you are scary, wrong, nasty, awful, and horrible, then you are going to listen to other people, and clearly their decisions are not going to be as useful to you as your own insight and inspiration.

So if a patient believes in a negative, destructive god, then my big challenge is to get him or her to see that God is actually a loving, caring, forgiving, understanding, trustworthy energy. Usually most people have had at least one experience in their lives that has been supernormal or very unique, in which they felt a god presence inside of them.

My Own Story

Even as a 5-year-old, all I wanted was to help people. I went to medical school with the intention of learning as much as possible so I could be of as much service as possible. But at that time, medical school was a dehumanizing experience. There was little concern for the patient. The only concern was to battle the disease by knowing what tests to run, what drugs to give, and what surgery to do. It was appalling to me. When I finished my training at Jackson Memorial Hospital in Miami, Florida, I realized that even though I'd learned what science had to offer, my desire to help people had still not been addressed. It was frustrating to see 20 people an hour refill their blood pressure medicine and then go back into the same unhappy lives. The medicine helped them survive, but their quality of life was no better, and they continued to suffer even though they were living. I knew I had to find some other way.

One day while I was in the surgeon's lounge at the hospital, I picked up a medical journal. It contained a picture of a Chinese man with 200 needles in his face. The caption read something like: "In China this is what they use for pain. In America, we use aspirin with codeine." A light went on. I realized the Chinese had been treating the same kinds of problems we have today for thousands of years.

Then in 1972 my brother-in-law, Stanley Milstein, MD, who is an ear, nose, and throat surgeon, invited me to an acupuncture symposium in Phoenix, Arizona. At the meeting were four Chinese doctors—acupuncturists—most from a family tradition where the knowledge is passed down from generation to generation. The symposium was at the Association for Research and Enlightenment Clinic (founded by William McGarey, MD, and Gladys McGarey, MD), which is the medical research division of the Edgar Cayce Foundation. These doctors said that we were physical, mental, and spiritual beings. I listened as they talked about the need for connecting with your own spirit and soul. They talked about the inner relationship of mind, body, spirit, and nature, and the purposefulness of physical life. I became very excited, and 3 weeks later I was working there.

I began studying the Edgar Cayce readings. Cayce was a psychic who died in 1945. He gave about 15,000 readings, more than half on physical conditions. I found them interesting because we are used to dealing with things at the chemical, electronic, molecular level. We are also used to dealing with one organ system at a time. Cayce didn't do that. He had the ability to go into a deep state of hypnotic sleep in which, according to his description, his subconscious mind had the power to interpret information it acquired from the subconscious minds of other individuals. He was able to attune and then discuss what was wrong with the person, how it got to be that way, and what needed to be done to restore health. The most exciting thing about the readings, other than the vastness of the information, was that there was always a direct connection between a person's attitudes and feelings and his or her physical health.

Cayce also discussed how the body's various systems related with one another—how the mechanical, musculoskeletal, and nervous systems interacted; how the nervous system influenced the rest of the body's organs; and how the circulatory, respiratory, lymphatic, and elimination systems were dependent upon one another to function well. I got a sense of how it wasn't a single cell and not just chemistry, but it was 300 trillion cells in the body all organizing into a particular order and set of functioning systems and all dependent upon one another to be healthy and functioning.

So the physiology of these readings opened my eyes to the realization that you can't just treat a physical symptom, because that symptom is not the cause. The symptom is the result.

Probably 70% of the readings contained as a cause of the disease or disorder what Cayce called *blockages* or *subluxations*. Basically, they are restrictions in joint motion. When joints get restricted, especially the spinal joints, you lose some capacity for cleansing. Cleansing and nourishing of the 300 trillion cells comes by circulating and exchanging the fluids that surround these cells. But if the joint is restricted, muscle-pumping action is impaired, and the soft tissue area around that joint does not get cleansed, so you begin to build up toxins. When this motion loss happens in the thoracic cage structure, it affects the sympathetic and parasympathetic nervous systems' ability to communicate with the internal organs. What you find on physical examination is hard, tight, tense tissues—hypertonic muscle. The skin becomes dry and irritable or excessively moist in the area of semistasis. These are signs that there is congestion or stagnation present.

Over the past 30 years I have found that a good number of physical complaints—not the diseases we can identify but the more vague complaints such as headaches, digestive problems, breathing troubles, and heart problems—restore themselves once the autonomic areas that control those organs have been released; the mechanics have been restored; the muscles have been relaxed, stretched, and balanced; and the person begins a regular program of movement. The body then heals itself.

You can restore the balance and movement of fluids with very basic techniques. We use moist heat and massage. When the system is not able to cleanse itself well, we have to physically move the extracellular fluids, and stretch and relax the hypertonic muscles. There are many, many different kinds of techniques that can be used to mobilize joints and muscles. The end product, regardless of style or technique, is a full, pain-free range of motion in postural balance. We use a variety of manipulation techniques, from counterstrain to muscle energy and myofascial release. Then you get into the restoration of "joint play," the high-velocity thrust manipulations that chiropractors use commonly and osteopaths use as a last resort. Sometimes if the hinge is totally rusted you have to give it a little tap.

Lots of manipulation is done, but the problem is that the practitioners do not routinely examine their patients afterward. Physical examination by motion testing is important to determine which joints are restricted and which directions and movements are restricted. Once you have treated the restriction, you need to reexamine it to see whether motion has been restored.

In the mid-1970s, I went to a conference in Florida put on by what was, at that time, the North American Academy of Manipulative Medicine. This was an academy founded by, among others, Janet Travell, MD, who was President Kennedy and President Johnson's doctor and a world authority on musculoskeletal problems; John Mennell, MD, an English orthopedist; and Paul Kimberly, DO, head of the Department of Manual Medicine at Kirksville Osteopathic School. I had had a serious car accident in the middle of medical school and had been suffering with musculoskeletal pain problems. I had been to all of the physicians and specialists available to me with no real result. So at the meeting I listened.

When you hear a very accomplished person speak about his or her subject, it's like hearing Pavarotti or Streisand sing—you can sense if there is excellence. When I listened to these three people speak, I knew that what they were saying was true. So being 28 and bold, I went up to Dr. Kimberly and said, "I am really interested in what you are doing. Would you consider giving me a treatment?" He said, "Sure kid, come on over here." He had a table set up and before too long there were 50 people standing around watching him work.

I surrendered to the process. He worked on me for about 40 minutes. Afterward I was about 60% better. Knowing from my own experience that it worked, I asked Dr. Kimberly and Dr. Mennell individually to come to Arizona. They brought their materials and their skeletons and their slides. It was like having a one-man show. We saw one patient in the morning and one in the afternoon for weeks at a time. They were training me all the while. Once I gained some degree of knowledge and a bit of skill, I began to work with Dr. Mennell. By then he had retired from practice but was still teaching. He invited me to help train physicians and physical therapists in his style of manipulation. So I worked with Drs. Mennell, Kimberly, and Travell and with the North American Academy for 12 years. Shortly after that, Philip Greenman, DO, from the Michigan State University College of Osteopathic Medicine, invited me to come and teach at Michigan State. I have now been teaching with him for several years.

Five Element Acupuncture

My acupuncture training came first. One day in the early 1970s I was sitting in our office at the clinic and in pops this little Englishman. He was an acupuncturist, and his idea was to spread information about acupuncture to the Western world. Our clinic was the only one at the time that was doing acupuncture because we had learned from the Chinese in San Francisco.

We had been trained in symptomatic or formula treatment. For instance, if you have a certain type of migraine that happens at a certain time of day with nausea associated with it, it leads you in a certain direction with respect to particular acupuncture pathways. Professor J.R. Worsley had a college of acupuncture in England, and—as with Mennell, Kimberly, or Travell—he had a command and depth of the knowledge. But even more than that, he had an excellence and eloquence in his ability to convey information from a totally different culture. Again, I knew right away that here was a person from whom I wanted to learn.

He talked about the fact that there is an energy and that this energy materializes as the Five Elements, which then materialize as the acupuncture pathways, which are the framework or the blueprint upon which the energy of the body forms. He said that this energy must flow in harmony with nature—the cycles of nature, the times of day, the seasons of the year—because everything waxes and wanes. You breathe in; you breathe out. The tides come in; the tides go out. Everything is changing. It is always moving and cyclic. The idea is to be in balance and harmony with nature outside of you and with your nature inside of you. He spoke of the spirit of man and the way he conveyed it touched something inside me that goes beyond the defenses and the intellect. And once that little spark was opened I realized there was more understanding to gain.

So off I went to England in 1975 to study at the College of Traditional Chinese Acupuncture in Oxford. It was the most enlightening experience. I had learned information before, but this information had the body-mind-spirit underneath it. My previous learning in medical school had been physiological and mechanical, with no sense of concern for the patient. Here I was taught that you must relate and connect to patients, and that if you touch their spirit with your spirit, their mind with your mind, their body with your body, then the spirits can commune and healing can occur.

Most people have some kind of complaint, whether it is physical, mental, or emotional. In Five Element acupuncture, we are all a manifestation of nature. We are a part of nature and not separate from it. We are totally dependent upon nature, just like we are totally dependent upon one another, and the energy that is us and "all that is" materializes the physical world. In order to maintain a healthy balance of life force, the energy must be balanced. So the idea in Five Element acupuncture is to discover the imbalance.

First, we have qi energy, which is really the unorganized energy of spirit. When qi energy is acted upon by the guiding force in the universe, it separates into the opposing cooperative energies—the yin and the yang, the positive and the negative, the male and the female, and the manifestations of the Five Elements: Fire, Earth, Metal, Water, and Wood. The Five Elements contain the 10 organs and 2 functions, which are represented in the 12 meridian pathways of acupuncture.

In the Fire Element there are two organs (the heart and the small intestine) and two functions (the heart protector and triple-heater). When someone gets a serious emotional shock—such as when the fiancé says, "I don't want to marry you, and I am running off with someone else"—it is the heart protector that buffers, surrounds, and protects the heart. It is also called the pericardium, which is the name of the sac that covers the heart physically. The second function is called the triple-heater, which is the body's thermostat. There are three heaters or burners, three *jiao* as they are called (upper, middle, and lower, located on the anterior chest and abdomen) that determine the temperature in the different organs. If you are put into a room that is 40° F and are asked to do a series of tasks, you are not going to be as good at it as you would in a 74° F room. In other words, the temperature has to be right. Everything has to be right. When you bake a cake it has to be the right time, the right pan, the right heat. So the triple-heater is the organ that maintains the body's thermostatic control.

But if you performed surgery on a patient, you wouldn't physically find three heaters because they are energies. But you can feel them. Place your hand close to the skin in these three areas of the body, and you will feel the emanations of the energy and warmth that are emitted from the body. They are supposed to be equal. So the triple-heater can be physically examined, but it is not a physical organ. It is an energy that you can feel.

The organs have their own areas of responsibility. Of the 12, the heart is considered to be the king and rules over the other eleven. But each one has its own area of expertise. The small intestine, for example, controls the ability to separate pure from impure, whether physical or mental. So people who have disturbances in the small intestine's ability to separate may end up manifesting behaviors that are unclean or sexually improper behavior. Gallbladder energy makes decisions and judgments—so these people don't make good decisions because the energy that is formed there is not pure. The liver energy has the responsibility of future planning and vision. People will come in and say, "I can't see where to go; I don't know what to do. Everything looks hopeless, and I have no sense of direction." The planner is off.

People manifest physical disorders related to their mental and emotional disorders. In the Five Element system, the mental and emotional disorders are the keys to determining what we call the *causative factor*. So at one point in a person's life, something became imbalanced and he or she was not able to restore health with his or her own system. One of the 12 energies was damaged so much that it was not able to recover. From that point forward, everything else has to adapt to accommodate it. This imbalance leads to another imbalance, and it goes down the line until we end up with diseases and death.

The key to Five Element acupuncture is to find the causative factor—what happened to which element and what within this element was damaged—so that we can use the acupuncture points to treat the gate of hope when a person has lost all hope or the spirit gate if the person is not connected with herself. If you can stimulate the body's energy to heal and correct the causative factor, the original source of the imbalance, then the body-mind-spirit will heal itself.

Once you have chosen the points to use, the needles are going to do one of two things. They are either going to sedate the energy or revitalize it. If the person is running around doing crazy things, making awful decisions, throwing things, acting manic, and so on, that could be due to desperation of being weak or to a hyperactivity without any control. You would sedate this energy to make it peaceful or revitalize to allow it to come up to normal.

The needles revitalize and redirect the energies of that particular meridian pathway. Each point has a physical effect—put a needle here and a needle here, and the runny nose goes away. The points also have mental and emotional attributes as well. For instance, panic, fear, and anxiety are often allayed if you put the child to the mother's breast and she holds it. So if the problem is in that area, we may treat the anxiety with a point to connect the patient to this source of security and safety, to the mother energy. Each point also has a spiritual nature. Take point eight on the circulation-sex pathway called the Palace of Weariness. It is in the spiritual aspect that we come to the Palace of Weariness when the patient expresses rejection or sadness and is not getting enough joy. This point can be used to warm and enrich that patient.

So there are different levels of treatment depending on what the problem is. The acupuncture needles are used to reroute the energy, transfer it from one place to another, stimulate it, or sedate it or revitalize it. They allow the spirit within the practitioner to be conveyed to the spirit-mind-body of the patient. This allows the patient to harmonize with this healing energy and raise his or her vibrations to a point where he or she can then take over and move along in life.

What Heals

I have learned that it doesn't matter what you do. It doesn't matter what technique you use or what system you use. It doesn't matter if it is a pill or a surgery or whatever. You can convey the same energy using the needle or doing manipulation or taking out a person's appendix. You can influence and impact that same place depending on your intention, your connection, your centeredness, and your caring. You can give that same comfort and support with a pill too. So there is value in all giving, regardless of what you give. Some are much more expansive than others, but it turns out that it is the individual's ability to relate to and connect with and gain the trust of the patient so the patient accepts the fact that she is deserving and worthy. You can set up an environment that will help the patient receive the healing energy that is everywhere all the time—we deny ourselves because we don't think we're good enough to receive it.

To be honest, I think 50% of the world's chronic physical pain, illnesses, and complaints would disappear if the structural mechanics, biomechanics, nervous system limitations, and restrictions were eliminated. If everyone had regular exercise and stretching, regular breathing exercises, a good diet, massage therapy, and a proper evaluation for mechanical restrictions and would go on a program of restoring those, I believe that half of the illnesses on the earth would disappear. And the body's ability to resist and to heal itself for the remainder would be far better. So whether it is colitis or gallbladder disease or whatever, so much of the time the primary causes in the Cayce readings were structural restrictions and bad alignments irritating the nervous system. I don't think we can ignore this part of medicine anymore.

I once had a patient in her mid-50s who was referred to me by a neurologist. She was complaining of pain in her arm, an inability to move her fingers, and numbness and tingling, all of which were a result of a stroke she had had about 5 years before. Her pain was getting worse, and she was not able to control it with the drugs. The neurologist referred her to me to see whether acupuncture could offer anything. She was unable to use her left arm for anything functional, particularly because it had spasms and was painful to touch. I did my acupuncture examination and looked for the imbalances.

Under the belly button is an energetic pulsation that we conceive of as the ancestral energy, the energy that comes into you from your ancestors and makes you who and what you are. That energy has to be centered, meaning that when you examine it, when you press down on the belly button, the pulse should come and hit you right in the middle of your fingers. If it doesn't, if it is off to the side or somewhere else in your belly, then you have to physically move the pulse back to center. If that pulse is off center, the body's energies cannot be balanced. So in Five Element acupuncture, the first thing you do is center that energy.

The second thing you do is look for the imbalance of energy from left to right. You can test this with heat. You see how much warmth it takes before the person is consciously aware of it. It should be equal. This woman's lower extremity pathways were all balanced, but her upper extremities had an imbalance of the lung pathway. Her right side took six passes for her to feel the heat. The left side took 40 passes. And that is a great discrepancy. All of her other energies were balanced from left to right and seemed to be within one or two passes of one another.

In Five Element acupuncture, we are not treating the symptoms. We may add points to help influence symptoms or help the person be more comfortable, but we are not trying to get rid of the headache. We are trying to get rid of the energetic imbalance that manifests as a headache. So in the testing, I found out that this patient was greatly imbalanced on this one pathway. The treatment was to use the acupuncture point that connects the right side with the left side of the meridian, much like lifting a dam on the river to allow the water to equalize. In her situation I did a neutral treatment. I didn't stimulate or sedate it; I just connected it and let it be there for about 30 or 40 minutes. We didn't see anything happen during the treatment. She came back a week later and said that about 24 hours after the treatment, her symptoms began to disappear. The tingling went away; the pain went away; and she began to be able to open and close her hand.

In her case, the blockage was an imbalance from left to right. Once that was released, the energy flow restored itself. That was all she required, and I never did another treatment.

The other case is a little more complicated. A 37-year-old woman was referred to me from a psychologist. She had injured her knee a number of times over a 7-year period and had had 12 surgeries, beginning with her knee and then down in her calf, ankle, and even into her foot because of pain and inability to bear weight on her leg. Some of the surgeries had made her better for a short time, but she would always re-injure herself or some other pain problem would show up in her leg, requiring another surgery. By the time she got to me she was barely able to walk and was on 300 mg of narcotics a day. She was desperate and considering an amputation. I told her that I had no idea whether I could help her or not, but she and her husband were willing to listen and hear what I had to say.

First, I prescribed the use of castor oil packs on her leg twice a day for an hour, which she started at home. She and her husband weren't being very conscientious about their diet, because food was the only pleasure left, so we talked about the need for the body to cleanse itself. I put her on a predominantly vegetarian diet and started her with biomechanical treatment. Over time she had developed problems in her lower back, thoracic spine, chest wall, and neck and shoulders. We didn't touch her leg for 2 weeks. We simply began restoring the mechanics of the rest of the system.

After 2 weeks you could begin to touch her leg on the surface. The swelling had reduced a bit so I began doing gentle surface, lymphatic massage for the leg every day. I also used Five Element acupuncture during the whole process, even though I never put a needle in her leg until the end. Her main problem was severe pain in her knee, calf, ankle, and foot. Little by little, we were able to go deeper with the massage. However, they were reluctant to admit that anything was better. But one day I said, "Of course she is better; I can hold her leg now." And she admitted that there had been an improvement. That was a big step. Something had changed.

Little by little I got her to do stretching exercises, mostly for her neck and shoulders and back and hips. We kept up with the massage. The leg got softer, less sensitive, less painful, less hard. About 4 weeks into the treatment, she went to California to visit friends. When she came back she had reduced her drugs from 300 mg to 240 mg a day and had begun to sleep. You could see a spark coming on in her. During the fifth week of treatment I did manipulation and acupuncture. When I examined her knee joint, I saw that it was functionally healed. The pain had been eliminated from the knee and upper calf and was now localized in the lower leg, ankle, and foot.

There are 26 bones in the foot and more than 30 joints, but there are 3 specific ones at the ankle. These had a certain hardness rather than the soft resiliency we like to see when there is a problem. I manipulated her ankle and her pain immediately disappeared. She got off the table with no cane, stood on that leg, went up on her toes, back on her heels, and jumped up and down. She had a couple more little restrictions in her ankle that I manipulated, but she walked out of the office without a crutch. The effect lasted 1 hour.

Once that pain was gone for an hour, the gate of hope was opened. She knew it could be healed. I never had any attachment to the outcome because I simply did not know. I do the best I can and pray. I manipulated her ankle again, and the pain went away for 3 hours, and she went down to 80 mg. The last week she was here she was hiking in the mountains, her bowels had returned to normal, and she was sleeping through the night. She was on 30 mg of narcotics but could not get down any lower because she was having withdrawal symptoms from the drugs. I told her to go on liquid narcotics and have her doctor wean her down until she was off it completely. The last time we talked she was down to 15 mg. No one in her world could even believe she was the same person because she was a functional, vibrant person again. Now, 3 years later, she is not on any medication and is working, hiking, bicycling, dancing, and continuing to exercise and stretch as well as receive massage to the affected area. She is reexamined and receives maintenance treatment once every 6 months.

It is incredible that the body has the ability to heal itself regardless of what is wrong with it. I feel grateful that we were able to do it. It was a growth experience for all the staff at the office to observe this transformation over time.

It is a miracle just being here. It is a wonder to be able to help people. The knowledge available in the alternative medical field can transform health in this country and the world—if only the healthcare providers will open their minds and develop their skills.

Part Eight

Conversations About Medical Education

"If we consider our obligation to the health of people now and of future generations, we must be open to alternative, complementary, and integrative approaches simply because we don't know and will never know the scientific basis of everything."

—RALPH SYNDERMAN

CHAPTER 30

TRACY GAUDET, MD

Transforming Medical Education

A major component in healthcare is the education of the practitioners. In early 2000, the editors of *Alternative Therapies in Health and Medicine* wanted to highlight the changes that were beginning to take place in medical schools around the country. So in the spring of 2000, I traveled to Tucson, Arizona, to meet with Tracy Williams Gaudet, MD, who was, at the time, serving as Executive Director of the Program in Integrative Medicine at the University of Arizona Health Science Center, the first postgraduate program in the country to focus on integrative medicine.

One of the youngest female physicians to distinguish herself in academic circles, Dr. Gaudet is currently the Director of the Duke University Center for Integrative Medicine in Durham, North Carolina. Gaudet received her medical degree from Duke University School of Medicine in Durham, North Carolina, in 1991 and completed her residency at the University of Texas Health Sciences Center at San Antonio. She was the recipient of the Merck Manual Award for Outstanding Performance in Medical School in 1991.

My background is in psychology and sociology, and while I always planned on pursuing a health profession, I did not anticipate going through medical school. It seemed that medical education was a fairly unhealthy system, and it was perplexing how such a system could produce people who were supposed to facilitate healing in others. But ultimately, I realized that if I wanted to have an effect on the system, I needed to be a product of it to have credibility. So I began my medical training with some sense and intention of transforming physician education.

After graduating from Duke University, I did my residency in ob-gyn at the University of Texas, San Antonio. While there, I received a newsletter containing a notice about the concept for the Program in Integrative Medicine. It sounded great, and I thought I should check it out because it was consistent with my passions. Dr. Andy Weil's conference schedule was in the same newsletter, and it said he was giving a conference in Montana. So I took a week's vacation and went.

The attendees at the conference were mostly what I call "Andy fans." We introduced ourselves and explained why we were there. When it was my turn, I said, "First of all, I have to say that I don't own any of your books." There was this gasp like, "Who let her in the room?" Of course, Andy was totally fine with it. Then I told him that I had heard about the concept of his fellowship program and was interested in it.

My original intention was to do the fellowship program and return to Duke. But the program wasn't open to ob-gyns, so I contacted the University of Arizona Medical School and explained why I thought that restriction should change. Meanwhile, Andy encouraged me to keep in touch. Time went by, and then a very odd set of events happened.

I had joined the faculty at the University of Texas and wasn't looking for another job. But I knew the University of Arizona had initiated a search for the position of medical director. I poked around and got the sense that they really were looking for a full professor. Although I was in the academic mainstream, I was young so did not apply. The search committee went through a national search and narrowed the pool, but in the process they started to realize that if they took someone who had spent his or her entire career within the current system, then what would be produced would be very similar to what already existed. I was still in conversation with them at the time, so I sent my resume.

Then it became synchronistic. I had never been to Arizona before but already had a trip scheduled. So they said, "If you are out here anyway, we will talk to you." I have to give Joe Alpert, the head of the Department of Medicine at the University of Arizona, a lot of credit because when I met with him he said, "I have reviewed your CV, and you are great but I can't hire an ob-gyn within this department." They had a very traditional system, whereby the person at the top knows everything and disseminates the knowledge down the organization. His construct was that the clinic had to run the same way. I couldn't function in that capacity, both because I was young and because my training was as an ob-gyn. So, to make a long story short, I asked him how he envisioned running the clinic. We brainstormed about what it might be like to have a collaborative (rather than hierarchical) clinic situation and to learn from one another. At one point he said, "Let me get a pencil and write this down." So in the context of that conversation, he totally reframed what he was thinking. Most people couldn't do such a thing, and I give him a lot of credit for that.

Things happened quickly after that and they offered me a position. It was—and is—a great opportunity to turn my dream and passion into reality.

The Fellowship

The first fellowship started 9 months later in July of 1997. So everyone teased me about how I am an ob-gyn and that was a good gestational period.

We use the term *living laboratory* to describe the fellowship. It drives the Fellows nuts, but for me that is exactly what it is. It is the concept that within this laboratory, we can be partners with the Fellows and design something new. They have all been through conventional education, so we have the freedom to ask "If we were going to do this in a different way, what would it look like, and would that make a difference?"

When people come to the program they don't anticipate the personal transformation that is going to occur. That is the seed of what we are talking about. I use the analogy of medical education being a big, dysfunctional, abusive, alcoholic family system. If you look at the roles that people play within academia, the ruling by intimidation plays like the role of the abusive parent. You watch students come in fresh and new, and then their spirits get lost in the educational process. And the nurses typically play the enablers—they are the ones who make you feel better when you have been trashed in rounds, and so it propagates itself. Part of the structure is that, to the outside world, you pretend everything is fine.

This isn't healthy. Here is part of my dream: medical education should require a serious personal commitment to a person's own inner growth. It should be as important as learning organic chemistry. And the educational process should support that. If this were central, then so much of what isn't working in medicine today would just fall away. Even the closed-mindedness about other systems would fall away, because it is the educational process that makes you think you are supposed to have all the answers. That mindset is simply part of your training.

There is a joke that goes like this: A team is making postoperative rounds. The attending physician says to the chief resident, "What is the patient's postop hematocrit?" The chief doesn't know, so he asks the resident who doesn't know, who asks the intern who doesn't know, who asks the student. None of them know. So the student says to the intern, "I forgot to look." The intern says to the resident, "It is stable." The resident says to the chief resident, "It is mid-30s." And the chief resident says to the attending physician with full confidence, "It is 37."

Anybody who has been through medical education laughs at this joke because that is the process. You learn that it is your job to know everything, and if you don't know, you pretend. All of this sets up a dynamic with patients. You can't sit with a patient and not know. That is failure.

The other place where this manifests is around death and dying, because that is the ultimate failure. If you are supposed to know everything and your job is to cure disease, then death is a failure. So a typical response to a dying patient from a physician's perspective is that they "turf" them. Once they think they can't help them, patients get sent to hospice and the physicians remove themselves emotionally. I think so much of what is not working is because we have built these walls around the physicians who are on pedestals but who aren't in touch with their own suffering. How can they possibly be present for someone else? So a big emphasis for me is the personal commitment to one's own growth.

But how do you instill these concepts in a medical curriculum, and how do you do that in a way that is replicable? We are learning, of course, but we got lucky, as we have with many things in this program. Just at the time when we were asking, "How are we going to do this?" something drops from the sky.

One of the things that dropped from the sky was John Tarrant. John is a psychoanalyst and a Zen Roshi from Santa Rosa, California. I posed this question: How do you take physicians and get them comfortable with not knowing and sitting with suffering? John thought with us and consequently, he has been a part of the program from the beginning.

The first week the Fellows are here, we spend 3 days in retreat with John. Most people have never had the experience—at least in their professional world—of the process of doing personal work with a group of peers. We—Andy, the fellowship faculty, the Fellows and myself—go up on Mount Lemmon, outside of Tucson. We do meditation and personal sharing. Truly, for most people, this has never been a part of their professional lives. Rachel Remen, MD, talks about this. One of the exercises she has her physicians do is to think about the most painful experience they have had in their professional training and share that with another physician in the group. Rachel said that none of the physicians participating in the exercise had ever told their story to another professional. It is the culture of medicine to put up walls, and if you have a patient die, your success is judged by how quickly you move on to the next patient.

John also holds a 2-day retreat every month with the Fellows throughout the entire 2 years they are here. Within that context, many things start to shift. At the end of the first year, we asked, "What is working? What is not working?" The thing the Fellows were most surprised about was the degree to which this process affected who they were personally and how they lived their own lives. They also pointed to the process as a critical part of what changed the way in which they interfaced with patients. So it wasn't just the fact that they had new tools that was important—it was the way in which they interacted with patients.

We encourage them to journal as part of the process and to live in their own lives. One does not have to do it perfectly, because that gets back into the "I-am-always-supposed-to-be-right" syndrome, but one should be committed to the process—flaws and all. We also have yoga once a week and we often cook together. As much as possible, we try to embrace what we are speaking about. And that is unusual for physicians.

This is a huge shift from normal practice. One half-day every week—Wednesday afternoons—is blocked for "reflection." It is not always sitting around and meditating; sometimes we go for a hike. Basically, it is about invigorating and replenishing our own humanness. There is something about the system of medical education that knocks that out of people. So our quest is: How does one instill humanness again, and how does that change the way physicians practice medicine?

It is related to alternatives in the sense that once you get into that place, it is absurd to think that you wouldn't be inclusive of other approaches. I look at it as the roots from which everything else comes.

Changes

Here is a great illustration of how this program affects the Fellows. At the end of year 2, for research purposes, we asked each of the Fellows to select two cases they felt had results and provided an experience—whether they understood why or not—that would have not happened prior to their training here. The one that was most profound to me is the one Russ Greenfield talked about.

He selected a story about a woman who was dying. As I listened to him talk—and this was in a research meeting—it hit me that before this program, there was no way that any of us would have ever said, "One of my greatest success stories is about a patient who died." That, just in itself, made me say, "Wow, something is shifting here." He spoke about the whole distinction between curing disease and facilitating a patient's wholeness and healing, which can happen in death as well as life. That is what happened with this woman, and for him to be present with that—to be an active part of that—was profound.

There are many great stories, but that was really profound. The value system had shifted. What matters had shifted.

An Average Week

We call the first 2 months *orientation*. The Fellows are not in the clinic. The retreat takes place; they do a lot of guided imagery work; and there is much philosophical discussion and education.

Guided imagery is one of the things we have them learn up front in large part because it facilitates the personal process. It gives them a practical tool, if you will, that they can use to achieve results quickly. But another reason we put guided imagery up front is that it is a window into their own personal work. So they spend these 4 or 5 days together with the educators, doing imagery with each other under supervision, learning a lot about themselves and further developing the group process that we initiated in the retreat.

During the first 8 weeks, there is a whole design focused on getting the personal process started and turning paradigms upside down so that new order and new learning can happen. For instance, one of the courses they take is the philosophy of science. Basically, people leave the first lecture realizing that they don't really know what they thought they knew.

Once we are through this part, there is a predictable pattern to their schedule. Monday mornings they are in the clinic—usually with Andy—seeing new patients. Each patient is seen for about an hour, and they take a history that is whole-person in its orientation.

Monday afternoon there is a patient conference, which addresses the question "How do you teach people the process of integrating all these things?" Who is to say that you should make this recommendation over that one, and how do you begin to learn that skill? That involves not only Andy, myself, the Fellows, and the medical director but also a Chinese medicine practitioner, a mind-body person, an osteopath, a homeopath, a nutritionist, a pharmacist—and the list goes on. It is within this context that the Fellows discuss a patient.

When we started this process it was the first time that the homeopath had ever talked to the Chinese medicine practitioner, because their job isn't to integrate the different systems. So this is part of the challenge. How do you design integrative treatment plans that are consistent with who the patient is, as well as what any of these systems—conventional medicine included—can do?

On Tuesdays, they have the morning block to further develop the treatment plans. They have a lot of thought and discussion during the conference, but it is really up to them to think about the patient and put it all into some cohesive package. Tuesday afternoons the Fellows are in clinic, and for 1 hour of the afternoon they are with the mind-body practitioner seeing patients in follow-up. So they are working with an "expert" and seeing this therapy applied to their own patients. On Wednesday morning, they are in clinic with the Chinese medicine practitioner.

Again, another major distinction we made is that they need to understand and have respect for the various systems and what they can do. They need to understand some of the language. The nice thing about this is that they see the same patients they just saw in the new patient evaluation, and they go through an entirely different system with them. This helps them understand some of the distinctions. To be able to describe tongues and talk about pulses in a Chinese fashion helps them understand what that medical system can do for patients.

Wednesday afternoon is reflection time. Thursday morning is research. We have research education as well as the program research that happens. Thursday afternoon is follow-ups with the osteopath. Friday is "didactics," which is a misnomer because we try to make it very experiential. But there is structured teaching for the 12 different areas. The first year is quite structured. The second year is more open.

We've clustered the 12 areas. One cluster is philosophical in nature because we need to shift the philosophy within which we practice medicine. Part of philosophy is about healing-oriented medicine, which is really a phrase that Andy has popularized. But I think it is a good distinction because I was trained in disease-oriented medicine. If you understand what it means to come from a healing perspective everything changes.

There is a cluster on self-healing. What can we as practitioners do, and what is it we should be paying attention to in our own lives? Much of it is about lifestyle—how we take care of ourselves mentally, spiritually, and physically.

One piece of all the core subject areas concerns the complementary and alternative modalities, which means learning about the modalities, what they are, what we know and don't know about them, and when they are effective.

The last piece, which is more the focus of the fellowship, is the whole part about leadership and facilitating change. The Fellows are selected, in part, as leaders who will have a vision and an ability to help things shift at the national level. This comes from the expectation that if the Fellows graduate and start programs somewhere else, they would need to know how to do things like business plans.

We hope the Fellows will start programs at universities or become deans of medical schools or work at a policy level. At this stage, given the mission of the program, it is really about redesigning medical education. We thought if we could produce a couple of people who would go into academia or academic-like positions and facilitate change at a broader level, then we could make a real difference. So the fellowship is focused at that level. But we also offer continuing education, and we are about to launch an associate fellowship.

The Associate Fellowship

The associate fellowship is modeled after the curriculum that we have developed over the last $2\frac{1}{2}$ years within the fellowship but is designed for the clinicians. It is a big undertaking. The program is designed for people to stay in their practice. Throughout the 2 years there are only 3 weeks onsite. The rest is distance learning—primarily web-based.

Our first class starts in August 2000. Again, the material, the information, and the way we are modeling the program is an extension of the fellowship but designed for people in practice.

The first class will be 40 people. I believe this will be a huge test. There is no doubt that you can teach botanical medicine in an extension program, but can people shift their orientation and the way they practice and how they live their lives through this kind of an educational process? It would be much easier to bring them to Tucson for 2 years, so that is the challenge.

Before our residential Fellows start in the clinic, they go through an integrative medicine assessment as patients. We do that the first year, and it is a very dynamic process. While they are in didactics and getting "lectures," they are also having the experience of these systems. So that is what we are attempting to do with this associate fellowship.

We'll see how it works. Rich Liebowitz, MD, just started as the director of education in July of 1999. He is now supervising and coordinating the educational efforts between the fellowships. The intent is that the fellowship is the laboratory and then we carry it out through CME (continuing medical education) and the associate fellowship.

Medical Education

I was perplexed for the longest time about why no one else has created something like this. Even though academic institutions are getting more and more interested in this approach, no one seemed to be focusing on education. People were more than willing to open clinics but without any thought of who would be running them. If your construct is all about the tools—that just as you learn about pharmaceuticals you can learn about herbs—then you don't need to address education because nothing in education needs to change. So it is only if you get the bigger picture that education becomes an issue.

But other universities are starting to ask, "What are you doing?" It's interesting because what brings people to ask the question is not always the same thing they leave with. But I have to tell you the most exciting part. There is a web that has been woven in the way things work in the world. Our dean, Jim Dalen, was at the University of Massachusetts as the head of the department of medicine when Jon Kabot-Zinn hadn't even published yet. Dalen discovered Jon's work and did with Jon what he did with us, which was to give him a chance. He moved Jon out of the college of nursing and put him in the department of medicine and said, "I am giving you a year. Do your stuff and then present at grand rounds." So there is a real connection because Dalen opened the doors for Jon in the same way that he gave us an opportunity.

Then Jon was at Duke University and connected with chancellor Ralph Snyderman. I have a Duke connection so there seemed to be this little triangle forming. Jon thought it would be great if we brought together deans and other high-level people who were interested in the conversation on education to see if we could work collaboratively.

Jon understands completely what we are speaking about. I always say that you can't have integrative medicine without integrative management. It is a different way of functioning and relating to one another. So Jon, Marty Sullivan from Duke, and I started talking. We planned for what felt like an eternity and then the meeting actually happened in July 1999, at the Fetzer Institute in Kalamazoo, the first meeting of the Academic Consortium of Integrative Medicine.

It was beautiful. We invited eight institutions. The concept was that, to be invited, they needed to be mainstream academic colleges of medicine, and they needed to have high-level support. There are many interesting efforts happening on the fringes of universities, but there needed to be somebody—a chancellor or a dean or someone in a position of power—who said, "I am behind this." So we invited Harvard, University of Massachusetts, University of Maryland, Duke, Arizona, Minnesota, University of California-San Francisco, and Stanford. The only institution that couldn't send a representative was Harvard, although they wanted to. There were three people invited from each institution—the "power person" and the program people. So from our institution it was Andy, Dean Dalen, and myself. From Duke it was Ralph Snyderman, Marty Sullivan, and Redford Williams.

The first night—which by the way was the hottest day in the history of Michigan—the power went out. We were sitting in this room with no lights, so we lit candles. People were sweating and had their pant legs rolled up. Jon facilitated a meditation, and we asked people, "Why are you here?"

We all had our own stories about why we went into medicine in the first place and how that seemed to be getting lost. The first night the conversation naturally went in the direction of what was happening in medical education that took bright-eyed students who wanted to help people and killed their spirit. We asked, "Is there a way for us to identify what is working and not working and put forward recommendations around a healing-oriented clinical education and competency?" We also thought that doing this as a group of institutions would have a lot more effect than if one of us did it alone.

We are now looking at how we should expand membership. Ralph Snyderman is the president of the Dean's Council of the American Association of Medical Colleges this year, so he is steering the boat for all the deans for the medical schools nationally right now. That is really exciting, especially if a critical mass within the leadership of academic medicine can get involved and help.

We are finalizing the dates for the next meeting now, which will be in September 2000 here in Tucson. So who knows where this could go?

Patient Stories

One of the things we're learning about is the magic that can happen when you give patients the right and the opportunity to be their own healers. Part of the shift that happens is this sense of partnership.

One of the first patients I saw before the Fellows started was this wonderful woman who had dealt with obesity all of her life. She was a very intelligent, wonderful, talented person. I asked her if she would be open to guided imagery. She said yes, so for a couple of months I did imagery with her. I don't think it necessarily mattered that it was imagery versus some other approach, but the dynamic that happened was, again, a returning of her own sense of power about who she was and where she was in her process and about her ability to do something. The locus of control went back to her. It was no longer my job to fix her, but it was "our" job to work together. And the last time I saw her, this woman had lost 60 pounds.

What the imagery did was to allow her to gain access to her own subconscious or unconscious. She could list all the reasons why she should lose weight—it wasn't about that— so what was the underlying dynamic? That's what the imagery unlocked.

We see this pattern in many of the patients. The other thing we hear all of the time is the power of just being heard. So many patients say that they have never had a physician listen to their stories. It is sad, but it is true. On my first day of conventional clinic as an intern, one of the upper-level people pulled me aside and said, "Okay, let me tell you truly and honestly the key to success in clinic. Never ask a patient an open-ended question. Because the second you do, you are screwed. You will hear the whole story of their life, and you will never stay on track. Only ask 'yes or no' questions."

So, the shift to listening and hearing patients' stories is as important as anything else.

At the case conferences the patients aren't there, so the Fellows bring pictures. Andy always asks, "Did you have a sense of who this person was?" It's the human connection. And that's the theme that runs through a lot of the patient's stories—it's the first time they have been listened to, the first time they have had the opportunity to tell their stories, the first time they were seen as whole people.

Anyone can come to our clinic, but we have a huge waiting list. Part of what determines who gets seen is driven by the fact that it is an educational program, and we need to categorize the patients by their main concern. So our longest wait, unfortunately, is with cancer patients because that has the greatest demand. But if we accepted patients on demand only, the Fellows would see only cancer patients.

We also limit the percentage of people we see from out of state because we feel like we should be serving this community.

The Clinic Process

Initially, if you were a patient, you would be sent information so you would know what is going to happen before you come. We like to make sure people don't think Dr. Weil is going to be their physician, so they get information and a bio and a picture of the Fellow who is going to be their primary doctor.

You get the information that you will not leave the first day with a treatment plan. Then, unless there is something emergent, on your first visit we take your history and do a physical examination. You are told about the patient conference and when to come back for discussion of your treatment plan.

The clinic is within the university hospital, which is a challenge. We are trying to create a healing environment, but what exists now is that you walk in and there is steel and fluorescent lights everywhere. The stirrups are up and in view. Just walking in the room can make you feel like you'd better protect yourself. Now we have renovated five of the rooms, and the Fellows are reporting a different experience when they see the patients in the renovated rooms. The Fellows feel more comfortable; the patients feel more comfortable; and the conversations tend to be deeper.

The renovated rooms look like what you would expect if you went into an alternative clinic—lots of wood, music, fresh flowers, incandescent lighting. There is a homey feel that is much safer and more comfortable.

But back to the patient—your Fellow would spend at least an hour with you on the initial visits. You would talk about your conventional surgical/medical history as well as what you love in life and what makes you want to get out of bed in the morning and whether or not you are doing that. You would also talk about what your greatest sorrows are and what makes you tick and your sources of stress and what you do to relax. So it's a much fuller history. And it is at this point that most people say, "Nobody has ever asked me these questions or just listened to me before."

There is still a white coat phenomenon, however, even though the Fellows don't wear white coats. Our culture still gives power to the role. So part of the quest is how we can utilize that to benefit the patients and the system. At the end of the first visit, because this is a training, the Fellows present the patient to the attending physician and Andy, if he is there. Then the patient would go on his or her way. The patient would be scheduled for a return in a week or two because the case would be discussed the following Monday afternoon.

When you return, your Fellow will have a typed report for you that is probably three to five pages long and contains the recommendations from the patient conference. Part of the conversation will center around your options and what we thought might be helpful. Then we try to understand where you want to start, what resonates the most, what are your beliefs, and what makes sense.

In the first visit the Fellows ask, "Why are you here? What is it that you want to get out of this?" Five people with breast cancer could have entirely different goals. This is one of the huge shifts. It is not just looking through our lenses as physicians—what can I do for you—it is understanding and valuing what you are there for and what you want done and how you want to be a partner in that.

Bumps in the Road

There are certain patients who come to the clinic because they are in the same conversation. But there is also another group who comes because the people are looking for a magic bullet— they don't want an integrative approach or to be partners—they just want the magic herb to cure them. So the challenge with this group is defining who we are, what we do, and what the expectations can be.

The other challenge is that there are patients—for example, a woman with inflammatory breast cancer and a man with testicular cancer—who absolutely refuse to believe they have cancer. "I don't believe in cancer," they say. Both patients could have been effectively treated, but they were refusing all treatment. And we see a lot of patients who come hoping we will support them in writing off all conventional medicine. This is challenging. Our hope is that we can be in enough of a relationship with these people that we can help get them to the place where they will see it differently and take a treatment we think is effective.

But to what degree do you support the patient's views? Here we are, saying people have a right to their belief systems and have a right to live in accordance with that, and then we don't agree with them. So when you come face to face with a situation like that, it is very, very difficult. There have been a lot of conversations regarding how we manage these patients because everyone in the program would deal with it differently. Andy is more willing to "fire" patients than some of the other people in the program. If what they are doing, in his mind, is not the right thing—if it's something pretty black and white—he will say, "I can't take care of you anymore." But do we do that, or do we stay in relationship with them with the hope that we can still support them some way?

We haven't made any fundamental decisions. Each time it is case by case, and each time it is a huge issue. We were recently accused of taking all our patients off chemotherapy and giving them herbs. I knew we weren't doing that, so I reviewed the first 60 cancer patients. It was interesting to document that, in addition to not taking people off conventional treatments, there were 10 patients who came to us refusing conventional treatment. Then, because they felt a level of trust with us that they didn't feel with their oncologists, they initiated conventional treatment. This, to me, was a sign of success.

Again, it is integration. So that is a big challenge. But whenever you are pushed, that is where your old stuff just comes right up. You feel that if the patient is not taking the treatment you think should be taken, then you are failing. So we also pay attention to the physicians. We spend a lot of time talking about how it is for them. What is coming up, and how are they processing it? It is a good illustration of how it is an interrelated system and that we need to pay attention to all the parts.

Self-care and caring for each other in the community is a huge aspect. The program started a wellness team. Their job is to pay attention to our wellness as a program and as individuals. We made a commitment as a community that this was important to us.

We also have a research arm. The challenges for research are the same challenges that exist in clinical practice and education: How do you get away from it just being another modality that you are randomizing? Most research would look at St. John's wort versus Prozac. That is important research, and I think we need to do it, but that is not testing whole patient care or integration. It seems like most research right now is at the "this-versus-that" level.

So how do we move beyond that and test what we are hypothesizing, which is that this is a different approach to medicine and healthcare? We have some interesting things under way. We received money to look at cancer care and integrative approaches. My hypothesis is that if we use an integrative approach, then the patient will end up feeling healthier, more balanced and whole, and more content with his or her life whether we cured the disease or not. That is what success would look like.

Another piece of our research is designed around our mission of education. The hypothesis here is that there is a different way to educate people and that a different process of education will result in a different kind of practitioner. We need to test that. It has been our anecdotal experience and has been the feedback we get from the fellows, but we need research. We received a grant to look at our 3-hour miniconferences to see if we shift practitioners' perspective in that short time or not and whether that ultimately results in a different healthcare with different outcomes. That is the real question.

But the thing that I am most excited about stems from the academic consortium, and the future directions of healthcare and education in this country being refocused in a way that the culture is seeking. I talk about Andy's career as an illustration of the culture. He has been saying the same thing for 25 years. What puts someone on the cover of *Time*? It is not because suddenly he said something different. It is because the culture is ready for that. That is why I love the John Astin study. People aren't saying, "I'd rather have an acupuncture needle than a pill." They are saying, "These are my philosophies about life and wellness, and that is what I care about."

So the most exciting thing to me is the consortium and the possibility that healthcare could be about health again and be a manifestation of the belief that a person's life is so much more than just the body. That is really exciting. That is what makes me happy.

CHAPTER 31

RALPH SNYDERMAN, MD

CAM and the Role of the Academic Health Center

Ralph Snyderman, MD, is chancellor for health affairs, executive dean of the Duke University School of Medicine, and president and CEO of the Duke University Health Systems. His list of distinguished positions includes Senior Vice President for Medical Research and Development, Genentech, Inc; Frederic M. Hanes Professor of Medicine, professor of immunology, and chief of the Division of Rheumatology, Duke University Medical Center; and director of the Laboratory of Immune Effector Function, Howard Hughes Medical Institute. He is currently the chair of the Council of Deans for the Association of American Medical Colleges.

Among his many awards, Dr. Snyderman has received the Lifetime Achievement Award from the Arthritis Foundation (1997), an honorary doctorate of science from the State University of New York Health Science Center (1996), the Alumni Citation Award from Washington College (1996), the Bonazinga Award for Excellence in Leukocyte Biology Research (1993), and the Ciba-Geigy Morris Ziff Award for lifetime achievements in inflammation research (1991).

The author of more than 300 journal articles, Snyderman is the editor of *Inflammation: Basic Principles and Clinical Correlates, The Academic Health Center and Health Care Reform,* and *The Academic Health Center in the 21st Century.*

In the summer of 2000, I traveled to Durham, North Carolina, to interview Dr. Snyderman at his office at Duke University.

My question is: What obligation do academic medical centers such as Duke have in improving healthcare for everyone? We need to look at the delivery of healthcare from all aspects and ask what works and what can be improved. What do we have to offer?

I am a firm believer that the scientific basis for the practice of medicine has delivered a form of healthcare that improves outcome or prevents disease for a vast number of human illnesses. I also believe that the continued application of science to the practice of medicine will improve our quality of health and well-being. I think the opportunities coming out of the Human Genome Project are going to open doors that will lead us into areas of health enhancement that we can barely imagine. I strongly support the scientific practice of medicine. Having said that, I am fully aware that scientific methodology is not the sole answer to all of life's questions.

If we consider our obligation to the health of people now and of future generations, we must be open to alternative, complementary, and integrative approaches simply because we don't know and will never know the scientific basis of everything. It is important that institutions such as Duke keep our eyes open to what we can do to benefit the people we serve and to have an open mind and open eyes to other strategies. We should not have a knee-jerk reaction in thinking that the traditional way is the only way or think that anything not discovered by academic medicine isn't good. It is our obligation to look at other approaches. In addition, we must be mindful of what patients expect of us. In the area of alternative strategies, the public is far ahead of conventional medicine in its exploration of the field. So, if for no other reason than to better understand what our patients are doing—often without telling us—we ought to know more about complementary and alternative strategies.

My paper on integrated healthcare systems addressed the broad scope of services that Duke and other such institutions should be providing to the communities they serve. In my view, we have had a very rapid and dramatic transformation in academic medicine. When I first came to Duke as Chancellor for Health Affairs about 10 years ago—and up until 5 years ago, in fact—we were an institution that delivered high-intensity specialty care. People came to us after they had already seen their primary care physicians and, in many instances, had already seen a specialist. If those efforts hadn't helped, then patients came to Duke as a last resort. My thought was that we owe our community a lot more than that—we ought to provide a full continuum of care. Based on this premise, we have developed an integrated healthcare system that provides services from disease prevention to hospice care. Once you take on the obligation of providing better forms of overall healthcare for the entire community, I believe it is the obligation of the institution to begin exploring alternative strategies.

Duke is currently delivering a fairly broad range of alternative and complementary therapies. Historically, we have had strong programs in behavioral psychology, which is the forerunner of what many now call *alternative strategies*. One of the larger programs developed at Duke 20 years ago dealt with primary and secondary prevention of cardiovascular disease. Those who were at high risk for coronary artery disease or who had already had heart attacks would come to us for preventive or therapeutic measures. Part of that program included approaches that would be considered "alternative" strategies—exercise, nutrition, stress reduction, and behavioral modification.

My initial entry into "integrative" approaches began five years ago when Larry Burk and others at Duke introduced me to anodyne imagery, which is basically a form of self-hypnosis. They wanted to offer it to patients undergoing stressful procedures at our medical center. I thought this was intriguing. We found that the strategy was eagerly accepted by patients and nurses and—once they understood it—by physicians as well.

We now have many stress reduction strategies, most often practiced at our Center for Living, which is a wellness center focusing on sustaining health and treating those who are ill. People with cardiac disease come to engage in rehabilitation within a robust environment that encourages them to think of themselves as healthy again. People with pulmonary disease are often seen walking around the track with oxygen tanks right beside those who are healthy and working out. People with asthma and arthritis who can't otherwise exercise use our walking pools. We also have a mindfulness meditation clinic, a t'ai chi program, and various other strategies to get people to reduce stress and feel good about themselves. This is an important part of healthcare at Duke.

Integrated Medicine at Duke

Last year we credentialed two individuals to do acupuncture. We selected two physicians who had medical degrees and were already trained in acupuncture. It's amazing because credentialing requires the approval of the executive committee of the medical staff, which is the most conservative bastion of our medical practice.

We are using acupuncture for pain and have agreed to use it in dealing with certain types of addictions, particularly smoking. So acupuncture is now offered to patients as a choice.

We have also just developed a formal program in integrative medicine. There are a number of areas in which conventional medicine has not addressed people's needs. There are certain things that we do incredibly well, like treating bacterial pneumonia and trauma. But there are other things that we don't do very well at all, such as treating chronic pain syndromes of virtually any sort. As a rheumatologist, if somebody came to me with gout, I loved it because I knew exactly what to do. The same is true for infectious arthritis—you really wouldn't want to go to an herbalist for that. But for something like fibromyalgia, which is an incredibly common pain condition, we don't treat that well at all. What I am really getting at is that conventional medicine has a spectrum of problems for which our remedies are very, very good. However, there are other situations in which conventional techniques sometimes do more harm than good. It is in these areas that we need to be open to other possibilities. So it is in these cases (where conventional medicine doesn't work well) that we have introduced alternative strategies at Duke.

We are also exploring opportunities in integrative medicine for students. In addition to the usual curriculum, our medical students meet together in small groups, initially 1 day a week and then every other week for several years. In these small group sessions, they deal with societal problems. The group leader has taken a course in handling stress from Redford Williams, MD, author of *Anger Kills*, and knows the most effective strategies for stress reduction, understanding stress, and dealing with stress. So all the students learn how to deal with their own stress upon entry to our medical school.

In addition to that, we have a number of elective courses in integrative medicine. One of them is offered through our Department of Community and Family Medicine. Other courses are offered by the Department of Psychiatry. Our students love them; they flock to them. The students have also organized an integrative medicine study group that meets biweekly. I have actually talked to those students and loved it. It seems that no matter what room we choose, we always have standing room only. You teach physiology and rarely does anyone show up; you teach integrative medicine and you have standing room only. So, obviously, the students want it.

The Profile of Future Physicians

There have been very dramatic changes in who is entering medical school. We now enjoy the presence of women and diversity among the student population. I came through Duke as an intern many years ago. One of the reasons that I came to Duke for my internal medicine training was that it had been known—and still is known—as one of the most rigorous programs in the country. I likened it to the Marine Corps of medical training. When I was on the house staff, I don't recall that we had any women in the group and very few of us were married. Our classes today are much more diversified, with women representing nearly half of all classes.

As to lifestyle, we were here virtually all the time. It was a male bonding thing, and, as with many types of male bonding, there were pecking orders. People were always jostling each other for where they were within the pack. It was a hard-nosed approach to medicine. The discipline and commitment were tremendous. There was no such thing as "I cannot do this" or "I will not do this." It was total commitment. Every other part of your life was secondary to the practice of medicine.

When I became an attending physician, a house officer, who happened to be a woman, told me she couldn't do something. She said she didn't have time. I was shocked because I had never heard a house officer say anything other than "Yes, Sir."

More and more, students are saying, "I want to practice medicine; I love medicine, but I have a life. I have a family, and I have other things. The practice of medicine is something I do, but it is not everything to me." I wouldn't trivialize their commitment to the practice of medicine, but they are not willing to sacrifice other parts of their life. This option would not even have been discussed 20 years ago. More importantly, the entire nature of rounds has changed from an almost military, highly disciplined structure to a much more open, interactive, kinder, gentler learning process.

Medical Teaching Rounds

When a person is admitted to the hospital, we take his or her medical history, do a physical exam, do a series of tests to determine the problem if the diagnosis isn't clear, and then create a therapeutic plan. In a hospital such as Duke—or any of America's teaching hospitals—the final responsibility for the patient is with an attending physician, but the ongoing care is often given by a physician in training or a supervised medical student. Once the workup is complete, the diagnosis and therapeutic plan or the diagnostic plan for the patient is presented for advice and final signoff by the attending senior physician. An attending physician is generally responsible for many patients on a clinical unit. When the attending physician's patients are presented to him or her by the house staff (i.e., interns, residents) or students or reviewed for daily progress, that is called *making rounds*.

In days past, rounds occurred in big open wards and the team would literally walk from bed to bed around the ward. There was the professor in a starched white coat, who was usually a brusque and firm individual, and a coterie of individuals at different stages of their training, the lowest being the medical student, then the intern, then the resident. The attending physician would generally stand on the right of the patient's bed, and the presenter would always stand on the patient's left so they would be face to face. A bag of medical instruments was placed at the foot of the bed. Everybody else gathered around the patient, standing up straight and not touching the bed. God forbid that anybody would ever sit down on the bed. Then the case would be presented to the attending physician in front of the patient.

In today's world, the whole process is more informal. There is also far greater sensitivity to what is said in front of the patient and more attention paid to the patient's modesty. Indeed, the consent of the patient to be visited by the team for teaching rounds generally is obtained beforehand. That didn't enter into the equation 10 years ago, but it does now. One of the most profound changes is that rounds and interactions with patients are more sensitive, more caring, more nurturing, and there is more sensitivity about the patient's point of view.

I believe that this softening up of formal activities such as rounds, as well as the enhanced understanding of the feelings of people, has been driven in part by the increased presence of women in medicine and their greater emotional sensitivity.

I was very struck by something that happened just a couple of years ago on rounds. There was a patient who had a tragic problem. The physician who presented this patient was a woman, and after the presentation, she cried. I had never seen that happen on rounds before. It was appropriate, and it was the way we all felt. Several years ago, that would have been unimaginable. It used to be thought that there should be a veil of professionalism to prevent the exposure of emotions. There is no question that physicians need to control their emotional feelings, because they shouldn't unduly influence the standard of care. But having said that, we are all people, so I thought her tears were wonderful. As a matter of fact, they were shared by many in the group.

We don't really understand why we even have emotions. We have not answered that question adequately on a philosophical or biological basis. Likewise, I don't think there have been careful, thoughtful discussions about the role of the physician's emotions in the care of patients. It has just been taken for granted that we ought not to let emotions get in the way of the treatment. But by not letting emotions get in the way of treatment, are we getting in the way of treatment? One of the most important aspects of patient care is actually caring for the patient and having the patient understand that we care. I don't think the medical profession has spent sufficient time reflecting on how we can develop more caring relationships with our patients. Specialization, technology, and time limitations imposed by managed care have severely limited ideal physician-patient relationships. Nevertheless, given the importance of caring and trust in the healing process, we must raise the debate of this issue to the highest level.

Opposition to CAM

There has been surprisingly little resistance to what we have done so far. At the entrance to our medical school, there are always posters announcing lectures that are scheduled. I generally scan all of them. I remember about 5 years ago when I walked into the building, I saw a large poster announcing a session on therapeutic massage and the importance of "healing hands" sponsored by the mind-body study group. I remember looking at it and thinking, "What the heck is this? Who are these people, and what are they up to?" I found out who the sponsor was—it turned out to be Dr. Larry Burk—and called him. I think this scared him, but what I found out was that there was tremendous interest on the part of our faculty in complementary and alternative medicine.

When I became an advocate for teaching anodyne imagery, we had to make an investment of $20,000 to bring a team of instructors in from southern California to teach us how to do it. When it became public that I was spending money in this way, I got an e-mail from the chair of psychiatry that essentially said, "Ralph, we have always been a little concerned about you, but now we know you have really gone off the deep end and are totally crazy." That was the initial (tongue-in-cheek) response. But within 6 months, people were clamoring for it.

So whereas the resistance hasn't been great, I think there has been appropriate skepticism. I was very proud of the discussion at the executive committee of the medical staff regarding the credentialing of our acupuncture staff. They openly acknowledged the need to be aware of these strategies and to bring them into the medical center. But they restricted the application of acupuncture to those things such as pain or substance abuse where there was some evidence that it would work.

Council of Deans

The Association of American Medical Colleges (AAMC) is the formal organization for all medical schools and teaching hospitals. One of the governing bodies of the AAMC is its Council of Deans. I happen to be chair of the Council of Deans this year. In several weeks we'll be having our annual spring meeting. Being the chair gives me certain influence over the programs, including the choice of keynote speakers. This year, for the first time in the history of American medical education, we are devoting a significant part of our meeting to integrative medicine. The keynote speaker is Dr. Andrew Weil. We've titled his talk "From Genomics to Ginkgo Biloba." The next morning we are having our main session on integrative medicine. We have the dean from the University of Maryland, the head of the National Center for Complementary and Alternative Medicine at the NIH, the dean of Harvard, and the dean of the University of California–San Francisco as panelists. Conventional medicine is putting its toe in the water and seeing what it is like, and I love it.

It is history in the making. When I contacted Andy Weil, he responded within an hour. He knows the power of integrative strategies. We can help make a positive transformation of American medicine at this time. The door is open right now. But it needs to be done right. There is a real danger of going overboard and bringing in a lot of things that will confuse the issue. We need to learn about the role of complementary strategies, but we cannot give up the rigor of the scientific approach to medicine.

There are some popular radio shows that deal with alternative strategies. They often have so-called experts on and are widely listened to throughout the country. Recently I heard a show on the herbal treatment of gout, and people were pontificating on the most abject nonsense. I am totally sympathetic about reaching out for better solutions for treating diseases that are very difficult and for which conventional medicine is not effective, but to advocate an unproven alternative in lieu of safe and effective strategies is offensive to me.

Many people are jumping in and calling themselves experts without really being experts. I wish people would be more humble about their approaches to healthcare. There is so much we don't know. Getting conventional medicine to start looking at complementary strategies will be good for everybody.

Vision for the Future

We are going to be moving to a broader array of strategies for dealing with health problems. People will also get more involved in learning about their own health. And I think there will be a stratification, at least initially, as the more educated, more affluent individuals who have computers spend more time on the Internet learning about health-related issues, so we will have a far more informed public.

As a country, we must understand the importance of education. Beginning with the most elementary education, we need to teach children about the importance of health and human biology.

I think, as we lay out the range of health-related problems, there will be a spectrum of remedies. Conventional medicine will dominate certain areas because the pathophysiology and therapeutics are understood and the therapeutics are generally effective. Then there will be other areas in which conventional medicine will be unsatisfactory. In these other areas, I hope that with experience and observation, we can learn which, if any, of these problems are better treated through, for example, herbal techniques, physical manipulation, stress reduction, or other modalities like acupuncture.

As far as the Internet goes, it is a whole new world and initially there will be many players; some will survive, and some won't. Right now it is very difficult to differentiate quality information from junk. Duke is actively engaged in exploring our role on the Internet. We are part of an entity called WebEBM (evidence-based medicine), through which we are developing what we call "best practices." Let's say there are 100 illnesses ranging from diabetes to rheumatoid arthritis. The question is: What is the best practice for treating these right now?

Along with several other academic institutions, we have developed a company to put these best practices on the Internet, primarily for caregivers. Patients will have access as well, and the data will be licensed to other healthcare institutions. Caregivers and patients will know that these are the best practices from healthcare institutions such as Duke, Vanderbilt, Emory, Washington University, and the University of Oregon.

We are also very close to completing our own web site, which will be a comprehensive site with lots of information and access for patients who want to come to Duke. It will also have clinical content. One of our interests in the area of complementary and alternative strategies will be to provide statements as to the credibility of different strategies. We would indicate whether any given strategy was subjected to scientific testing and clinical trials or was unproven.

Concerning how healthcare might look 10 years from now, I think one of the biggest unknowns is what are we going to be dealing with in regards to health insurance. This is currently a mess.

Right now most alternative strategies are not covered. I can understand the health insurers not wanting to cover procedures that have not been proven effective, but what is proved and what is not proved is a big question. Even within conventional therapies there have been many tugs between medicine and the insurers. For example, insurers initially were very resistant to bone marrow transplantation for breast cancer, saying it was experimental. Then, after a number of lawsuits—which they lost—the coverage became much more common. The irony now is that some new medical studies are questioning the effectiveness of bone marrow transplantation for breast cancer patients. So this is a muddled area.

Should stress reduction be covered in a health plan? Should t'ai chi? Should massage? I don't know the answers. Obviously it costs money to do these treatments, and if it can be shown that a particular therapy is effective, then it should be used. If it can be shown that the therapy is more effective than other more expensive, unhelpful, and sometimes detrimental therapies, the ones that work certainly should be paid for.

Virtually every teaching hospital in America, including Duke, is vulnerable to tremendous economic stresses and pressures. What is happening today in healthcare funding is an unseen but major danger to our healthcare system. Its impact on the future of conventional or alternative medicine is a big unknown.

Let me go off a bit on a tangent here. Andy Weil makes the point that if we could better educate the public about self-help for healthcare—particularly about the prevention of diseases for which conventional medicine offers only expensive or ineffective therapies—and if the public would deal with these issues more effectively through, for example, herbal strategies, who would be against it? If fibromyalgia is treated more effectively through physical manipulation, t'ai chi, or mindfulness meditation, I would love to see that funded by health insurance.

It is important to focus on the currents of change in healthcare and what an exciting time this is. It is a time of tremendous opportunity and vulnerability. The vulnerability is largely economic, with the public demanding more but insurers and the government paying less. The population is getting older and smarter. People understand the value of their own health. They also understand what the health system can do for them. However, this is incredibly expensive.

The current mechanisms of funding healthcare are not sustainable, either from the federal government or business. The current system is getting more and more expensive, so the negative aspect is that we have a healthcare system and infrastructure that are in danger of crumbling. In addition, we have a potential lack of discipline about what is good healthcare. It's difficult to tell whether the information on the Internet is coming from a sound study involving hundreds of thousands of people or from somebody in a garage claiming that some snake oil is good for a particular problem. With the dispersal of therapies on the Internet and all types of alternative strategies, it is becoming difficult for the public to know what is good anymore. That is the downside of public interest and increased access to nonvalidated information.

The good side is that progress in medicine has brought us to a time when science and alternative or complementary techniques—which historically have been on divergent pathways—are coming back together. One of my most amazing "Eurekas!" occurred during a conversation I had with Andy when he was talking about his botanical approaches for the treatment of various illnesses. Andy said that botanicals, rather than being a single specific chemical (which we call a drug), contain a series of similar chemical derivatives. In herbal medicine, you don't have a single active agent because nature produces a number of chemically similar versions in the aggregate that have a medicinal effect. He was talking about how, in some ways, nature is more gentle. Rather than hitting you with a very high dose of a single chemical agent at a level 100 times greater than your body has ever seen it, botanicals contain, say, 10 similar compounds at a much lower dose. Andy contends that botanical remedies may be more natural for the body.

I have a research laboratory that is funded by the National Institutes of Health where we do molecular research. I am working in the area of receptors, or how cells respond to the chemical environment. What hit me during the conversation with Weil was that we were finding there were multiple receptors for certain specific chemicals. We have found that there are arrays of receptors that respond to certain chemicals and that, influencing the activity of each other, receptors act in an interrelated fashion. I told Andy that his statement about botanicals was interesting because our research was totally consistent with the fact that there are arrays of receptors that cross-talk to each other. That may explain why a single pure chemical compound in a drug may have a different effect than a botanical product with multiple derivatives of the drug.

I run at least 4 days a week—this is part of my mindfulness meditation. I try consciously to get into where I am and let my mind drift and not get too focused on anything in particular. On a recent run through Duke Forest, I was thinking that over the course of human evolution—let's say a million years—up until the last 100 years the only pharmaceutical effects we could experience were based on what we ate. So our whole evolution was based on a therapeutic array that is very different from the pharmaceutical therapeutic array. The therapeutic array we have evolved from is botanical rather than pharmaceutical. This doesn't minimize the benefits of drugs from any clinical situations. However, there may also be powerful calls for herbal remedies as well. We really need to think about that.

One of the beauties to me as a person who aspires to be a scientist is that if science has an open mind—an open, gentle, compassionate mind—then we can look at some of the alternative approaches and say, "There really is a context for this." We could embrace them and try to understand them better. That is a point I am going to make when I speak to the Council of Deans. Andy and I have come at this from almost 180 degrees apart, yet we are converging in our thinking.

There is one additional point I would like to make. I think there is going to be a merging of understanding the physical basis of some of the complementary and alternative approaches. A lot of it is going to come from hard science—genetics and neurobiology and all the neurosciences. On the other hand, we will never understand the scientific basis of everything. We must be open to approaches that work even when we don't understand how or why they work. I find our times to be extremely exciting. I think we are going to enter a whole new world of understanding about health and the practice of medicine.

Part Nine

Conversations About Healing with Hands

"We use our hands diagnostically, perceptually, and therapeutically—that's how simple and profound this is."

—JAMES JEALOUS

CHAPTER 32

JAMES JEALOUS, DO

Healing and the Natural World

There's a reason that people drive from neighboring states to see James Jealous, DO, at his clinic in Vermont. It is the same reason that students line up to take his classes and that the University of New England College of Osteopathic Medicine founded a scholarship in his name—the James Jealous Scholarship for Excellence in Osteopathic Medicine. Dr. Jealous has dedicated his life to exploring the natural world in its most essential, fundamental form, and it is this knowledge and the resultant skill that makes him one of the most respected osteopathic doctors in America today.

Dr. Jealous graduated from the Kirksville College of Osteopathy and Surgery in 1970 and is certified by the American Osteopathic Board with special proficiency in osteopathic and manipulative medicine. In private practice since 1971, he currently lives and teaches near Franconia, New Hampshire.

I had the honor of interviewing Dr. Jealous at his clinic in Milton, Vermont, in the fall of 1996.

Let's start by looking at the conditions in medical education. The whole process of becoming a physician is largely contradictory to the principles of healing. Students are not nurtured, nor are they encouraged to explore, nor are they communicated with as fellow travelers in a remarkably beautiful journey into the mountains of life. The healing arts have become quite sterile, and the biomolecular view of healing has distinct limits that trim off the "individual." This, of course, is a reflection of the educational ecosystem. The growth and development of a physician should be nurtured by the most loving and perceptive environment that is humanly possible to create. This is paramount to bring a complete picture of illness into focus.

Osteopathy, in its conception, contained a philosophy as well as a science. Osteopaths were asked to consider questions of the soul, death, transcendence, and to use only their hands in healing. The background in which life occurs has meaning. I believe that any healing art needs to help individuals find the way to a deeper reality than a biomolecular model of health.

It is interesting to me to see how many alternative medical models are slowly becoming biomolecular. Many "natural" cures are really biomolecular remedies and are used like traditional medicine uses drugs. From my perception, that's not necessarily alternative because an alternative medical practice would be of a larger vision and be very individualized in its application. It would not have a remedy for each symptom or disease but a unique option for the patient. The deeper questions about life need to enter into the picture and be part of the inquiry about healing. We are oversimplifying the art and losing the essence of what healing is about. Holistic is not using a variety of "cures;" it is seeing the Spirit, Soul, Body as a Whole. The treatment is not subdivided; if it is, then one must see one's position relative to the Whole and not try and "destroy the disease" (allopathic) but support the health of the Whole. This was osteopathy's beginning. It remains barely alive and is practiced by only several hundred DOs.

The idea of Whole—a unit, the undivided—is foreign to our culture and is slowly vanishing like an aboriginal form that is viewed as primitive by the intellect. Each one of us faces the reality in ourselves and must meet that responsibility first; then the perception will follow. For our culture it's a "deep" question; for the aboriginal soul it's a natural state. We need to focus not so much on cause and effect but on the priority of the Whole as it moves in relation to a Great Mystery. Teaching requires an effort in the same direction, a view of the Whole individual moving into new dimensions of life. We need to protect the ecoreceptive perception that is our natural state of being. This is slowly being trimmed away, and as a result, people are more sick than necessary. If they become ill, their inner balance and peace of mind are not juxtaposed to the causal event, and as a result, suffering is increased. The same process is present during education.

If we are seeking an alternative system of healthcare, then training must reflect that difference. Philosophy is not enough. We must try and live the principles. Physicians must not prioritize their relationship with the patient around time. This is a serious problem. An office call for an acute illness requires at least a half hour. I'm not bright enough to practice medicine in 7 minutes. Taking longer is necessary and prudent, but also it's economical.

I mention this because alternative medicine should not be more expensive. An osteopathic treatment is usually applied once (for an acute illness). Patients have a perception on why they got ill and how that effects their essential goals in life and recover more quickly without medications. Long-term patients begin to "manage" their inner balance and learn about staying healthy. All this requires remarkably less healthcare. Healers are teachers, fellow travelers, and explorers. Patients are in similar roles within the sphere of their lives. We are here to free people from needing routine healthcare—not to create dependence. Short, quick office calls leave patients frustrated and dependent; they either keep coming or break away and find their own way. The medical care in the United States is trying to "herd" people like cows. People are essentially spirited and will find their way forward on their own. Routine healthcare is becoming less and less sensitive.

This type of thinking is at the foundation of osteopathic medicine, but is it the status quo? No. Like all schools of healing, the deeply essential core is the least evident. The individual is still the key answer; we can't blame who we are on anything. Some people just desire to serve as much as possible the Health in each of us—not fight diseases. Most DOs have bought into the status, materiality, and fear of the mainstream medical model. The exceptions that we find prove the potential of our philosophy, but only a small number of DOs continue to explore our foundations.

The Foundations of Osteopathy

Our aim is to learn about the natural laws using the perceptual skills that we develop in our training and practice. The core of this work is perceptual. The concept grew out of repeated observation until the laws of nature became more clear. We learn to sense the Whole.

When one meets a patient, one sees the Whole—a very unique and rare event in our modern world. One does not divide life into soma/psyche/visceral, etc. This is an event contained only in the moment one is in. It's extraordinary. Patients are very much aware that a different attention is present. They comment on it. It's not intellectual or intuitive. It's aboriginal, instinctual.

There is no immediate conclusion or diagnosis—that's much later. The moment is filled with the effort to be present with the Health in the patient and the story as it unfolds into its own answer. Sometimes this requires a distinct form of patient, slow observation without focusing on a need to conclude. The process is foreign at first, but after a time one finds it quite natural, as it essentially is. We learn our skills by apprenticeship to something that has no name but that teaches us a great deal. We learn sensory perception without conceptual overlay, but it runs deeper than one can imagine. Learning this is different and demanding.

We use our hands diagnostically, perceptually, and therapeutically—that's how simple and profound this is. We are not listening for symptoms but for a preestablished priority set in motion by the Health in the patient. The founder of osteopathy, an MD surgeon, had a vision and followed his insight. He trained physicians to use their hands for healing, along with very simple and natural remedies—diet, rest, meditation, prayer—nothing was added but "hands-on healing." And it works!

The Natural Laws

First of all, the natural laws are not manmade. They are not conceived by research other than observation. Secondarily, we are aware that many laws exist and operate in healing that we are completely unaware of, and yet they still enter profoundly into the process. The interesting thing is that our perception can sense the intention of natural laws, the intention of the Health at work, where priorities are being established. Usually, once this is communicated, the patient is already aware of it but may have discarded the information. Our motive and our skill is to understand the intention of the Health in the patient as it works undivided in pursuing balance and harmony. As I said earlier, this is not limited by terminal disease.

After being trained to sense this reality in a hands-on practice, one feels very blessed to be an osteopath. The natural world is endowed with a consciousness that extends in all directions. It takes years and then some to learn this. It's a way of life, really.

My idea of alternative medicine is an alternative perception of the world, not just disease. Alternative medicine, to me, is about a different view of life, a more reverent and deeply informative beauty. Giving tea tree oil for nail fungus instead of a potentially toxic chemical is a much more natural remedy, but it's still not an alternative view of healing. Any form or mindset that goes after the disease to override it is only partially alternative. What supports the Whole at its interface with the wisdom of the natural world is alternative. It supports the Health, the nondivisible, the transcendent wisdom of life, first. In ordinary illness, rarely is more required.

About 80% of all common illnesses will heal with this approach, if the patient is able to let it work (i.e., time, perception). Otherwise, a more direct allopathic approach is required. Most alternative healthcare is still refocusing into an allopathic model. The purity of tradition is dying because very little time is being given to a deeper relationship with natural laws. We are fooling ourselves, and in some cases we are being fooled by persons interested in financial gains under the banner of the alternative, but the depth and commitment aren't there. One must know for oneself.

Let me tell you a story about a patient who died but was healed and at peace.

I had known John for 15 years because I was his family doctor in a small rural town. He was 52 years old and a workaholic. His wife and son were very anxious and chemically ill. He was driven. I saw him for years, episodically.

At 52 he developed lung cancer from exposure to chemicals at work. We referred him, as he wished, to an oncologist. He was treated with chemotherapy and pain medication (narcotics). One day he called my office and came in, asking for a treatment. I agreed. This request was out-of-nature for him. He came every week. I never pushed or inquired why, just treated him following the purity of Health, not trying to engage the disease, which I felt was far beyond curing.

Over the next several months, something felt different. Remember, he was really unreachable before. Finally, I asked him why he wanted these treatments. I could feel a deep change under my hands, something had emerged out of the suffering. He told me that without the treatment he needed lots of pain pills and with the treatment he did not need any! I was shocked but not surprised by this. He continued, "I am more peaceful after the treatments."

Where was this change coming from? We sent him to no psychiatrist, no Zen monastery. From where did the flower bloom? He died easily and at peace, loving and with his relationships in balance.

He helped me understand what I had only sensed before. The Health in the patient cannot become diseased or die. You can't kill it. It's transcendent. All we need to do is listen, use our hands in a skilled fashion, be patient, have the time and follow the Health. Then the natural laws—not "framed by human hands"—will reveal to us our role in the moment. The intellect remains in check. It's really none of my business how the process of healing is occurring.

All I can do is help life come into balance in the way it intends to. This is the key phrase; the way it intends to. I saw John a couple of days before he died, and it was like putting my hands on the healthiest person alive. I know this sounds strange, but there was a beautiful balance in him. He was happy.

Healing is not about getting rid of symptoms. It's about an individual wholeness that we remember instinctively the moment we touch it. The treatments help us recall and reintegrate what does not need to be learned. In some people death is a doorway to a perception our culture has trimmed away.

When a patient comes into the office we are always beginning, each moment, just waiting and perceiving the purity and sensing Health at work. This requires years of training and a love for the gift of our natural essence. We are listening with our hands to a story unfolding into the consciousness of each of us. How many doctors get told the whole story?

Healing with the Hands

It's not easy to explain in any way other than what it is, of itself, so I hope this is not confusing for people not associated with the perceptual skill. It took me 20 years to begin to understand. I still feel like a beginner. It's a lifelong journey into every possible corner of living in relation to natural laws. I'm learning more all the time. Really, it's a profound life that we are endowed with. Some new relationship is always expressing itself; this comes during treatment. The patients bring the learning with them. It's unspoken, but our senses know it, clearly. Increasing skill is not a predictable event. New skills arise from the direct association with the natural laws of healing. One learns things completely unexpected, not found in books, not extensions of known skills, but fresh. I never know what the next "fact" will be. I trust completely that in following the principles of my training, the understanding will grow.

What happens when I put my hands on a patient? That's a deep question. My answer will be personal. I can't speak for my fellow osteopaths or my students. It's a question of integrity with one's own health and a deep relationship with the gift of living.

I teach about the skeleton, and I teach bones; it's part of a continuum. One must understand and work with bones a long time. It grounds the senses and helps one understand disproportion and balance in the Whole. It's the early sensory model. One learns all the techniques usually divided into manipulation, counterstrain, myofascial release, cranial, etc., and years of anatomy—years of understanding motion until you sense a normal unit of life. One begins to sense the healing forces. At first our minds are confused because it is not a mechanical or hydraulic model. Many people stop here. I think it's too hard to believe what one senses.

We study embryology, the laws of our formation, "never missing perfect proportion," as one embryologist put it. We perceive this wisdom and the precision it demands from us. We need extensive training. Some people really believe in shortcuts, but life wants us Whole—not a part of us, all of us. We have to have the patience to tolerate our ignorance and not hide it. We have to believe that we are "special." I don't mean better, but a conscious creation of a higher Intelligence, like anything beautiful. We are part of nature's art.

Teaching requires one-on-one training and real respect for the Health in the student. We are not teachers but fellow travelers on a road of choice. It's not slavery. I teach at the pace set by the student. This applies on all levels, undergraduate and many years past postgraduate. It's heart-to-hands. The hardest lesson to teach is to work at the tempo of the Health. We don't hack away at disease. You know, 3 minutes of waiting is torture for some people. We need time, "free" time.

Students learn that they already are "skilled," perceptive. We allow what is natural to emerge; they surprise themselves. Very few teachers try and help us see the dynamic life we are. We don't need to become enlightened; we are enlightened. We need to sense our wholeness; we relax into this beauty and begin. Life by itself is beautiful. I'm not blinded by the violence and suffering. I see it, and I see something "other" sustaining us. In medicine this focus is missing. My experience with mainstream medicine is not a pleasant one because of its focus.

Fifteen or so years ago I had a swelling in my thyroid. I saw several specialists and was told that I had cancer. They were all very nervous, excitable, disturbed; they lacked insight and were afraid of my cancer. They laid out a morbid picture. I was very scared. I told them I was not coming back because I realized from their fears that I was afraid of dying. It surprised me because I thought I loved life enough to die without fear. I decided that I needed to come to peace with death and not work out of fear. The doctors were angry. I never told anyone. I just decided that I wanted to be free of the fear. It was a question of integrity with the gift of living.

I did not touch the growth for $1\frac{1}{2}$ years. I did this because it really was frightening to feel it and think about death, cancer, and a "void." I worked at not letting myself forget how afraid I was of death. Then I'd go about my day. Nothing else. I really tried to see my fear and help it through this misunderstanding.

It went away. The growth went away and never returned. I'm not claiming a self-cure. I have no idea what happened or why. But I had a choice between my spirit and fear. I am proud to be part of nature. I love nature. I am proud to be mixed in with the trees and the sun and everything. This feeling of wholeness was violated by the fear. I could not stop loving what gave me form and consciousness. I took my fear along with me and continued. We are enlightened. We know we belong intimately to life, and it's precious; it keeps giving each of us 100% without reservation. It's simply true.

The Force and the Form

The founder of osteopathy, A.T. Still, MD, said, "The body is a second placenta." I guess the question is best answered by saying death does not exist. I don't superimpose my understanding on my patients. I support all their decisions once they are clear about their choice of healthcare. I have patients from all sides of the issues. My job is to remain aware of the "undiseasable" Health in them and support it.

Patients are skilled; it takes humility to come for help. When I place my hands on a patient I begin by sensing the wholeness, the transcendent, not as an idea or as an immortal truth but by waiting until it is evident. I see the fear; I feel it in my hands. I sense the disease, the lesions, the history, and I wait. I'm looking for what I don't know—not a diagnosis; that's later. Now in this moment the Health is interfacing with disease. This priority must be seen directly, not by deduction.

Healing is the emergence of originality. Let's take a look at this one sentence for a moment. The breath of life comes into the body. We can sense various rhythms that are created from it, and we can perceive this process taking place. We're not interpolating it. We're not analyzing it. We can actually perceive the breath of life come into the body, come to the midline, and from the midline, generate different forms of rhythms in the bioelectric field, fluids, and tissue. Essentially, what's happening is genesis. It never stops. Moment to moment we are building new form and function. And one senses this, directly.

When I was reading the embryology literature, I found the research done by a German man named Blechschmidt. He was a scientist in love with embryos. His question was about the biodynamics and biokinetics of human development. How does this thing work? What happens? He never got his answer. He wrote that the cause of the origin of the embryo is held within the consciousness of the embryo itself. That's not a direct quote, but there was a secret, a mystery, that must remain. One can sense its genesis. It is at the center of the healing process.

Blechschmidt was fascinated by the fact that there was a force inside the fluids of the body that was not coming from the genetic field. This force inside the fluid actually contains the idea of the form of the human body—whether it's a kidney or vertebra or eye—and it brings it into manifestation. Then the genes modify it. So we have genetic, cultural, and race modifications. Before these modifications, there is divine form. It coexists during our whole life. There is a moment when we're all perfectly held in the matrix of a much finer Intention, a moment of healing.

Blechschmidt described six different ways in which fluids will interact with each other inside the body. William Sutherland, who is the founder and genius of osteopathy in the cranial field, perceived these forces in the fluids, yet the two men had never met or read each other's work. When I read that this embryologist was describing the same forces in the fluids as one of the great teachers of osteopathy, that's all it took.

Since then, I've spent a lot of time just looking at pictures of embryos in the first 6 weeks of life, before the genetic field takes over. Many people won't agree with what I'm saying, or perhaps they will misinterpret it, but these forces exist. Many old cultures recognize this truth. But how did they know it? They knew it because it was something they perceived directly—a natural occurrence.

Now, are we just taking a philosophical trip, or is there some practical knowledge in the perception and understanding that there's a force breathing into the body 24 hours a day? It's on watch, on call, working for the patient. It cannot become diseased. It's before that. All it does is carry the original form into that person. And it's the thing that emerged from the man that had cancer when he knew he was dying. It's what we would call "his spirit." Why it came the way it came in that moment in time, we don't know. But it interfaces with every moment of our life—the air pollution coming in our nose, the good thoughts we have, our hair, our age, how much we have to urinate. It interfaces with every moment, and if it stopped being there, you wouldn't die; you'd dissolve. You would have no matrix for your consciousness, even after death.

Let's say, 3 years ago, you hit your head, and ever since you've had dizziness. You've had all kinds of medicine, and nothing worked. You've still got the vertigo. If you walked into my office and I put my hands on you, I would not be looking for the strain pattern in your body. I wouldn't look at your disease. I observe the breath of life, this force in the body that's unchangeable, and look at how it was trying to help you. Your illness was precognitive. It knew you were going to walk into that wall before you did, not in a psychological way, but perceptually, something knew.

I'm not talking about premonitions. If you talk to enough people who have automobile accidents, just milliseconds before it happens, they know it. I'm talking about how the body is set up to receive the shock, whether it was emotional, biochemical, genetic, or physical. So the treatment program is set up almost before—and certainly during—the process of the insult to the body, or spirit, or soul.

The blueprint to get the patient well is there because the thing that made the body is the thing that sets up the blueprint. It creates compensation, to hold balance—what we call home-ostasis—as long as possible. Now I know that a physician hearing this would say, "This is crazy." Some ideas of health are extremely narrow-minded, so death is an insult to a physician. But it's much bigger than that. We can feel the movement of this force inside the body, unchanged in the adult from that of a newborn, and for 2 or 3 days after death. Then it seems to disappear. Now, I won't go into that, because that's getting on the edge and there are a lot of things I don't know about it. But I think Elisabeth Kübler-Ross has done a great service for humanity. She made us wake up to the fact that there was more to life than just what was apparent to us. She put love on the front line. It wasn't emotional love. It was an unconscious awareness of a bond that exists between every human being before you even meet the person. It's very much a reality.

The Practice of Osteopathy

The patient comes into the office. He's banged his head; he's got the vertigo. It's been going on for 3 years. So if we put our hands on the patient's body, the first thing we do is we open our senses to the peripheral space in the room and extend it to the horizon, by its own force. Not by intention. A lot of people like to use their intention, their attention, and they like to visualize. I know enough anatomy to know that if I tried to visualize anatomy, I would be making a terrible mistake, because there's so much variability. For me, those elements of inten-tion, attention, and visualization don't enter into this therapeutic process. They have places in other motifs but not in this.

Just like your lungs breathe in and out, attention breathes in and out. You know how you can relax the abdomen so you're not breathing up top all the time, so what would happen if your mind was allowed to breathe?

Instead of working with breath or air, we work with the breath of life. We let the mind breathe. This takes hard work. Some people start crying after they do it for the first time because they realize they were handmade, on purpose, by an artist who loves his work. They feel com-pletely embraced by life, and they get the magic. Then one struggles to get it to come back. That's when they fail because you have to let go of it. The first step in feeling this breath of life is not about palpation or poking around looking for lesions. You're feeling the Health of the patient first. You're feeling the breath of life as it comes into that living organism, into that person, and you're feeling the body, soul, and spirit as a complete unit of function. One does not partition. If you divide the body, soul, and spirit, even conceptually, under your hands, you're not doing what I'm talking about. You're doing something else.

I'm not talking about putting your hands on a person and saying, "This person is nervous" or "he's having a bad day." That's intuition. This is a totally different thing. You feel the breath of life come into the body and up the midline. The midline is a bioelectric line that's a remnant of the notochord formed in the embryonic plate. It's a primary line of orientation for all spatial dynamics. The breath of life comes in along that line, and then it creates changes in the body. It creates movements, fluids, tissues, and so forth.

This Health in the patient has been trying to heal him since the disease was imprinted. So in the case of the person with the vertigo, the Health has been working on it for 3 years. It has the blueprint to heal it. Now, the most common question I get right now from students is, "Why doesn't it heal the patient without our help?"

When you get into the vortex of the interface between the healing forces and distortion, there could be 100 pounds per square inch of pressure being held in the distortion. The force of the insult set up vectors in the body. I don't wish this on anyone, but let's say you saw a friend run over by an automobile. How many pounds per square inch do you think that shock is putting into your system? A lot. Enough so that if you had to, you could lift an automobile off the ground. Let's suppose that this healing force could balance out that hundred pounds per square inch in your body. If you put a hundred pounds per square inch of force into the body, you would rupture every artery, vein, and lymphatic. If it generated the force necessary to heal it directly, its own architecture would collapse.

So there's no gain. In other words, it has to heal through transubstantiation, which is changing the physical force into another form of force that it can deal with. At a certain point of softening, very quickly, just like the snap of a finger, it switches into another form of energy. The information for that change is coming from the breath of life. So the disproportion of the lesion or injury or disease is bounded on all sides. The disease process is an intelligent decision made by the breath of life to protect the organism from destroying the whole of itself. Disease is not the enemy. It's an intelligent, wise decision to come into balance.

Think about death. What do you reclaim at death?

You reclaim your original form. It's incredible when you see it. Do you know how many times, after a couple of treatments, a patient will say, "I feel more like myself." They will say, "I can see light moving across the surface of the leaves after it rains." I say, "It's always been there. That's not a mystical perceptual field. It's normal." We are naturally quite gifted.

What would happen if you claimed your original form? Wouldn't it be interesting to know who you were? Wouldn't it be interesting to know the intention of the breath of life when it made you?

This type of conversation, on a less detailed level, goes on with my patients most of the time. I'm not trying to talk them into it. I can't say I love them in the usual sense of the word, but I see something in them and I know it's coming out, and I ask, "Why not right now?"

Why don't they all get better? It's just not time. And that's the only answer. The patient should not be blamed for not getting well. If the standard medical people make mistakes in not giving patients enough time to understand the body, soul, and spirit as a unit, alternative healthcare practitioners make equally bad mistakes when they make the patient responsible for not being conscious enough to get well. It's no one's fault. It's more about tempo and "healing-time."

People aren't stupid. Most people are very bright. Some doctors think they're smarter than everybody else, but it's not true. We are all very human.

Teaching Students

I tell my students that they can practice any way they want, as long as it's safe, effective, and intelligent. They may not choose to practice the way I do. So they watch me treat patients, and I teach them based on their questions. Eventually, they want to imitate what I'm doing. So they imitate it a couple of times, and it works, and they think they have it, and then it doesn't work any more. So they get self-critical; their self-confidence level drops.

I try to convince them that they are already completely skilled. I try to get them to uncover something extraordinary in themselves. It's just a matter of time. If they let their minds relax and sit and listen to the patient the same way I do, they come up with answers. It usually takes about 2 years for them to accept this, before they'll try it with one patient. They may see 700 or 800 patients on their own during that part of their training, but usually it's 2 years before they'll try it. Then they wait and begin to find the Health.

I received a letter from a student yesterday. I trained her for 5 years. She spent 400 hours intermittently with me before going into a conventional family practice residency. She was recently assigned to a 92-year-old woman who had been in good health until she developed a growth on her neck, which was a squamous cell carcinoma.

My student wrote, "While the patient's physical condition quickly deteriorated, she was obviously fearful about what was happening to her, as was her family."

Now, here's an intern in a hospital, taking care of a terminally ill patient with a squamous cell cancer. I think it's pretty good she noticed that the patient and her family are frightened. Anyway, to make a long story short, she wrote, "I found myself alone with the patient, which was a rare moment. And while I was listening to her heart, I realized what I was really trying to do. On one level, I could feel the fear inside of this woman, almost a hum inside of her nervous system. But underneath it was a sweet, shapeless sense of certainty and health."

Then she wrote, "While I stayed there, I felt a huge shift."

Now, that means that the partition between the fear and the sweetness let go. The autonomic nervous system, the parasympathetic, and sympathetic came more into balance, probably through the effect of the treatment on her limbic system. She felt a shift, which she couldn't describe. She then wrote, "The patient seemed to relax. She had a quiet, peaceful night, which was very unusual, and when I checked with her this morning, she seemed very comfortable. She died a few hours later."

An extraordinary story. We don't know, but there's a good possibility the treatment let her slip across easily. Did she hasten the process of death? No. She helped the patient come into balance, and then the system went in the direction it would naturally go. We didn't make that decision, and that's what makes osteopathy a natural science.

The moment when someone perceives the sweetness, the ineffable original force, is a key moment. The recognition of the Health is a moment that's always there. You come to a conclusion about what the blueprint is and what it's trying to do, and you actually help it go in that direction.

This may be a very subtle force. You have to be right there at that interface, and you have to have watched and watched and watched it so that at the point where it interfaces, you can be present with the action of the blueprint. When you read the blueprint, you read the tone, the texture, the intention, the intensity, and the tempo as one thing. You've got all those five elements, plus. When they all balance, you accent exactly what is there. There are other ways to treat that are effective, but we're talking specifically about the breath of life and its effect on the body.

In Summary

I want to summarize the things I think are important. First is that the whole is real. Holistic medicine doesn't mean that you do homeopathy, acupuncture, and osteopathy, and give them antibiotics. Holistic medicine means that the patient is indivisible. A person cannot be broken down. Holistic medicine means you have the ability to perceive the whole, and not partition it, which is a big responsibility.

We talked about the laws of generation and healing; healing as the emergence of originality, and that it can happen at any moment.

Another thing is perceptual training. You have to own the gift you are given. Sir Laurens Van der Post wrote some great books on perception. He is an extraordinary teacher. If you want to understand instinctual perception, his work with the aboriginals in Africa is a great resource.

In David Abrams' book *The Spell of the Sensuous* he talks to some medicine men who know about the six directions of perception. It's a good book to help a person explore reality. Three years ago I gave a lecture on perception, about the importance of the horizon in our perception. It was completely from my own experience. When I read Abrams's book, it was a good affirmation for me.

For me, the essence is to allow your attention to breathe over the edge of the horizon, set it free, and then wait for it to come back on its own. There's a perceptual bridge here that we can teach people.

The other thing that we talked about was that the treatment program for the patient is prioritized by the forces that form the body so that when the patient comes in, the treatment program is already set up. We don't create the treatment process. We have to uncover it. That is a big sentence, and it should be explored.

We talked about transmutation and about how death is not a disease. It's important not to limit the patient to your practice.

If you don't feel like you're helping the patient, get some help. If the patient doesn't want to go anywhere else, then find out why he's afraid. But keep expanding the influences on that patient's life, and don't hold on to the patient.

It's very interesting that the natural healing community has taken on the allopathic approach to medicine. The patient comes in with symptoms, and he gets symptom remedies. It's like prescribing prescription drugs. They're caught up in an intellectual format, and they're not even aware of it. Natural medicine is natural medicine. Now, what does that word mean? Nature means everything that lives or breathes or is. So starlight? I bet a lot of people would get well if they just went for walks at night and could see the stars. All therapy is unique to the conditions of now, not the disease.

What good is it to start giving patients all kinds of things until we really understand the whole process? A real healer is not going to give exactly the same remedy for the same disease twice. So if we want to practice alternative medicine, we have to get rid of the menus. We have to look at the menus as a support system to buy time, but it's not the end of the road. We are not all on the same timing.

Traditional osteopathy is not about episodic healthcare. It's a long-term relationship with people wherever you practice. It takes years to get to know another human being. Some of the people I've treated for 30 years. I'm not threatened by their diseases, and I think that's important.

The other point that is important is that the student-teacher relationship is a long-term thing. We have to accept the responsibility of being taught. One of my greatest teachers was an old man I met on the river one day. I was way up country fishing and there was this incredible storm. He got in his car and headed back to town to his home. I didn't have anywhere else to go, so I asked him if I could come in his house. The storm came, and his house trailer was rocking on its foundation. The electric wires were down in the road, and there were sparks all over the place. There were ambulances and cars coming from everywhere.

I sat there with this old man at the table, and he never moved. We just sat there. Inside this trailer was a hovering stillness. It was incredible. We were just sitting in this trailer with all this chaos going on. After 20 minutes, everything calmed down. He looked at me and said, "I never could understand why people would rush around to make an emergency out of life." Then he just sat there. Twenty minutes later, he got up and started cooking a meal. He knew how to let the moment be the source and center of his temple; he was a living reminder.

I subsequently became good friends with him. That was an important moment, because I realized that it's not just osteopaths who are doing this kind of work and who can understand what's happening in the moment or be awake to that breath of life and that stillness. We all are aware of something greater and need to remember our Originality.

The health maintenance organization that we're all looking for is what makes an embryo. It generates and maintains life. I don't think there is anything wrong with centering your general practice on the whole human being. Not everybody is going to be interested, and not everybody is going to think that you're doing a great job. But that's not what it's about. What it's about is whether or not there's a general pattern to your practice that's useful to people and their well being.

And the last thing, in big black letters—***it's hard work.*** So prepare to really live! Thank you.

CHAPTER 33

JANET QUINN, RN, PhD
Therapeutic Touch and a Healing Way

Nurses have played an important role in the increased use of alternative and complementary medicine in schools, clinics, and hospitals throughout the world. The therapeutic value of caring, healing relationships is well known in the nursing community, as is the value of touch. One of nursing's leaders who has helped to bring this knowledge forward to a larger community is Janet Quinn, RN, PhD, currently an adjunct associate professor at the School of Nursing, University of Colorado Health Sciences Center, in Denver.

In addition to teaching, Dr. Quinn conducts research, lectures, writes, and maintains a private practice in spiritual direction in Boulder. She received her PhD in nursing research and theory development from New York University in 1982. During her career she has received many awards, including the Healers Award from the Nurse Healers and Professional Associates; the Edgar S. Wilson, MD, Fellowship Award from the International Society for the Study of Subtle Energies and Energy Medicine; and the Holistic Nurse of the Year award from the American Holistic Nurses Association.

In 1996, I interviewed Dr. Quinn at her office in Boulder, Colorado.

The turning point for me was in graduate school. As a new nurse, I walked into the intensive care unit (ICU) for the first time and was appalled at the way human beings were reduced to lumps of flesh lying in a bed. Patients were not covered. There was a tube in every orifice. People were talking back and forth over the patients like they weren't there. I was horrified and swore I'd never become like that. Several years later, I realized that I had become just that, so I left the ICU. First I taught in a diploma program in nursing, and then I went to New York University to get my master's degree.

Martha Rogers was teaching "The Science of Unitary Human Beings," the basic premise of which was that human beings are energy fields. It was unlike anything I'd ever heard, but I went through the program. The last semester the elective I took—and I took it because it was offered at the right time on the right day—was a course on Therapeutic Touch, taught by Dolores Krieger.

I have to tell you, it did not sit well with my Western scientific orientation. I thought it was preposterous. I sat in class with my arms folded across my chest thinking, "It's only a few more weeks." Then Dolores used me in a demonstration one day, and while I won't bore you with the whole story, at the end of that experience there wasn't any question in my mind that something had happened.

Shortly after I graduated, my mother was diagnosed with metastatic colon cancer, and I moved to California to take care of her. I used therapeutic touch and had many experiences that shattered my worldview. It left me in the position of either deciding that I couldn't trust my experience or changing my worldview. I chose the latter, which was to accept that there are dimensions in life other than those we can see and measure.

Therapeutic Touch

The simplest definition of Therapeutic Touch (TT) is that it's the use of the hands on or near the body with the intent to help or heal. The most critical part of that definition is that it's done with the intention to help or heal. This is what makes Therapeutic Touch different from casual touch or a procedural touch or even a back rub. The practitioner is completely focused in what we assume to be a meditative state, on this intention to help or heal. So the consciousness of the practitioner is very important.

Researchers prior to me looked at outcome. Their questions were, "What happens?" and "Is there an effect of this process?" I was interested in "How is there an effect?" I reasoned that if it was an energy exchange, we shouldn't have to touch people to get the effect. And if practitioners went through the same motions but didn't have the intention, they shouldn't get the same effect.

To study both of those issues—the issue of touch and the issue of intention—I developed a mimic treatment. In the real treatment, nurses first shift into "a centered state of consciousness." Centering is about quieting down, stilling the mind, and getting present in the here and now. It's about leaving all other distractions and demands aside, being completely present with this one person, right now, and in that state of consciousness, to formulate in one's own way the intention to be an instrument for healing. These two shifts happen in the consciousness of the practitioner before anything else happens.

Then the practitioner goes through a series of steps, moving the hands from head to toe over the body of the patient, attempting to perceive the quality of the energy flow. There is a step that clears the energy field, and a step that directs energy for healing. (Because the assumption is that it's energy, all the steps are framed in the context of energy, but this is a working hypothesis.) I developed a mimic treatment in which nurses were taught to go through exactly the same motions, but instead of centering and focusing on the intention to heal, I taught them to mentally perform serial sevens, which is a process of subtracting from a hundred by sevens.

Sixty coronary care patients were assigned randomly to one of the treatments. We looked at state anxiety before and after these treatments, and found that in the group that had received the real Therapeutic Touch there was a dramatic drop in anxiety. In the group that received the mimic there was no change in anxiety. The only thing that was different in these two groups was the intention. They went through the same steps for the same amount of time. Patients were given the same explanation. So the critical variable, from our perspective, is intention and consciousness.

But it absolutely confounds things if you try to use an experienced practitioner to do the mimic. That doesn't work. That's what I did in my second study, and it totally confounded the whole study. Once you've learned how to do it, you can't not intend to do this. You can't separate the intention to help and heal from these movements. They've become integrated, somehow, in the body/mind of the experienced practitioner. It was a great learning experience. It told us that the idea of intention is not necessarily just about a conscious decision that resides only in the aware mind. In an experienced practitioner, intention literally becomes embodied, becomes part of who that person is and he or she can't separate that anymore.

The theory is that in a healthy person the energy field is balanced, and in illness, at some level, the energy field has lost its balance. Therapeutic Touch is useful in helping the system restore itself to wholeness and balance. It stimulates the individual's natural healing response. We assume the healing response is intrinsic and resides in the individual and is not applied from the outside.

Clinical Experiences

When I first learned Therapeutic Touch, I felt nothing. I couldn't sense the changes in energy fields or temperature changes, but I knew it was important to have intention and to go through the motions with intention. I remember working with a postoperative patient who had knee surgery. She was in so much pain that she was crying, but her pain medications were not due for another 2 hours. I felt such a sense of compassion for her; I thought, "Let me try Therapeutic Touch."

So after explaining to her what I was going to do, I centered myself, assessed, felt nothing (as always), then went through the process of clearing and trying to help that pain move through her system. In about 5 minutes, the patient fell asleep and slept for 3 hours. When I saw her later, she said it was the first full relief she'd had from pain since the surgery. To me, that was another one of those turning points.

One of the things that I've experienced over the years is that pain responds very well to Therapeutic Touch. I'd even go a step further and say that from my clinical experience, the more acute (versus chronic) the pain, the better the response to Therapeutic Touch.

What is really ailing people when they finally come to the physician's office? They have whatever it is that they have, but they are at a point of frustration and hopelessness, or need some kind of connection. The studies are pretty clear. About 80% of what people come for is going to be self-limited. Instead of writing a prescription, what would it be like if the physician said, "Let's do 10 minutes of Therapeutic Touch"? But people have to make a decision about what kind of practice they want to have. It's a huge decision because it means that they have to shift their model of reality about what really helps and who we are. Once that shift happens, integrating the techniques is not a problem.

The Meaning of Holistic Medicine

The important shift is the shift in perspective and philosophy. Otherwise—and this is my observation about a lot of what we're seeing in alternative medicine—we take these techniques out of their context, which is a holistic, whole-person context that takes time, energy, attention, and intention, and we put them into the little black bag of tools, using them in the same old way that we do our techno-cure approach to healing.

There is an assumption that gets made by lots of people—patients and providers—that if you're using some kind of alternative therapy, you're providing holistic care. Nothing could be further from the truth. The fact that somebody's using something that's alternative to the mainstream means this tool is not usually found in the toolbox of mainstream health providers. That does not automatically make it holistic.

Our goal should not be to keep adding alternative practices to the same little black bag. The goal should be to change bags, to create a true healthcare system. Because what we have right now is really a sick-cure system. The focus is on the curing of disease, which is great, but it doesn't go far enough. So how do we create a true healing system, where healing is understood as meaning "to become more whole"? How do we create—in our individual practices, in our one-to-one relationships with patients—environments that facilitate the healing of the whole person? Those are the questions.

I call my practice "Haelan Work™." Haelan is the root form of the word *healing,* and it means to be or to become whole. Haelan Work is based on three fundamental assumptions. The first is that we are not responsible for our illnesses, but we are called to be responsive to them. The second is that all curing and healing emerges from within our own unique body/

mind/spirit, at times assisted by medication, surgery, and other therapies, but not due to them. And the third is acknowledging that as whole people, we are body, mind, and spirit; that spirit is always about mystery unfolding; and that healing is therefore fundamentally mysterious, beyond our control and manipulation, yet open to our conscious participation and intention.

These three assumptions are radically different from the assumptions we find in traditional Western medicine. But they also are radically different from what you find being discussed now as *holistic* or *alternative*. My point is that neither of those models (conventional or alternative) is appropriate because both assume that the healing power resides with the practitioner.

Some practitioners say that we are responsible for our illnesses, that we create our reality, and that we choose our illnesses so we can learn the lessons that the illness has to teach us. I find this position offensive. I would even go so far as to say that I find it immoral. It increases suffering for people who are already deeply suffering by telling them that their suffering is their own fault and their own choice. Now, the seductive nature of this reasoning is that the assumption that we've created our illness gives us the illusion that, "If I create it, maybe I can change it." It works great when it's working. When people do get better and go into remission, they have this tremendous sense of power and control. The problem is when the exacerbation occurs. The person is left with nothing but having to face or feel that they've failed. That's what I consider immoral—this totally needless suffering. Death is not a failure. Death is the most natural thing there is.

There is no answer to the question "Why did this happen?" But there is an answer to the question: "What can I make of this?"

Sacred Spaces

The first thing to remember if we want to create a healing environment is that we are the environment. We are the most present, most influential part of that environment for our patients when they're sitting in our office. All of the colors on the wall, the pictures, the lighting, the windows, and the plants are beautiful; they nourish us. But we are the biggest part—we fill that room for that patient at that time.

This is hard to face because it brings a whole other set of responsibilities. It's not just about making the office nice. If we accept the basic premise that we are energetic and that at some level we are not separate from each other—that we are one—then the question becomes: "What are you doing with your energy while you are with this patient?" How can you become a healing energy with which this patient interacts so that healing happens? Just by being in your space with you, does healing happen? How do we do that?

At least part of the answer is that we have to do our own work. We have to become whole people and live an authentic life. We have to become healed. Instead of saying, "How can we change the environment?", we must ask, "How do I change myself?"

It doesn't have to be so big. It can be a simple thing. The first step of Therapeutic Touch is learning how to center. It's a simple shift in consciousness. It's a breath in and a breath out and getting present. So it doesn't have to be this huge, dramatic thing, where we all undergo a huge personal transformation to become enlightened before we see another patient. We can begin simply by being conscious of our effect on the patient's environment; understanding that we are it for that patient at that time. And then out of that awareness, begin to work with our own energy.

Ritual is important, too. It doesn't have to be anything anybody else can observe. A ritual should focus attention and consciousness. For instance, the one thing that nurses do the most each day is wash their hands. So what would happen if they attached a ritual to the hand-washing so that when they finished with one patient and washed their hands, they imagined that they were letting go of the whole interaction with the first patient? The words I use are "I release you. Go in peace." That's how I end every Therapeutic Touch session. Let the water wash over your hands, take a deep breath, and let go. One can begin to see how working from a place of center is actually good for the caregiver, rather than being another demand.

Therapeutic Touch is definitely as good for the practitioner as it is for the patient. I see Therapeutic Touch as the most basic energetic therapy. In my mind, if people want to do energy work, Therapeutic Touch is the place to start. It's the most basic approach to working with energy. I just wonder why some people tend to dismiss Therapeutic Touch. If you're willing to use acupuncture, why would you dismiss Therapeutic Touch? It's the same theoretical system. Instead of using needles or pressure, you use touching. Something about it must be threatening. Acupuncture is more like medicine. You have a tool. You can still remain one step removed from a more personal interaction.

The predecessor is the laying on of hands. That's probably the oldest and most basic healing technique. You'll find laying on of hands in the Bible, and you can find references to some type of laying on of hands in the earliest recorded histories. The difference is that the laying on of hands is typically done within some kind of religious framework. It's linked with faith. The hands are laid on, and (supposedly) the faith of the recipient is what allows the healing to happen.

In Therapeutic Touch, there's no assumption that the recipient must believe anything. They don't even have to know that it's happening for there to be an effect. It need not take place in a religious or spiritual framework. It may, if that is the belief system held by the practitioner, but it need not, which makes it applicable across the board.

With the laying on of hands, there's an assumption that God is acting through the person, that it's a special power. That is another distinction between these two. We assume that the ability to use Therapeutic Touch is a natural human potential that can be actualized with compassion, and the person doing it has no special powers.

Holotropic Breathwork

In 1986, I was doing a lot of Therapeutic Touch with counseling. I found that my patients and I would sometimes get into very different states of consciousness, and with some, there would be a release of deep feelings and old memories, and sometimes there would be experiences that would happen that they couldn't even describe. They felt like they were regressing to young childhood states. I was fascinated by that but not particularly well prepared to handle it. There were times when I would have a sense that I was beyond myself and the patients were beyond themselves and that we were meeting in some other place.

Months later, I got a flyer in the mail about transpersonal psychology. Then I found out about Stan Grof and Holotropic Breathwork. I thought it would be a wonderful complement to the work with Therapeutic Touch because they have very similar understandings. So I studied with Grof and became certified.

Holotropic Breathwork was developed by Stan and Christina Grof. It is a technique in which people lie down in a very protected space, both psychologically and physically, and increase their rate of breathing until it is faster and deeper than normal. Very loud, evocative music is used to assist the desired shift in consciousness. It is an approach to accessing nonordinary states of consciousness with the belief that healing can emerge spontaneously if the person accesses these other nonordinary states.

Therapeutic Touch and Holotropic Breathwork are similar in philosophy but radically different in approach. What is similar in their philosophy—and what underlies all of the "techniques" that I use in my practice—is the assumption that the wisdom and healing comes from the person, the patient. In Holotropic Breathwork, the assumption is that the psyche knows exactly what it needs to do for its healing and that the job of the facilitator, once again, is to be a midwife and not the person doing the healing.

The centered state of consciousness in Therapeutic Touch could be called *nonordinary reality*. We could define *ordinary consciousness* as that state of awareness in which we find ourselves most of the time. When you're racing through the airport trying to catch a plane—that is ordinary consciousness. Therapeutic Touch asks you to leave all of that and come to a place that is more inward and very quiet and focused.

My Patients

Often the reason for entry into my practice is physical, because I'm a nurse and my emphasis is on Therapeutic Touch and healing. It is often people with cancer. I also see AIDS patients, and then some people will come just for Therapeutic Touch for an acute injury. Some are short-term. I only see them two or three or four times, and they are gone. Other people are working on their healing process, and that's a long-term relationship.

One of the questions I ask when people want to work with their cancer is: "Do you want to live?" It seems obvious. "I'm here, aren't I?" But it's not. Sometimes they don't want to live, but they're doing this because of their significant others.

If their answer is "Yes, I want to live," the second question is "Why? What is it that you want to live for?" Then I really try to listen to what part of them is talking to me. Often the first answer isn't their heart speaking. It's their "shoulds" and their "ought-tos." But when people can begin to feel what part of them is unlived, it's often quite different from what they think they should be living for.

The process varies. Some weeks we might just talk. Some weeks we might talk and then do Therapeutic Touch. Sometimes I might be teaching them meditation or Centering Prayer.

Centering Prayer

For some time now, my spiritual practice has been "Centering Prayer," which comes out of the Christian contemplative tradition. I was introduced to it by a monk named Thomas Keating at the Snowmass Monastery in Colorado.

I was raised Catholic but promptly left the church at age 18. Meanwhile, I learned Therapeutic Touch, and since 1974, I have been asking to be used as an instrument for healing. Therapeutic Touch, at its core, is the offering of unconditional love and compassion, and so for years I asked over and over again to be an instrument for unconditional love and compassion. This, of course, was spiritual practice, but I did not realize it. Then, quite suddenly, while I was a visiting fellow in immunology at a university by the ocean, I had an ongoing series of spiritual experiences that, at the time, were terrifying to me. I thought it was happening out of the blue, out of nowhere. But my sense of it now is that it was the natural product of years of spiritual practice by another name. All of our careful language, our conceptual frameworks, the way we describe things, cannot constrain the Divine.

During this process I found Thomas Keating's *Open Mind, Open Heart* and discovered that there is this whole extraordinary tradition within the Christian church that I knew nothing about, even though I was raised Catholic. I wasn't taught these things, but they exist nevertheless. There is this rich tradition of contemplation and meditation and spiritual practice that I had looked everywhere else for. Discovering this really helped me cooperate with the conversion experience and return home to my Catholic roots.

The experience is difficult to describe. I was drawn inexplicably and beyond my will into this little church on the island. I tried to ride by on my bicycle, but I could not ride by. When I went in there, I shook. I'd go in for 5 minutes and run out and bicycle home in a panic. This went on for days, every day. One thing led to another and little tiny steps brought me in more and more. But the most profound part of it was finally sitting in the mass and listening to the gospel. The reading at the time was the story of when Jesus was asked, "What's the most important commandment?" And Jesus said, "To love your God with all your heart, with all your soul, and all your mind. And to love your neighbor as yourself." And when I heard those words, I heard them not with my ears and mind, but I heard them as if they were being spoken inside my own heart. There's no way to describe this, but I heard them inside myself, and I heard the absolute truth of them. That is it. That's the kernel of what happened.

Thomas Keating once said to me that the only point of life is to become a more and more transparent manifestation of the love of the Divine. He looked at me, and his eyes were sparkling, and he said, "You're not here alone, you know." And that's the point. We're here for service. We're here to love other people. It's not just about us as individuals. So this is my passion now. Not to convert people to Catholicism but to help people recover that sense of connection with the Divine. How can I help touch a part of them the way those words touched inside of me, so that they know they are loved—that every single creature is loved completely and deeply and held with utter tenderness by the Divine? How can I help bring people to that place? Because when that happens, we'll stop killing each other.

I have no idea how this path is going to unfold or what it's going to look like, but I know that's the purpose.

This is hard to talk about because there's a real hesitancy to bring God into our discussion. It's like we can't quite talk about it in a public forum. It's not popular. We won't even use the word *God* in polite company. Maybe you can get away with it if you talk about *the one*, or *the divine*—if you use a little *d* instead of a big *D*. Maybe this would be okay. It's a fascinating problem because if you ask most people, "What do you think is the most fundamental longing of the human heart?", they answer truthfully, "Is it not for union with the Divine?" It is a tragedy. We're lost, with more and more knowledge, and less and less wisdom.

Healing

When I say all healing is self-healing I mean that all healing is a process of emergence. It emerges from within the wholeness of the given individual, the body/mind/spirit of the particular person. The way we typically think is that we give the drug and the patient gets better, so we have cured him. The cure comes from outside. My understanding of it is, even when we're talking about drugs and surgery, the healing comes from within. We have plenty of cases in which we give people medication and the expectations are that they should do well, but they don't respond. And we have cases in which people shouldn't get better—it's really clear they're going to die—and they do fine. *So something else is going on besides what we're doing.* It's the person doing the healing who must be able to use the drug; he has to be able to take it in and metabolize it. It has to happen within the person.

But when I say all healing emerges from within, I don't assume that it's under the control of the person. That's a critical distinction. It is a misunderstanding to say, "Healing comes from within; therefore the person is responsible for it." The mind, body, and spirit are one, so this is the question: Who decided the mind is in charge? Why have we made that assumption? It's a Western, intellectual, elitist assumption that the mind is the best. But maybe the mind is not in charge. So, to assume that because healing emerges from within, that it's under control, is illogical.

To me, the question of how healing emerges is part of the fundamental mystery. I struggle with this and lately have been struggling with it almost daily. Does the Divine break through in healing physical illnesses? Certainly there are people who believe that. It's a mystery to me. I don't understand it. And part of my conflict, my struggle, is that if God can break through, why would God ever choose not to break through? This God is infinite mercy and compassion. Would this same consciousness choose to leave one person suffering and another person not, simply because the latter had the right words? Said the right prayer? Had the best healer? I can't see such arbitrariness or capriciousness in God. I don't have the answer to this. I don't even have a theory about it.

Therapeutic Touch was developed in a secular framework and continues to be practiced in a secular framework. However, every person has her or his own belief system, and everything one does is filtered through it. I would ask to be an instrument of the Divine in my own work. That might be different from the way an atheist practices Therapeutic Touch, but an atheist could do it because it's simply a technique, a tool.

Florence Nightingale said that the nurse's job is to put the patient in the best condition for nature to act on him or her. That's what Therapeutic Touch is. It is an attempt to get this system in the best possible place so that a person's natural healing capacity can emerge. If I take it a step further and ask, "How does the Divine break into that?" I could say, "Can you imagine a better condition for healing than feeling held in the lap of the Divine in unconditional love and compassion?"

All of our years of accumulated scientific knowledge tell us that people who are loved and relaxed heal the best. Social support literature tells us that our connectedness with each other is primary, not secondary, to our health and our healing. So we know that there is something about our shared humanity on which our very survival is contingent. If we as practitioners can make that kind of connection with people and hold them in that place, somehow, whether through energy or with information, at some level these people can drink in the sure knowledge that they are loved, and this is a profound healing opportunity.

But again, in our culture, it certainly would be the last thing anybody would consider valid. They'd say, "Oh, isn't that nice! That caring. How nice." And we not only dismiss it, we demean it.

I remember one of my AIDS clients. I'll never forget Joseph. We worked a long time together. I was leaving for a trip and was very worried about whether Joseph was going to make it. So I decided to do a little ritual. On the last visit before my trip, I brought a little stone rose-quartz heart with me. He had brought me a card. As we sat together, he looked at me and got a little teary. He said, "I really love you. I never knew I could love anybody, but I really love you."

I said, "I really love you, too." And I gave him the little heart. When I came back, I saw him only one more time. He was very debilitated, lots of dementia. We sat together, and his sisters said, "He's been waiting for you." He looked at me and said, "I feel like I'm losing my mind." And I said, "You are losing your mind, Joseph. Don't struggle with it. It's all right." He died a few weeks later.

The point is this man was dying, but this man was healing. He had the experience of unconditional love and connection that had always eluded him.

You see, people get worse all the time. Many of my patients get physically worse, but that's different from not healing. To me, healing is about the emergence of new or right relationships at one or more levels of the human experience. So if people are coming to me, somehow, something happens. You know, it's not necessarily a big process. It's not like their life is necessarily transformed. But I think I know what you're talking about. There clearly are people who die of cancer, screaming and fighting, and have no sense of peace about it. That's reality.

Again, my position is to realize that I am the facilitator of this person's process and not the one to judge. There's no way that I can judge if that's a wrong way to die. Maybe that's just the best way that person can die for now. Mothers are like that. If a woman who has a couple of little kids is dying of breast cancer, she is not someone who's going to move to acceptance and letting go without absolutely fighting with every cell in her being. And I support her in that.

Many doctors and nurses burn out and feel like failures if their patients die. But that's because in the traditional model the measure of your success is, ultimately, whether you prevent death. So how can you ever be a success?

We should change our measure of success. If the measure of success is going to be the prevention of death, we're ultimately going to fail 100% of the time. The goal must change to healing. When we focus on healing, instead of curing, or along with it, we can be 100% optimistic, right up to and including death.

Some traditions call death *the ultimate healing*. So there's reason to continue to be able to work in a way that is hopeful and optimistic. Healing can always happen. Okay, we had a bad session today? Healing can still happen. Because the door is never closed, something new and creative can always emerge.

Angeles Arrien talks about the "Four-Fold Way." The last step is to "let go of attachment to the outcome." I see that as a basic principle of healing practice. We must let go of our attachment to getting a particular outcome. As soon as we decide what outcome we think we must have, we effectively preclude all other possible outcomes. If we really see that healing comes from within the person and we understand that it's going to be a mystery unfolding, there's no way we can know what the outcome's going to be—so what's the point of staying attached to any particular one? We can have our hopes and work toward them. Yet we must be willing to shift as the process unfolds.

I would say that once all this is grasped deeply by the practitioner, it is ultimately liberating. We can bring our full humanity into service to this person, with unconditional love and compassion—fearless, because we know the ultimate outcome is not in our hands. Perhaps it is here, in the depths of our shared humanity, that the Divine breaks into our lives and into the healing moment. Everyone will die. But will everyone die knowing love?

CHAPTER 34

DOLORES KREIGER, RN, PhD

Healing with Therapeutic Touch

Dolores Krieger, RN, PhD, is a registered nurse, researcher, theorist, and author. In 1972, with colleague Dora Kunz, Dr. Krieger developed Therapeutic Touch, a system for healing primarily using the hand chakras. In the last 25 years, Dr. Krieger has personally taught more than 52,000 healthcare professionals the use of Therapeutic Touch. Therapeutic Touch is now taught in 90 countries worldwide.

Dr. Krieger received her PhD in nursing science at New York University and is professor emerita of nursing at New York University, where she taught at the master's and doctoral levels for many years. She is the author of *The Therapeutic Touch: How to Use Your Hands to Help or to Heal, Therapeutic Touch Inner Workbook: Ventures in Transpersonal Healing, Accepting Your Power to Heal: The Personal Practice of Therapeutic Touch,* and *Therapeutic Touch as Transpersonal Healing.* She also has a tape series called *The Audio Series in Therapeutic Touch,* produced by Sounds True Recordings.

In the fall of 1997, I drove 10 miles on a dirt road up the side of a mountain to interview Dr. Krieger at her home, "The Rockery," in the Rocky Mountains of Columbia Falls, Montana, where deer, bear, and mountain lions also live.

The reason anyone comes to the health professions is out of a sense of compassion for humans, but nonetheless, I never thought I would be able to "heal." By chance I was exposed to the research of a religious group called the "Layman's Group." These were people from various religions in the United States—scientists and clergy—who wanted to scientifically test certain biblical statements. They decided that laying on of hands could be objectively tested, so they brought in many healers and studied what the healers were doing and how their patients were responding.

Fortunately for me, I happened to see some of this because I drove a friend, Dora Kunz, to the meetings. They had invited her because she has had very unusual perceptual abilities since she was a child and could perceive what was happening energetically during the healing process.

At the time, Dora and I were on the board of trustees for the Pumpkin Hollow Foundation, so we invited one of the foremost healers, Oscar Estebany, to come to their site in the Berkshire Mountains and do his healing work. The idea was primarily to help people and also to take the study into more depth. Dora, Mr. Estebany, Dr. Otelia Bengsten, and I—simply because I was a nurse and a PhD—made up the core of the study group. Mr. Estebany saw patients at Pumpkin Hollow Farm for about a week for three consecutive years. It was amazing to watch. He was by no means an ostentatious person. He was like somebody's grandfather, except that he had a very sharp, well-waxed mustache and was extraordinarily kind. He had been an officer in the Hungarian cavalry. At one point, when his own horse became injured, he was faced with having to kill it. Instead, he stayed up all night with the horse's head in his lap and tried to do whatever he could for the animal. In the morning, the horse was back in the field. That's how he found he had healing abilities.

For a while he thought all he could do was heal animals, but one Sunday a neighbor's child became very ill. There were no doctors around, so the father picked up the child, ran to Mr. Estebany, and asked him to do to his child what he had done for the horses. At first, Mr. Estebany refused because he thought that it would be sacrilegious. But finally, out of compassion, Mr. Estebany did what he could for the child. And the child got well.

After that he decided to spend the rest of his life helping people, so he retired from the cavalry and emigrated to Canada.

As I watched him, I kept thinking to myself, "Wouldn't it be wonderful if nurses could do this?" I knew that I needed to study the phenomenon of healing in some way that would exert control and be substantive. Eventually, as I reviewed my notes on hematology, I realized that one objective way of seeing whether anything significant was occurring physiologically during the laying on of hands was through the hemoglobin and the hematocrit ratio in the patient's blood.

We did the first study, and the hemoglobin and hematocrit ratio significantly increased in the patients who had laying on of hands, whereas in the controls, it remained the same. It was the first substantive and truly objective study that had ever been done on healing in the U.S. Now, the study has been replicated all over the world. It has been found to have both acceptable validity and reliability, and its findings are considered to be a matter of fact.

Dora felt that she could understand the healing process well enough to teach it. We had about 50 health professionals in the group at that time, so she began teaching the laying on of hands, and I was one of the students. Patients told me that they felt an energy flow from my hands. Once I realized that I was having an effect, nobody was safe—the slightest cough, the suggestion of headache, and there I was. As we gained experience, we realized we were teaching more than laying on of hands. We sharpened and formalized our technique and named it "Therapeutic Touch."

In the early 1970s, a group from the Menninger Foundation held annual conferences on healing consciousness. They invited about 90 researchers on human consciousness. I was one. They also invited Dora because of her unique abilities. The man who ran the conference is the granddaddy of biofeedback—Dr. Elmer Green. One day he called several of us together and said, "You eight people are into healing. We wonder whether you would be willing to do a spontaneous study." He explained that we would work on a patient, and then a panel of five medical doctors would judge what we had done.

We were standing in a circle outside the breakfast room, and I happened to be on his right-hand side. He was going around the circle from left to right, asking each person if they would like to take part. Only two people before me had agreed to participate. They were Dora and another man, who also had clairvoyant abilities. I thought to myself, "This is going to be like the white hats against the black hats because of their extreme differences," and when it came to my turn, I found myself saying yes just to add diversity.

Each of us had 15 minutes with the patient. A scribe took down whatever we said. We could ask the patient anything except what was the matter. Then we were asked to make a diagnosis. The panel compared our information to the patient's records and scored us. Dora, Jack, and the other clairvoyant got 100%, and I got 80%, which really awakened me to the reality of what we were doing.

I hadn't realized how objective the process actually was. That's what gave me the courage to go forward. I began to realize that it is not the faith or the specific religion of the individual that is important to the healing process. It is important to the person but not to the process;

healing occurs in every culture in the world. Other factors, in addition to one's belief system, are significant, which is why Dora and I decided to develop Therapeutic Touch, which does not have a religious context.

Then, in 1975, I was teaching nursing science at the master's and doctoral levels at New York University, and I thought to myself, "Therapeutic Touch is doing so much good, we really ought to be teaching it here." So I developed and proposed a formal curriculum at the graduate level, and it was accepted by the Dean's Advisory Council. I originally thought that the nurses in pediatrics and medical-surgery would be the most interested in taking the course, but, to my astonishment, the people who have been most active are nurses who work in the intensive care unit (ICU)—particularly in the neonatal ICU—and in the emergency room. The other group that I'm delighted with are the people in hospice. So that's how Therapeutic Touch got started. It's been 30 years since we developed Therapeutic Touch, and that class still continues to be in the curriculum at the master's level. The university named it "Frontiers of Nursing."

Then and Now

I don't know that the basic premises have changed so much as they've shifted. One thing that has grown stronger is the realization that Therapeutic Touch is a process, and another is our understanding of the dynamics of that process. One element that differentiates Therapeutic Touch from other healing modalities is that you begin by centering your consciousness. Many people do that, but the unique thing we do is that we stay on center throughout the entirety of the Therapeutic Touch process, so you are using that centering milieu as a background against which you do the techniques. In trying to form a liaison with one's higher orders of self and under the urge of compassion, you can make a deeper contact with the patient, and that contact may be transpersonal in nature.

It's not easy to describe, but it seems that what happens is that, if you are actively—e.g., consciously—engaged in being on center, that engagement can change your worldview. If that happens, you begin to find that your lifestyle must also change. Further, if your worldview and lifestyle change, you are edging into a nice definition of transformation of personality. This is what can happen to people who use Therapeutic Touch. It's a dual process. One aspect involves helping and healing the person who is ill, the other concerns what happens within the therapist, her inner work.

Frequently, the person who is being healed admires the healer. What we do, once we realize that this has occurred—and if the healee wishes to learn how to help others—is teach the healee some of the basics of Therapeutic Touch. I call it *peer therapeutics*. When we're sure the patient is competent in Therapeutic Touch, we select a person who has the same problems or illness that the first patient had. Now, that first patient has changed roles. He or she is now playing the role of healer on a patient who had the same experience. What invariably happens—this is the "aha"—is that these novice healers often get a tremendous insight into what their own problems had been when they, themselves, were ill. And, of course, that's the purpose of teaching them Therapeutic Touch in the first place.

In the mid-1980s, I did a study in which I taught "pregnant husbands" how to do Therapeutic Touch on their pregnant wives. That study worked out so well that many people in the experimental group continued Therapeutic Touch after the completion of the study, frequently involving their whole family in it. We even have second and third generations now who do Therapeutic Touch *en famille*. In some cases, it went into the community. People told their neighbors and relatives about their use of Therapeutic Touch; they saw the effects and became interested and communicated this to others. Thus Therapeutic Touch has the potential of becoming a social dynamo.

Of course, the other thing that has happened is that Therapeutic Touch therapists have diversified tremendously. They range from medical doctors to professional actors. One of the things that actors and actresses find in using it is that they begin to develop a greater sensitivity for the audience's reactions. Their rapport with the audience actually gets better. Of course, that's one of the things that happens with Therapeutic Touch, for the healer-healee interaction is essentially the art of relationship. We're really teaching the therapeutic effects of a vital human energy, and in the process, you understand yourself and other people better.

A Story of a Healing

By and large, we find that it's not the individual illness that tells us about the validity of Therapeutic Touch, but to ask the question, "What systems are most sensitive to Therapeutic Touch?" And the system that is most sensitive is the autonomic nervous system. Next would be dysfunctions of the lymphatic, genitourinary, and circulatory systems, and then musculoskeletal problems. You see, there are certain systems that are very sensitive to Therapeutic Touch, some that sensitive under certain conditions, and others that are not at all sensitive to Therapeutic Touch. For instance, the female endocrine systems—dysmenorrhea, amenorrhea, problems with conception, the whole process of pregnancy—are much more sensitive to Therapeutic Touch than are the corresponding male systems.

One of the things that surprised me was Therapeutic Touch's effect on manic-depressives. We are very good at bringing a person down during the manic stage in bipolar disorder. And we've had success with people at the other end of that scheme—in catatonia, for instance. Strangely, in many cases, once catatonic persons regain their normalcy, they somehow know which nurse it was who did Therapeutic Touch on them. In one case, after the patient came out of his coma, he called the nurse by her nickname, which only her friends knew. He had somehow picked it up when everybody thought he was not aware of his surroundings.

One of the things the autonomic nervous system controls is the process of urination. In one case, a hospitalized man was not producing any urine whatsoever. The medical team finally left the patient's room to schedule the surgery to remove his kidney because they felt there was nothing more they could do. But the nurse assigned to the case decided to do Therapeutic Touch. Within an hour, the man urinated. Not much, but he urinated. However, he then urinated again a little bit later, and the urination kept up so that by the time the doctors came back to tell the nurse when the operation was to be scheduled, the man had urinated so much it was startling, since he was thought not to be able to urinate at all. The end result was that he never had that operation. Because urine can be measured, the scheduled operation was canceled, and all of this is in the records. This is a concrete example of the value of Therapeutic Touch.

So these are the things that excite me. It says two things: one is that we have by no means reached the outer limits of Therapeutic Touch; the other is that we really don't understand human consciousness, as occurs in the case of catatonia in the previous example. Something similar to what I've related above also occurs with healees who have had a cerebrovascular accident (stroke) and been in a coma, during which time they've been treated with Therapeutic Touch. They, too, have known which nurses were doing Therapeutic Touch with them and were aware that Therapeutic Touch was being done with them.

Here's another story. There was a woman named Patricia who had a type of cancer from which she was going to die in a very short time. We gave her Therapeutic Touch, and she was so moved by the experience that she learned Therapeutic Touch herself, became a volunteer at a hospice, and, to this day, does Therapeutic Touch to help hospice patients in their final days. That was 12 years ago, and she has taught many volunteers how to do Therapeutic Touch during that time.

These are not just isolated instances. One commonality among those who do Therapeutic Touch is that they say their life changes dramatically. It's not the Therapeutic Touch; it's that they, in the process of compassionately using Therapeutic Touch, change themselves. It's very potent in that regard. Of course, the empowerment comes from the act of sustained centering— that is, the process of staying on center during the entire Therapeutic Touch process. It becomes ingrained in your life, and, because of that, you change. Your perceptions become different. You develop the chakras in your hands, and as you begin to get that sensitivity, you realize that you don't "stop" at your skin. You literally don't stop at your skin. Over time comes the realization that not only don't you stop at your skin but that your neighbor doesn't stop at his or her skin. Once that happens, you begin to understand more clearly that relationships are something very different from what we think they are. You now look at all animate beings, whether people or trees, as completely different experiences from what your culture taught you to expect. You know that your human energies are constantly and dynamically interacting with the vital energy fields of others in a manner not thought of in Biology 101.

Centering

We use the term *centering* in three different ways in our culture. One use of the word refers to grounding, in the psychological sense of getting oneself stabilized or centered. But that's not what I'm talking about. Another kind of centering is called *centering prayer*—getting oneself into a state of grace. I'm not talking about that, either. The centering I'm talking about is an in-turning in the sense of trying to find the center, the locus of dynamic equilibrium, of your own consciousness. When you do this, at first there's a sense of quietude. Then, as you begin to use Therapeutic Touch as an act of compassion, something else happens. You have a person whom you want to help, and you want to understand how you can bring that help about, and this forces you to try to understand what is deepest within you that could span that breach. So the practice of Therapeutic Touch forces you to begin to understand the nature of your own interiority, and that, in turn, forces personal transformation.

In the process of attempting that, instead of perceiving outward—the sun is in my face, the wind is on my body—your perception is inward. This is what you explore, and your perceptions themselves change. It'll happen in a comparatively short time, and it captivates your attention because it's all about you. It's your consciousness examining itself. You become aware of the fact that there are "potentials" within yourself. And as you begin to test them out, you learn how to actualize them. And in that actualization—because the original goal was helping that other person and so you could do this objectively—you begin to sharpen your own skills as a human being.

I'm saying this in very simple terms, but it is not simple. It's hard work. It demands an ability to concentrate. One of the greatest allies that we have in this process is compassion, and the fact that the act of compassion can carry you far beyond yourself. In Therapeutic Touch we appreciate that transforming process. In the teaching of Therapeutic Touch, we help people recognize what is occurring within themselves, and much of our teaching is geared toward fostering that inner ability to perceive. On the average, it takes about $2\frac{1}{2}$ weeks. I've taught well over 52,000 health professionals by now on that basis, and I can tell you that it does, indeed, take about $2\frac{1}{2}$ weeks, assuming the person actively practices it. If it's just a head exercise, that's different. But if they consciously work at it, such people find their own abilities sharpened and potentials being actualized, most of which they were previously unaware.

The Process of Therapeutic Touch

Therapeutic Touch is a conscious process. Briefly, after centering yourself, you explore the vital energy field, using the hand chakras, attempting to find the imbalances in a person's vital energy field. Then you try to get whatever it is that you encountered back into balance again. After you have rebalanced the energy, you do another assessment to see whether you have done any good and to plan the next session, if that is still needed.

If you can, imagine yourself on center during all of this process, using those "inner perceptions" to make sense of the data coming from the chakras. You're trying to understand a whole different language here—a language of human energetics—and you come across an area of imbalance that talks to you with something as simple as a tingling sensation. However, most frequently, what people feel are temperature changes, like heat or cold in a particular area of the vital energy field. Let me give you a personal example with cold. Cold can have several meanings, depending on the type of cold you feel. There's one type that means—for me, anyway—that the endocrine system is out of balance. Another type of cold, which feels like a frigid vacuum, tells me there is a malignancy. It's very different from the cold that tells me it's an endocrine gland that is the problem. It has distinct characteristics of its own, and so I'd never mistake one for the other.

In the end, you just don't find out that a person has a headache—you also get a sense of that person as an individual, because you are working in her personally "designed" vital energy field, which is in constant flux and dynamic movement. It's constantly translating its inner self to you. So it doesn't surprise me that one of the faculties that you're developing while doing this is, for instance, telepathy, as a study I did some years ago pointed out. This ability, telepathy, is not dramatic. You will simply begin to recognize it in little things. And as you begin to realize that you have that ability, you add that to the armamentarium of skills you bring to the healing process.

The life force is very difficult to describe because we don't have the appropriate words in our culture. Strangely enough, there are 94 cultures in this world that understand that you don't stop at your skin. But not in the Western culture. We have no difficulty understanding that the way my voice is getting into the cassette is through a kind of energy we call "the electromagnetic field." We have no difficulty taking measurements with lab instruments and saying, "That electromagnetic field extends this far." But we have difficulty realizing that the same fields play through us as well, eliciting the behaviors that mark us as human beings.

It shouldn't come as any surprise either that the major happening between the two of us that's occurring right now is on a nonphysical level. You see my hand waving in the air, but what you're listening to is more than my words. It's the tonality, the pitch. It's the meaning. But it's very difficult for our rather mechanized culture to understand that what's being transmitted, energetically, is meaning. Let me change the metaphor for a moment. Imagine that a boy and a girl are at a cocktail party. The boy is at one end of the room, and the girl is at the other end. They suddenly look at each other, and something happens between the two of them. We call this "love at first sight," but we cannot forget that "something" nonphysical occurred, and whatever it was, it transmitted itself through a crowded, noisy cocktail room, and on target.

We think of that as happenstance. We don't realize that it's part of the way we work. The greatest part of our understanding of our consensual reality is through the kinds of interpretations we are willing to accept about what's happening beyond our skin. That's what we call reality.

From our point of view, such things as emotions are also energetic. Now, how can I demonstrate that? Imagine the following scenario: a husband and wife are violently arguing with one another. There's a little child, four or five, who is in the same room, watching his parents fight. Now, you could hook up that child to a meter and you would find everything from an acceleration of heartbeat to a dramatic galvanic skin response, all of which could concretely measure the emotional upheaval that's going on in the child, who really isn't part of that violent argument. You could translate that incident into almost any one of a thousand situations that you might want to examine in the laboratory, and what you will be forced to recognize is that, indeed, something nonphysical is occurring in that emotional atmosphere that provokes the child's physiological indices to change.

These things tell us that we are creatures of the nonphysical more than the physical. The physical just gets us from place to place, but the nonphysical allows us to dream and imagine and become fully human, if you will. And it's in that urge to become fully human that we really find our place, our meaning in life, whatever that may be.

Now, to get back to the realm of healing, what we find in Therapeutic Touch is that there are certain ways of either influencing or actually moving these energies. In terms of pure physicality, there is something one can do that turns out to be quite dramatic when it's done well. Take the case of somebody who has high blood pressure. If you do a Therapeutic Touch assessment on the vital energy field of this person, you will find that around the neck—there is a nerve plexus there that regulates the blood pressure to the brain—the energy flows feel absolutely crazy, chaotic, without rhyme or reason. Moreover, you will find that the "feeling" in the chakra at that site is one of tension and pressure, like a balloon filled with water beyond the point where it should burst. But you can do a very simple maneuver that in Therapeutic Touch we call *unruffling*. You bring your hand quite close to the body where the phrenic nerve is and then bring it out—both hands, bring them out. It's almost like you are pushing a pressure front ahead of your hands, and then you just let it dissipate. You gently "push" it out, and then let it go.

But it's not just a mechanical process. You are combining this with specific intentionality, and when combined with intentionality, it's not "just" pushing out. You can actually dissipate that confusion, that chaos, that intense pressure. Lo and behold, not only will the person feel better, you can take a blood pressure reading and find that it has gone down significantly.

Now, that's something that even a person who's a novice in TT can learn how to do. And it has been done so many times and tested so many times that I can talk about it freely. So here is a good instance in which it's really crucial that you understand what you're doing—because, if I just went through the motions, it really wouldn't happen. Understanding the power of the intentionality and being able to gauge it by this state of sensitive interiority can have a considerable, measurable effect.

The Nature of Reality

We don't understand reality. Let me give you something that may make this a little bit clearer. These ideas, incidentally, did not originate in Therapeutic Touch. My best definition of Therapeutic Touch is that it is a contemporary interpretation of several very ancient healing practices.

If you really understand what's happening in the martial arts, it's not the fact that you wear black pajamas or that you're pretty good with your feet. It's not the physical impact, you see, but rather it's the knowledgeable tearing away or tearing into, the injuring of, the vital energy field overlaying these crucial points known as chakras that is your objective. So you begin to realize that this is something that is part of the humanness of us, energies that are subtle and nonphysical that pattern themselves into human functions and that is what you seek to injure or make dysfunctional.

Our difficulty is that in our culture, we're always looking for a gimmick. There has to be some technological thing, otherwise it's not real. No matter how liberal or how progressive or how conservative we call ourselves, we want something substantial there. We don't realize that this thing, the individual's vital energy field, is right here, now—it's just of a different nature than our expectations.

I have always thought that one of the most humane of all human attributes is the ability to heal or help another person. But I think we forget about the self-healing that also needs to happen. One of the things I realized early on was that many people come to healing because they, themselves, have a need to be healed. And within the process of helping others, their own self-healing occurs. And I think that we forget that people who are ill need to be able to do that, to somehow help themselves, as well as have you as healer, or myself as healer, help them. They need to be helped to realize their own capacity for self-healing. This is one area I have become interested in and am currently studying.

I also want to point out that there is so much to human energetics we have yet to learn. It seems there is a whole universe of possibilities out there that we've hardly begun to grasp. It's really important to keep an open mind, to realize that it's not a particular technique, that you don't touch this and turn that or do some other maneuver, but rather that there is a whole universe of possibilities for learning out there for us, and we can always learn something new about the way we work.

We get up in the morning and go through our day, then go to sleep at night, and we say, "Ah, finished the day." But that's not true. We've participated in so much more than we realize. If we could make that understanding conscious, if we could effect such realization, I think we could help ourselves and others so much more significantly than we permit ourselves.

Part Ten

Conversations About Indigenous Medicine

"Mother Nature is a deep, deep well of... wonderful mysteries, some of which hold answers to questions that we can't answer on our own."
— MARK PLOTKIN

CHAPTER 35

MARK PLOTKIN, PhD

In Search of Plants that Heal

Ethnobotanist Mark Plotkin, PhD, has spent much of the past two decades in the rain forests of South America learning about indigenous curative plants and medical practices from tribal shamans. Through his work with tribes in Brazil, French Guiana, Suriname, and Venezuela, he has categorized more than 300 shaman plant cures.

Plotkin studied ethnobotany at Harvard, Yale, and Tufts, and is the first botanist to receive the San Diego Zoological Society's Conservation Medal. He previously served as director of plant conservation at the World Wildlife Fund and as vice president of Conservation International. Founder of the Shaman's Apprentice Program, which encourages younger tribal members to apprentice under the aging shamans, Plotkin currently devotes his time to curative plant research and consultation, lecturing, writing, and fundraising for his new organization, the Amazon Conservation Team. He has published numerous scientific articles and is the author of the popular book, *Tales of a Shaman's Apprentice* and *Medicine Quest*.

In early 1996, I met with Dr. Plotkin at his home in Virginia. As we sat in an office full of jungle artifacts, I quickly found myself enchanted with his tales about plants that can, when threatened, evolve new traits seemingly at will, and of shamans who sing patients back to health.

I'm an ethnobotanist, which is a scientist who works with indigenous peoples and studies their relationship with local plants. My typical day in the jungle starts with climbing out of my hammock at the crack of dawn, jumping in the river to scrub off, and then heading into the jungle with a medicine man or shaman, followed by a couple of shaman's apprentices. In my life outside the jungle, there is no typical day because I'm a fundraiser, the director of a nonprofit organization, a consultant, a writer, a lecturer, and something of a missionary for getting the word out about the importance of complementary medicine.

When we (Europeans) first made contact with indigenous peoples 500 years ago, there was a tendency to dismiss them as not having a soul, which allowed us to demonize them. They weren't really people so it was okay to stick swords through them. But it turns out that they have an incredible culture, not just in terms of the plants and medicines, but also in terms of their religion, legends, music, and philosophy.

When I first went to the rain forest in the late 1970s, I could see that the indigenous cultures were eroding as soon as they came in contact with outside civilization. I wanted to collect their information about plants before it disappeared, but it was like trying to catch rain in a paper cup. There was no way any one person or any group of people could gather this information before it disappeared. There are always things these people hold back or things that you're not there in time to see.

For instance, for 14 years, a Tirio shaman by the name of Nahtahlah told me that he never used insects for medicine. But I was in the bush with him a year ago and watched him stick a twig into an anthill and apply it to his back. After he'd been bitten five or six times, he knocked the ants off his back. "What's that for?" I asked. And he said, "I use this for back pain and when my joints ache."

There's another shaman who is referred to as *The Poisoner* in my book *Tales of a Shaman's Apprentice*. When I met him, he smiled and said, "A white man, huh? You know, I've killed about 20 of them in my time." He then spent 12 years telling me that he didn't know anything about medicines. But he turned out to be the paramount shaman, and now every time I go, he shows me a new medicine.

The Shaman Apprentice Program

The point of the shaman's apprentice program is to ensure the knowledge is passed on to the next generation. However, the goal is not simply to teach the younger tribal members a list of medicinal plants; it's also to teach them to value and use the old culture.

Here's an example—I just returned from the jungle a few months ago. While I was there, I worked with a Mexican physician who was providing treatment for diseases that the traditional (ethnic) medicines aren't effective against. This fellow comes into the clinic in his breech-cloth and says, "I've got an eye infection; can you fix it?" He had standard conjunctivitis.

The physician says, "So many people have this that I'm out of the cream, but there's a plant growing outside the hut that's been tested in the laboratory, and it's safe and effective for treating conjunctivitis, so let's give it a whack."

I asked the fellow if the local Indians had a name for the plant. "Nolo-pakan," he said. And when I asked what they used it for, he said, "To treat eye infections."

So through the shaman's apprentice program, we are trying to reconnect the Indians to their traditions. We've succeeded in teaching them which plants were used, what they were used for, and what the dosage was, but we haven't made that total connection to get them to use the medicinal plants. I want to emphasize that we're not trying to say, "Western medicine's no good, and you've got all the answers." We're trying to say, "Look, what you knew had value. If you use your traditional plant, which is safe and effective for eye infections, then you will have more money to buy polio vaccine, which you can't make from plants."

This program has caused a sea of change with the Tirios Indians. Some of the shaman's apprentices are going to other tribes to work with other shamans. They have started a medicinal plant garden to teach the children. They're starting to sing the old songs and to dance the old dances. But there's one hurdle we haven't gotten over: we've created a generation of shamans' apprentices. In fact, we've created a new generation of shamans' apprentices' apprentices, because the guys who were in their early 20s when I started working there now have kids who are 14 and 15 who are joining the program. But what we haven't been able to do is create a new generation of shamans, and that's the ultimate goal.

I'm trying to raise enough money to take the three most promising shaman's apprentices to Mexico to spend time with the Huichol and Mazatec shamans. There, shamanism is thriving and the tradition is unbroken because the missionaries did not destroy it. Outsiders have done such a job on the shamanistic traditions in the northeast Amazon that the shamans just don't have the powers to turn the apprentices into shamans. At least they haven't expressed the willingness to do so. That's why I need to bring in outside help. I want the shamans themselves to teach these guys. Maybe it'll work, and maybe it won't. But if you don't stick your neck out, you don't succeed.

Can Plants Think?

As you mentioned, in my work I talk about "chemically inert" plants. Lettuce is a good example of this. When you eat it, you don't hallucinate; you don't go to sleep; you don't throw up. It doesn't have a major effect on the human body. Everything you take in—whether it's the air you inhale or the food you put in your mouth—causes some change, but it's "inert" if it doesn't exert a powerful biodynamic effect.

But other substances, like alkaloids, do cause powerful reactions. An alkaloid is a class of chemical compounds that figure largely in Western medicine. Codeine, strychnine, caffeine, morphine—all of these are alkaloids. They have certain biodynamic roles in plants, probably to repel attacks by insects, and they have a major effect in the human body. Anybody interested in this "bug-to-drug" connection should read a brilliant chapter in *Tropical Nature* by Adrian Forsyth that explains why plants would evolve these compounds and what these compounds do to bugs.

The industrial revolution was made possible by natural rubber, but that's not why the Hevea tree evolved it. It's because when the beetle bit into the bark; it got a spray of this stuff that gummed up its mouth and taught it not to bite into the tree any more. The message was: go to the next tree over. But as soon as one tree comes up with something that repels an attack by insect, if you're the next tree over, then you'd better come up with something even better to convince that bug to move on to the next tree or back to the first tree.

I like to think of plant intelligence in a broad sense. I don't necessarily subscribe to the idea that plants have hidden brains and can outthink us in the sense that you try to outthink the person who's haggling with you over the price of something in the marketplace. It's just how evolution works, which is, if you don't have your act together in terms of being able to reproduce and distribute your gametophytes, you don't make it to the next generation. If you don't come up with something new, you get eaten and you're not there.

So, in that sense, plants are brilliant. Otherwise they wouldn't be here. But that means that every other living species is brilliant as well. So if you open it up in a broad sense, you can talk about the intelligence of plants.

Medicinal Plants

You must remember that ethnobotany has long been criticized as essentially being the compilation of laundry lists. They use species A for this, species B for this, species C for this. But so what? It's when you find patterns that it gets interesting. I was in the Peruvian Amazon a year and a half ago, working with this old shaman. On the way back to camp one day, we passed this plant called *una de gato*, or cat's claw. He said, "People from all over are coming here to be treated for HIV with this stuff." In my line of business you hear these claims all the time, so you have to be skeptical. But 6 months later, I'm in Suriname in northeastern South America, and another old shaman shows me the same plant, which he used to treat coughs and colds.

What's the common denominator? It's viruses. Widely separated people using the same plant to treat viruses. I immediately called a friend at the National Cancer Institute, and he said, "We get this call all the time. We've tested it in the laboratory, and it does not kill the AIDS virus. So we don't know what's going on. Perhaps it's an immune-system stimulant." I researched the literature and found out there was some laboratory work on this plant that showed it stimulated the production of white blood cells. But as I understand it, white blood cells aren't particularly effective in killing viruses.

The point here is, who knows? But it's something worth following up in the laboratory. It wasn't all that long ago that people turned up their noses at Echinacea, and now it's been tested in the laboratory. It is an effective immune stimulant, and everybody's buying it and putting it in their medicine chests.

These are the types of leads that point you in interesting directions. It's not to say that all of the plants will prove effective. It's not to say that plants that are only used by one small group—or even a single shaman—aren't effective. When you're doing this type of work, you have to set your priorities, so you look for these patterns. Another priority is: Do you want to find a good cure for headaches? Suppose you do. Nobody is going to spend $120,000,000 to bring it to market because there's an excellent cure for headaches already—aspirin. It's cheap, effective, and doesn't have horrible side effects. However, if you find a cure for migraines, then you're going to have people knocking down your door because there is no effective cure for migraines.

You ask why do local peoples use compounds that test as ineffective? Well, there's no question in my mind that when you remove things from the cultural context, something is often lost. Maybe if you don't have the shaman with the rattle standing over you, it doesn't work. Maybe it's because you are from a culture that believes you're going to get better if you have that shaman there, so it's the placebo effect, or maybe it's some sort of synergistic effect between the placebo effect and the chemicals in the plant. People look down their noses at the role of the placebo effect in shamanistic medicine, but it's the cure in at least 30% of the cases in Western medicine, and some people say it's the cure in 60% of the cases. So if you can bring in the placebo effect, I'm all in favor of that.

By the same token, we have magic bullets, and these magic bullets work whether you have a shaman standing over you or a midwife standing over you. Some of the best magic bullets are alkaloids, because when we went back and found the original curare collections that Waterton made in the early 1800s and tested them in the lab over 150 years after they were collected, they were still as lethal as the day the Indians made them. When Professor Schultes went to Kew Gardens, the Royal Botanic Gardens in London, and found the original ayahuasca collections made by Richard Spruce in the 1850s and had them tested in the laboratory, they were still as hallucinogenic as the day they were collected. You didn't need a shaman standing over you, and you didn't need to be sitting in the middle of the Amazon; it still worked.

But then there are trees in which, if you take your machete and slash the bark, the sap turns red to yellow to orange to white as it drips down the bark. There's no question that the chemical composition is changing before your eyes. So the race is on to set up laboratories in the rain forest and collect the plants in a form in which the chemistry doesn't degrade. When Schultes did his classic work, he'd collect the specimens, dry them, and maybe 6 months later, if the plane didn't fall out of the sky with the specimens, or the canoe didn't turn over and the plants went over the waterfalls and were lost forever, maybe they would make it back to the lab. And they'd say, "Gee, there's nothing in this stuff." But the point is that it was dry, and it had been collected 6 months earlier.

Right now, if a plant doesn't have a chemical effect, our culture says it's not a medicine. But time after time we see how ignorant we are of the chemistry of the human body, and of healing. An immunostimulant can get dismissed because you put it in the test tube with the AIDS virus, and it doesn't affect the virus. By our standards, it doesn't work. But maybe it stimulates the immune system. If you take the human out of the middle of the equation and you take the plant and the virus and put them together, nothing happens. But if you run it through a human, maybe it does work.

We have to get away from this attitude that because people are poor or naked or living in the jungle or illiterate, there's nothing we can learn from them. Technology, used well, can help us learn more about the secrets of the rain forest and of the shamans, and of these different types of healing, rather than be something that is going to replace them. But the way that so much of this cultural exchange is done now is that technology moves in and crushes these people, these cultures, and these forests, and we're left with nothing.

A good example of that is curare. These admixtures, the things that the Indians put in with the curare plant itself, such as inert plants and insect parts, have long been dismissed as mumbo jumbo because when you test them in the laboratory there's nothing in them that has biodynamic properties. But recent research has revealed that even though these things are not poisonous on their own; they potentiate complex reactions that make the curares more toxic or make the hallucinogens more hallucinogenic. So it turns out that these guys in breechcloths are better chemists than we are in this case.

However, it's important not to over-romanticize these people and make them out to be noble savages with all the answers. I agree with the concept that these people have medicines we don't and that we need to learn from them. They don't have stress-related heart disease. You don't see the typical symptoms—people worn down, can't sleep, reflux—that are so common in our culture that tell us there are some things wrong with the way we're living our lives. But one of the things that has killed a lot of them in the past— and still does to some degree—is infection. And our culture has cures for this.

On Replicating the Rain Forest

One of the reasons synthetic drugs took hold in our culture is simple—would you rather have something that you can make from scratch in the laboratory, or would you rather rely on a supply from Nicaragua or Colombia, where there are all sorts of political and transportation problems? However, even though we can synthesize just about anything these days, it's still cheaper in most cases to get the plant to produce it and extract it, or to get the starting blocks from the plant.

But creating artificial environments in which to grow these rain forest plants here in America isn't that easy. For instance, there are 80,000 species of higher plants in the Amazon, many of which have never been seen studied in depth by Westerners. The same species in one area may have a different chemical composition than in another area. So the idea that if we just make a big enough greenhouse in Marin County or here in Washington, DC, then to heck with the rain forest—well, it doesn't work that way.

Living in and on these 80,000 plants are somewhere between 20 and 30 million species of insects, which have at least as much medicinal potential as the plants. And we know a lot less about those insects than we do about the plants. Further, we don't know about the life history of these plants, so even if we took two or three of them and planted them, it might be that we couldn't grow them in our soil or that the insect that pollinates them isn't there.

The point is the symbiosis. Here's a story. The sloth lives in trees in the Amazon and only comes down every couple of days to defecate. It digs a hole, usually at the base of the plant it is living on, and craps into the hole. Some people see that as laziness. It is a sloth, after all. But I see it as essentially the birth of agriculture.

Then there are the ants that live in these trees. All you have to do is brush against the trees, and the ants come pouring out and bite you. The tree, in turn, produces a starch that the insects eat. So here you have the symbiotic relationship where the plants are being protected by the ants and feeding the ants in return.

There's a fungus called Cordyceps that lives on the forest floor. When insects or arthropods come past this fungus, the fungus attaches itself to their body. Once it does that, the fungus exudes a compound that burns a hole in the insect's exoskeleton. Then it inserts itself into the insect body and proceeds to eat virtually all of the nonvital organs in the insect. Once it's done that it invades the insect brain, which causes the insect to climb to the top of a tree in the rain forest. Then the fungus eats the insect brain, thereby killing the insect and causing the exoskeleton to split open, allowing the fungus to release its spores 120 feet above the forest floor.

And people dismiss fungi as lower organisms!

Mother Nature is a deep, deep well of these wonderful mysteries, some of which hold answers to questions that we can't answer on our own. We all know about taxol from the yew tree in the Pacific Northwest. A lot of people don't realize that it was left to rot by loggers because it was regarded as having no value. But they tested it at the National Cancer Institute and found that it was effective for treating certain forms of ovarian cancer. My colleague, Jim Duke, an ethnobotanist at the United States Department of Agriculture, found out that indigenous peoples had been using the Pacific yew for medicines for many years. If we'd paid attention to what the Indians were telling us, maybe we'd have looked at the yew tree a lot earlier.

Favorite Medicinal Plants

My absolute favorite medicinal plant is Virola, because that's the one I studied in Professor R.E. Schultes' first class at Harvard. The Indians of the northwest Amazon call Virola the "semen of the sun" because they believe that it's holy and comes from the land of the gods. Professor Schultes saw Virola used in the northwest Amazon for two purposes: to paint on fungal infections of the skin and as a powerful hallucinogenic snuff. I went to Suriname almost 40 years later and found them using it to paint on fungal infections of the skin. Then I went to the Yanomamo Indians in the northeast and found them making the same snuff. It's also an important timber tree. It produces oils used to make soaps in other parts of the Amazon. It's just a wonderful, all-purpose, beautiful, effective, healing tree.

But you can't get it here because it doesn't work dried. This is why people need to push their senators and representatives to make sure there's more funding for this type of research.

Mysteries of the Jungle

I was just down in the jungle working on treatments for diabetes, and I was with Kamanya, who is the head of the shaman's apprentice program. I was sitting with him in the middle of the village. Everybody had gone to sleep. We were surrounded by houses that had little cooking fires inside that burn all night and have a wonderful smoky smell. It was a full moon, so the whole village was lit by this silvery glow. We were talking about our times together in the jungle and how things had changed for the better in terms of the young kids interested in the old ways, when I felt a presence behind me. I didn't look. I just knew there was somebody behind me. A voice spoke up, and it was the Sikyana, the poisoner. He sat there and said that we'd known each other a long time and how at first he thought that a lot of the stuff I was asking about was none of my business and how he wanted to look into my eyes and my heart to find out what kind of a person I was and to lead me by the nose a bit. But he said that now he wanted to teach Kamanya, his son, and myself the old ways, to make sure this knowledge would be passed on, and that the medicines that he had taught us, which had already blown us away, were just the tip of the iceberg compared with what he knew. A shiver went down my spine. I'll never forget that moment.

The jungle is part of my life. I have a foot in that culture, in that place, in that time, in that ecosystem. I'm not a person who wants to pack up and run off to the jungle and live there happily ever after. I am a red-blooded American boy. I love my country and my culture, for all its problems. But I also love these people and that culture and that ecosystem.

Things happen there I can't explain. In my book I talked about how I encountered the Jaguar Shaman in a night dream and then discovered the next day that the Jaguar Shaman was completely aware of the same encounter.

Schultes has always talked participatory science. He said that if somebody aims the snuff pipe at you, you don't say, "Oh, no, I'll lose my objectivity." Your response should be, "Pass it on over."

I know people who have a real problem with that, who say, "It's not science if you're talking to the little men in the trees." But if you are talking to the little men in the trees, then you understand why the Yanomamo say that when you take the snuff you see little men in the trees. Because you do!

Despite all these experiences, however, I'm still very Jewish. There's a great Jewish tradition of the healing arts, stretching from Maimonides in the distant past to Andy Weil today. So I see myself as part of that tradition. Secondly, there's that intellectual quest of Judaism. Three of my four grandparents were immigrants, and the thing they pushed on their kids was education, learning the written word. Part of what I do as an ethnobotanist is not the old "rape and run" approach to ethnobotany, which was, "They've got plants; they've got knowledge; let's get it and find the cure for 'X' and make a zillion dollars." It's "what's in it for the native peoples?" And what's in it for them is putting this stuff down on paper in their language so they have a record; they have appreciation of their culture. I want to see their culture endure just like I want to see my culture endure.

There's also a Jewish concept called *Sedaka*. I owe the fact that I have a nice house and was able to write a nice book and have a nice job essentially to what these people have taught me. And I want to pay them back for that. A portion of the proceeds from my book go to help them through the Shaman's Apprentice Fund. I want it to be a two-way street.

A Moment of Enlightenment

I had a moment of enlightenment when I was there. Everybody has their own reality. You don't see the world through the same eyes that I do. So why should I think that some guy living in the Congo is going to relate to the world that I do? The witch doctors who can turn themselves into jaguars and shamans who can travel hundreds of miles through the air to throw curses are as real to the people in the Amazon as VCRs, mortgages, and lawyers are to us. So why is our view right and their view wrong? I've seen stuff I can't explain. I've heard about stuff I can't explain. Does that mean it's wrong or it does not exist? Absolutely not. And that's what I mean about different realities.

I think my acceptance of things is what broke the ice and allowed me to get into the indigenous cultures. People make the mistake of thinking that either you're accepted by these people or you're not. You're one of the guys, or you're not. But it's an evolutionary process. It's like the Chinese box puzzle. You open a box, and inside, instead of the answer, often it's another box. So you open that box, and just when you think you've gotten to the smallest box possible with the answer to the ultimate mystery, you open it up and there's another box inside. That's why the Jaguar Shaman started coming across with information the day I met him, and Sikyana waited 12 years.

A colleague of mine, a physician, just came back from the Ecuadorian Amazon, and he is still shaking his head. Do you know what a botfly is? It's a fly that lays its eggs in your arm, and the egg hatches into larvae, and the larvae eat your flesh, and it essentially has to be dug out of your arm. So this guy came into the clinic with a botfly larva, and the doctor was getting out his scalpel to cut it out, when a Jivaro shaman came in and said, "What are you doing with that scalpel?"

The physician said, "I'm going to cut this thing out."

And the shaman said, "No, no. You don't need to do that. I'll handle it." So then the shaman leaned over the guy's arm and sang a song, and the botfly larva crawled out and dropped out on the counter.

Now, who would you rather be treated by?

So there are these things that happen that are unexplainable by Western science, and they keep happening. I'll give you another example. A colleague of mine, Silviano Camberos, is a Mexican physician. He was visiting a Huichol Indian peyote ceremony when one fellow got stung by a scorpion. Now, the scorpions in this area are deadly. So Silviano said to the shaman, "I'd better get my bag and shoot this guy full of antivenin because he got stung by one of the bad guys."

The shaman said, "No, no. He's taken all this peyote; it won't affect him." And it didn't. He had no negative reaction whatsoever.

How would Western science explain that? Western science would say that the scorpion didn't inject any poison or that it wasn't one of the toxic scorpions or that the guy didn't really get bitten. But the point here is that we don't understand everything.

My colleagues and I have started a nongovernmental organization called the Amazon Conservation Team, which is bringing together like-minded people to say that conservation hasn't come up with all the answers yet, and we need to find better ways of working at the grass roots level with indigenous peoples and indigenous healers, because that is where much of the battle will be ultimately won or lost. I'm interested in reaching out to like-minded people who regard the earth as a sacred place, who are interested in complementary healing traditions, and who want to protect the resources that can end up in our health-food stores, our pharmacies, our medicine chests, our laboratories.

I'm a great believer in that old saying of Margaret Mead's: "Never be afraid to cast your lot with a small group of people committed to change the world, because indeed, that's often the only way that change takes place."

CHAPTER 36

STANLEY KRIPPNER, PhD

Medicine and the Inner Realities

Stanley Krippner, PhD, who received his doctoral degree from Northwestern University in 1961, is on the faculty of the Saybrook Graduate School, where he has taught since 1972. Previously he was the director of the Maimonides Medical Center's Dream Laboratory and director of the Child Study Center at Kent State University. In addition to his position at Saybrook, Dr. Krippner holds faculty appointments at The International Holistic University in Brasilia, Brazil, and the Institute for Medicine and Advanced Behavioral Technology in Juarez, Mexico.

Dr. Krippner is the author and coauthor of many books, including *Exceptional Dreams* (with Fariba Bogzaran and Andre de Carvalho), *The Mythic Path* (with David Feinstein), *A Psychiatrist in Paradise: Treating Mental Illness in Bali* (with Denny Thong and Bruce Carpenter), *Spiritual Dimensions of Healing: From Tribal Shamanism to Contemporary Health Care* (with Patrick Welch), *Dream Telepathy: Experiments in Nocturnal ESP* (with Montague Ullman and Alan Vaughan), *Healing States* (with Alberto Villoldo), *Human Possibilities: Mind Research in the USSR and Eastern Europe,* and *Song of the Siren: A Parapsychological Odyssey.*

In 1997, I interviewed Dr. Krippner at his offices at Saybrook Graduate School in San Francisco, California.

In the mid-1960s, Montague Ullman initiated a dream laboratory at Maimonides Medical Center in Brooklyn, New York, and he needed a director with a parapsychological background. Several prominent researchers—experts who knew about dreams and electroencephalographic technology—turned him down because there was no guarantee of continuous funding. But I was either naive enough, foolish enough, or wise enough to accept the job. So that's how I entered the field of dreams. I learned by doing. I knew nothing about dream technology when I arrived.

Our research demonstrated that anomalous dreams—telepathic, clairvoyant, and precognitive dreams—could be studied in a laboratory setting. We made the case that this type of dream deserves to be taken seriously. The results of our experiments are not easily repeatable, so we cannot claim that we demonstrated the existence of anomalous dreams, but we certainly gathered enough data to indicate that these dreams should no longer be brushed aside as mere coincidence, falsification of memory, or deliberate lying. If anyone is interested, the summary of all of our work appears in Gackenbach and Sheikh's *Dream Images: A Call to Mental Arms* (Amityville, NY, 1991, Baywood).

The way my interest in shamanic healers developed was serendipitous. A musician friend, Mickey Hart, a drummer with the Grateful Dead, knew Rolling Thunder, an intertribal medicine man from the state of Nevada. Mickey lived in Marin County when I was working in New York, and I would stay with him when I visited California. One weekend he flew Rolling Thunder to San Francisco so we could meet. We got along quite well, and I later observed many of Rolling Thunder's healing sessions, both in California and Nevada.

A few years later I made my first visit to Brazil with my former student, Alberto Villoldo, where I spoke at the InterAmerican Congress of Psychology. We met some of the Brazilian healers with whom I had corresponded, and upon returning, Alberto and I gave a talk about the Brazilian healers and Rolling Thunder. There was a publisher in the audience who thought our lecture could be expanded into a book, and that led to our coauthorship of *The Realms of Healing*. In the meantime, I had met Olga Worrall, one of the most intensively studied healers in the United States, and once *The Realms of Healing* was published, other healers began to come out of the woodwork.

I have had a long-standing interest in indigenous people and also had a childhood interest in dreams. So when I travel, I ask my contacts to put me in touch with the local shamans. I went to South Africa in the 1980s, met a dozen Zulu shamans, and was able to observe many of their healing ceremonies. The same thing happened during a trip to Mexico when I met María Sabina, the most famous shaman of the 20th century.

Working with Shamans

Rolling Thunder was remarkable. Typically, he was eclectic and used everything he could come by if he thought it would be beneficial to his clients. He took me into his medicine trailer once in Nevada, and there were literally hundreds of paper bags, each with the name of an herb written on them. There were Chinese herbs given to him by Chinese physicians as well as allopathic medicine samples, with instructions on how to use them, given to him by allopathic physicians. He told me, "I will use anything that might be of help."

In 1979, Rolling Thunder had timed a healing treatment to coincide with my arrival in Nevada. The client, Robert, was a young Native American who was severely alcoholic. I was supposed to hypnotize him. I wanted to do some preliminary tests, but Robert was in retreat, in solitude. So the first time I met him was when I arrived at the campfire. Our introduction had been preceded by an hour and a half of drumming and singing. We were surrounded by some 50 people, and I was expected to hypnotize him with no preliminary interview, examination, or opportunity to develop rapport.

I decided to use mental imagery with Robert. I asked him to imagine what it felt like to crave alcohol, and then to transform that feeling into an image. His image was of a terrible monster who was out to destroy him. Then I said, "This community of people who cares for you and loves you is going to give you a gift. What gift are they going to give you?"

Robert said, "They are giving me a bow and an arrow."

I responded, "They're giving you a bow and an arrow, which represents your native traditions, so you now have the power to kill the monster. Imagine yourself destroying the monster."

He imagined himself shooting the arrow into the heart of the monster, and it collapsed. Then I told him to imagine something to drink that would be healthier than alcohol. He chose fruit juice and native teas. I had him imagine drinking these beverages, and he complied. Then I suggested, "Whenever you have the urge to drink alcohol, close your eyes and transform the urge into a monster. Use the bow and arrow to shoot the monster, and immediately drink something healthful, either in your imagination or actually."

After I finished my guided imagery session, Rolling Thunder appeared in a white buckskin suit and feathers and performed the traditional "cupping and sucking" ritual. He took an eagle feather, poking and prodding Robert's body. Whenever Robert winced, Rolling Thunder would put his hands around the spot, put his mouth between his hands, and symbolically suck the poison out of Robert's body and spit it into a pail. Rolling Thunder was very careful with his words. He never said, "This is the poison." He said, "This represents the poison." The viscous-looking, dark red fluid that appeared, which was probably tobacco juice, was taken off and buried.

Rolling Thunder had drawn the group's attention to a hooting owl. He said the owl was symbolic of death, so this was Robert's best chance to transform himself. The owl had hooted seven times, which Rolling Thunder said was a lucky number, so this was a favorable omen. Frankly, I didn't hear an owl hooting, but the group members swore that they could remember that owl. Shamans are masters of drama and they are also tricksters, literally tricking people into getting well.

The next morning, a tearful and grateful Robert thanked me. And in a follow-up inquiry I conducted about 3 years later, he was still sober.

Like many Native Americans, Rolling Thunder had a cyclical notion of time and paid more attention to the seasons than to the years. It's very naive for people to think that consciousness is the same the world over, in all times and places. Consider the Spanish conquest of Mexico. The consciousness of Native Americans was very, very different from that of most Europeans. The Spaniards had a very linear perspective on history: beginning, middle, end, emphasizing cause and effect.

Another example is the presence of spirits. If you reported seeing or hearing spirits in Europe, you might be burned at the stake for sorcery or witchcraft. But the native shamans entered altered states and frequently talked to the spirits. From the perspective of the Spanish Inquisition, they were heretics deserving of punishment or even death to purge them of their sins.

Among North American Indians there was a curious balance of the collective and individuality that, as far as I know, has not existed anywhere in the world for such a lengthy period of time and in such a dynamic equilibrium. Even the vision or dream of a child could be taken seriously by an entire community. Shamanism is an open system, and new insights are incorporated into a tribe's ongoing mythology as they are needed. The Western religions would never have allowed that. For them, the holy dogma was embedded in such sacred texts as the Bible, Talmud, or Koran. The dictates of these texts—and the associated writings of the religions' founders—comprise a closed system.

When the Spaniards came to Mexico, they outlawed the use of sacred mushrooms, morning glory seeds, and cacti. But in some places the old traditions managed to survive. Oaxaca, Mexico, is one place where these traditions were practiced for hundreds of years. María Sabina was a sabia, or shaman, in the Mazatec tribe. Gordon Wasson, a New York banker, had heard rumors that the Oaxaca Indians were still using the sacred mushroom. So, with his financial resources, a good heart, and a great respect for native people, he went to Mexico to investigate these reports.

María Sabina claimed to have had a dream that this would happen; this dream directed her to reveal the secret of the sacred mushrooms to Wasson. But some people in her village felt that this disclosure would prevent the magic in the mushrooms from working for the Indians, so they burned down her store and killed her teenage son. María Sabina paid a terrible price for divulging the secret, but she was true to her dream.

Some of the principles María Sabina felt she needed to promulgate were respect for the earth and the importance of spiritual life. Wasson ingested the mushrooms with María Sabina in a sacred ceremony. It changed his life. He focused his studies on what are now called entheogens—plants that allow a person to have contact with divine sources. She was almost 90 years of age when I met her. We had two interviews. She admitted that she was now too frail to use the *hongitos*, the "little ones," the sacred mushrooms. However, she still believed it was Jesus Christ who spoke through them. She told me that during Jesus Christ's ministry on earth, he visited other parts of the world, walking through the villages and countryside, healing people and doing good deeds. The sharp stones would sometimes cut into his bare feet, but he would take saliva and slap it on his feet to stop the bleeding. And where the red of the blood and the white of the saliva combined, a little sacred mushroom later sprouted, and Jesus Christ was in the mushroom. So, when María Sabina and her client ate the mushrooms together, it was Jesus Christ who told them the nature of the problem and how it should be handled.

Long before the Spaniards arrived in Mexico there was a similar myth in which Quetzalcoatl, the legendary feathered serpent and lord of the sun, gave up his throne and wandered among the ordinary people, doing good deeds. And when his feet were cut by the stones, the saliva and blood would mix together to produce a sacred mushroom.

This syncretism demonstrates the adaptability of shamanism. The conquerors came and brought the new religion, and Quetzalcoatl became Jesus Christ. The myth lived on: there is a deity within the mushrooms. The mushrooms are the flesh of the gods.

Yemamja and the Brazilian Traditions

When the slaves came from West Africa to Brazil, they found that the Roman Catholic saints resembled their own deities. In some of the West African tribes there was a minor deity, Yemamja, goddess of the salt water, to whom they prayed when they traveled in slave ships across the Atlantic ocean. Those who survived the terrible trip venerated her and she became a powerful deity in Brazil. When the Portuguese forcibly converted the slaves to Catholicism, the slaves matched Yemamja with the Virgin Mary. They kept praying to Yemamja, but when the slave masters or priests arrived, the slaves quickly switched to "Hail Mary, full of grace." The slaves were more clever than the Portuguese realized; in this way, they preserved part of their tribal culture.

Yemamja was one of the original deities. According to one of the tribal myths, Yemamja married her own brother and gave birth to a son, but she did not give birth to a daughter. So when the son reached manhood, what could he do? His grandmother was too old, but his mother was still very attractive, so he chased Yemamja around the world, captured her, and ravished her. She immediately gave birth to 12 children, as well as the sun and the moon. There was no guilt, no shame. I've often said that psychoanalysis would have been much different had Freud discovered the Yemamja myth instead of the Oedipus myth.

Practitioners in the African-Brazilian religions are what we would call mediums, rather than shamans. Both practitioners access altered states, but the medium is under the control of the deity or spirit, while the shaman retains control. A shaman will allow the spirits to speak through him or her, but he or she also can converse with the spirit. However, there are some practitioners who behave more shamanically on some occasions, more mediumistically on others. Also, some practitioners have bureaucratic duties—such as running a church or a temple—so they're actually priests and priestesses as well. You cannot make general statements about spiritual practitioners without noting that exceptions abound.

Paulo Xavante is an Indian from the Xavante tribe in the southwestern plains of Brazil. I spent some time with him during an ecology conference in Brazil. When he performed his ceremony, Paulo was wearing a commercially designed T-shirt decorated with a scene from the rainforest, shaking his rattle, and wearing a beautiful feather headdress.

Paulo Xavante specialized in treating soul loss. This is a practice that most shamans perform under one name or another. It's a problem you do not find in the psychiatric manuals, though a psychiatrist might say, "What they are talking about is severe depression." From the shamanic point of view this trivializes the problem, because worse than being killed, worse than dying, is losing one's soul. The soul can be stolen or misplaced. Sometimes people leave their body during a dream, and their soul stays in the other world when they wake up. People can also lose their soul to a sorcerer, a practitioner who operates outside the community, selling his or her healing and hexing services to the highest bidder. In some societies, you can have two or three or four souls, depending on the belief system. Sometimes part of the soul can be stolen or damaged. Sometimes several souls can get lost.

What Paulo Xavante does is alter his consciousness by drumming. He will then enter the "other world," look for the lost soul, and bring it back. Once the soul is restored, the person feels better. But sometimes Paulo Xavante has to fight a battle against the entity that is holding the soul and it may take more than one session to bring back the soul. Finally, Paulo Xavante gives his clients instructions so that their soul is not captured or lost again.

One of my students at Saybrook wrote her dissertation on Fawn Journeyhawk, a Native American shaman living in the American Southwest. Soul loss is also Fawn's specialty. She often works with posttraumatic stress disorder, especially as experienced by Vietnam veterans whose souls were lost in Vietnam. She claims to "journey" to Vietnam and plead with the dead Vietnamese who have captured the soul to forgive and release it so that the veteran—who is now filled with remorse and new understandings—can get on with his or her life.

Fawn also has worked with both males and females who have "lost their souls" to the spirits of alcohol, cocaine, or heroin. She told me that one can't bargain with these spirits because they're too ruthless. So she fights the spirit of cocaine, whom she describes as a very seductive, beautiful woman, or the spirit of heroin, who is a crass and ruthless man, or the spirit of alcohol, who is very complex and can be either male or female. Once she has found the spirit who controls the addict's soul, she must engage in a fight. She's always at risk when she initiates the battle, so she takes her power objects and power animals with her as she "journeys." Also, before Fawn goes into battle, the addict must participate in sweat lodge ceremonies, which include fasting, praying, and purification.

Why Native Healing Works

Indigenous societies have their own classifications. They have diseases that don't appear in the *Diagnostic and Statistical Manual of Mental Disorders* or the *International Classification of Diseases* and that most allopathic physicians know nothing about. For me, there is a difference between disease and illness. Disease is closely aligned with biological processes. Certain diseases exist all over the world, such as measles and diarrhea. But some ailments are not the same all over the world because social construction changes the disease into an illness. In rural Japan, there is an illness called *wagamama*, where people go berserk and rip off their clothes. People in the United States say, "We don't have culture-bound syndromes." But we have anorexia nervosa and bulimia. You don't find these illnesses in most indigenous societies, because they don't emphasize style and slimness as an ideal to the extent that characterizes U.S. society.

Some years ago, I was a member of the National Institutes of Health study group that surveyed relaxation and cognitive-behavioral treatments for chronic pain and insomnia. We surveyed hundreds of studies showing that these techniques often work and published the review in the July 1996 issue of the *Journal of the American Medical Association*. We found that (for some disorders) meditation does work. Biofeedback does work. Hypnosis does work. Cognitive behavioral therapy does work. Relaxation techniques do work. Mental imagery does work. In other words, inner reality can affect outer reality when used as part of medical, psychotherapeutic, or counseling practice. We also studied data on many of the native healing practices. And I would agree with the psychiatrist E. Fuller Torrey that there are four basic reasons why they work—at least some of the time.

First, they work best when there is a shared worldview. If the practitioner and the client can agree on what the problem is and what needs to be done, the healing effect is potentiated. María Sabina and her client both ate the sacred mushrooms, both received the prescription from Jesus Christ, and then both set to work, doing what had to be done.

A shared worldview is not mandatory. Sometimes a native person will be dragged kicking and screaming to an allopath to get an injection of penicillin. He may not believe it is going to work and may think that this is the worst possible treatment. Nevertheless, it does work. So if the shared worldview is not always present, one or more of the other key ingredients must achieve salience.

For example, the personal qualities of the practitioner are important. Some practitioners are so kind, loving, and friendly that the client wants to get well to please them. These qualities may differ from culture to culture. In some cultures, the practitioner is so stern, dogmatic, and authoritarian that the clients feel they must get well. So the personal qualities of the practitioner are another healing ingredient.

The third factor is the expectation of the client: the trust, faith, and expectation that the procedure will work. This is probably the reason that placebos work as well as they do.

The fourth component is the treatment itself, the potential ability of the treatment to empower the client. I really can't think of a better word than "empower," whether the healer empowers the client biologically by eliminating microorganisms with antibiotics and other medicines, empowers the client by repairing a broken bone, or by helping him or her cast off the guilt and shame that have been fomenting negative self-images that foster the ailment. One of these four components must be present. And the more that are available, the more likely it is that the client is going to recover.

In this regard, we can make a distinction between healing and curing. Curing is basically an allopathic, biomedical concept. To cure something, the physician gets rid of the symptoms and sends the patient on his or her way. But healing is more complicated, more holistic. The practitioner not only alleviates symptomatology but heals the spiritual aspects of the ailment. The client is taught how to prevent the ailment from recurring. The practitioner also attempts to heal the society, the family, the clan, or the social group. Sometimes the client will die, but he or she will die a healed person, reconciled to death, and be ready for the next step of the journey. Even though I champion and respect allopathic medicine a great deal, it focuses on curing rather than healing, and by focusing on curing, the social and spiritual matrix of treatment is almost entirely lost.

Religion versus Spirituality

I attend the Glide Memorial Methodist Church in San Francisco, but I have a variety of affiliations. I started out as a Lutheran because my mother was a Lutheran; then I became a Presbyterian because my father was a Presbyterian. I was even an elder of a Presbyterian Church. When I was at the University of Wisconsin, I taught at a Unitarian Sunday School. I'm currently a member of the Universal Life Church (which enables me to perform wedding ceremonies) and the First Church of Humanism in New York City. But I also have been allowed to pray in the Dome of the Rock, which is an Islamic holy site in Jerusalem. I have participated in many Jewish ceremonies and have been initiated in a Hindu temple on Bali. I have had two Buddhist initiations and helped set up a Taoist sanctuary in the southeastern United States.

Several "Mothers of the Saints" in the African-Brazilian religions have told me that I am of the *linha* or "line" of Oxala, the deity of purity and truth. Swami Radha once suggested that I contemplate the image of the White Tara, symbol for the quest for knowledge. Finally, my day of birth makes St. Francis of Assisi my patron saint. I have small statues or paintings of these three spiritual figures in my office for inspirational purposes. As you can see, I'm very much at home in a number of religious institutions.

On the other hand, I am aware that institutionalized religion is all too often racist, sexist, homophobic, and has blood on its hands: Eastern, Western, Northern, and Southern religions are all imperfect, yet most of them claim to have the final word. So it's important for me to separate out spirituality from religion. Religion is institutionalized. Religion consists of a body of believers, a set of rituals, and an articulated dogma. Spirituality can be public or private; it can be social or individual. Spirituality is an attitude and a practice that involves a transcendent reality and assumes that there are different activities and behaviors that provide an encounter with that transcendent reality, whether it be the Great Spirit, the Tao, the Ground of Being, the Earth Mother, the Heavenly Father, the March of History, the Unity of Humankind, Heaven, or Nirvana. One can be spiritual without being religious, and religious without being spiritual. One can be both; one can be neither.

More to the point: there is religious healing, which occurs within an institution, and spiritual healing, which does not necessarily occur within an institution. Shamanism is a spiritual practice. It's never been a religion. I have met Roman Catholic shamans like María Sabina, Muslim shamans, Jewish shamans, Hindu shamans, Buddhist shamans, and Pagan shamans. All of them work within their own framework, yet many seem eager to accommodate allopathic perspectives.

For example, when Europeans introduced the notion of germs, many shamans remarked, "We believe that there are invisible spirits wandering through the body, causing problems. This is what the Europeans call 'germs.' It's the same thing. We just have different names for them."

Many years ago, I introduced Rolling Thunder to his first Western physician, an osteopath, Irving Oyle. They spent several hours talking privately and came out of their conversation arm in arm. Dr. Oyle said, "We had a long talk and figured out we do pretty much the same thing. Rolling Thunder said that when a sick person comes to him, he listens very carefully, observes very carefully, makes a diagnosis, goes through a ritual, gives the client some herbs to restore health, and the client usually gets well. When a patient comes to me, I listen very carefully, observe the patient very carefully, make a diagnosis, go through a ritual called 'writing out a prescription,' which will provide the patient with some medicine to restore health, and usually the patient gets well. In both cases, a great deal of magic is involved—the type of magic called 'faith.'"

Without romanticizing shamanism or any other type of indigenous healing tradition, there is something to be learned about the cultural context that shamanism constantly emphasizes. In one study, U.S. cancer patients who participated in group meetings lived longer; if replicated, this may be an example of how social support can actually extend people's lives. But shamans have known this for millennia and have emphasized the involvement of the community in their healing practices.

Imagination and Postmodern Thought

In June 1965, when I was working at Maimonides Medical Center, conducting dream telepathy experiments, I was hospitalized with several bleeding ulcers. It became very serious. I had been misdiagnosed before I came to New York City, and when I came down with mononucleosis, the ulcers simply popped. I was bleeding to death. One of my friends phoned Shirley Harrison, a well-known medium living in Maine. Before she knew the diagnosis, she said that I was quite ill and would need an operation, that I'd be operated on before Monday afternoon, and that I would survive.

During the operation, the surgeon removed a section of my stomach and my large intestine, then sewed me together. I had a rubber tube coming out of my side to drain the waste material. But the wound wasn't healing, and the surgeon was puzzled as to what the problem could be. Shirley Harrison came to see me in the hospital—she had flown to New York to join my friends in prayer and to work on my behalf. She brought out her Ouija board and put it to use. The planchette skipped over the board. Finally, Shirley remarked, "You're not healing because there are four stitches that have come loose, and they are causing the infection. But you will be fine in 3 days."

Each day, in 20-minute segments, 3 times a day, I imagined that those stitches were coming out of the tube. On the morning of the second day, two double stitches came out of the tube. On the third day, no more waste material drained from the tube. It was removed and the opening closed.

I have great respect for allopathic biomedicine because it has saved my life time and time again. I was very fragile as a child, with severe allergies and many respiratory problems. I had wonderful parents who would often spend the night with me while I was coughing up blood and could hardly breathe. Some years ago, I was hit by a van and almost killed in Spain; all the healers I knew tried to help me, but I also had a marvelous surgeon. More recently, I survived prostate cancer, using both radiation therapy and herbal preparations. I have never found any conflict between allopathic biomedicine and complementary or alternative medicine.

However, one of the basic problems with the Western perspective—and allopathic biomedicine is part of the Western perspective—is its incomplete nature. What allopathic biomedicine explains and what it works with, it does quite well. But what we call the *modern Western tradition* is embedded in linear rationality and a type of science that tries to predict and control. To predict and control, one must have explanations, and one must produce data that are repeatable.

Most of Western science is logical and linear. It rarely takes a systems perspective that appreciates the complexity of the universe. For example, the parapsychological phenomena that are appreciated by indigenous cultures and many spiritual traditions are ignored by Western science because they are not easily repeatable. The Western scientist proclaims: "If I can't duplicate it, it doesn't exist."

What is often called *postmodern science* responds that perhaps there are some events that we will never be able to control or predict, but that doesn't mean we cannot study them; it doesn't mean we cannot describe them. This is one of the contributions of chaos and complexity theory. Sometimes we simply have to be satisfied with describing phenomena. The "other" world is the marginalized world, the world of parapsychology, of synchronicity, of complexity. It is those aspects of reality that the modern worldview simply refuses to acknowledge, but it is still part of the whole. The driving forces in the Western world are medicine, science, politics, and business. They all deal with concrete, tangible phenomena. And they construct reality. Earlier in the modern era, religion constructed reality. Now religion has faded as a power broker, but medicine, empirical science, politics, and business construct reality. I do not believe that we create our own reality, but we certainly construct it with our attitudes, our belief systems, and our mythic narratives.

According to postmodern thought, language can never completely represent reality. But language constructs people's experience, so the power players who control language control people's experience. That's why the power players in biomedicine, with their diagnostic categories, control the way people experience their sickness. Once an ailment is put into a category and given a name, most people accept that expectation and have the experiences that the diagnosis implies. But if some people do not get well, it is possible that they have a condition that does not fit into the categories of biomedicine. At this point, practitioners might look to the complementary and alternative therapies to see whether they have categories that are more adequate descriptors.

By appreciating the potential contributions of native and indigenous traditions, we can develop broader and deeper perspectives on more of the phenomena of the universe, and ultimately this will help us to become better caregivers, better health practitioners, and better counselors and therapists than we are at present.

David Lukoff, one of our Saybrook faculty members, was a member of a team that worked on what has become the "religious and spiritual problem" category in the fourth edition of the American Psychiatric Association's *Diagnostic and Statistical Manual of Mental Disorders*. Recently, Etzel Cardeña, Steven Jay Lynn, and I coedited a book, *Varieties of Anomalous Experience*, for the American Psychological Association. Jeanne Achterberg (another Saybrook faculty member) and I wrote the chapter on anomalous healing experiences.

These are crucial issues because the United States, Canada, and many other Western nations are becoming multicultural. The new immigrants, especially those from Southeast Asia, have their own belief systems and their own categories of disease and illness. Practitioners need to know about these beliefs and categories if they are going to treat these people adequately.

Before the end of the current century, there will probably be no ethnic majority in the United States; everybody will be part of an ethnic minority, Euro-Americans included. Thus it is essential to appreciate diverse worldviews and to realize what harm can be done through misdiagnosis. In one celebrated case, a well-meaning psychiatrist was interviewing a 70-year-old Native American woman. Going down the symptom checklist, he asked if she had ever "heard voices." She answered affirmatively, referring to the voices of the earth's spirits. The psychiatrist immediately classified her as a schizophrenic and institutionalized her, not realizing that everybody in her tribe was expected to "hear voices." These are the mistakes that are made if one does not understand and appreciate other cultural points of view.

Like this Native American woman, people who do not have authority or power become the "other" and are labeled and categorized as being, in this case, "mentally ill," because their social context is ignored. Eventually, the woman's "voices" instructed her on ways to obtain a release from the mental hospital.

What Is Medicine?

We often conceive of the human body as being the same all over the world, but even the body can be shaped, decorated, stretched, or compressed in different ways. The body image is constructed differently in different times and places. The human body in Chinese medicine is not the same as it is in allopathic biomedicine or even in Ayurvedic medicine. The body is treated differently with different medicines from culture to culture; the Chinese "triple burner" system and the Ayurvedic "prana" concept do not exist in Western biomedicine, yet they serve as a basis for diagnosis and treatment in their own systems.

There are many legitimate human experiences that are ignored by biomedicine. Examples are out-of-body, past-life, near-death, and peak experiences as well as precognitive dreams and cosmic consciousness. Currently, biomedicine is a part of the power establishment, the financial establishment, and the political establishment in most of what is called the *developed world*.

In biomedicine, medical students learn to construct their reality through the verbal practices of seeing, writing, and speaking. This is often called *biological reductionism,* and it is the central vision of medical students. This is how they learn to tell stories to their patients and how they shape the experience of their patients. But where is the use of metaphor? Where is the use of symbolism? Where is the use of social and spiritual resources?

There is no such thing as "a medicine." There are many medicines, many therapies. Stories are fundamental to all of these medicines and therapies. All of them establish categories by which health is normalized and by which illness is contrasted with what is considered normal. All have narrative structures that synthesize complaints into culturally meaningful syndromes. The patient describes a complaint or a symptom, and the practitioner, following an examination, gives a label that becomes culturally meaningful. Also, all therapies and medicines use what we can call *rhetoric.* This term has been introduced in this context by Jerome Frank in his classic book, *Persuasion and Healing.* Rhetoric is the voice of authority and it becomes the means by which the efficacy of the treatment is evaluated. Also, all medicines and therapies establish healing "roles" and caretaker "careers." The practitioner has a "career," while the patient and family have "roles." And all medicines have interpersonal engagements of some sort—sometimes a 5-minute engagement, sometimes a 5-day engagement—but there's always an interpersonal interaction following, which a panoply of therapies and treatments are put into operation to control the symptoms and their causes, hopefully to prevent worse things from happening and to provide relief in some form.

All medicines must be considered in their historical and cultural contexts, so I like to say, "All medicine is existential." You have to look at a medicine in its given time and place to really understand it.

Biomedicine, in all fairness, does contain a holistic, humanistic element, but it is not the dominant stream; it's not the stream that has obtained power. Alternative and complementary medicines, like Chinese and Ayurvedic, are more corollary, more at ease with the uncertainties of human existence, and certainly more holistic. But they, too, can become closed systems, sacrificing client welfare to their own dogma.

Here is one way to contrast medicines. In biomedicine, nature is physical and knowable. Patient narratives are devalued because the physician knows more than the patient. In some complementary and alternative medicines, the story the patient tells is listened to very carefully and physical concepts are expanded to cover spiritual concepts as well. For instance, biomedicine encourages heroic measures to keep people alive. Most complementary and alternative medicines are more focused on providing the patient a good death. The notion of the good death doesn't seem to be a priority in biomedicine. In Salvador, Brazil, I visited the Society of the Good Death, a group of spiritual practitioners devoted to helping their clients make their passage comfortably and peacefully.

I've had many relatives and many loved ones who have died within the past several years, but few of them had good deaths that were facilitated by their physicians. If they had a good death, it was facilitated by friends and family members. We have to realize that biomedicine has a disenchanted worldview. It lacks the concept of the vital force, of qi, of prana, of what the Malaysian shamans call the inner wind or the *angin,* and, as a result, there is no such concept as soul loss. I think we need to conceptualize health in systems terms: the whole is more than the sum of its parts, and according to complexity theory, the whole also is different from the sum of its parts. Once we realize this, we'll be on our way to revitalizing Western medicine without bringing in concepts that are superstitious or counterproductive.

Conclusion

As I mentioned, biomedical physicians do not acknowledge soul loss, but when a study was made of rural Mexicans who believed in soul loss, or *susto*, the people who had been diagnosed with soul loss had higher mortality rates than did those who had not been so diagnosed. The two different groups of rural Mexicans were equally sick from the biomedical point of view. Was the diagnosis a self-fulfilling prophecy, or did the local practitioners have insights that alerted them to the severity of the condition?

In biomedicine, you're dead when you are braindead. But even death is socially constructed. Among the Huli of New Guinea, breathing and heartbeat may remain, but if *Bu*, the life force, is gone, that person is considered dead and treatment stops. So the concept of death varies from culture to culture, just as the concept of life. Hence social constructs can save people's lives or condemn people to death. Cultural and personal myths cannot be overlooked in our discussion of health, illness, and disease.

We don't have all the answers to the pressing problems of health, illness, and disease. We can learn not only from Western biomedical science but from the study and observation of alternative and complementary practitioners. The study of human experience is a critically important part of science; the observation of indigenous and native practices is also a part of science; the use of nonlinear, systems-oriented methodologies is becoming a part of science.

One can enhance personal mythology by learning about and appreciating the mythologies of other people, other ethnic groups, other cultures. This is a challenge for the 21st century. As for the biomedical establishment, it retains its power, but research studies show that one in three people go to alternative or complementary practitioners, spending billions of dollars. This should be a wake-up call. Practitioners and researchers need to realize the implications of this trend and be sure that these alternative and complementary practitioners are humanistic, holistic, and responsible regarding professional standards and training. In the postmodern twenty-first century, there will be room for a greater variety of healthcare practitioners, counselors, and therapists. But Hippocrates's dictum—"First, do no harm"—is one of the few pieces of rhetoric that I believe will retain its applicability across treatments, even when medical and therapeutic authority and power are more diversely distributed.

CHAPTER 37

MICHAEL HARNER, PhD

Shamanic Healing: We Are Not Alone

Michael Harner, PhD, anthropologist, shamanic practitioner and teacher of shamanism, is the founder of the Foundation for Shamanic Studies, an international nonprofit organization dedicated to preserving shamanic knowledge as it survives on the planet and to teaching the basic principles of that knowledge for practical applications in the contemporary world.

Harner, who has practiced shamanic healing since 1961, received his doctorate at the University of California-Berkeley. He is a former professor and chairperson of the department of anthropology at the Graduate Faculty of the New School for Social Research in New York and has taught at Columbia, Yale, and UC-Berkeley. His books include *The Jívaro, Hallucinogens, and Shamanism,* and the classic, *The Way of the Shaman*. In the course of his study of shamanism, Harner lived and worked with indigenous peoples in the Upper Amazon, Mexico, Peru, the Canadian Arctic, Samiland, and western North America.

I first met Dr. Harner when I took a basic course in shamanism in the mid-1980s from the Foundation for Shamanic Studies. Dr. Harner happened to be the teacher and the course had a profound effect on my worldview. So I was delighted when I was asked by the editors to interview him for the journal. In 1996, we met in his office in Mill Valley, California, during an intense storm, and after the power was knocked out, we finished the interview by candlelight.

The word *shaman* in the original Tungus language refers to a person who makes journeys to nonordinary reality in an altered state of consciousness. Adopting the term in the West was useful because people didn't have preconceptions about what it meant. Terms like *wizard, witch, sorcerer,* and *witch doctor* have their own connotations and ambiguities associated with them and don't always refer to shamans. Although the term is from Siberia, the practice of shamanism existed on all inhabited continents.

After years of extensive research, Mircea Eliade, in his book, *Shamanism: Archaic Techniques of Ecstasy,* concluded that shamanism underlay all the other spiritual traditions on the planet, and that the most distinctive feature of shamanism—but by no means the only one—was the journey to other worlds in an altered state of consciousness, which he called *ecstasy*. There are generally three worlds recognized cross culturally in shamanism: the Upper, Middle, and Lower. We reside in the Middle.

From a shamanic point of view, it's often very important to get out of the Middle World when journeying for spiritual purposes. In the old days, shamans often journeyed in the Middle World to see how relatives were doing at a distant place or to locate the herds of migratory animals. But most of our work today is in the Upper and Lower Worlds where shamans have voyaged since ancient times. Going to the Upper or Lower Worlds, one reaches spiritual beings of compassion, power, and wisdom.

Shamans are often termed *people who know* in their tribal languages because they are involved in a system of knowledge involving firsthand spiritual experiences rather than beliefs. Shamanism is based on personal experiments conducted to heal, to get information, or do other things. In fact, if shamans don't get results, they will no longer be used by people in their tribes.

The practice of shamanism is a method, not a religion. It coexists with established religions in many cultures. In Siberia, you'll find shamanism coexisting with Buddhism and Lamaism, and in Japan with Buddhism. Shamans are often in animistic cultures. Animism means that people believe there are spirits. So in shamanic cultures, where shamans interact with spirits to get results such as healing, it's no surprise that people believe there are spirits. But the shamans don't *believe* in spirits. Shamans talk with them, interact with them. They no more "believe" there are spirits than we "believe" we have a house to live in, or have a family. This is a very important issue because shamanism is not a system of faith.

I might say something more about "spirits," because it's a disconcerting word for many people. What is a spirit? In 1961, when I was with the *ayahuasca:* using Conibo Indians in eastern Peru in the Amazon, I was training with a shaman, many nights. I worked with the anaconda spirit, the black panther spirit, the freshwater dolphin spirit, various tree spirits, and so on. They would come; we would see them; and so on. Then one night I got introduced to the outboard-motor spirit. And then the radio spirit and the airplane spirit. I came to realize that anything that you see in complete darkness or with your eyes closed is technically a spirit. That makes it sound like it's just an image in the air, but shamans find out which spirits have power and which don't. They discover what spirits can help and in what ways. It's very important to recognize that whatever you contact in nonordinary reality is technically a spirit. It's a spiritual reality.

Shamanism is also not exclusionary. They don't say, "We have the only healing system." In a holistic approach to healing, the shaman uses the spiritual means at his or her disposal in cooperation with people in the community who have other techniques such as plant healing, massage, and bone setting. The shaman's purpose is to help the patient get well, not to prove that his or her system is the only one that works.

Shamans are often given gifts for their work, but in some cultures, they will return all the gifts if the patient dies, which I think is a commendable innovation that might help us with the costs of health services today!

Shamanic Healing

Shamans talk with plants and animals, with all of nature. This is not just a metaphor and they do it in an altered state of consciousness (ASC). Our own students rapidly discover that by talking with plants in the proper ASC, they can discover how to prepare those plants for remedies. Shamans have been doing this since ancient times. They typically know a great deal about plants, but it's not essential. For example, Inuit shamans don't have access to a lot of plants, so they work with other things. But in the Amazon, shamans know the songs that go with the plants, which they commonly learn from the plants themselves.

One former student of mine in the United States developed a practice of discovering and using healing plants based on his learning directly from the plants. He found that the pharmacopoeia he developed was very close to the ancient, classic Chinese pharmacopoeic knowledge of how to prepare and use these plants for different ailments. Another former student in Germany worked with minerals and found how they could be used in healing. It turned out that her discoveries were very close to what has been known in India from ancient times.

You ask what happens when a sick person asks a shaman for a healing? Well, a shaman might make a journey to another world for diagnostic purposes, to get information about the person's problems from a spiritual point of view. It doesn't necessarily matter what the diagnosis is from an ordinary reality point of view. There's no simple one-to-one concordance between spiritual illness and ordinary reality illness. You can't just say, "This equals that." So the shaman will often make a journey to find out what the spiritual causality may be and, according to that causality, decide on the treatment.

From the shamanic point of view, people who are not spiritually power-filled are prone to illness, accidents, and bad luck. The shaman may decide to restore a person's linkage to his or her spiritual power. This spiritual power is something analogous to a spiritual immune defense system, but I wouldn't make a one-to-one equivalence. It's an analog. The power makes one resistant to illness. If somebody is repeatedly ill, then it's clear that they need restoration of a lost power connection. A healthy person who is not sick might go on a vision quest to get this power connection, but one of the shaman's jobs is to help people who are in no condition to do that for themselves.

Today in our culture many consider it avant garde if a person talks about the mind-body connection, but the fact that the brain is connected to the rest of the body is not really the most exciting news. It's been known for hundreds of thousands of years. The shaman, more importantly, knows that we are not alone. By that I mean, when one person compassionately works to relieve the suffering of another, the helping spirits are interested and become involved. When somebody who is disinterested, who is not an immediate family member, out of generosity and compassion helps somebody else to relieve illness or pain and suffering—this is when miracles occur. So the big news that shamanism offers is not that the head is connected to the rest of the body, but that we are not dependent solely on ourselves for healing—there are powers to help us.

Soul Retrieval

Anyone who has had a trauma, from a shamanic point of view, probably had some loss of his or her soul. By soul we mean the spiritual essence possessed throughout one's life. Healing soul loss is done with soul-retrieval techniques, and one of the classic shamanic methods is to go searching for that lost portion of the soul and restore it, something I learned to do among the Conibo Indians of the Amazon in 1960-1961. Today it is an impor-tant aspect of shamanic healing practices here in the West. My colleague, Sandra Ingerman, had written about the application of this work to our contemporary society in her book *Soul Retrieval*.

Indeed, if you ask a group of people, "How many of you feel you've lost part of your soul?" it's typical that almost everybody raises a hand. At some deep level, there seems to be a natural awareness of this problem. By the way, even a minor trauma can result in some degree of soul loss and can be treated.

Extraction

Another major technique in shamanic healing work is extraction. Extraction involves removing a spiritual intrusion. Just as there can be infections in ordinary reality, so there can be spiritual intrusions. We don't have to mean that "evil" spirits have entered. It's more like termites in a wooden house. If you've got termites in your house, you wouldn't say those termites are evil; you'd say, "I'd just like to get them out of the house." In this same way the shaman works to remove things that interfere with the health of the body, such as spiritual intrusions, and extract them. This is not done through journeying. It's done through working here in the Middle World in an altered state of consciousness.

In about 90% of the world, the altered states of consciousness used in shamanism have been attained through consciousness-changing techniques involving a monotonous percussion sound, most typically done with a drum but also with sticks, rattles, and other instruments. In perhaps 10% of the cultures, shamans ingest consciousness-altering plant substances to change their states of consciousness.

I began participating in shamanic work more than 40 years ago among the Conibo Indians in eastern Peru, with the aid of the psychedelic *ayahuasca*. When I came back to the United States, where there was no *ayahuasca*, I experimented with drumming. Much to my surprise, it really worked. It should not have surprised me, because drums and other percussion tools were reportedly used by perhaps 9090 of shamans worldwide. Almost everything you find in indigenous shaman-ism is done because it works. Over tens of thousands of years, shamans developed the most time-tested system of using spirits, mind, and heart for healing. So if healers in 90% of the shamanic cultures are using the same methods, we pay attention and call them *core methods*. And, of course, we find they work.

To get back to the extraction technique: it involves an altered state of consciousness and seeing into the client's body. Much shamanic work, including journeying and extraction, is done in darkness for a very simple reason. The shaman wishes to cut out the stimuli of ordinary reality—light, extraneous sound, and so on—and move into an ordinarily unseen reality. The shaman learns to look in the body with "x-ray vision" and see the illness and its location and then to extract that illness.

Depossession

Shamans who do another type of healing help the dead as well as the living. These shamans are called *psychopomps*, or conductors of souls. From a shamanic point of view, when you're comatose, you're "dead." So the shaman, in the case of a comatose person, would seek out the person and see if he or she wanted to come back. Shamanism is not a system that intends to keep people "alive" in this ordinary reality whether they like it or not, because the shaman knows that this is not necessarily the best reality. You make the journey for people who are comatose or deceased to find out what they want. If they want to return, then the job of the shaman is to help bring them back. But if they want to go on, then the job of the shaman is to get them to a place where they will be content and not leave them adrift in the Middle World.

So now we come back to this business of possession. Most cases of possession of humans are by other humans who are dead, who are here in the Middle World and don't know they're dead. If people are disempowered or have soul loss or power loss, they are like an empty vessel into which these confused entities can come. This is involuntary possession.

Shamans can conduct the entity—with its permission once it realizes it's dead—to a place beyond the Middle World where it will be reunited with people it loves. With this done, so that the clients are no longer possessed, shamans restore their full soul and lost power connections so they are again whole and resistant to further possessions.

Depossession work has slightly different forms in different cultures, but the basic principles are the same. I hope that one day our culture will recognize the need to permit shamanic practitioners to work with such spiritual aspects of illness in cooperation with health professionals who do not deal with spirits, for the methods are valuable in dealing with alcohol and drug dependency and multiple personality disorders.

Unfortunately, when science started, partially as a reaction to the Church in Europe, it ordained that souls and spirits have no reality and therefore could not be considered in scientific theory and practice. That's an *a priori* position; in other words, ironically, a "scientific" statement of faith enunciated in the eighteenth century. In fact, however, science has never disproved the existence of spirits.

I would submit that now, at the beginning of the twenty-first century, it is time to stop having a science that's based on faith (the faith that there can be no spirits).

Origins of Illness

From a shamanic point of view, all people have a spiritual side, whether they recognize it or not. When people get angry, jealous, or have a hostile emotional attitude, they can vent not only verbal and physical abuse but spiritual abuse without even knowing it. In other words, if somebody is ignorant of shamanic principles, they can do damage to other people on a spiritual level.

Among the Untsuri Shuar or Jívaro people of eastern Ecuador, with whom I lived for quite a while, they call these intrusions "magical darts." There were many feuds and wars, and sometimes healers would get angry, lose their discipline, and use their powers to get even. But it is important to know that this is a big mistake, not just ethically, but in terms of self-preservation. No matter how justified an angry person feels emotionally at the time, those spiritual powers who are representative of the great, loving, hidden universe will disconnect. It's like we're rechargeable batteries. We still have some power, and we can do damage, but the power source is no longer charging us. I've seen this many times in the Amazon. The shamans, in their anger, can do harm for a while, but eventually everything they send out comes back in on them. In their depowered state, this often results not only in their own death or pain, but their immediate family can also be affected disastrously.

This doesn't mean you shouldn't get angry at people. It just means that you should have shamanic knowledge and discipline and know there are parameters. You can get angry with somebody and verbally let out steam and, at the same time, control your spiritual power. For your own self-preservation, be aware that if you don't work to relieve pain and suffering—and especially if you work in a contrary way—you'll soon lose your power protection and become ill or even die.

Self–Healing

A problem with the concept of self-healing is that it excludes the spirits by calling itself *healing*. From the shamanic point of view, nobody has lived into adult life without spiritual help, whether he knows it or not. The self-healing concept is a secular concept, and that's fine as far as it teaches people to take some responsibility for their illness. But it also teaches them to take responsibility for their own death. With that approach, everybody's a failure at the moment of death, because he or she is responsible for the whole thing. From a shamanic point of view we are not that important. We are not necessarily the biggest thing in the universe. The shaman has a more humble point of view, that we, not being alone, can get help from spiritual sources. And the shaman has the role, of course, of accelerating that possibility.

I don't want to rule out self-healing, but it is a very limited secular view of reality, just recognizing that the brain is connected to the body.

Ordinary Reality and Nonordinary Reality

The terms *ordinary reality* and *nonordinary reality* come from Carlos Castaneda. Ordinary reality is the reality that we all normally perceive together. It's the reality in which we can all agree that there is a clock on the wall. Nonordinary reality is the reality that is associated with the shamanic state of consciousness—that is, when your consciousness is altered and you're able to see what you normally don't see in an ordinary state of consciousness.

The term *nonordinary reality* is useful because it permits one to be reminded that access to these worlds is related to the degree to which you have entered the shamanic state of consciousness. It clarifies our thinking. For years, many people were confused when a shaman said, "I made a journey and was away for 3 years, and such and such happened." Now that person in nonordinary reality had the experience of living somewhere else for 3 years but might have been gone only a half hour in ordinary reality.

Ordinary reality is something that virtually everybody agrees on. In contrast, nonordinary reality is very person-specific. The information obtained in nonordinary reality is tailor-made to the individual—other people may not perceive it at all, as opposed to the information obtained in ordinary reality, in which everybody gets the same thing.

Nonordinary reality is also an empirical reality—that is, the person interacts with it, sees it, touches it, hears it, feels it. And the shaman also sees with the heart. In nonordinary reality, for something to be the same for different persons, it has to be the same in the heart. Here (in ordinary reality) for something to be the same it doesn't matter what your emotion is; you'll see it, for example, as a door in the room. If I showed you a picture of my mother, now deceased, you and I would not have the same emotional relationship with that picture. But if I said the word "mother," and each of us saw our own mother, the emotional feeling in the heart would be closer—not identical—but closer. So to see things exactly the same in the heart, they have to be a little different for each person, because each person has a different personality and a different life history.

Divination

Work in shamanism also involves divination. People can journey for themselves or have somebody who's a shamanic practitioner journey for them to get an answer to a question. What's really interesting is when somebody who's a complete stranger—about whom the shaman knows nothing—asks for an answer to a question, the shaman then journeys or uses other techniques and gets miraculously detailed information that's valid for that person's life. This can happen because these things are known by the spirits. The shaman doesn't need to know anything except to communicate the messages of his or her own spirit helpers.

Foundation Activities

Sometimes I informally call our foundation the "University of Shamanism." I say this because our primary purpose is to return spiritual authority to the individual by training people in shamanism. Many of these people are doctors and other health professionals. After our training, it is they who must discover how to integrate what they are taught into their practices. To help with this, in 2002, the Foundation for Shamanic Studies cosponsored a conference of health practitioners who have studied with us, to exchange information about how they have used these methods in their practices.

Our applied health research is investigating certain matters regarding shamanic journeying and drumming and health. My wife, Dr. Sandra Harner, is the director of the Shamanism and Health Project. Her research involves two major aspects, one of which is the effect of shamanic journeying and drumming on one measure of immune response and on emotions.

In connection with this work, she has gotten some hints that people with certain profiles of psychological descriptors respond much more effectively in terms of the immune response than others. This is a subject, obviously, of considerable interest. She has also found that there is a tremendous increase in the sense of well-being as well as decreased mood disturbance and stress in people working with shamanic drumming and journeying. But to say more would be premature.

It's ironic that a system of healing that—other than using herbs—is the oldest known system of healing in the world, should have almost no research going on in it at all, other than what we at the foundation are able to do with our meager resources. I look forward to the day when the possibility of spiritual causality is not ruled out of research, so that science, in fact, can be completely scientific.

We also have what the medical profession would call *anecdotal accounts*. People often come to the shamans when everybody else has failed. We have many cases in which, once people start getting shamanic treatments and laboratory tests are continued, the tests turn out negative, whereas they previously were positive. The assumption from the medical profession, of course, is usually that the previous diagnoses were incorrect because there's been a reversal or "spontaneous remission." After all, it's virtually impossible, on a case-by-case basis, to prove causality. However, if you practice shamanic healing for years, the positive track record becomes unmistakable.

My primary interest right now is in miracles. I've devoted some years now to finding out what principles are involved to have miracles happen. I think we're making significant progress. Almost everything that anybody's ever read about in the shamanic literature or the miracle literature is something that we have some knowledge of how to do now. And this includes miracles of healing.

Starting in 1997, I moved forward on this project with some of our most advanced students.

Once a shaman contacts the spirits, there's a crossover of the power from nonordinary reality to ordinary reality. The two realities are conceptually discrete, but the shaman is able to move the power of one over to the other. When this is done successfully, that's how healings occur and how we have what is called miracles.

When you start shamanic journeying, if you're the kind of person the spirits feel compassion for and want to help you, you're going to get lots of teachings you never asked for and never expected. Because once you go through those doors to nonordinary reality—whatever those doors are—the spirits will teach you according to your preparation and needs, and your life will change. Even one journey may start changing your life.

CHAPTER 38

ALAN DAVIS, MD

Shamanism in Medical Practice

The use of shamanism among medical and healthcare practitioners has been increasing for the past 10 years, enough so that when I was asked if *Alternative Therapies in Health and Medicine,* in conjunction with the Foundation for Shamanic Studies (FSS), would like to produce a conference on "Integrating Shamanism into Medical Practice," I readily agreed. The person who asked was Alan Davis, MD, PhD. Alan had organized a group of seven physicians trained through the foundation who were using shamanism in their day-to-day lives and practices. This "Group of 7" became the faculty for the conference, which was held in the summer of 2002 in Santa Fe.

When he isn't organizing conferences or skiing, Dr. Davis is an assistant professor at the University of Utah School of Medicine, Division of Physical Medicine and Rehabilitation and the medical director for Quinney Rehabilitation Institute at Salt Lake Regional Medical Center. His medical practice focuses on inpatient medical rehabilitation. He completed his physical medicine and rehabilitation residency at the University of Medicine and Dentistry of New Jersey and then completed his neuroscience PhD by investigating how yoga-like breathing exercises produce a relaxation response. Dr. Davis has been apprenticing with Sarah Sifers, PhD, a graduate of the FSS 3-year program, and has completed the 2-week FSS intensive course in advanced shamanism and shamanic healing directed and taught by Sandra Ingerman.

In the fall of 2001, I traveled to Salt Lake City to interview Alan. We met in his hillside home, took a shamanic journey together for insight, and then sat down to talk. The monologue that follows is a result of that conversation.

I initially developed an interest in shamanism to do my personal work. I'd been through a lot of counseling and reached the point where I had insight and an intellectual understanding of my own personal issues. But even though I thought I'd peeled the onion to the very core, there was still something missing. Someone recommended I see a shamanic counselor named Sarah Sifers, PhD, and through her, in the context of doing my personal work, I was exposed to an entirely new world of healing on a spiritual level that I found totally engrossing. I quickly became interested in trying to work with other people in this way and so began an apprenticeship with Sarah to learn shamanic healing technique and practice.

A few years later, while at a medical conference in San Francisco, I met Michael Harner, PhD, founder of the Foundation for Shamanic Studies. I talked to him about the need for bringing this type of work into medicine and was totally surprised to find out how many physicians had actually completed some type of training through the Foundation for Shamanic Studies. Every group in their most advanced training program has 5% to 10% physicians. I found this heartening.

Using Shamanism in Medical Practice

I'm a hospital-based physician in a community hospital. Specifically, I'm the medical director of an inpatient medical rehabilitation unit, so most of my patients have had major medical problems requiring lengthy hospital stays and rehabilitation therapy to bring back some level of lost function. Our goal is to maximize the person's functions so that they can do as much as possible without help from others. The people I see have had orthopedic problems such as hip replacements or amputations or neurological problems, particularly from strokes. Some have brain injury, spinal cord injury, multiple sclerosis, or they have significant debility from illnesses such as heart attack, advanced lung disease, or brain cancer. It's a traditional rehabilitation hospital population, and my clinic is a very traditional medical office.

But bringing shamanic spiritual work into a conventional setting brings up a number of issues. One immediately thinks, "How can I actually do this on a practical basis?" For example, many of the healing techniques use drumming or rattling as a way to clear away the ego in preparation for the healing work. But in a hospital setting, beating on your drum and rattling rattles as you see your patients is not the accepted behavior. So there are two questions: "What's it look like to the patients, and what does it look like to the hospital or clinic staff?"

Another big question is "Even if I could modify these techniques, is this something that I'm supposed to ask permission for, or do my patients expect that I will automatically use all of my talents to help them?" It's a significant issue. If you say to yourself, "Patients expect me to use all of my talents and want healing on every level," then one can rationalize the use of shamanism in a hospital or office practice.

Physical medicine and rehabilitation, or physiatry, is arguably the most holistic of the medical specialties. Every person has a team of therapists. They have physical therapists to work on their mobility and occupational therapists to work on their ability to take care of themselves. If they have cognitive issues or swallowing issues, they have a speech language pathologist. There's a social worker, a rehabilitation psychologist, and a physiatric physician assigned to every patient. Certainly the people providing counseling to the patient will touch on different aspects of the patient's life. But you could also ask, "If we're truly holistic, shouldn't we look at the whole person, which means the spiritual part of the person as well?"

For myself, I've come to the conclusion that I'm not comfortable with just modifying the techniques and doing them in a way that the patient would never know or suspect. When I see a patient who I think really may benefit from healing work on a spiritual level, I'm up front with them. I simply say, "I also do some other kinds of healing techniques that address things on a spiritual level. Would you be interested in exploring that?"

I've had patients say, "I don't think I'm ready for that." And I've had patients say, "Yes, I'd like to know more." If they say yes, then I explain what issues we could consider from a shamanic framework. Then I give them the logistics of the process so that they can make a decision on whether to proceed or not. Of course, I have to be very sensitive to the person's own beliefs. I live in Salt Lake City, and there's a significant religious culture here with the Church of Jesus Christ Latter Day Saints. Some people don't separate their inner spirituality from their religion. But regardless, it's important to honor the patient's perspective and beliefs. I don't present shamanism as a religion, and I haven't had any patient define this as a religious conflict even though it is something profoundly and deeply spiritual.

Some people undergoing rehabilitation just aren't ready for addressing the spiritual. They are learning how to walk again or how to control their bowel and bladder again or how to eat food or talk again. They may not be able to add one more thing to their plate. So they say, "I'm not comfortable with it." But what frequently happens is that after the patient has gone beyond his or her most basic needs, he or she comes back to see me and says, "When you talked to me in the hospital about shamanism and spiritual healing, I couldn't even think about doing anything. But my life is settling down, and I'm functional now, and I can think about it."

Using Shamanism with Patients

I have actually taken out my rattle and done journey work in the hospital setting. The drumming issue is less of an issue now because I conduct a therapeutic drumming circle with my patients on a regular basis with my psychologist. This is our pet project and predates my interest in shamanism. Once or twice a month we ask all the patients if they want to come and drum with us. We usually have good participation. We hand out drums and other percussion instruments and just have jam sessions. It fills the patients with energy and is a very special experience. Even the hospital administration and the nurses have come to watch the drumming, and everybody who sees it just smiles. They accept the eccentricity of it.

So shamanic work can be done in the hospital setting. But you have to explain to the patient what you're going to do and why you're going to do it. For example, take a patient with a brain injury. A brain injury is typically due to a car accident, and people with brain injuries frequently just aren't the same. A person with shamanic training says, "This person may need a soul retrieval." Or you may hear from your patient, "I don't have any energy and feel powerless and depressed. I constantly feel like there's something wrong that I can't quite name." That, from a shamanic perspective, suggests that they may need a power animal retrieval. Many of the physical things that manifest in these patients suggest extraction work. Extraction work is removing energy from a person's energy field that doesn't belong there.

Now, I have to say one thing. From a shamanic perspective, the shaman is really just a conduit for the healing. You have to be able to put aside your ego to do this type of healing work. You, as the shaman, are just the catalyst for the healing to take place. A lightning rod doesn't do anything to the lightning; it just collects the energy and grounds it in the earth. In the same way, a shaman is a conduit for spiritual energy that does the healing work. In the beginning, you spend a significant amount of time trying to become an "empty bone" or "hollow reed" so that spiritual energy can come in and do the work. The better you do this, the more effective you are as a healer.

The process goes something like this: I give the patient an overview of shamanism. It's an ancient healing technique—probably the first healing technique—that was used tens of thousands of years ago by indigenous cultures. And in the modern world, we can still use these techniques. Then I explain what the process will be like. First I diagnose the patient for spiritual illness. I can do this with the patient in front of me or at a distance without the patient there. But my results are definitely better when I do it with the patient present.

In the diagnostic journey, you contact your power animal or your spiritual teacher, whoever you work with for healing techniques. You ask, "What healing needs to be done for this patient?" Then you have a dialogue with your spirit helpers about what is needed. But if you come to it with an agenda, because you feel very attached to the person, that's usually an impediment. It means ego is getting involved. You don't want to do the wrong type of healing technique, so you always listen to your spirit helpers.

The answer may be as simple as "John with the brain injury needs a soul retrieval and power animal retrieval." If so, I might do a small journey at the bedside with the patient or in my office downstairs in the rehab unit. I have a small rattle that's shaped like an egg. I tell the patient, "I'm going to sit by your bed, and you're going to be lying in your bed, and I'm going to shake this rattle as I go to a place and look for your missing life essence."

I tell the patients that I'm going to go find their life essence and bring it back. In the hospital setting, there are a number of ways to do it. Commonly we blow soul parts back in through the crown of a person's head or into their heart. But the soul parts can be collected and put in something and just given it to the patient. You could collect the soul parts and put them in a crystal or even in a piece of chocolate, if you want. Whatever works, but you always check in with spirit about what is recommended.

A power animal retrieval is done in a similar way. You journey to look for power animals that will volunteer to be helper animals to give back to patients some of their power and to relieve some of their depression and feelings that they can't rise to life any more. The techniques are very simple and don't have to be drawn-out endeavors.

Another very practical thing that I've done with this work is that in my morning journey I go through the list of my patients in the hospital and ask, "What does John need today? What does this patient need today?" I take an inventory of what I could possibly offer them. But I don't do any treatment covertly.

Some results are profound, and some are subtle. There's also a point where you're not sure which of the many things you're doing have had an effect on the patient. In the rehabilitation setting we're addressing so many things from so many different perspectives, sometimes it's hard to say. Here's one example that comes to mind. I had a brain-injury patient, a young man in his thirties who fell asleep driving and was ejected from his car. He had a significant bleed in his brain, not a subtle injury, and was comatose and on a breathing machine for quite a while.

He came to my inpatient rehabilitation unit and did really well. His tracheostomy was quickly removed, the catheter in his bladder was quickly removed, and in less than a month he was walking and talking. I didn't even broach the subject of shamanism while he was here in the hospital because his initial rehabilitation was such a special experience. When I started seeing him in my clinic, he had done as well as any brain-injury patient could hope to do and was actually transitioning back to his previous job. The job required a fairly high level of thinking on his feet and very good interpersonal skills. This may be a lot to expect of someone who has had a brain injury, but he did well even though he wasn't able to do it fulltime. He would come to my office with his wife and talk about how wonderful he felt and how this whole experience had been so incredible for him—except that he couldn't pick up his guitar and play any songs. He said that the words would get stuck in his throat. And sometimes he tended to be disorganized and had trouble communicating his thoughts. So even though everything had gone really well, he was a bit depressed and felt like something wasn't quite right.

He was functional, but he wasn't where he wanted to be because he still wasn't himself. Of course I thought, "Sounds like he needs a soul retrieval." Now, a soul retrieval is a very common thing when someone has a major physical or emotional trauma because one experiences soul loss as a self-preservation measure. If you're steaming toward a wall at 55 miles an hour, a part of your soul leaves as a self-preservation measure. From a psychological standpoint we call this dissociation. From a shamanic perspective, it's soul loss or loss of some of the life force. So I broached the subject with him and his wife and gave them some written material to read about soul retrieval. But I left it to him to decide if he wanted to pursue this type of healing.

After a couple of visits, he brought up that he would like to consider doing some of this work. Since he was a patient in my clinic, I asked him to come to my house because I have a special place in home where I like to do this work.

First I did a diagnostic journey to find out what healing needed to be done. The answer was that he needed a soul retrieval and a power animal retrieval. So we proceeded to do the soul retrieval and the power animal retrieval, and I could tell immediately after that he was very energized by the experience. But even so, I didn't know what was ultimately going to happen.

A few months later he contacted me to tell me that he was able to sing his songs—they didn't get stuck in his throat. And he felt like the piece that was missing had been given back to him. He said he felt more whole, more able to focus, and better able to interact with people without feeling that he was just talking in circles. He had more energy for his work and had returned to some of his previous recreational activities—mountain biking and wind surfing and playing his music.

There's another story I'd like to tell. A young woman in her thirties had a stroke right after she gave birth. It was a terrible thing for her. She was completely paralyzed on one side of her body, and her speech was very slurred. She was with us for rehabilitation, but she was not able to put her full effort into it or into her own personal goals of being able to walk again and being able to hold her baby. Her effort was halfhearted. She was in the rehab unit for quite a long time, and after watching this for 2 months, I brought up the fact that I might be able to help her. I offered to retrieve a healing song for her. This is a very simple healing technique that frequently has very profound results. To retrieve a healing song you go on a journey and talk with your power animal or your teacher. You ask to retrieve a healing song for the person in question.

I retrieved a song and taught it to her. I also gave her a rattle so she could do it just the way I did it. When you do a healing song, you keep singing it until the person has it memorized. In her case, since she had some memory problems, we did it for a few days in a row. I also wrote it down for her. After we did the healing song for a few days, she was able to put her full effort into her rehabilitation. You could see her come back to life. There was a spark in her eyes and she was motivated. It was a very simple song but it had incredible results.

To be honest, the complexity of techniques has absolutely no relation to the results you get. For example, you don't even necessarily do any of the healing yourself. You can go on a journey and ask your teacher or your power animal to provide whatever healing is needed for that person and ask them to do the entire thing. You're not involved at all. You can get incredible results just from that.

Other Shamanic Healing Techniques

There are techniques that we all learn such as power animal retrieval, soul retrieval, extraction work, depossession work, and, in the case of death and dying, psycho pomp work. And there are also many other healing techniques that one just learns from teachers or power animals. Sometimes they gift you with something special.

For instance, this last year I had eczema in my hands for the first time in my entire life. The dermatologist told me that many doctors get it because we wash our hands all the time. But I said to myself, "Well, maybe there's a spiritual part of this that I should explore." So I journeyed on the meaning of my hand eczema. It turned out to be a gift from spirit. My hands are like spirit eyes. When I'm examining my patients, I can, with the proper focus, activate these spirit sense organs in my hands and use them to help in diagnosing what's happening on a spiritual level.

The eczema still comes and goes—it's part of maintaining the sensitivity. The journey wasn't a healing for me, it was a realization of this gift.

Sometimes we don't get answers. When this happens, I explain to the patient that in this point in time, I can't answer his question or address his problem. It may be that we try again at another time and the answer is there. That happens. But also, sometimes someone may come for healing and I'm not the person who should do it. It just may be that I am told that, yes, this person needs some healing, but I'm not the one who's supposed to do it for him or her. You may or may not get a recommendation of another healer or of a different kind of healing.

Frequently in those situations, you aren't given enough information to even understand why—it's just the way it is. And I don't push when those situations come up.

I always get the techniques I need from the power animals and teachers I work with. Having done the work for a while you have a sense for what's needed, but I would never just go ahead and do that work alone. You always follow your teacher's guidance.

Now, this is not the normal way a physician works. Physicians are taught to engage their brains and use their diagnostic abilities and make a treatment plan based on their intellect and knowledge. So as a physician, you really have to work at letting your ego go in this kind of situation.

But let me make one thing perfectly clear. I give my patients every single normal medical thing I would give them, no matter what, from the start. Shamanism is something I do as additional treatment for those who want it. I don't substitute my spiritual offering for my medical treatment. In addition, I do not have a separate spiritual practice for shamanic work. This is only for my regular patients.

Shamanism's Value to Medical Practice

The physician who explores shamanism can learn a few special things. One is that to really do this work, you have to do it from your heart. For me, the overall biggest lesson of all has been how to open my heart and have love and compassion for my patients. The day-to-day work of a physician frequently shuts down physicians' hearts. I would say, as a whole, most busy, overwhelmed, overworked physicians are relatively heart-closed. The most wonderful thing that's happened to me is that I'm able to have a more open heart and more compassion and love for my patients.

To do this work, you can't just do these techniques in a mechanical way. In the process of getting ready to do any healing work, you raise your power and fill with spirit, and that filling also happens to the heart. The heart is the dominant organ in this type of spiritual healing. So even though you may initially learn the techniques and do them in a choreographed way, to really bring them into your life and live them, you have to open your heart and let that part of you that connects with the other person and connects with spirit be totally wide open and nonjudgmental. Your brain and your ego are set aside and you accept the fact, as a shaman, you are not the one doing the work.

I think shamanism is very needed in medicine right now because most physicians who have been in practice for a number of years feel like something is missing. We're not taught how to be a healer in medical school. We're taught how to intervene in a disease process and how to look at disease as the enemy. We are taught to look at the body in a very mechanical way. Shamans look at the body as a vehicle for the soul or life essence.

A major lesson that medicine can learn from shamanism is that to be a healer you have to accept the fact that you are a catalyst, a conduit, a hollow bone, an empty reed that's going to let that which really heals people come in. This is a very important lesson in medicine. By accepting that healing comes from another place, you truly accept your own humanness because there comes a point where you realize that you can't do it all. We all have had patients that we just don't know what to do with. Medicine can deal with the basic disease processes, but when you look at the whole person, traditional medicine only deals with a very small part of the problem. True healing does not come from working on a diseased organ system or body part; it comes from another level.

We are all taught in medical school that we are the one. It's doctor as hero; doctor as knight in shining armor with the pulled sword, fighting disease to the death. Shamanism has richness when addressing death. The shaman embraces death and understands it. It's part of the process. To this end the shaman may carry out psycho pomp work.

Psycho pomp means conductor of souls. This is the process whereby the shaman makes sure or even assists a person's soul to cross over into the light after death. Sometimes a soul doesn't want to cross over. They may be too attached to their habits, or relationships, or they may feel that they have unfinished business. They perpetuate their existence in a filmy reality that looks like a shade of their previous life. Sometimes someone can't let go of them fully. The shaman goes to the place or person and convinces the soul to cross over voluntarily. I knew a person who drank himself to death. I found him in his apartment with bottles all over the place still wondering what was going on. When his departed relatives came to see him he chose to cross over. There's also a whole group of experiences on the other side!

Spiritual Intrusions and Extraction Work

One shamanic healing technique is extraction work. Extraction work removes intrusions, and intrusions are like energies that are in the wrong place. It's not your energy. There's something in your body that shouldn't be there and it's causing malfunction. Extraction work is taking out that intrusion to promote normal function.

The diagnosis to look for intrusions involves scanning the whole body, from head to toe. Now, you don't find that the person is missing his or her angel wings; you find some very practical things. You'll sense that there's something wrong in the person's ankle. You can sense a person's back pain. There are three different techniques for scanning. One technique is using your hands and feeling changes in the person's field around his body. It's not aura work particularly; you're actually physically sensing temperature changes that magnetically pull you toward them. Another technique is merging with your power animal or your teacher, and you look through their eyes and hear with their ears and feel with their hands. A third technique is to use the tunnel that you go down in your journey as a diagnosis zone with the beginning of the tunnel being the person's head and the end of the tunnel being the feet. You know this tunnel like the back of your hand because you've traveled through it thousands and thousands of times, and so you look for things that aren't normally there.

I used this technique on someone recently and found rocks and pebbles on my path that aren't normally there. And over the area that represented the patient's pelvis, I saw these sickly white things. When I asked her about it, she said, "I have polycystic ovarian disease. I have a lot of pelvic pain all the time, and my ovaries don't work right." So this is an adjunct diagnostic technique that could be used also to find other ways of looking at problems. Extraction work frequently finds spiritual things that are physically manifested in people's bodies.

Once you find something, you extract the energetic intrusion—you remove it and neutralize it. One common way of neutralizing it is to put it in a body of water. You can have an actual bowl of water right next to you or you can visualize it going into a pond or river or lake. But you don't collect the intrusion and drop it on the floor. Then it can just go to another person. This is also one situation where you really have to be filled with spirit because you don't want to take the extraction into yourself.

Spiritual intrusions can come from a number of sources, and one of them is negative thoughts forms. All of us send spiritual intrusions to other people. When you're mad at someone, you can send him or her a spiritual intrusion unintentionally. It's so common that we don't even realize it. But when you do the extraction work, you don't know where the intrusions come from. I don't try to have an understanding of what it was that brought it on. I just do the work and get rid of it. There's a lot of negative thought forms floating around, particularly now.

There's a lot of fear in this time of war. We're in a soup of positive and negative thought forms, and the intrusions can come from all kinds of sources.

In a similar vein, in our society, instead of being soul stealers, we are soul givers. Let's say you're in a relationship with an alcoholic. If you're the kind of person who wants to cure that other person then you're constantly giving of yourself. Of course, many types of people aren't interested in fixing themselves, so what happens is that you're constantly giving your soul essence to them. That's why being with a person like an alcoholic is so draining. You're giving pieces of yourself away, and at the same time, you're trying to control this other person and force him or her to do your will. Dominating someone or manipulating someone can promote soul loss. And in our society, we do this unconsciously all the time.

Shamanism's Effect on the Shaman

Has shamanism changed my life? Well, I think that in some ways I'm the same, and in some ways I'm profoundly different. I've always been a happy, gregarious, outgoing, energetic Pied Piper type. That's always been Alan. But I would say that for me, the gift of shamanism has been the opening of my heart.

When I look back, my heart was open on one level, but this work has opened my heart on a deeper level. It's had a profound effect on my closest relationships and on my ability to really listen in a therapeutic relationship. Because I *can* listen now. I'm not just churning on what this person needs. I'm fully present and being fully present with my heart open allows healing to occur. There's healing just from the therapeutic relationship of being focused with my heart open and fully listening to the other person.

The other thing has been a profound spiritual awakening. My whole life has been a spiritual pilgrimage, starting with investigating my own religion. As a teenager, I learned transcendental meditation in the 1970s and delved into yoga. I pursued a religion major in college even while I was premed and made my own religious pilgrimage by leaving my own religion and exploring other religions. Then, after medical school, I did research on the physiological effects of different breathing techniques. When I look back on my pilgrimage, I realize I was looking for the I/Thou relationship. I wanted connection with the spiritual, and all my exploring was about trying to get closer to the spiritual. More than anything I've ever done in my life, shamanism as a spiritual practice has fulfilled that. It's a very simple, approachable, and non-intellectual way of connecting with that other.

So in actual fact, there are two things going on—I have the practice of shamanism that I use as healer of other people, but I also have a practice of shamanism as a spiritual practice. The two are inseparable. And like any spiritual practice, it's constantly evolving. At this stage in my life my shamanic practice looks like this: I try to journey every day. The journeys may be journeys on personal questions and issues on my own behalf or about things in my life. What do I need to know today? What is my lesson for this day? It also involves connecting with nature on a deeper level. When you walk this path, you look at nature very differently. Everything is spirit—the rocks have just as much spirit as the plants and animals and that makes you want to listen. All these things have lessons. So when you walk the land, you're listening and trying to connect. You become more in tune with creation, the earth, and those things in it. It opens you up to that.

I have learned core shamanism from the Foundation for Shamanic Studies. This means I didn't learn indigenous culturally-based shamanism that has been handed down from grandfather to father to son. Ritual is something that I have retrieved in a journey because I needed something. For example, here's a ritual: If something is bothering me a lot and I'm having angst about some issue, then I do a ritual to let go of it. I'll do a journey and say, "What do I need to do? I need some way of letting go of this." And they'll say, "Go to nature, and ask for volunteers from nature to take this for you." So I'll go outside and some rock or plant will say, "Take me." I'll collect them in a piece of cloth and then ask my teacher or power animal to fill the collection with my angst. Then I'll hide it in a field and let go of it.

Another thing that's changed is that I understand reality differently than I did before. I see our bodies as vehicles for the soul. I see that each one of us has a life essence that comes to this earth by choice. We choose to have the experiences we need in this life. I see creation—that we, as conscious beings, are constantly cocreating. The way that we think—something in our attitudes—will manifest in this world in one way or another, both positively and negatively. And I feel that sense very profoundly.

I sense that everything is very connected, and I see the connection on more levels than I did previously. I see the earth having both a physical dimension and a spiritual dimension. It has many more layers than it did before, and it has a consciousness that is approachable. I see what we call God, not as something that's just abstract and out there, but as something very approachable. And I see spirit as all of these different aspects—all of these power animals and teachers are different aspects of the One. It's not a question of a leap of faith to a god that's out there as this intellectual concept. It's very approachable and real.

You have a relationship with the spirits—you talk to them, you dance with them, you learn from them. They are real. You learn from the earth. You can learn from the moon. The moon has a consciousness with specific things to teach. The sun has something to teach. The chameleon has something to teach; the bear has something to teach; and they all have different lessons. If you want to learn from them, you ask.

That's the view to a shaman.

CHAPTER 39

DAVID CUMES, MD

South African Shamanism and the Tree of Health

It is an interesting phenomenon that as we move forward in time and expand our base of knowledge, we often go back in time to the most ancient texts in search of information and wisdom. David Cumes, MD, recently created a Tree of Health, which helps people envision and attain the different aspects of health. But its conception is based on the ancient Jewish Tree of Life from the Cabbala, which Cumes studied at length. The Tree, however, is not the only modern/ancient aspect of Cumes' life and work. Born and raised in South Africa, he received his medical training at the University of the Witwatersrand, Johannesburg and is a Fellow of the Edinburgh Royal College of Surgeons, the South African College of Surgeons, and the American College of Surgeons. Yet he also recently completed an apprenticeship to an elderly Zulu medicine man (*sangoma*) during which time he learned to dispense plant medicine and "throw the bones," two ancient healing traditions. A trained wilderness guide as well, Cumes has led many healing journeys into wilderness areas of Peru, South Africa, and the Sinai Desert and is president of Inward Bound—Healing Journeys. He is the author of *Inner Passages, Outer Journeys* and *The Spirit of Healing* and has a private surgical practice in urology in Santa Barbara, California.

In the winter of 2002, I traveled to Santa Barbara to interview David Cumes in his home, which some might say was a "house with a garden" but is perhaps better described as "a garden with a house." I know his skills as he has thrown the bones for me several times. For this interview, I asked him to talk about his experiences with South African shamanism and his creation of the Tree of Health.

My interest in indigenous healing systems started when I was conducting wilderness journeys to Peru in the late 1980s. I became involved with Alberto Villildo from the Four Winds Foundation and took part in numerous shamanic rituals with him, including ceremonies with *ayahuasca*. At the time, I knew there was something to these systems, but I couldn't quite put my finger on it. And although I benefited from this experience of shamanism, I didn't think it was my way.

Obviously, being South African, I knew about the *sangomas* and *nyangas* and their abilities and had respect for them. In fact, whenever I was in South Africa, if I had decision-making to do or was at a crossroads in my life, I would check in with the *sangomas*. But in the early 1990s, something strange happened. I was in South Africa visiting a friend, and a *sangoma* man threw the bones for me. He said, "You're a doctor in your own country, but it won't be long before you are doing my kind of medicine." He was very specific. A few years later, when I was on a retreat in the bush, on a game farm of a friend, I went to see a female *sangoma*. She threw the bones and said, "Your grandmother's bone is saying you have to do this work."

I had read Ray Graham's book *White Woman Witch Doctor*, which is about her initiation into becoming a *sangoma*, so I called her and asked what she thought. She said, "No, you live in America. All they're picking up is that you're a healer because you conduct wilderness healing journeys. If you want to do something, study with a Native American back home."

I felt "off the hook" after that. So I came back to the States and looked into Peruvian shamanism and Native American shamanism and all of that. I even looked into Ayurveda. But nothing fit. I was thoroughly in limbo.

Then about 4 years ago, when I was in South Africa again, I visited another healer who went into a trance and channeled the ancestors. First, she told me about my migraines and that I'd just pulled my back out, and she indicated where my back pain was located. This certainly got my attention. Then she went into a trance. She became possessed, which is where an ancestral spirit comes into the body and talks through a native tongue. Her spirit talked in Zulu even though she was a Sotho woman. She said, "Your ancestors are calling you to come back and do this work, and until such time as you do this, you will have headaches." She then gave me very strict instructions—I had to build a hut in South Africa and buy certain cloths and a cow and all kinds of things.

Again, because I wasn't certain, I went to someone else for a second opinion. This other woman threw bones for me and confirmed everything. "The bones fall as if you are already *sangoma*; all you have to do is complete it," she said. Since that time, I have taken my study with the *sangomas* very seriously.

The Work of a *Sangoma* Healer

The work of a *sangoma* is the same as any shamanic work and also like some of my wilderness work. But the *sangomas* have their own passwords for getting into the field (the spirit world), and their model is somewhat different. They believe in ancestral spirits. They believe that dead people are not dead and that if we come into a relationship with our dead loved ones, they can be of assistance to us and help us in our lives.

Now, anyone's ancestors can help them, but in a few instances, there is something more going on. This is particularly true for someone who's called to be a healer. These people will usually be connected to somebody in the spirit world who wants to complete the work that they never completed in his or her lifetime. It might be a grandmother or grandfather or great-grandmother or great-grandfather. In my case, it is a black woman who worked for my grandfather on my mother's side. This woman was a *sangoma* who was very attached to my grandfather and grandmother and wanted to work through me. So this woman is really the one who is doing the work.

There are three main ways of accessing the spirit world in this tradition. One is possession, which means that with drumming and dancing, your ego steps aside, and the ancestral spirit comes in and starts channeling. It's very dramatic in African context, unlike the trance channeling you would see in California where the person goes into a meditative state and then suddenly something comes through.

Another way of accessing the spirit world is through the bones. The idea is that there's a field of intention set up between the healer, the spirit, and the patient. And there's an assigned meaning to each bone. By throwing the bones—it's the spirit who actually throws the bones—and by knowing what each bone means, the *sangoma* can interpret them. Much as spirits have energy that can move objects, they can also move bones and make them fall in a nonrandom fashion. I find this the most easy and objective way because I can't always have 5 or 10 people drumming for me and be in that kind of ceremony.

The third way is with dreams. The dream world will tell you what you need to know or do. In the context of the African practicing in the African bush, he might dream of a plant. The *sangoma* may not have ever seen the plant before, but she would know that the next day a patient was going to come to her, and she would have to find that plant for that patient. Or she may have seen a patient and then dreamed a plant for that patient.

As far as my own personal dreams are concerned, they relate to my day-to-day activities because I'm not dealing with plants. So I dream about patients or my kids or my relationships or other issues that are current and practical. My dreams guide me. Now, the dreams and the bones speak in metaphor, so you can interpret them incorrectly, and you have to be careful not to put your own projections in the way. But that's how the healers work.

They dispense plant medicines and conduct rituals that often include sacrifices. Their idea is that the ancestral spirits are the ones who do all the work so the spirits will tell the *sangomas* what plants are needed, what medicines are required, and what's wrong with the patient. They might also intervene directly with the patient. Personally, I think what's going on is that the *sangomas* are channeling universal healing energy, and they do it through the medium of ancestral spirits.

I've now used these rituals with some of my patients here in Santa Barbara. For instance, if you had migraines and came to me in my office, I might throw the bones for you. The bones would tell me about your psychosociospiritual profile and probably give me a good idea about where your headaches were coming from. But I want to make an important point. Many medical intuitives will say, "Your headaches are from this." I'm more cautious. Modern technology is incredible, and I prefer to have my patients get a full medical workup, just to make sure there's no physical problem. So most of the patients I see already have a medical diagnosis. And, yes, they might have migraines, but we also know that they do not have meningitis or a brain tumor. Then I can look at the migraine in terms of their psychosociospiritual being and can say, "The trouble with the migraines is that you have a dysfunctional relationship with your boss or you're having trouble with your younger child or your ancestors are angry with you." But in terms of identifying organic illness, I'd much rather use Western technology.

Within this system there are specific rituals for everything. Obviously, the context in which you do them in a black, South African culture would be very different from what you might do in middle-class America. So any ritual I design and use here is tailored for Western culture.

Some rituals have to do with purification—with bathing or steaming, both of which can be done with special medicines. Clearly sacrifices are not culturally acceptable in the West, but you might do something similar in terms of making an offering to your ancestors by cooking them a meal, offering libations, or just getting in touch with them to solicit their support. Then there are medicines for just about every eventuality. There are love potions and medicines for a woman who has had an abortion and wants to cleanse herself from the spirit of the child. Or maybe a man has lost his wife—there is a ritual and medicine for that as well. My understanding of the rituals is that not only does the medicine do the work, but the ancestor also does the work. So there's a plant effect, and there's a spirit effect.

The Field

These techniques are all ways of connecting to the field. I could go into all the evidence that shows the field exists—the medical studies on distant healing, prayer, distant intentionality, etc.—but I think the people reading this book will probably agree that the field exists. In terms of the *sangoma* model, there are three ways to connect with the field—through trance (which comes with drumming, dance, and chanting), throwing the bones, and dreams. But in a Western sense, the field is like a triad. First, there's the divine spirit or the big Kahuna. But truthfully, I think that people who believe they're connecting with God are not actually doing that, even though it may feel like God. That's my own personal bias. Moses may have connected with God, but he was terrified and had to close his eyes. And the Cabbala tells us, "You shall not see my face and live." That's because it's too much for us. We need mediators.

The second part of the triad is the ancestors or spirits. The *sangomas* believe that the ancestors are the intermediaries between the living and God. But "ancestors" are not just blood ancestors, they might be spirit gods or angels or a whole plethora of different forms. In Buddhism, it might be enlightened beings. In Catholicism, it's the saints. The African model is more practical—the ancestors are not enlightened in that sense. The Africans simply connect with spirits that are not bound to the space-time continuum and can therefore be helpful because they can see things that are coming in the future. They can see the past; they can see the present; they can move things around; they can influence your life; and they can protect you. If they see that you're going to have an accident, they'll give you a flat tire—that sort of thing.

The third part of the triad is the higher self. Often we get information from our own subconscious, our own godlike self.

Sometimes it's hard to distinguish what is coming from where. The occasional person may have a message from God, but most of us are prone to relating to the higher self or to these other spirit helpers. There are ways of knowing when it's not your higher self, because you will get a message that is clearly out of the bounds of your own knowledge system. A message that contains archetypal information in the African context is usually spirit information.

For instance, I frequently get clarity about what to do. It can be very simple, and it happens in meditating, in yoga, in the wilderness, or when I'm just waking up from sleep. Something goes off like a light bulb. But it's coming from me; it's not coming from another source. Then, every once in a while I hear a voice. That's different. Or I'll get an image in a dream, which doesn't feel like it's coming from me. It's coming from someone else who is sending me a message.

Let me give you some examples. I've written two books, and I dreamed both the titles. And there are many scientists, such as Einstein, who get inspirations in their dreams. I think this type of information comes from some higher source that is divine but isn't directly God.

But the field is a big mystery. I can only speak about the tiny bit of understanding I have from my own encounters with it. Do I identify it as vast and immeasurable and incomprehensible? Absolutely. Do I know what I am talking about? Absolutely not.

The important thing is that something is there and we have the option of relating to it or not. Most people don't relate to it, either because they're scared of it or they don't believe in it or their culture or religion forbids them to believe in it. But they're missing out on a huge component of living. If we are aware of the fact that there is a huge mystery out there and start to learn a few of the passwords, we can begin to get into the mystery.

Encounters with the Field

I was once on a trip in the Peruvian jungle. We'd spent the night in one of those houses on pedestals, and in the early hours of the morning I woke up and decided to wake the boat crew so we could get an early start for Cuzco. It had been raining that night, and as I was going down the stairs, my foot slipped, and I fell 6 feet down to the ground. When I landed, I snapped my wrist. So there I was in the middle of nowhere with a broken wrist.

While I was nursing my wrist in the boat on the way to Cuzco, I realized that I had had a dream that night. It was really an apparition. Such dreams are usually important ones for me, and this one was just the face of a friend I had worked with in South Africa when I was a surgical resident. He was a traumatologist from Spain and had lots of experience with fractures. He also had a very unique way of fixing a particular fracture in the wrist.

Now, I had not seen Paco in 20 years but if you said to me, "What did you know Paco for?" I would have replied, "Paco taught me how to reduce a Colles' fracture." So first I see an apparition of him, and then a few hours later I have a Colles' fracture. It's because of this and other incidents that I now pay close attention to my dreams.

Another example of connecting with the field is when three colleagues wanted me to join them in their urology practice. I had a dream that I was in the office they had designated as mine, and as I was sitting there, I started feeling very uncomfortable. There was a noise going off in my head like a jackhammer. Up until then, I thought it might be expedient to join them, but after having the dream I called them and told them no.

So these encounters are often not gigantic. They're just little things that are there to tell you what to do.

Of course, sometimes you can get dreams that come through friends. Once, I was thinking of buying a 40-acre parcel of wilderness here in Santa Barbara. I was very keen on it, but my secretary had a dream that she was driving along the property, and when she looked at it, there'd been an avalanche. As she came down to the bottom of the hill, she saw me underneath all the rocks and dirt. I was bloated and dead and buried by the avalanche. So I didn't look at that piece of property again. Sometimes when you're not listening, the spirits might choose to send the dream to someone else who will relay it to you.

I think if you're in touch with the field then you can channel universal healing energy, just like anybody can do Reiki or healing touch. But some people are more powerful; some people have their fingers plugged into the main more so than others. My feeling is that the bushmen of the Kalahari are very powerfully connected with the field when they do their trance dance. They actually travel out of body up to the spirit world and almost have a near-death experience. When they come back and put their hands on someone, there's an incredible energy there.

I'm just starting to incorporate this type of hands-on healing in my practice. Usually I'll pray to the ancestors to help the person while I do some ritual wherein there might be some hands-on contact. The point is to generate healing energy.

Obviously I'm still in my internship phase and still a junior in this area. Ninety percent of my time is dedicated to my urology practice or the wilderness journeys. I'm not in full time *sangoma* practice. Most of the work I do is simply sitting down with patients in the yurt and throwing the bones to give them clarity. It can be incredibly healing for someone to discover something that he or she has been in denial about or hasn't paid attention to or for a person to have an insight into a relationship that's been ignored, whether it's with a deceased grandfather or a living relative.

The nice thing about *sangoma* work is that it's very down-to-earth and practical. It's not too esoteric. So it could be something as simple as a woman asking, "Should I be with this man?" If, when you throw the bones, the two relevant bones are together, then the answer is clear. You can't read it any other way. Or it might be that a man is having difficulties at work. When you throw the bones for him, it looks as if somebody is bothering the man at this office. So you ask, "Is there somebody bothering you? There's a malevolent energy surrounding you at work." The man may not have been aware that his secretary was working a form of witchcraft on him, even though it's not witchcraft in the Western sense. But intent can be malevolent. So once the man sees it for what it is in the display of bones, he can take action.

Sometimes spirits come up repeatedly, like a grandfather on the mother's side, and the person will burst into tears and say that the grandfather on his mother's side was the best thing that ever happened in his life. He'll say, "What should I do about this relationship?" And I will say, "They're not gone, they're still there for you." Then this person may start to relate to that relationship and begin listening to his dreams, and/or start giving offerings to that grandfather.

I'd say 90% of the people I see in my yurt come for advice with regard to therapy and which way they should go. Should they have chemo? Should they have surgery? And the bones can be very helpful in these circumstances.

One prostate cancer patient of mine, on whom I had operated, subsequently came to me and had the bones thrown. According to the bones he needed to give up his business and retire. The bones basically said that his work was quite toxic to his health. So he made these major changes, and his whole life turned around. Now, would he have done that without the bones? I don't think he would have.

The Tree of Life

The other aspect of my work is that I have spent some time studying the Tree of Life, which is an energy system similar to the chakra system. But instead of seven chakras, there are 10 sephirot. And like the charkas, the sephirot are also centers of energy.

The chakras go directly up the spine. Then there are two energy channels that circulate around the spine, which in yoga are masculine and feminine, the sun and the moon. And there's a polarity implicit in those channels. The Cabbala and the Tree of Life have a similar model, but it is slightly different in that the left side of the tree is feminine, restrained and restrictive, while the right side of the tree is masculine and expansive.

Each sephira, like each chakra, has a different quality to it. *Malkhut*, which is at the bottom, is the sephira that connects us to earth, and, like the first and second chakras, it incorporates all the basic elements. The next sephira, *Yesod*, represents ego and foundation and is equivalent to the third chakra. These are the lower energy centers that make us who we are in the world—survival, flight or fight response, regeneration of the species, who we are as a person, and what our ego tells us to do.

When you get above *Yesod*, you come to *Tiferet*, which is the heart of the tree. *Tiferet* is like the heart chakra, and once the student of Cabbala gets to *Tiferet*, he can go beyond and study on his own. It's the same with yoga—once you've moved the energy above the diaphragm to the heart chakra, you're in the higher centers.

If you keep going up, the next one is *Daat*, which is not a true sephira, but this is where knowledge can be put into the Tree of Life directly from God. It's like a portal where God can come in and say, "I'm going to come in and fix this because something is not going right." When this happens, miracles like spontaneous healing can occur. This is also where grace can come in.

At the top is *Keter*, the crown, the place of "I am that I am." It's like the crown chakra. It's bliss consciousness, unity consciousness, the oneness experience. In the Cabbala, it's where you come into recognition that you're actually experientially part of God. When you get to *Keter*—and I'm not an expert by any means—you get into eternity, nothingness, something like the Buddhist concept of emptiness.

On either side of the Tree of Life are the two poles of the tree—the feminine and the masculine. *Binah*, the topmost sephira on the left is receptive, intuitive, feminine intelligence—as opposed to *Hochkma* on the right, which is more cognitive, intellectual, masculine intelligence. They are always polarities. If you go down a little lower you get to the *Gevurah*, which is the feminine version of judgment, much more severe and restricting compared to the masculine version of *Hesed*, which is mercy and more expansive. The other two sephirot, *Hod* and *Nezar*, are hard to understand.

The Tree of Life is originally from Jewish mysticism, from the Zohar, and probably started way back with Solomon. It was fully developed during the golden days of Judaism in Spain.

The yogis conceptualized the chakras and the Jews the Tree of Life. They've given their system different names and slightly different manifestations, and the cabbalistic one is a bit more complex. However, it has since become a universal tool, as have the chakras. So it's no longer unique to the Jews.

One other thing—there are four Trees of Life. The first Tree is the tree of calling, of emanation, of the word. God called the universe into being. So it's intention. The second Tree was the tree of creation, which is where God formed the blueprint for creation, the design, the plan. The third Tree is the tree of formation, where he put all the ingredients together, like making a cake, and the fourth Tree is when he baked the cake. He actually made it. This final tree is the cycle of making.

If you think about it, things happen in four stages. Take a building—first you have the intention, and then you make the blueprint or the plan, which is the creation. Next is formation, the contractor putting everything together, and then you actually build the building. I could never work out why words were so powerful, but it's because everything starts with emanation. The word is the thing that starts the process going. So in that lies some of the complexity of the Tree of Life.

In the old days the cabbalists would use the tree as a structure for esoteric practices to move energy up the tree beyond *Tiferet* to *Keter*. They would use prayer, meditations, dancing, and singing. This is interesting because it's very much like the African model. The Blacks and Bushmen pray by singing and dancing and drumming, which is an incredibly powerful means of prayer. So really, the Tree of Life is just an intellectual structure to make sense of the universe.

The Tree of Health

One of the important things for me about the Tree of Life was that I was able to make a Tree of Health out of it.

All of healing has to do with polarity, as does everything. I think the yogis and the cabbalists were right about that. There is a universal law of polarity and balance, and it's inherent in the body system.

On the left-hand side of the Tree of Health are all the things that would inhibit, restrain, constrict, and hamper the life force. And all the things on the right side of the Tree of Health will enhance, facilitate, or augment the life force. The inner healer is in the center of the Tree of Health.

If we think in terms of the life force, which would be prana or qi or ruach, if you were talking in Hebrew, then the life force is critical to the inner healer. The two are interrelated. If you have a very vigorous life force and you're happy, your inner healer is stronger, and your immune system is enhanced. So in the center of the tree of health, in addition to life force, there is will and balance, as well as the four polarities—the calling, the creating, the formation, and the making—because even healing has a plan. Inner practices such as yoga, meditation, nutrition, and so on enhance the life force.

There are certain key components that are universal, that everybody knows are important but rarely does anyone do something about them consciously. The first one is hope, trust, faith, and belief. If you look at patients who have spontaneous remissions of incurable diseases, the one common thread is incredible faith that things are going to be fine. They have faith that something else that's bigger than they are is going to help.

On the left side of the tree, things that hinder, would be no faith, no trust, no belief.

The next one down is resignation versus surrender. Resignation really is hopelessness. It's, "There is nothing I can do about it. I've 6 months to live so I might as well get on with the job of dying." Surrender, however, means whatever is going to happen is great because it's been sent to me from a divine source, and I'm going to make the most of it. It's an attitude of surrender to a higher force as opposed to a hopeless, head-down, depressed, and anxious demeanor. Those are two different energies. One will restrict the life force, and the other will actually enhance the life force. Surrender doesn't mean that you're not going to have medical attention. It means you'll have whatever it takes, but in addition, you know there's something good coming your way. You know that even if you die, it's going to be good.

This has to come from within—it can't be something you impose from the outside. I think we tend to underestimate death. The Buddhists say that of all the meditations, the meditation on death is the most powerful because like the elephant leaves the heaviest footprint in the sand, the meditation on death leaves the heaviest imprint on your subconscious. And I think that's where the shamans are way ahead in the game because many of them have had near-death experiences. So if someone can bring the idea of surrender to the healing process, it can have a huge impact.

The next polarity, of course, is fear versus love and courage. Clearly if one is fearful of death, fearful of threat to life, limb, and function, we know that this may overwhelm the immune system and inhibit it. The opposite is love, which gives one courage to continue, whether that love is from a pet or a loved one or a close family group or even a support group. We just have to find a way to channel the love. There's also the universal healing energy, which basically is love. I think when a true shaman connects with a patient, it's much more likely that they will be connecting through the love force, through this universal healing energy as opposed to what we do in Western medicine, which is to connect through technology.

The next polarity is guilt versus no guilt. Guilt and shame are underestimated in terms of healing. Many people feel guilt about what they've done. There's sexual guilt, parental guilt, relationship guilt, and guilt regarding your community. For instance, many people with very rigorous religious upbringings feel that they do not deserve to be well. Or maybe they feel they've brought the illness on themselves as a punishment for not being "good." But guilt is something that has to be taken out of the equation. It has no place in healing.

Then we have denial versus truth. You need to come to grips with your problem. You have to have a plan, and if your plan is unrealistic for the challenge ahead, it's not likely that you're going to prevail. If you think you've got some minor upper-respiratory infection and you've actually got lymphoma, you're in for a big surprise. If you have to have an appendectomy, that's no big deal, but if you have a complicated health problem, you need to be able to go through the four stages of calling, creating, forming, and making to have an overall comprehensive plan. The inner healer is divinely inspired; it's part of the higher self. And the higher self needs to know the truth, and the inner healer needs to know the truth of the diagnosis. But truth has to be kind, and it mustn't be brutal. And truth is relative, so you shouldn't tell people "the whole truth and nothing but the truth so help me God" if it's going to be harmful to them. They should be told in a way that is helpful and supportive.

Toward the bottom of the Tree of Health is ignorance versus knowledge. The more you know about your condition, the better choices you're going to make. Knowledge is power, and knowledge also gives you confidence to tackle the thing.

And then, of course, there's action versus inaction. Right action is what we're talking about because eventually you're going to have to take action. You're going to have to find the oncologist and the surgeon and the radiation therapist and the nutritionist and the psychotherapist and the yoga teacher and the meditation teacher and bring it all together in a comprehensive health plan that speaks through all these polarities and actually addresses you individually.

People can look at the Tree of Health on a regular basis and see where they are in terms of truth or hope or action. Then they can do whatever it takes to put those things right, because those are the things that will make the difference. If they don't cure themselves in this process, at least they will heal themselves. And with a regular inner practice, they will gain a sense of the field. They will understand that they're not alone, that they are supported by something, and maybe they'll have dreams from loved ones that have passed on. Funnily enough, one of the qualities of spontaneous remission is having dreams from ancestors who have passed on just before the patient miraculously has the remission.

Kundalini

In all of this, you have to understand the basics of energy polarity. How does energy move in the body? What is the life force? What is kundalini, and how do we make this energy move? How do we find balance? The Tree of Health only works in the context of this whole gestalt of energy balance.

Kundalini is very much tied in with the life force. If we can activate our life force, we can activate our kundalini. In terms of the hierarchy of chakras, if the kundalini is mobilized through the different esoteric practices; it moves up the chakra ladder and energizes each chakra as it goes up. The whole idea is polarity balance. When the sun and moon channels are balanced with meditation, exercise, nutrition, etc., the energy that courses along the spine deviates from the sun and the moon channels into the central channel where it stimulates the kundalini.

The Zulus talk about the *umbilini*, and the bushmen talk about *num*. These are basically kundalini. They mobilize it with dancing and singing and drumming. The bushmen use rattles around their legs and do this monotonous dance that can go on all night. We're not so blessed, so we have meditation. We have more subtle practices that are, in my experience, not as powerful. Psychedelics is another way to do it but with less control. But the more diligent we are in our spiritual practice, the more likely we will find energy balance in the body going up the chakra ladder all the way to the top.

Kundalini, the feminine energy at the root of the spine, is similar to the divine aspect of the goddess that is at the root of the Tree of Life. When the kundalini moves all the way up the Tree of Life or all the way up the chakra hierarchy, it meets Shiva, the male principle of the crown. The experience is of fusing to oneness, unity consciousness, whatever you want to call it. It is ultimate healing because you are directly in contact with the field.

It would be great if we could do it, but for most of us, nothing happens. For me, every now and then when I'm in wilderness, I have a very brief oneness experience. But it's very brief. And while I don't think it's important for us to aim to be in *samadhi*, it is important to aim to be in balance, and as much as we can in context of all stresses of our daily life, to put aside at least 30 minutes a day to some enjoyable inner practice where we move this energy, balance our chakra system, and at least experience a sense of harmony, wondrousness, and awe. When the kundalini is most active, the life force is most active. And the more active the life force is, obviously the more powerful the inner healing.

Part Eleven

Conversations About Cross-Cultural Medicine

"[U]ltimately what heals a condition and what promotes well-being in a human are not medicines, foods, or meditation techniques, but rather what we call in the West the vital energy of an individual."

—SCOTT GERSON

CHAPTER 40

HARRIET BEINFIELD, LAC, AND EFREM KORNGOLD, LAC, OMD

Eastern Medicine for Western People

When you walk down the San Francisco street on which Harriet Beinfield and Efrem Korngold live, it appears to be an ordinary modern-day neighborhood, meaning it is full of things manmade—asphalt roads, houses, concrete sidewalks, fences, metal cars, stuff. But then one comes to a high wooden fence surrounding a wooden house, and when the gate is opened, trees, plants, shrubs, flowers, paths, and wind chimes abound. Clearly, this house is an oasis.

In 1998, I walked through these gardens to interview Harriet and Efrem in their home and share tea with them in their kitchen.

Harriet Beinfield, LAc, and Efrem Korngold, LAc, OMD, have practiced Chinese Medicine for 30 years. They were among the first Americans to be trained at the College of Traditional Acupuncture in England. Together they have written two books—*Between Heaven and Earth: A Guide to Chinese* and *The Chinese Modular Solutions Handbook for Health Professionals*—as well as many articles. They both lecture, teach, and maintain a private practice—Chinese Medicine Works—in San Francisco.

After becoming a licensed acupuncturist, Korngold studied herbal medicine at the Kunming Traditional Chinese Medicine Research Institute and the Shanghai College of Traditional Chinese Medicine. He received his doctor of Oriental medicine degree from the San Francisco College of Acupuncture and Oriental Medicine in 1986. Beinfield received her licentiate acupuncture degree in 1973.

The overarching goal of Chinese Medicine is to cultivate people's capacities and to correct whatever underlying disturbances are causing distress. In order to achieve this, it is useful to investigate how a disorder arises so the process can be disassembled and reorganized, not merely masked. This noble goal is not always attainable, but the medicine compels us to strive for it. In Chinese medicine, everything is linked with everything else—not just as an idea but in actuality. Health and illness coexist and arise out of the same conditions. Disease is not a random event—it emerges from a lived life. Simply put: Chinese medicine not only focuses on the content (the disease) but also on the context (the person who has it).

Everybody exists within a matrix that includes a family; job; home; neighborhood; geographic area; and psychological, social, and cultural milieus. Chinese medicine considers the impact of all these influences. We attended a workshop recently with the late Dr. John Shen, an admired elder of the Chinese medicine community, who was in his eighties. Reflecting on more than 50 years of practice, he said that while the medicine is good—the herbs are potent and the acupuncture is effective—the ultimate success of any treatment depends on how a person accepts and uses it. He talked about what he referred to as "taking care of your life," which is something that medicine can't do for you. In the Daoist-Confucianist tradition, physicians were also instructors who helped people learn how to live.

Dr. Shen told a story about a 38-year-old woman who, even after two surgeries, had unremitting uterine bleeding. She asked Dr. Shen if he could help. He looked at her, felt her pulse, and talked to her a little bit. Then he said, "I think I can help. But first I need to do a test to figure out why you're bleeding. You need to go home and stay in bed for 2 weeks."

She panicked and said, "I can't do that. I'm an attorney—I'm too busy."

To which he replied, "Then I can't help you."

She was incredulous and asked what he meant. He explained, "I can't decide what to do for you until I figure out why you're having the problem. It's possible that you're bleeding because of the surgery. On the other hand, it may simply be due to your body condition. But they require different approaches."

He suspected that she was bleeding because she was debilitated. She was a young woman but was already exhausted. She finally agreed to the test; after 2 weeks, the bleeding stopped.

This is Chinese medicine. An intervention not only provided diagnostic information the doctor needed to confirm his hypothesis but also treated the patient. She got better. Equally important, it educated her about the nature of her condition. She realized that a major component of her problem was the fact that she was chronically exhausted, even though she didn't think of herself that way. Dr. Shen was effective by thinking and acting through the mind of Chinese medicine, even before he used acupuncture or herbs.

There are several legitimate languages to use in talking about Chinese medicine—the scientific one of measuring electrical skin resistance at acupuncture sites, the release of peptides and hormones stimulated by the needles, the pharmacology of herbal compounds. There is also the qualitative, clinical language of how people feel they've been helped—outcome studies. On the one hand, Chinese medicine is a method of restoration and recovery; on the other hand, it's a systematic way of knowing, a medical epistemology that includes a method of self-exploration that helps people develop in less tangible ways than taking herbs, receiving acupuncture, or following a new diet.

There's an ancient Chinese medical text that names three levels of healing. The lower level asks us to address a person's complaints to diminish her pain. The middle level directs us to understand someone's nature. And the upper level charges us to assist a person in fulfilling his or her destiny. Most people automatically associate Chinese medicine with the lower level: can acupuncture relieve back pain or hot flashes? Can Chinese herbs improve immunity? What should I eat to make my acne go away? Complaints are what initially draw people to Chinese medicine, but what seems to keep them enrolled is that they feel they are being seen, heard, and helped within a broad frame of reference and that everything they are and bring with them is relevant to the process.

While working with people over the last 30 years, we've noticed that acupuncture can produce desirable side effects. Shifts in people's lives occur; dreams change; and they report elevated states of awareness. Some of this may be due to the release of endorphins, but our intuition is that acupuncture acts in ways for which we don't have a language. It integrates all the layers of our being, our invisible subtle bodies with our wholly palpable physical selves. The outcome is a sense of inner alignment that people deeply crave. The experience of feeling connected pleases them, and Chinese medicine's ability to deepen that feeling keeps them coming back. Acupuncture gives an authentic meaning to the term *integrative medicine*.

I saw a woman with a uterine tumor that had metastasized to her bones. Besieged with nausea and vomiting, she couldn't keep water down, let alone food, but wanted to avoid hospitalization and IV feeding. She had extreme pain in her legs and hips, but morphine made her feel groggy and tired. A combination of acupuncture, an herbal fomentation on her abdomen, powdered ginger under her tongue, and rectal injections of herb broth halted the nausea within 1 day. She progressed to sipping herb broth and rice gruel. Acupuncture every 6 hours enabled her to discontinue the morphine. She had complained of feeling that her upper body was disassociated from her lower body. Minutes after the needles were in place she felt as if her abdomen and lower limbs were rejoining with her upper body, returning the sense of coherence she wanted. The acupuncture altered not only her perception of pain but seemed to soothe and lighten her consciousness. She felt more charged and a greater sense of calm.

It is ironic that within Chinese society, which highly values the collective good, the medicine cares for the individual. Yet in America, where individuality is so highly regarded, the medicine tends to overlook the unique needs of the person, instead seeking to find a collective cure. This has been especially problematic in designing research, because people are focused on determining the best acupuncture points for migraine or rheumatoid arthritis. Typically, the Chinese medicine practitioner will answer, "It depends on the person."

If the arthritis is due to an invasion of heat (inflammation), it's different from that caused by cold (reduced circulation) or dampness (accumulation of fluids). In the first case you would administer cooling herbs; in the others you would use warming or diuretic herbs. And sometimes the kidney, liver, or spleen networks require strengthening, so you need to include herbs to correct their deficiencies. Every person is an original ecosystem. You assess the individual terrain to design the most appropriate intervention. But usually Western researchers want standardized treatments for similar complaints.

The vocabulary of Chinese medicine preceded Western medical language by several millennia, so the same words, like *kidney* or *liver*, have different meanings. The organs are called *networks* because they are functional physiological and psychological domains, not discrete anatomical structures.

Chinese Herbs versus Western Herbs

Pharmacological research demonstrates that astragalus and echinacea both have immune-modulating properties, so in the sense that they both help to protect the body from the cold or virus, they're similar. But Chinese medicine tends not to use herbs as single bullets: a single treatment for a single cause. Because the body itself is complex, the Chinese approach is multimodal to match that complexity. Herbs are usually used in synergistic combination rather than as specific agents.

If somebody is weak and pale, they lack qi (pronounced "chee"). If they are also restless, have dry skin and trouble sleeping, this suggests depleted blood. In this case it makes sense to give herbs that replenish qi and blood. But often when someone is weak, she doesn't have the capacity to distribute the qi and blood adequately, so it's necessary to include herbs that mobilize and circulate the nourishment that the herbs contribute. That's a simple example of how herbs in combination are more effective.

Every medicinal plant has a complicated profile of constituents, properties, and effects. Investigators may be trying to isolate which polysaccharide fractions in echinacea and astragalus confer their immune-modulating effects, but herbs have many influences. And then when you begin to combine two, three, five, a dozen, or more ingredients in a formula, you have a level of complexity that is daunting to the Western medical research model. From the Chinese medicine point of view, echinacea is a cold, dry, detoxifying herb that counters inflammation and swelling, whereas astragalus is a warm, nutritive herb that strengthens resistance by invigorating the body. Echinacea is used in times of illness, whereas astragalus, like ginseng, is an adaptogen that restores the body's capacity not only to resist illness but to work, reproduce, and store energy.

Let's use another example, such as taking St. John's wort for depression. Some people respond immediately, others slowly, and some seem not to respond at all. This doesn't necessarily mean that the herb is not working—it may mean that by itself it's insufficient to achieve the desired result. In Chinese medicine we "listen" to the pulse through our fingers to "view" the ongoing process of the body. When we introduce a new influence like St. John's wort, even if the person doesn't feel a change subjectively, we can often tell whether there's been an effect by the alterations in the pattern of the pulse. Perhaps St. John's wort is having an effect but not enough for the person to notice, and other herbs must be added to the treatment to potentiate it.

By asking questions, feeling the pulse, looking at the tongue, and examining the body, we learn the characteristics of the problem and the nature of the person. For instance, depression is just a symptom—a signal that something isn't right. We want to investigate what deeper disturbances are responsible, like which of the organ networks and body constituents are not functioning well. The same symptom, depression, can have different sources. A disharmony of the lung and liver or of the kidney and heart can produce feelings of hopelessness, irritability, and apathy.

On the other hand, a disharmony between the kidney and heart could variously be experienced as a panic attack or as a recurring urinary tract inflammation. So people with different symptoms may have the same underlying problem, requiring similar treatments, yet people with the same symptom may need completely different remedies. St. John's wort by itself may work better for a kidney-heart disharmony and not as well for a lung-liver disharmony.

Here's another example. Take a group of people with digestive problems—one person will get migraine headaches, another sinusitis, another irritable bowel symptoms, and another will have bad breath. Diagnosis may show that they all have a spleen disturbance characterized by heat, dampness, and qi stagnation. Despite the variety of symptoms, these people would basically require the same herb formula and many of the same acupuncture points.

The pulse and tongue and signs and symptoms supply the clues. Then we evaluate the symptoms according to the person's constitutional type—the self-organizing pattern that forms the milieu within which these signs and symptoms arise. The idea of types is a universal concept in the West and East. In the Hippocratic era, the four types were phlegmatic, bilious, sanguine, and choleric. We introduced the notion of five types—based on the Chinese theory of five phases—that both describe a person's styles of being and help to predict past, present, and future dispositions toward illness.

Fire, Wood, Metal, Water, and Earth

The connection between psyche and soma is seamless. When we encounter a patient, we receive information globally. Then we use the categories of Chinese medicine to decode it. In our book we describe how five-phase thinking elaborates five broad classifications into which people can be grouped: fire, metal, water, wood, and earth. So we immediately begin figuring out where they fit, according to their most obvious and striking idiosyncrasies.

An earth, fire, or wood type may come more than halfway to meet me, spilling over boundaries, even invading my space. But this would be completely out of character for a metal or water type. Metal types live carefully within their bodies, contained, respectful of boundaries, prudent and restrained. They stay in their own space. They are methodical, love-of-logic people who enjoy rituals and are willing to follow rules. So if a patient were a metal type, it wouldn't surprise me if he or she began with questions in the service of clarifying the relationship: "How much is this going to cost? How often will I need to come? What should I wear? Can I read you the list I've made of my complaints?"

If a wood type were to have questions, it would be out of a sense of urgency and impatience. The motivation would be different: "How long will this take?—I need to get back to business. When can I expect results with my asthma? How soon will I get regular periods without cramps?"

So how people are, the way they carry themselves or walk, their "body language," and their level of animation are all diagnostically relevant, not just their medical records.

One of my patients, a physician, is a water type. He is a deep thinker, skeptical, empirical, and reluctant to put himself in someone else's hands. A water type is organized at his core by the kidney network, which governs the ear. He wanted to see whether Chinese medicine could reverse his progressive hearing loss or at least retard its progress. Meanwhile, he also complained of chronic irritable bowel syndrome and prostatitis. We made little impact on his hearing, but his prostatitis, digestion, and overall health improved considerably.

By identifying him as a water type, I knew my approach could not be aggressive and that it would take him time to become comfortable. When he felt better following acupuncture or after taking an herbal prescription, he'd say, "I think that helped me, but how do I know? I could have gotten better by doing nothing." Yet he continued to come back for several years, suggesting that he felt as though he was deriving benefit.

Once I recognize someone as a metal type, I know a lot about them. Their internal climate predisposes them to dryness and heat and their nasal and respiratory lining is sensitive to irritation, so herbs that are moisturizing and cooling can compensate for their vulnerability. They are also likely to need loosening up or relaxing. This will show up in their relationships with other people, their jobs, how they inhabit their physical spaces, and how they feel within themselves.

This is not about changing someone; it's about helping her be better at being who she is. Usually our strengths are linked to our weaknesses. Sometimes metal types are so good at adhering to familiar patterns of behavior that they have difficulty initiating exploratory adventures. Yet sometimes that's exactly what's going to be helpful to them. A metal type will also be predisposed to problems related to tension in the neck, shoulders, chest, or abdomen. Metal is expressed in the body through the functions of the lungs and large intestine. The polar dynamic between the lungs (metal) and the liver (wood) creates the possibility of conflict: the lungs are responsible for dispersing qi and blood downward and inward, and the liver is responsible for pushing qi and blood upward and outward. If there is undue friction in this relationship, a rhythmic flow is disrupted. Sometimes the liver thrusts more blood and qi up than the lung can send down. When circulation is blocked above the chest, this causes tension in the shoulders and neck. If these forces collide in the chest, it causes a feeling of tightness in the chest or wheezing.

One clue leads to bigger clues, and these clues are multivalent. Our job is to generate a complete picture, using pathology, ontology, and personality as the palette with which to paint a meaningful portrait.

The idea that your strengths are your weaknesses means that there's always a duality at work—there's always yin and yang. You can't definitively say, "Men are yang and women are yin or that anger is hot and fear is cold" because all things exist in relation to each other. In other words, these types are not shallow, rigid, or simplistic. They're not static pigeonholes; they're characteristic strategies, more like verbs than nouns. We're equally endowed with our basic parts—lungs, heart, kidneys, liver, and so on. But our way of coordinating all of this is individualized, becoming even more complex as we grow and mature. The essence of how we put ourselves together moment to moment is quite unique and characteristically us.

You catch a cold differently than does your partner. There are many circumstantial factors that come into play, depending on your age, the status of your immune system, but still, there is a characteristic way that you get sick that is different from your partner's. So we can't treat you both exactly the same and expect you both to get well in the same way or at the same rate.

The Language of Chinese Medicine

The conceptual language—as is true for other medical paradigms—is simultaneously descriptive and heuristic. There are distinct and complementary categories for the underlying processes such as the body constituents (qi, moisture, blood), the organ networks (liver, heart, spleen, lung, kidney), eight parameters (yin-yang, cold-hot, depletion-congestion, interior-exterior), five phases (wood, fire, earth, metal, water), three burners (chest, diaphragm, abdomen), three treasures (mind, qi, essence), developmental cycles (7 years for women, 8 for men), five seasons, and more. What this represents is something like "all roads lead to Rome." Each of these means of describing and interpreting the data leads to a deeper insight into the nature of the organism and its unique *modus operandi*, its *dao*.

If I start by evaluating qi and blood, that will lead me into an exploration of how the organs are interacting, which will uncover emotional and existential issues, which will illuminate behavioral habits and interpersonal styles. When these separate stories are woven together into a unified moving picture, I will be led to an understanding of how, where, and when to intervene, and even though it may be small or discreet, it will reverberate throughout the organism and provoke a shift in an individual's physiology, awareness, and behavior. Through that, his or her innate mechanisms for repair, recovery, and maturation are mobilized.

The life of the body continually reveals itself to our gaze, and Chinese medicine teaches us how to see it, how to seek it out, how to expose it, how to remove obstacles from its path, and how to nudge it back into the current of its own destiny.

Sometimes it's challenging to know where to begin explaining Chinese medicine—in a sense it's arbitrary because Chinese medicine informs us about how organs, body constituents, behaviors, eating patterns, and emotions are interrelated. So it doesn't matter whether we're talking about a sore throat, irritability, fibroids, or cystitis, because what we're always looking at is a multidimensional dynamic at play within the body and between the key team members responsible for a given manifestation. It's not linear, nor is it confined to one layer.

There can be a kind of tug-of-war, or processes moving in opposite directions. A person could have chronic diarrhea due to cold in the abdomen and acute bronchitis due to heat in the chest. Dampness and dryness can coexist—the mucous membranes can be dry in someone with edema. This person will feel lethargic, chilly, and heavy all over—all signs of dampness and cold—and at the same time feel thirsty, itching, and burning in the nose, throat, and chest—all signs of dryness and heat. A deep, chronic (yin) problem like diabetes can be the backdrop for an acute (yang) problem like healing a wound. People try to oversimplify with either-or thinking—is it yin or yang? Am I hot or cold? Wood types can be well organized, sharing characteristics with metal types. Extroverted fire types also need the solitude that water types hunger for much more of the time.

Chinese medicine trains you to develop yourself as an instrument. You don't keep your subjectivity neatly outside the treatment room door. You use your senses and emotional responses to read the patient.

This is completely different from Western medicine, which stresses detached objectivity or noninvolvement. In Western medicine, the doctor is the servant of the technology, the emphasis being on the replicable effects, independent of the agency of the doctor. In traditional medicine, techniques are an extension of the doctor's intentions, his or her qi. So state of mind and relationship with the patient matter.

Western medicine focuses on defects, how to repair a torn ligament, how to excise a malignancy, how to reduce cholesterol or annihilate bacteria. It concentrates single-mindedly on pathology. Chinese medicine is also concerned with relieving pain and reversing disease—but not solely. It also has the capacity to reinforce optimum function by coaxing the kidneys to perform better, by activating the circulation of blood, by encouraging tranquility. Chinese medicine enhances the good in order to constrain the bad. It seeks to recreate a harmonious internal milieu.

There's a famous paragraph in the *Nei Jing*, an ancient text that's quoted over and over again: "The superior physician doesn't allow the patient to become sick." The quote goes on to ask: "What's the point of digging a well when you're already thirsty or of forging weapons when the war has already begun?" Then it's too late. The good doctor maintains the reservoir so it doesn't dry up. That's prevention. The idea of prevention in the West is undeveloped—medicine is organized around the treatment of pathology; doctors are the generals who vanquish disease as the enemy. But then again, there is no absolute dogma. I have been personally grateful to Western medicine. My father just had successful coronary bypass surgery, and when my son was an infant, he had holes in his heart surgically repaired. Aggressive intervention is sometimes called for, but deliberation should be generous.

There are several metaquestions: Who are people, and what is their purpose? What is the mission of medicine? If you understand life as a material phenomenon, you look at humans as physical, biological, chemical entities, and you define medicine as the attempt to correct pathologies within those physical, biological, chemical domains. But if you define the purpose of life as being able to experience happiness, to overcome ignorance through the development of the mind and you see the mind as developing in a long-term sense, perhaps not even confined to one biological lifespan, then the goal of medicine is to help somebody fulfill that purpose.

It's critical to help someone understand who she is and to identify her blindspots. In our ignorance lies our suffering. By helping someone become a careful self-observer, cultivate her mind, reflect upon and adjust her actions and habits, you're serving her. And this is the sphere of healing that may or may not relate to the realm of cure.

Acupuncture

Many Western scientists, such as Bruce Pomeranz, have studied acupuncture in relation to pain. And they have made an enormous contribution. For instance, Pomeranz has refined—through his experimentation and research—what is already part of the tradition of Chinese medicine, because he investigated the phenomenon called *De Qi*, which is a particular kind of subjective event that happens when the needles are inserted and manipulated to produce the analgesic effect. He has been able to replicate this electronically without needles and has identified that there are certain deep muscle fibers that are part of the endorphin mechanism—both locally and globally in the body—that mediate this response.

But this type of phenomenon in Chinese medicine is only one of the recognized and very well-defined aspects of qi. There's another acupuncture technique called *Dao Qi*, which means that by using the needle in a particular way, you can produce in the individual a sensation of something traveling from one place to another pretty much along the pathways of the meridians. So an adept practitioner can make the qi run wherever he or she wants it to go. This is particularly useful in treating pain and conditions that are associated with pain, such as bursitis or back pain. The basic principle is that pain is the result of blockage, a lack of circulation of important constituents that not only nourish the tissue, but also provide a medium for the elimination of metabolic wastes. So when this circulatory system isn't functioning, two things happen: there isn't nourishment, and there isn't elimination. The outcome is discomfort.

Essentially, what you are treating is circulation—pain is usually the consequence of disturbed flow. So the technique called *Dao Qi* is a very precise method of inducing circulation in a particular part of the body. That's how acupuncture works, by influencing the circulation of qi.

The question "What are the meridians, and where are they?" is a good one. Nobody has dissected the meridians. The medical scientist Robert Becker mapped the channels electrically. He showed that there are electrophysiological loci on the skin and within the muscle layers that correspond exactly to the points on acupuncture charts. He concluded that the meridians are an alternate regulatory system in the body that has to do with electromagnetic currents and electromagnetic organization of tissue growth and repair and that this has a lot to do with how the body heals when there's an injury. So now we talk about a "current of injury." When tissue is traumatized, there's actually a depolarization that occurs. In the process of restoring the electromagnetic field and current to normal, the tissue heals. And it appears that you can manipulate this electrically, as well as with acupuncture needles.

Clearly there is an aspect of our functioning that is intangible but still demonstrable. We now have the technology to identify these very subtle fields and currents. They are very, very small, but we can measure them and see how they fluctuate. Acupuncture influences these events. It also influences hormonal secretions. You can measure hormonal changes in the blood as a result of acupuncture. You can measure circulatory changes. Acupuncture seems particularly to affect microcirculation. The vascular beds that surround every organ and tissue are affected almost immediately by acupuncture. It changes the pulsatory activity of the capillaries so that one of the most common effects of acupuncture is the appearance of an erythema around the needle, indicating an increased vascularity at the locus of the point. But that increased vascularization is also taking place in the deeper tissues and organs of the body.

In Chinese medicine this phenomenon relates to the saying "where qi goes, blood flows."

Qi and the sensation of qi are different from nervous impulses because the sensations of qi travel more slowly. A certain percentage of the population—12% to 15%—are called *acupuncture sensitives*. These people will tell you precisely where the sensation is going, corresponding exactly with the recognized meridian pathways. The meridians traverse the surface of the body and penetrate its interior. They organize and regulate all other systems including the circulatory, lymphatic, and neural networks, linking them so they function in a coordinated way.

Qi

Qi includes consciousness. Qi is everything that has dynamism—anything that moves or changes is a manifestation of qi. Qi is said to have been born from the division of *dao*, of the undifferentiated whole becoming yin and yang. Qi is the motivating force, and anything that has to do with actualization, movement, and change is qi. So the mind, a process of the organism in continuous dialogue with itself—sensations, images, and thoughts in constant flux—is an expression of qi. It *is* qi.

That's why you can use your mind to regulate your body. That's the basis of qigong, which is a system of self-regulation for developing our mental and physical capacities. Qi is the fundamental reality. It exists along a continuum, just like visible and invisible light. We say things are subtle (mind) at one end, and solid (body) at the other. But they are all part of the same continuum. Mind is simply one end of that spectrum. You could use the analogy of water. At one end of the spectrum water is frigid, hard, and dense; at the other end it's a sublime vapor. But it's still H_2O.

The Chinese use water repeatedly as a metaphor for qi, because it's so mutable. It can assume any shape, constantly transforming from one state into another. So the body—we shouldn't just say "the body," we should say, "the life of the person"—is manifold. If we're paying attention to what's most deeply inside us, we call that *the mind*. If we're paying attention to what's most at the surface, we call that *skin*. But qi, as scholar Nathan Sivin says, is simultaneously what makes things happen in stuff, stuff that makes things happen, and the stuff in which things happen. Qi is what gives me my shape. It gives everything a form and a quality, and it's the thing that you and I share that's exactly the same.

There are three primary philosophical ideologies that inform Chinese medicine: Taoism, Confucianism, and Buddhism. They share a fundamental proposition that there is not an isolatable, immutable self that is wholly separate from the world. For practical purposes, there's what the Buddhists would call a "relative self," the sense of identity or continuity that we associate with our ongoing experience.

There is no absolute self; there is just Dao. And each of us embodies that Dao, just as we live within it. To the degree that we recognize ourselves as unique, we have a sense of a separate self. But clearly it's a transient, constantly spontaneous arising. Qi, which is universal, follows its own nature, its own laws, and is completely unpredictable. It could be anything at any time, in any place, and is, in fact, all things at all times in all places. But that's not really how we experience our day-to-day selves as Efrem or Harriet or Bonnie. The Taoist view is that the true essence of life is unknowable.

Lao-tsu wrote in the *Dao Te Ching*, "The Tao that can be named is not the eternal Dao. It is the unnameable that is eternally real." A name is a confinement, but Dao has no limits, no boundaries. So that which I name *Dao* is not the real Dao, but it's as close as I can get.

It was the poetry, the cosmology of Chinese medicine that appealed to us 30 years ago, and it still appeals to us today. We feel that so many of the delusions and ignorances, so much of the suffering that we encounter today, are a result of our false perception of ourselves, the ideology of *me*-ism, and our false perception of what our purpose is as a culture and a society. Chinese medical thought, like Buddhist thought, affirms the interconnectedness of all things—that our relationship with all the parts of ourselves and with each other is what's significant. The absolute division between self and other is a false division, just like the division between mind and body is false.

Pediatricians at the Centers for Disease Control have declared gun violence an epidemic. It's a social disease that is treatable and preventable by eliminating the underlying cause, the unbridled proliferation of weapons for profit. These physicians unwittingly voice the integrated thinking of Chinese medicine: health is not attainable without changing the underlying conditions that produce disease.

We were dedicated to social justice and change when we became engaged in Chinese medicine. We saw this medicine as a model that could be helpful—not only in alleviating suffering but in helping to reorient us, to provide another way of imagining ourselves and improve our world. One of its messages is that without healing each other, we can't truly, deeply, heal ourselves. We can't be well.

The main focus in our culture is whether something works. After 30 years of practicing Chinese medicine, we see that it does work, and we see when and a glimmer of how. But it's the values that remain critical to us—the knowledge and the wisdom embedded within it.

CHAPTER 41

SCOTT GERSON, MD

Fundamentals of Ayurvedic Medicine

Ayurvedic medicine arose in India over 3000 years ago within a tribe of contemplative people. Recognizing disease as an obstacle in the pursuit of enlightenment, these people devoted themselves to this issue and in their contemplations, discovered a way of living that could keep a person healthy for a normal 100-year life span. Until recently, the West has known very little about this remarkable body of knowledge. Since one of the goals of our journal is to bring the evidence for other systems into the medical literature, in 2000 we planned a special issue on Ayurveda. Consequently, in the fall of the previous year, I traveled to Brewster, New York, to interview Scott Gerson, MD. We shared both conversation and tea in his office at the National Institute of Ayurvedic Medicine.

Dr. Gerson received his bachelor's degree in philosophy from Brandeis University in Waltham, Massachusetts. He then traveled to India where he met one of his early teachers, the highly renowned vaidya Dr. V.N. Pandey, director of the Central Council for Research in Ayurveda and Siddha Medicine. Through this friendship, Dr. Gerson began to study Ayurveda at the College of Ayurveda in Trivandrum and the Arya Vaidya Sala in Kottakkal. He was awarded his fellowship in Ayurveda from the Institute of Indian Medicine in Poona, India. He earned his Master's degree in Ayurveda from the University of Pune, where he is currently completing his Ph.D.

When he returned to the United States, Dr. Gerson received his medical degree from the Mount Sinai School of Medicine in New York and completed requirements for a specialty in internal medicine. He was recently appointed clinical assistant professor in the Department of Community and Preventive Medicine at New York Medical College.

Dr. Gerson founded The National Institute of Ayurvedic Medicine in 1982, and since that time has integrated Ayurveda with conventional allopathic medicine. He is the author of *Ayurveda: The Ancient Indian Healing Art, Ayurvedic Principles of Weight Management*, and *The Comprehensive Textbook of Ayurvedic Medicinal Plants*.

My journey into Ayurvedic medicine started when I was quite young and living in the Bronx in a predominantly Jewish-Italian neighborhood. An Indian family moved into our apartment complex. They were the only Indian family in the entire community, and everybody shunned them because they looked and spoke differently and the smells emanating from their apartment were different. But you couldn't keep me away. I was constantly there. They had a son who was a few years younger than me, and I remember sitting on his grandfather's lap—I was on one knee and his grandson was on the other—and listening to stories from the *Mahabarata*, a famous epic tale in the Hindu tradition. I also remember being in the kitchen while his mother was cooking and playing underneath her sari—both of us were under her skirt. This is my earliest memory of Indian culture.

By the time I was 10, I was very interested in Indian things. I had also acquired, inexplicably, an interest in hypnosis and was actually practicing hypnosis, albeit mostly on my little sister. At 14, I began to use one of the first biofeedback machines ever made. I still have it—it's now about 30 years old. So I was developing a dual stream. On the one hand, I was very interested in India and Indian culture; on the other, I was developing an interest in the mind and the tricks that the mind can play and how the mind affects the body. All of this manifested in my graduating cum laude from Brandeis University with a degree in philosophy.

After I graduated, my father looked at me and said, "What are you going to do with a degree in philosophy?"

I looked back at him and said, "I have no idea."

I took a part-time job as a writer for the now defunct *Soho Weekly News*. I was living my life when one day a friend said, "Did you know you could go to India as a courier for the price of the tax on the ticket?" Of course I went, but before I left, I contacted Benaras Hindu University in Varanasi and arranged to come as a foreign student to study Sanskrit.

About 4 days after my arrival, there was a welcoming party for the foreign students. During the party, I met a woman in her mid-70s who began talking to me about a system of healing in the tradition of Hinduism that used the ability of the mind to have effects on the body. She explained how they used herbs and plant-based medicines, metals, and, in some cases, heavy metals and gemstones. She also said that all things in nature had healing properties. I was fascinated. I trailed her, ignoring all the other people, trying to engage her in further conversation. Finally, she got tired of my questions and wrote down a name on a piece of paper. She said, "If you want any information about this system of medicine, call my nephew."

So I did. As it turned out, her nephew, Dr. Mohan Lal, happened to be the dean of an Ayurvedic medical college in Trivandrum, now Tiruvanathapuram. I visited him and he was impressed enough with my earnestness that we pulled all kinds of strings and I ended up enrolled in the Ayurvedic medical college. And that is how my journey began.

It took me 7 years to get my degree in Ayurvedic medicine. I completed the first 3 years consecutively and then, because of personal considerations, I came back to the United States and worked for a while before returning to India to finish. Toward the end of my studies, Dr. Mohan Lal sent me to meet a man in the northern part of India. When he realized that I had a deep interest in meditation and the relationship of meditation practices to Ayurveda and healing, he said, "Go visit this man." Little did I know that he was sending me to Shantanda Saraswati, the Shankasharia of Jyotirmath, who was a very important religious figure in India at that time.

I knew His Holiness Shantanda Saraswati for a total of 3 years before his death in 1982, and it was he who initiated me into the practice of meditation and eventually gave me permission to teach simple forms of meditation to my patients. It was also His Holiness Shantanda Saraswati who suggested that I return to the United States and obtain medical training in my own culture and tradition. He felt it would be important to have the respect of the society where I was going to be practicing if I wanted to import Ayurveda into that culture. So at his urging I undertook training as an American medical doctor.

In 1982, I founded the National Institute of Ayurvedic Medicine and dedicated my life in a very formal and deep way to the study and practice and scientific validation of Ayurveda in the West. I am mainly a primary care physician, and my main impulse is to remain as quiet as possible and treat my patients. That is what my life is about.

Fundamental Principles of Ayurvedic Medicine

In my over 20 years of experience and probing into the subject of health and disease in human beings, it has become clear to me that the fundamental defect in humans is that we have lost the memory of our true nature. According to Ayurveda, there are three aspects to all things in the universe: a material aspect, a subtle aspect, and a causal aspect. Another way of saying this is that we are made up of the body, the mind, and the spirit. And it is the body and mind parts of this trinity that are subject to decay and fragmentation. The spirit is not subject to decay or deterioration of any kind.

However, most people I meet are only aware of their physical structure and the material aspects of life. We don't appreciate the subtle parts of life, like the effects of the mind, not to mention the spiritual aspects of life. So Ayurvedic medicine is a system that seeks to reestablish the wholeness of a person, to repair the fragmentation, and to prevent and reverse the decay, not only in the body, but also in the mind and spirit. Ayurvedic medicine has very real and precise methodologies and modalities that focus on these aspects.

Ayurvedic medicine arose in India between 3000 and 5000 years ago. Archeological evidence from digs performed at the cities of Harappa and Mohenjodaro indicates through carbon dating that Ayurveda existed at least 3000 years ago and probably earlier. It arose within a group of very pious and contemplative people, who were the forerunners of Hinduism. This society was involved with rituals and ceremony and worship of natural forces—the wind, the mountains, the earth, and particularly the sun. Their main intent was to achieve full realization. It wasn't long before they recognized that disease was a formidable obstacle in the pursuit of enlightenment. You couldn't sit in meditation or reflection if your gastric ulcer was giving you distress. Realizing that they had to come up with a solution to disease, they devoted themselves to this issue. In their contemplations, they discovered a way of living that could keep a person—mind, body, and soul—healthy for a normal 100-year life span. They termed this system Ayurveda, which means knowledge of long life, or knowledge of longevity.

The first thing these ancient people discovered was that all things in the material universe, including human beings, are composed of five elements. This observation has become known as the five-element theory in Ayurveda. The sages looked around and within themselves and saw that all things are composed of the *pancha mahabhutas* or the five great elements: space, air, fire, water, and earth.

Another important fundamental concept in Ayurveda is the concept of the three *doshas*. According to Ayurveda, the five elements—space, air, fire, water, and earth—coalesce to form three fundamental biologic energies called the *doshas*. Space and air become an energy, or *dosha*, known as *vata*. Fire and water become an energy known as *pitta*. Water and earth come together and form *kapha*. These three energies control and regulate all the functions in human physiology.

It is interesting that almost simultaneously across the Himalayan mountain range in China, sages were formulating a similar idea. Both cultures saw this five-fold nature of the universe. However, it was these early Vedic priests who recognized the relationship of the five elements to the tripartite humoral forces that define and regulate biological processes. I usually tell people who are learning Ayurveda that these three words are the only Sanskrit that they really need to know: *vata, pitta, kapha*.

Vata, deriving from space and air, is the lightest and most mobile of the elements and is a bioenergy that, in the human body, is responsible for movement of all kinds. So *vata* moves everything, from the blinking of your eyes to the coursing of blood through your arteries and veins, to the movement of air gently in and out of your lungs, to the elimination of wastes from our body, even to the thoughts crossing your mind. Wherever there is movement of any kind, physical or subtle, there is *vata* energy powering and regulating it.

Pitta, being the only bioenergy that contains fire, is primarily concerned with the digestion and transformation of one substance into another. So when a person eats a carrot, which contains more than 350 micronutrients—vitamin A, beta carotene, alpha carotene, B vitamins, minerals, and various other trace elements—how does the body know to take the beta carotene and, after it has been digested and absorbed into the bloodstream, carry it preferentially to the lung tissue and the retina of the eyes? How does the body have the intelligence to selectively transport that nutrient to its proper locus? That, according to Ayurveda, is *pitta*. It is the intelligence of the body to know how to change a carrot into a human being in just the proper way.

Kapha, derived from water and earth, is the heaviest of the bioenergies. It brings solidity and stability to the body and mind. It brings resistance to disease. It brings immunity. Psychologically, kapha is responsible for tendencies and emotions that hold families, towns, cities, and entire cultures together. It is the cohesive force. *Kapha* is responsible for the impulses of generosity, compassion, empathy, forgiveness, and divine love.

The three biological energies combine in various proportions in all of us, and it is this unique proportion of *vata*, *pitta*, and *kapha* that makes us unique. Also, it is the unique proportion of the three *doshas* and how they combine in each of us that constitutes the next fundamental principle of Ayurveda. The unique proportion of the *doshas*, as it occurs in you, is known as your constitutional type, or *prakriti*. Everything in Ayurvedic medicine—every treatment, every dietary recommendation, every mantra—is based on an understanding of an individual's *prakriti*. An outward symptom or disease complex occurring in 10 different people could potentially be treated in 10 different ways. A headache in a *vata* person would be treated completely differently from one in a predominantly *pitta* or *kapha* person. This is one of the seminal contributions of Ayurvedic medicine to the history of healing. Ayurvedic medicine places a great deal of emphasis on the differences of individuals.

Because there are no cookbook approaches, Ayurvedic medicine is more complicated to master. There is no single herbal formulation that can be taken or no single acupuncture point that can be pushed to eradicate a headache. Rather, we look at everyone as a whole, as the entire trinity of body, mind, and spirit. We first try to understand what constitutes the individual. What are the elemental predominances? What are the energies that are excessive or deficient? Then, keeping that in view, we look at the symptoms. In Ayurveda, this dual form of assessment of both the individual and the disease is known as *rogi roga pariksha*.

So when a person comes to you with a headache you first diagnose who they are and how the three energies are working within them. You find out where is the balance and where is the imbalance. You don't worry about the headache until you get an understanding of the person because you want to understand the energetic nature of the person first. And that is accomplished through sitting together. There is no shortcut method. Ayurvedic consultations have no time limit. If it takes 10 minutes to understand the nature of a person, fine. However, if I am to any degree confused or uncertain, then I must take as much time as I need.

It is very important to practice Ayurvedic medicine with integrity and completeness, especially with regard to the initial assessment of the nature of a person. That must be firmly established in the mind of the doctor. Sometimes, in order to achieve this understanding, I will use certain techniques such as asking the person if he or she will excuse me for a moment and then purposely staying out for 5 or 10 minutes. When I come back, I immediately make observations. Is that person angry? Is that person insulted? Is that person afraid? What is the response and reaction to that particular situation? Because it is often by placing people in somewhat uncomfortable situations that you see their true nature.

So in Ayurvedic medicine we are given ways to prod and poke into the nature of an individual. When that is established, we turn our attention to the nature of the disease itself. I will give you an example. A person walks into the office complaining of a headache. In modern medicine, headaches are generally regarded as caused by tension, which has an effect on the state of vasoconstriction or dilatation of blood vessels in the head region. The treatment usually has to do with modifying the state of vascular flow. So this is considered to be the mechanism of headache in most people.

In Ayurveda we understand headaches to be a more individualized event. In a *vata*-predominant person, a headache could be due to the excess of *vata dosha*, which happens to be situated in the head region. So there might be an abnormal movement in the blood vessels. The treatment would be toward diminishing the *vata dosha* to normalize the blood vessels that are constricting with very little stimulus. However, the same headache in a patient of a *pitta* nature could have nothing to do with abnormal vasoconstriction. The problem in the *pitta* person is more likely due to heat rising up to the head region. As you know, in any container, including the human body, heat tends to rise. So a person's headache could have to do with heat that is being created lower in the body—in the liver or in the small intestines—that is finding ways to rise to the top of the body and situate itself in the head. The ideology in this case has nothing to do with abnormal constriction of the blood vessels. So the principle of treating a *pitta* headache would be to diminish the amount of heat in the body using everything from cooling breathing techniques to herbs with refrigerant qualities to cooling yoga postures to foods that have a cooling effect on the body. So for the same symptoms, there are two totally different causes and two different treatment approaches.

The Role of Consciousness in Ayurveda

According to Ayurveda, ultimately what heals a condition and what promotes well-being in a human are not medicines, foods, or meditation techniques but rather what we call in the West the vital energy of an individual. The object of Ayurvedic medicine is to promote the unimpeded flow of consciousness through every tissue and sinew of the body—and it is consciousness that brings the light and intelligence to every cell and subcellular structure so that it functions in the most optimized way. If consciousness is impeded in a particular region or organ or tissue, that area of the body will experience a distortion of its intelligence, which translates into some type of abnormal functioning and disease. Ayurveda seeks to reestablish and maintain consciousness so the body maintains its memory of how to function. It is really the most important modality of Ayurveda: never to forget that all things are structured in consciousness.

In Ayurveda we understand that the *doshas*—*vata*, *pitta*, and *kapha*—are the agents of disease. In other words, disease manifestations can be precisely and perfectly understood through an understanding of the *dosha* imbalances in a person. But what causes the *doshas* to go out of balance? If we could identify those factors then we would arrive at what we call *hetu*, or the causes of disease. So now we have arrived at the causal level of disease. Through contemplation and reflection about the nature of disease, the ancient *rishis*, or wise physicians, arrived at an understanding of these very factors. They enumerated three factors that are the causes of disease, all of which have a direct relation to consciousness.

The first cause of disease according to Ayurveda is known as *prajnaparadha*, which is translated as "blasphemy of the intellect" or "mistake of the intellect." Whenever one has a mistaken understanding of something in his or her environment, it is a mistake of intellect. For example, if you think that going outside with wet hair can lead to pneumonia, which it cannot, that is a mistake of the intellect. If you think it is not harmful to the physiology to eat a cold and heavy substance such as ice cream in cold and damp weather, such as in the winter season in North America, then you are mistaken. If you think that all women are emotional and undependable as business partners, that is a mistake of your intellect—you are not understanding something in its true nature. According to Ayurveda, a mistake of the intellect or wrong understanding of the true nature of the environment can lead to disease. In fact, it is one of the main causes of disease.

A second cause of disease is known as *asatmyendriyartha samyoga*, which translates as a wrong association of a sense object with the sensory apparatus. In other words, we have five senses: sight, smell, taste, touch, and hearing. There are appropriate and inappropriate inputs to these senses. According to Ayurveda, it would be harmful if one were constantly exposed to harsh sounds or loud sounds or if he or she constantly listened to gossip. If you walk to work every day and pass by a garbage disposal that has very noxious smells, this could violate the *doshas* and lead to disease. If you restricted your diet to only one taste to the exclusion of all others—if you exclusively ate things that tasted sweet and there was no bitter or astringent or salty or pungent flavor in your diet—this could lead to a vitiation or distortion of the *doshas* and hence to disease. So a proper and intelligent association between our sense organs and the sense objects is important. And not adhering to these principles leads to disease.

Finally, the third cause of disease that the ancient *vaijas* understood was *kala-parinama*, which means not paying attention to the cycles and rhythms of nature. So having sexual activity at sunrise or at sunset or during the woman's menstruation period is considered not paying attention to the cycles. Eating the wrong types of foods in the wrong seasons is another. If you go to Miami Beach you will see this phenomenon of *kala-parinama*. You see women in their late 70s dressed up in miniskirts, parading around and acting as if they were still in their 20s. That is an example of not paying attention to the cycles. These women are acting in a way that is inappropriate for their age and status in life as an elder.

If people understood that they have an energetic nature and that all things have unique energetic confirmations, the next step would be very easy. It would be obvious that certain foods are appropriate for certain people at certain times of the year. But the first step is to escape from the prison of our material vision of the world and to enter into this new subtle vision and understand the energetic nature of things.

The Art of Diagnosis

Diagnosis is intended to provide information not only about the function and state of the physical tissues and organ systems but also of the emotional, mental, and spiritual state of each person. We have diagnostic tools to address each of these facets. The physical diagnosis is based on the ability of the Ayurvedic physician to make very precise, minute observations about a person. So we use many different cues. We look at how many times a person blinks per minute, the setting of the ears (high, low, or intermediate), the thickness of the lips, the amount of frizziness seen in the hair, the body stature, the frame of the person, and how prominent the veins and tendons are on the hands. We will examine the amount of fat tissue versus muscle tissue in the body. We will look at almost every physical characteristic that you can imagine, including the shape and contours of the nails and the markings on the tongue. These things give us knowledge of the person. The diagnosis has to do with both understanding the nature of the person and understanding the nature of the disease. The person and the disease both have these material, subtle, and causal levels.

To examine the physical aspects of a disease, we look at physical aspects of a person, so it is important that we understand physically how a person is constituted. We will look at some permanent features, such as the color of the eyes, the thickness of the lips, the boniness of the joints, and the prominence of the veins. Features like this give us a good idea about the proportion of *vata*, *pitta*, and *kapha* in a person's nature. There are other physical features that give us some idea about the disease process. For instance, we can examine the markings and textures of the tongue, look at the shapes and signs in the nails, and examine features relating to the urine and the feces. These give us physical impressions of the disease process.

With regard to the subtle aspects of a person and the disease, we have other methods. We need to see how the mind works and processes information. What are the mental and emotional tendencies? So we engage a person in conversation and observe his or her reactions to various subjects. Often, we are able to discern which parts of a person's life are causing distress. So, while engaging a person in conversation often seems very casual, we are actually doing it in a sophisticated and intentional way. We are asking about work, the relationship with the significant other, the relationship with mother and father, and other facets of life that Ayurveda tells us to make a point of discussing.

One of the most interesting diagnostic methods in Ayurveda involves paying attention to the speech that a person produces with relation to different subjects. We listen specifically to the vowel sounds and their purity and to the consonant sounds—especially the terminal consonant such as the *t*'s and *d*'s on the ends of words—as a person speaks about particular subjects. The vowel sounds relate to the emotional content that is held in a particular subject, and the consonant sounds relate to the mental clarity that a person possesses about a particular subject. Speech changes according to a person's clarity on the subject and the emotional content that underpins that subject, because speech ultimately comes from the mind. Like I said a moment ago, the rhetorical question to ask is "Where does speech originate? The irrefutable answer to that question is that speech originates in the mind. In fact, in Ayurveda we understand four different stages of the origin of speech. The first three stages are in aspects of mind. It is only in the fourth stage that speech manifests through the vocal apparatus and out through the mouth and lips.

But that is only one aspect of subtle diagnosis of a person and disease. Perhaps the most famous aspect of subtle diagnosis is *nadi pariksha*, or pulse diagnosis. This is the ultimate form of energetic diagnosis. It has been brought to a very sophisticated level by many *vaidyas* practicing Ayurveda in India. The pulse is a sophisticated diagnostic tool that can be used to understand in a reproducible way the *doshic* balance in an individual. Through the pulse we can understand not only how the *doshas* are supposed to be in a particular individual, but we can understand their current state of proportions. And if what their *doshic* balance is supposed to be differs from how it is currently, we can confidently state that a person has an imbalance, whether it be an excess in *vata* or a deficiency in *kapha*.

So you first observe to know how the patient should be, then you observe to know how the patient is. We can achieve balance once we understand the discrepancies between the balanced state of the *doshas* for a particular individual—the *prakriti*—and the imbalances that exist in that individual currently—the *vikriti*. Then it is clear how we need to manipulate the *doshas* to reestablish balance.

Ayurvedic Medicine and Spirituality

Now, we have covered physical assessment of the individual and disease and subtle assessment of the individual and disease, but what sets Ayurvedic medicine apart from many other alternative modalities is its well-established approach to the spiritual basis of disease as well. In Ayurveda we also pay attention to the spiritual aspects of both assessing a person and diagnosing a disease. To do that we use several techniques.

First, in Ayurvedic medical schools throughout India, all Ayurvedic doctors are trained in Vedic astrology. We understand that there are often discernible planetary influences on the arrival, progression, and prognosis of a disease process. Many times, if we see a particularly malevolent aspect in a person's astrological chart, we will offer remedies in the form of gemstones or mantras. And, as a scientist and research-oriented physician, I can affirm that I have seen enough evidence to convince me that there is validity to this aspect of Ayurvedic medicine.

The other way of understanding the spiritual aspects of a disease is to sit down with a person and engage her in a discussion of her life story from beginning to end, starting with where she was born and how the events of her life have taken her from stage to stage. It is often possible to see recurring situations and lessons that a person still needs to learn at the karmic level. Very often, these unlearned lessons at the level of the soul are having a profound effect on the disease process that a person is experiencing. So that is the other way we incorporate the spiritual aspects of human beings.

In my book *Ayurveda: The Ancient Indian Healing Art*, I have a section on meditation and I want to read you the preface. It will give you some idea of the importance that I attach to the practice of meditation:

"The ancient sages have defined one supreme way to attain the final goal of a prosperous and happy long life free of misery. This way is through meditation. This is very simple and can be done by anyone, yet the effects are profound and direct. It has been said that anyone who meditates properly will receive all the benefits of every extant health system and spiritual teaching. Meditation is the key to unlocking and freeing human potentials otherwise condemned to wither and die. It is provided to mankind for self-realization."[1]

Meditation is the center of my life. As I told you, the instruction given to me more than 25 years ago was to remain quiet and take care of my patients. So, part of that instruction includes the constant practice of meditation. It is through this practice that I am able to be an instrument of healing.

---

[1]From Gerson S: *Ayurveda: the ancient Indian healing art*, Rockport, MA, 1993, Element Books Ltd.

CHAPTER 42

ROBERT THURMAN, PhD

Gifts from Tibetan Medicine

Robert Thurman is a scholar, author, and former Tibetan monk. After education at Philips Exeter and Harvard, he studied Tibetan Buddhism for almost 40 years. He holds the first endowed chair in Buddhist studies in the United States and is the Jey Tsong Khapa Professor of Indo-Tibetan Buddhist Studies at Columbia University in New York City.

In 1964, when he was studying to become a Buddhist monk in India at the age of 24, Thurman met the Dalai Lama. Since that time, Thurman and the Dalai Lama have maintained a lifelong friendship. Before returning to the United States and his academic career, Thurman also studied Tibetan medicine with Yeshi Dhonden, the Dalai Lama's personal physician. In 1987, Thurman and actor Richard Gere founded Tibet House in New York City, a nonprofit organization dedicated to preserving the living culture of Tibet. Thurman currently serves as its Director.

Thurman is the author of *The Central Philosophy of Tibet: A Study and Translation of Jey Tsong Khapa's Essence of True Eloquence; Inner Revolution: Life, Liberty, and the Pursuit of Real Happiness; Essential Tibetan Buddhism; The Tibetan Book of the Dead* (translation); *Wisdom and Compassion: The Sacred Art of Tibet* (with Marylin H. Rhie); *Circling the Sacred Mountain: A Spiritual Adventure Through the Himalayas* (with Tad Wise); *Worlds of Transformation: Tibetan Art of Wisdom and Compassion* (with Marylin H. Rhie); and *Mandala: the Architecture of Enlightenment* (with Denise Leidy).

I met Robert Thurman in the summer of 2001 at Menla, a retreat center in the Catskill Mountains of New York, while he was hosting a think tank on Tibetan Medicine, and interviewed him the next day at his home in the forest near Woodstock, New York.

This journey began for me in high school. I was pointedly nonreligious as a young person and was into science, in particular philosophy and psychology. But it seemed that the Western psychologies and philosophies were all "in the head" and didn't offer anything that could effectively change one's inner emotional structure. I wanted something better, so I began to read in yoga, Buddhism, Hinduism, Daoism, and Sufism. Then, in the middle of college, I hit a wall and decided I could no longer sit at Harvard listening to professors expatiate on Shakespeare and Wittgenstein. So I took off for Asia.

I liked the Sufi masters I met but felt they were back to theism. The same was true of the Hindu masters. But when I met the Buddhist masters of Tibet, I instinctively felt that this was it. But it wasn't just devotional. When I read the great relativist philosopher Nagarjuna—I would call him a critical deconstructive philosopher of the second century of the Common Era—my mind began to be satisfied. I started learning meditation and yoga without sacrificing reason or critical thinking. And I thrived on it. The idea of having a spiritual path that was also critical, intellectual, and scientific appealed to me.

I actually became a monk for a few years, but then I realized my limitations. I also realized that further development at a certain stage depends on relating to others with compassion. It's not something you can do locked away in a meditation room. You have to overcome your bad habits related with other people to be enlightened.

There are three aspects to the Buddhist path of enlightenment—ethical behavior, meditation, and critical wisdom, which is really science. Critical wisdom involves penetrating the surface of apparent reality and finding its deeper nature. Buddha was not just the founder of a religion; he was also a scientist in the sense that he looked into the human mind and body and discovered its nature. The good news is that it is possible for human beings to fully understand themselves and fully understand their environment. When I say fully, I mean to the degree that they can be free from suffering. Not just free from neurotic suffering yet subject to ordinary suffering, as Freud postulated—but free from all suffering.

So after I renounced being a monk, I returned to academia, which was very natural to me because discovering the nature of the world is the key drive for enlightenment.

Studying Medicine with Yeshi Dhonden

Let me backtrack for a minute. I returned to the United States from my first trip to India when my father died sadly and suddenly of a heart attack. I then met Geshe Wangyal, a Mongolian lama and spent a year and a half with him in New Jersey. He was a particularly remarkable lama who had been in Tibet for 35 years. He was the one who gave me a personal way of "getting at it," not just through the texts, although he taught me many texts and helped me with the language. However, he did not want me to be a monk.

He said, "Be like a monk. Study all the time and shave your head, just don't do the formality because I am telling you, you're not going to stay a monk."

"Oh, you don't know me," I said. "This is it. This is for me. I don't care about this other crazy Western world." But I was only 21 years old.

Finally, I kept bugging him so much that after a year and a half, in early 1964, he took me to India and introduced me to the Dalai Lama. I stayed for a year and became the first Western to be ordained as a Tibetan Buddhist monk. In the Tibetan culture, it's not a big step to become a monk. It's the best thing you can possibly do for yourself and everybody else and is much like a life-long MacArthur Fellowship. The Tibetans were still just newly in exile—this was in the early 1960s—and had, with Nehru's permission, recreated their culture in these little enclaves in India, which is actually how they saved their culture. So they didn't think twice about allowing me to become a monk, even though my mentor, who had been living in the West, knew that my own cultural background would make it difficult for me in the long run.

The thing that is germane here is that before my mentor left me in Dharmasala, he suddenly shows up one day at our little rooming house—in those days the town was primitive, with people living in shacks made of cardboard and tin—with this man who looked like a Garuda bird, which is a mythical eagle-human being, like those birdmen in Flash Gordon. My mentor said, "'You study with him."

I asked what type of Lama this man was and my mentor told me he was a doctor. So I said, "What do you mean, he's a doctor? I didn't come here to study medicine. I'm studying enlightenment. I'm studying voidness. I'm studying compassion."

"No," my mentor said, "You can do whatever else you want, and you can study other things, but I want you to study medicine with Yeshi Dhonden. You're going to need that."

I couldn't imagine what for. There were no doctors in my family, and I had been brought up ignorant of the human body, as were most western people. I didn't know anything—was the kidney something in my ear or in my brain? I had no interest and no idea. But because I respected my mentor so much and because I liked Yeshi Dhonden, I did study Tibetan medicine with him, and it was an incredible revelation.

I learned anatomy, but not exactly like the systematic anatomy of the west. The Tibetans have their own version of anatomy that focuses on the functions of organs, and their drawings emphasize the acupuncture meridians and other functional interrelationships between organs and sense faculties or organs and limbs. So I learned that tradition, memorized much of the data, and actually learned to read the pulses and look at the urine the way Tibetans do.

I also saw many patients. They accelerated my training because I was the only western student, and I had a good relationship with Yeshi Dhonden. At the time, he was very overworked reestablishing the medical institute in exile and seeing the many refugee Tibetan patients whose systems were deranged by the huge climate change. Many Indians in the neighborhood and many military people were also coming to see him. By the time I got there, he had already dealt with the local Indian health authorities, both western-trained and Ayurveda-trained, and they had come to trust in Tibetan medicine.

India has a model of medical pluralism to which our country should aspire. They have four or five medical systems that are allowed to operate in parallel and therefore the Indian medical consumer can go between the different ones for different needs. They have western medicine, Ayurveda, Unani (Greek), Rasad (Muslim), and Siddha (pulse). Tibetan medicine, which is related to Ayurveda and has some relation to Unani, became just another one of the systems.

So I learned Tibetan medicine even though I wasn't sure I was ever going to be a medical practitioner. I also learned Tibetan astrology because you have to learn it. And it introduced me to the whole Tibetan culture in a very powerful way. I began to understand my own body and nature in a different way that undergirded the philosophical, meditative, high, ultimate reality I was dealing with on my spiritual quest. It therefore fit in beautifully and made my spiritual quest more holistic. So it was a very good thing.

The Tibetan Medicine Vision

Tibetan medicine has a very fascinating history. Tibet is a place where some of the very ancient trends in Asia were preserved and refined by people who were 20% monastic and therefore into learning and the deep investigation of the nature of reality. Besides having a spiritual side from Buddhism, Tibetan medicine draws from ancient Greek medicine as practiced in Iran in the Persian court, ancient Chinese medicine, and ancient Indian medicine. It may have been one of the dominant forms of Buddhist medicine that we lost track of when Buddhism disappeared in India with the Muslim invasions at the end of the first millennium. Then, of course, it also includes aspects of Mongolian and Tibetan shamanistic medicine.

It is, therefore, very integrative, very literary, and very investigative. It has a huge botanical lore and a very sophisticated system of compounding herbs, minerals, and animal products. But, whatever Tibetan medicine is, it never was a fixed system. It was always open to all kinds of influences. And because Buddhism was pan-Asian, the Tibetans were always interactive with other Buddhist cultures.

In a certain way, Tibetan medicine can help unify Chinese and Indian medicines. Not that we're going to reduce everything into one homogenized medical system, but maybe some principles will emerge that will help people who are adept and devoted to a particular type of training understand the other types of training and frameworks. The point is that Tibetan medicine provides an integrative framework. And I think the Tibetan vision might be very valuable in the next decade here in the West.

The Tibet House U.S. in New York—there are Tibet Houses in India and Mexico and other countries—is the Dalai Lama's outpost here for trying to preserve Tibetan culture, to develop it, to see that it expands and eventually, to restore it in its home setting. To do this involves sharing any good thing about Tibetan culture—or even simply the love and appreciation for Tibetan culture—with the world. In that light, Tibetan medicine is an essential contribution.

Years ago, the Dalai Lama said to me that when Tibet could be itself in the modern world—whether as a satellite of China or independently—and when they could have true internal cultural and human autonomy again, he would urge that Tibet's national industry should be the medical industry. The two things that the Tibetans have done well in exile are the "Dharma industry"—teaching meditation and philosophy—and the medical industry. They have already made a big contribution in India. There are 42 Tibetan clinics in India that serve many non-Tibetans. And the one aspect of the Tibetan culture that the Chinese could not destroy, although they tried to take the Buddha out of it, was the medicine. They didn't kill all the doctors, even though many were monks, and they sent the medicine to China. Now there's a demand for it—the Chinese use the herbs and the knowledge. So what's happened in India and China shows that Tibetan medicine has value in other cultures. We would like to see this worldwide in a more formal way.

Misconceptions

The western audience has a tendency to think that the essence of the Buddhist message is that ordinary human life is bad—it leads to sickness, old age, death and then future lives in terrible conditions—and that the Buddha discovered a way to get out of life, to disappear to someplace where there was no pain. Of course, this is not only *not* meaningful; it is stupid. This distortion of Buddhism was presented early on by people who did not understand Buddhism and who were desperately seeking to escape from the world. However, the actual point of what Buddha discovered was different.

What the Buddha discovered was that human life can be happy and that human life is immensely valuable. Buddhists agree with Darwin in that human beings are interwoven in a whole chain of biological forms. The difference from Darwin is that we believe that we personally have been dogs and personally have been giraffes and personally have been bugs and personally have been any animal you can think of in an infinite past. But we have evolved through a lot of effort guided by altruism, empathy to other beings, generosity, tolerance, and a nonviolent response to injury and through developing intelligence, wisdom, and mental stability. In other words, through cultivating these virtues as other animals—which is very hard because their reactive responses are hardwired more than ours—we've become this type of being that is self-aware, self-critical, and able to deprogram and reprogram even instincts. From the Buddhist's view, there is no hardwiring to a human being. Therefore we are the beings who have the best chance of becoming really happy.

This was Buddha's great discovery. Really, the point is that Asians love Buddhism because Buddhism says that on top of being blessed with the Ganges River valley and the Indus River valley and on top of having a lot of good Chinese cooking, you are human and therefore you can become fully happy in such a way that even if an elephant stepped on your hand and you were injured, that wouldn't disturb your happiness. You would want to repair your hand, of course, and you would feel pain, but it would be in a way that you would be able to free yourself from feeling unhappy about the pain. In other words, there would be nothing that you couldn't deal with.

The Buddha said that being self-centered and ignorant about the nature of yourself and the world is guaranteed unhappiness. That's when people misunderstood him and thought he meant that everyone was unhappy. He said every *unenlightened person is unhappy*. Every self-centered person who thinks the world is there for them is going to be unhappy because the world doesn't think so. It is as simple as that.

The "epitome of Buddha's teaching" comes from a certain anecdote in history. It comes from one of his disciples who was approached by someone who asked, "What does your teacher teach? You have a certain light about you. I think I would like to meet this teacher."

First the disciple said, "I cannot tell you; I am just a simple monk." But finally he said this one little verse, and it has become famous throughout the history of Buddhism. He said, "All things arise from causes. What are those causes in specific cases and how to stop the negative among those causes—that's what the Buddha teaches."

Now, that's not religious. It is scientific. And this is the essence of the tradition.

The Medicine Buddha

This is what Buddhism believes: Shakyamuni Buddha was doing performance art, if you will, and at a certain moment he turned himself into a blue Medicine Buddha with a sapphire radiance. Then, in front of his audience, he transformed the whole environment into a magical universe where everyone simultaneously perceived everything as medicine. The grass, the trees, the chairs—everything was medicine. Even poison was medicine if you used a tiny amount or homeopathic trace. Within that matrix of seeing the universe as medicine—as benevolent, positive substances if it was known how to use and combine—he then taught what are called the four medical mantras.

The Buddhists believe that Ayurveda and all of the ancient medical traditions emerged more than 2500 years ago from this event. They call the medicine vision a *mandala*, which is a purified universe. What is great about this is that in Tibetan medical training, the physician learns that mandala. And in that mandala, all the medicines are there—the plants, the trees, the nuts, the minerals, and the waters. So you learn to memorize and see the environment that way. They even have a visualization yoga in which the physician learns to identify himself as the Medicine Buddha, to merge with the Medicine Buddha, and cultivate the compassion of a Buddha whose only aim is to help beings be well.

Buddhists have the theory that the human life form is superior to the divine life form. Humans are better off than gods or angels—which are beings they actually do believe in and interact with—because the gods and angels are more complacent. They don't have predators nipping at their heals. Humans are right there. They die easily, get injured easily, get old quickly. They know that things are serious and that their choices will make a big difference. Therefore they have a big motive to find out what's going on. That puts them in an advantageous position. So the Buddhist worldview is very human life–affirming.

Therefore the Medicine Buddha fits logically with the Buddhist message about the value of human life. To have human life disturbed by some minor cause like eating some wrong thing or catching some contagious disease is a real shame because then that human being loses his or her platform for higher evolution. Their life goes on, of course, but if they die unenlightened they have lost a fantastic opportunity, and it will be a long time before they will win their way back to being human again. And this is a big loss to an individual human being from a Buddhist point of view.

The Medicine Buddha, then, is Buddhism's most positive vision about how the earth itself is a good environment for the human being. Human beings have adapted to it, and if you know how to manage this environment—combine a blade of grass of this kind with a little herb of that kind if you feel this way—you will be in balance again. And that is not even the main thing—if you bring your spirit in balance and you bring your mind in balance, then you become enlightened. So the teaching of the Medicine Buddha is believed by Buddhists to fit right with the Buddha's own message of healing the whole world by helping beings understand their situation and become free of suffering so they can be happy and enlightened and help others.

The Physician on a Spiritual Path

The ideal Tibetan physician, of course, is an enlightened person. That doesn't mean that every Tibetan physician is fully enlightened; it means that any Tibetan physician is on that path. This is the way they prevent themselves from getting burned out or resenting or exploiting the patients. However, I am sure some still do because no tradition is perfect. We human beings can twist anything. But this is what we need to recover for western civilization—the physician on a spiritual path.

The Hippocratic oath is a spiritual path. It's just been too mechanized, industrialized, and commercialized. People take the oath without thinking about it. And there is no course. For example, in medical school they should teach a class in the Hippocratic way, what it deeply means and what Greek spirituality was about. Asclepius is the Greek god of healing, and the Hippocratic oath was to serve beings, to execute the will of Asclepius, and to help humans. It was not to be there for profit or fame or power over others but to help suffering beings.

I think almost anybody who goes into medicine has at least some component of wanting to help others. But it gets beaten out of them by the commercialization, the research emphasis, the drug companies, the corporatization of everything, and the heavy 19-hour shifts. So without needing to follow Buddhism, medical education could teach this from western resources, such as Jesus, Aesclepius, and Hippocrates.

The Four Noble Truths

The Four Noble Truths of Buddhism are the fundamental framework in which Buddha taught his first students. They are like a medical diagnosis about life. The first Truth is that the unenlightened life is going to be frustrating and therefore full of suffering. Because it's you against the universe, and then you lose, because the universe is going to outdo you sooner or later. That's not even complicated.

The second is the Truth of the "fact of the cause of suffering." The cause of suffering is my delusion that I am something separate from the universe and that I am more important than the rest of the universe. This puts me in conflict with the universe, which knows it is more important. So that delusion of mine, that misunderstanding, brings me into conflict with that which I don't need to be in conflict with.

So first I come to a better understanding about my relationship with the world and about my relationship with myself. The symptom is the suffering that I don't like, and the etiology is that the cause of suffering is delusion, plus actions driven by the delusion such as greed and hatred. I become greedy because I want more of the universe to be incorporated by me. I become angry when I perceive the universe to take something away from me. I become jealous when I think somebody has something that I want. I become proud when I think I have something they want. These are all of the vices that rise out of that delusion.

The third Noble Truth is the prognosis. Suffering can be ceased; the cause can be understood and stopped. Wisdom can replace ignorance and then suffering will cease and I will be happy. And the fourth Noble Truth is the method of curing it, the therapy. This "method of curing" is the eight-fold path, which involves ethical, spiritual, and intellectual physical, verbal, and mental methods.

Compassion

Compassion is a very important topic. It is crucial. This relates to what I said about the yoga that is taught to every Tibetan medical student, which could be paralleled in western thinking by something like "Hippocratic Oath Yoga." Western doctors could have a special course in medical school where they learn about the Eleusinian mysteries or Hippocratic yoga. They could learn some type of meditation, and they could evoke, like an ancestor, Hippocrates and other great doctors. They could visualize these famous doctors as present to them, and they could cultivate in themselves a desire to fulfill the selfless service to beings that all of these great doctors have had. They could do whatever would be inspiring—not just reading about it once in a book but meditating about it and trying to cultivate such qualities in themselves. So they might say, "I do hope to have a BMW when I have paid my debts and am a practicing doctor, but that is not going to be my motive. I am not going to twist my diagnosis in people. I am not going to favor the rich over the poor. I am going to try to be compassionate to all." In other words, medical students should be aware of the human failings and temptations and meditate against them as part of their training and study.

Compassion, of course, is very trainable. Let me talk about how compassion is developed in Tibetan Buddhism because that's the great gift in Buddhism. It has this wonderful developmental psychology. Compassion is defined in Buddhism as the wish to help others, which is a natural human wish.

Human beings have evolved because they are more compassionate than other animals. Human form is a life form that developed out of compassion. Most mammals don't carry a baby in their gut for 9 months and then watch it run around helplessly for 10 years and deal with its teenage freak-outs and then pay its college tuition—do you know what I am saying? An animal just dumps an egg in the sand some place and jumps back into the ocean. You have less connection with others if you have a hard shell. But the human form is a soft shell.

The militaristic anthropologists and biogrammarians in a militaristic country like America tell us that we got to be human by killing elephants and saber-toothed tigers on the savannah. But that is a bunch of baloney. We compensated for our gentleness—as compared with sabertooths—by talking to each other in a tree and saying, "Hey, let's get a spear." But in fact, we are more gentle. If I am really fierce by my nature, my human body is useless. Where are my fangs and claws? Sabertooth would make a meal of out me. So we were scared and hid, learned to talk to each other while hiding, and by talking we got to sharing minds, which is the advantage of the altruism of the human form. Once we shared minds, we came up with much more clever things than the sabertooth. We could imagine being a sabertooth and how to catch them and trap them.

Compassion is saying that the human being, therefore, has a natural empathy in their biological form. Of course, humans have the possibility to be absolutely vile and because of their greater cleverness, they can be much more destructive than a sabertooth who eats just one person for a meal. We can kill millions. We can deplete whole species and destroy the whole planet. So yes, we can be worse than an animal, but our basic nature is gentle, and our power came through our gentleness. We are building on that nature when we build compassion. And the way we build compassion is to celebrate our empathy and our interconnection.

The Motherhood of All Beings Meditation

There is a meditation that is very powerful called the Meditation of the Motherhood of All Beings. Mother-recognition is the first step. It comes from the idea of "infinite pasts, biological intertwinement of living beings." You could do this through a Darwinist view; you wouldn't necessarily have to have the former life idea of the Buddhist. You could be a cell or an atom or a molecule. You meditate on the fact that somehow the molecules that I have now have been the molecules of every kind of being that has been my mother in all my infinite pasts. It is the sense of cultivating and deepening that sense of entwinement. When we connect to the motherhood, we can develop a vision where we see every other being as our mother. It's a weird vision, believe me. I don't pretend to have attained it, but I have practiced it enough to know some of the symptoms, and one of them is that you start having a permanent *deja vu* experience with everybody you see because everybody looks familiar.

So medical students could easily be taught this. If they were Christian or Muslim, they could think, "We are all God's children, and we have an entwinement in God, so we're actually brother and sister." You could then meditate on the brotherhood and sisterhood of everybody. If you did this for 30 minutes a day for 2 years, by the time you were seeing patients it would be like seeing a brother or sister. That element might get lost in the emergency room, but it would still change your basic outlook. And so this is the way to compassion.

There is another meditation like the old proverb "put yourself in the other fellow's shoes." In this meditation, you think of someone who really irritates you and then meditate that you are him and looking at you. When you do this, you realize that you really irritate him, and therefore he is nasty to you, which is why he irritates you. But then you see something about yourself—you notice the way that you say things with some little inflection, or that you're Mr. Superior Whitey or Mr. Superior Blacky or that you're the male superior to the dumb female, or vice versa, or that you have more money, whatever. You become more sensitive to the interaction and eventually, you will find actual sympathy for someone about whom you felt jealousy. There are other meditations where you visualize yourself as the other person, and you realize how frustrated she is by something. You realize that even though she may be condescending toward you, she is actually in a miserable state, putting on a front that she is so cool and you're not. So you begin to feel sympathy for her and then you chuckle when she behaves in a funny way, because you are freed of the grip of feeling jealous.

These things really work but they don't work just by thinking through them. You have to spend time each day. So the medical school should have 30 minutes a day when the students do yoga and meditation in the morning. If they did that, the students would come back to their studies with greater enthusiasm. Actually, they would make more money in the long run by being better doctors but without having the motive for money. And even if they didn't make so much money sometimes, they wouldn't get all paranoid and compulsive and feel that they were going to lose everything. They would be relaxed about it all, and this would be better for them personally as well as medically.

Critical Thinking

On the critical wisdom side, parallel with compassion, people are taught to investigate their own way of holding their identities. It's like studying Erik Erikson or Jean Piaget but doing it more carefully and doing it more personally and viscerally by using meditation in relation to the study. It isn't just meditation or just study—it has to be study *with* meditation.

First, you are taught how you hold your identity. In Buddhism, we call this "the identity habit." In other words, "I'm a WASP," "I'm a male." But how is it that I feel that I'm that? I'm Bob. But where is the real Bob? This is a little complicated, but it's not that complicated or that difficult. How is it that I think I am Bob? Where is Bob? Do I have one of those high school bracelets with Bob written on it?

But we can change our names. For instance, I can be Tenzin, or I can be professor Thurman. And my Mongolian mentor used to call me Alexander, which is one of my middle names. So we learn how we hold our identity, and the key insight is that who we feel we are is something that we have to *maintain*. It is not automatically learned. In developmental psychology— Piaget type—the question would be: When do infants begin to think of themselves as "me" in a certain way? When you work with this, you begin to realize that being Bob is a kind of a job. And then you realize that identity is a work in process and that you don't have to have a certain identity. I'm a western male doctor, and I am stiff and rigid, but I *could be* a new kind of doctor who is connected to the patient and who is very scientific and technical and yet who also has a larger view of interconnection of things.

In other words, there is a meditative process for the erosion of the rigidity of the identity habit. It is also a study process. It is an analytic, critical, philosophical, and meditative process, which goes along with cultivating the positive and strengthening feelings of empathy, compassion, connectedness, and familiarity.

To become aware of just how rigid your identity habit is, you have to develop an ability to split your awareness. Psychosynthesis is a method that does this very effectively. Gurdjieffians also do this. You create what is called the *witness consciousness* or *spy consciousness*. It's like you were spying on yourself. This is not your main consciousness because if you put your main consciousness into watching yourself, into being self-reflective, then you're seeming solid self will disappear immediately because your main self has jumped into another angle. They say the best time to think about this is when you have been falsely accused or when you are feeling righteously indignant about something because that's when you are most assertive that "I am Bob, and I did not do it." The *I* seems to really come from somewhere and land on something.

So you develop this sliver of awareness that observes your solar plexus, throat, chest, how you feel a constriction here, and how you want to assert yourself in a certain way. You observe all the things that the feeling of righteousness mobilizes internally. And you say, "Okay, Buddha might have said that there is no such fixed, absolute, thing as self but I don't agree. On a visual level, I'm Bob. That's really what I am, and don't tell me that I am not." So you really know this clearly.

The second step is a very interesting one. It is self-acknowledgement of our own practical mentality. For instance, when we go shopping, we examine things; then we choose this car or this vacuum cleaner and buy it. We could go on examining these things forever, but we don't. We know that we haven't made a completely exhaustive analysis and that we might be wrong, but we finally decide the odds are with us and we act. That's how we work pragmatically. So when we realize that "I am me" in a very rigid and strong way—we say, "Okay, if I really am me and I make an effort to find myself, I should be able to do that." That's the quest. If I am so real, then I can find myself.

But when I start looking, things get very confusing, very vague, and very strange. I cannot find myself, or I have difficulty, or I feel that I am "just around the corner." Well, there is a limit to that. Finally, I've been around so many corners and I wasn't there that I have to decide at some point that, okay, I'm not there. Which might be against how I am still feeling. But I think: I am going to honor my dualistic, pragmatic, critical, rational mind, which is the mind I live by. So even though I undo my pragmatic mind so I can get it out of the way and be one with the universe, it is still there. So I honor that and I don't get lost in some place of never knowing or some mystic idea that there's a little Bob in a boat up there with a silver cord transmitting things to me. I'm not going to go off the deep end like that. This is considered very important because we are going into deep psychological areas.

The third step is that there are various ways of looking. Once we truly acknowledge how fiercely we hold self as opposed to the world and how pragmatic we are in our basic nature, when we get those two lined up, we start looking. There are many ways—sevenfold, fivefold, twofold. The simplest way might be what's called the *Royal Reason of Relativity or Relationality*.

We recognize from the first step that the feeling we have about the self is that the self is a thing in itself. It isn't related to anything else. It is an absolute, just there. But the way of relationality is: if I experience it, it's relational. So as I'm looking, whatever I feel, I'm relating to, so therefore it's relational. There is no nonrelational thing that relates.

That's an easy syllogism—it's almost a totality. But what that means is that we look and we look, and we look, and we say, "Ah, there I am," and then we keep going and get into a tight little circle where we look for the looking for the looking for the looking. It is hard to do. This is when you need to be a Zen meditator, to really go to the absolute limits of this. You have to be able to concentrate and focus.

If we remember the reason of relationality, we also remember that a discovery of any state about the thing itself will be relational because it will be an experience we will move into. It is *not* going to be like a big bang or a big this or a big that. Sometimes we will come up with a little feeling of fear, like we are dislodging something that we need, and sometimes we come up with a feeling of confusion like we are lost. But if we just keep relating to things, we realize they are not absolute.

Different people will come up with different results to a different extent. But we are talking about medical education, not necessarily about the quest for satori—although I think everybody should have satori. But you don't have to go to a Zen monastery for 20 years. I know a lot of people who go for 20 years and who don't understand this thing about the self. They don't get satori; they just get empty-headed. Meditation without being directed by understanding and study and by a certain focus is like taking a microscope and waving it around the room. You are not going to see anything. You have to have an aim. So this is the key essential aim.

What I am saying, in the context of medical education and compassion, is that the more self-knowledge that occurs, the basic insight ultimately is that what I am, I am responsible for because I am making it all the time.

It's a relational thing. I'm adopting a certain identity. I adopt it to relate to things in a certain way. I have learned a successful way in relating. I mobilize my limbs; I talk, I use the language; I memorize the table of elements and anatomy to pass the exam. I am making that self. It keeps getting made.

Now, if I go and live in the country club with a bunch of greedy people who don't care about anything and are materialistic, I am going to be more materialistic. I will be a bad doctor. If I associate with spiritual people, if I do it a certain way, I am going to become better. If I associate with compassionate thoughts or ideas—I don't have to be religious, I can be humanist—but if I cultivate that I will be more of that. The point is, whatever I am, I am responsible for it. It just didn't happen. It's not given from some place. My parents didn't make me the way I am. School didn't make me the way I am. I've used those things, and they've influenced me, but I am making myself.

The more erosion of the unquestioned absoluteness of the self there is, the more openness to the other. They say that final compassion comes when you have a satori-type of experience. But there is no one satori—the great masters had hundreds of them and then they lost track.

We absolutize everything, but there is no absolute moment when everything is going to be painted purple. That is not the case. It's a gradual process like butter melting in a bowl, like smoothing wrinkles out of a cloth that you're ironing. These are the metaphors of the tradition. Finally, you see through yourself, because you deal with the fact that if I really look, the absolute fades away. If I take my absolute feeling about me and look for myself with myself I won't find anything.

So when you do that, they say there is this experience in which you suddenly feel transparent. That's why they use the term "emptiness." It's like you are like a crystal. You are looking through yourself, and you are also looking backwards through the nerve in the brain that is looking, and everything is transparent. You feel at peace and calm in a vast space. You *are* a vast space. And you don't find anything.

But that is not the final state—it's a temporary moment because you are still being absolute looking for this absolute, and you have to be warned that the state of vast space is not the absolute. It is a metaphor because it is still relational because you entered it. You experienced it and therefore it doesn't get in the way of your new relationalities. It's as if you are looking through a piece of glass that is etched. When you look through it, you see stuff but you do not see the glass. Then you change the focus and see the etching and pattern of the glass.

The metaphor for wisdom is when you are seeing the glass and you see through it and don't see it as anything. You don't see any self. And compassion is when you notice that the glass has this etching and so you see yourself as transparent and at the same time you see all the other beings you're interconnected with. You see a much vaster vision with you and your interconnection with others because you are making a much less powerful bias toward yourself. You're still responsible for yourself and you know that you're operating yourself and not them, but you can also see their point of view almost at the same time as your own. Because you have this transparency. And also they're transparent. You can also see how they could be fine if they were free in their relativity, but then you see them knotted up in a certain way around a delusion about themselves. And then you're seeing them knotted up, and you are feeling their knottedness as if it were your own knottedness. That is true compassion.

But you don't even think you're special. You just feel their pain, and therefore it's like when your hand is hurt. When you burn your hand on a pot, you don't put on the medicine and salve and anesthetic and think, "Ahh, I am so nice to my hand." You do it because you are feeling it.

Medicine as a Spiritual Path

Now here is another tricky but important thing that I want the doctors to know. Because doctors deal with so much human suffering and such extreme situations and see so much death, I think they become highly realistic people. If they are oriented in this better way of not just rigidly being themselves apart from it all, and if they reinforce their natural human empathy rather than deconditioning it in a militaristic manner, they will become immensely wise in a lifetime. A lifetime of medical service to beings is just like a path to enlightenment. I don't think there is any difference. Not if it's exploitative and if you're just trying to make money and be important, but if it is truly a service, I think it is a path of enlightenment. There's no difference between that and being some monk on a mountain. It's perhaps even better than being a monk on a mountain.

So what I am saying is that if they start a little bit of this process, they will strengthen their compassion. And if they do positive things to reinforce it, and if they get this going as a lifelong process, they will recharge. Imagine the energy you get from many people's pain. It's like you have many hands that are hurting you and you are going to move quickly to overcome the hurt.

The last point I want to make is that Buddhism is not a simplistic psychology. Obviously, if you felt everybody's pain on even one ward, you would crumble. You couldn't do anything. If you were a surgeon and you felt the pain of the heart surgery patient, your hand would quiver and you wouldn't be able to make that incision and open up the breast bone. You couldn't do that. In other words, this is my message here: Enlightenment is not a simplified state. Not at all. It is the supreme tolerance of cognitive dissonance. It is a much higher-level tolerance of complexity. So you can have total compassion for that patient and you are going to do anything to save her heart, but you are going to ruthlessly cut in an absolutely expert manner. You're going to be clinically detached to do it, and yet you are going to be totally committed to the outcome. This is wisdom and compassion simultaneous. This is the key.

Part Twelve

Conversations About
Medicine as a Spiritual Path

*"There are potentials of body, mind, and spirit
available to us that far exceed conventional
limits, and there's a growing body of research to
support this."*

—ROGER WALSH

CHAPTER 43

CHRISTIANE NORTHRUP, MD

Medical Practice as a Spiritual Journey

Christiane Northrup, MD, a visionary pioneer in her field, is a board-certified obstetrician/gynecologist (ob/gyn) physician who helps empower women to tune into their inner wisdom and take charge of their health. She graduated from Dartmouth Medical School and completed her residency in ob/gyn at Tufts New England Medical Center Affiliated Hospitals.

But her journey as a medical practitioner did not end with degrees, licenses and a successful ob/gyn practice. Sensing a deep need for change in the way medicine dealt with people in general and women in particular, Dr. Northrup helped found Women to Women, an innovative healthcare center for women. With the same goal in mind, she wrote the best-selling book, *Women's Bodies, Women's Wisdom: Creating Emotional and Physical Health and Healing*. She is also the editor of the monthly newsletter *Health Wisdom for Women* and the host of four successful public television specials. Her newest bestseller, *The Wisdom of Menopause*, was published in March 2001. Northrup's work has been featured on *The Oprah Winfrey Show, Today, NBC Nightly News with Tom Brokaw, The View*, and *Good Morning America*.

In 1995, I traveled to Maine to visit Dr. Northrup at her clinic there, a most comforting space that just happened to be located on Pleasant Street. In the course of our conversation, Dr. Northrup had more to say about this type of synchronistic manifestation.

You know from my writings that I believe in the soul and in the fact that consciousness does affect shared reality. So how do we do the practice as soul work? For instance, we're in the middle of a renaissance within Women to Women. One of our partners left on disability, and at this point we have more debt than we're interested in. But this practice was founded on the vision of "what could be." Our overriding bible is the law of manifestation, which is that you attract to you what you dwell upon. You attract what resonates with your own vibratory rate.

Let's go back a bit. In 1984, we determined that the healthcare system was somehow wrong and that women should be cared for differently. So we decided to start a practice called Women to Women. There was prayer, hope, and tremendous enthusiasm, but the shadow of that enthusiasm was a belief that women had been victimized and that we ourselves had been victimized. That was the energy with which we created Women to Women.

Of course, this sets up the very same cultural expectations that we've been dealing with in the conventional world, which is that women are going to clean up after everything. Within 2 years, we were drowning in our own workaholism, in our own codependence, and in our own "be everything to everyone." We set ourselves up as the rescuers. We were going to rescue women and show them a better way. So what would you attract by the law of manifestation? You'd attract victims who needed rescue.

Many victim types have an internal structure that says, "Help me; you can't." And if you get a patient load of 40% of that kind of person, with that kind of self-defeating belief system, you will have a major energy drain on all levels: spiritual, emotional, financial.

Then 4 years ago, we decided that it was perfectly okay to fire patients who were abusive. Can you imagine? The customer service department at L.L. Bean would go bananas. But we learned that it was okay to suggest to people that this was not the practice for them. We now know that when people come in with the "help me; you can't" energy that we are not going to be able to rescue them, that no one can help them until they shift this energy themselves.

We all need to recognize that if you set yourself up as a rescuer for everything that's ever gone wrong with women, then implicit in that is the belief that somehow the women didn't participate on some level in the kind of life they have. We as a culture need to leave behind that victim mentality now. It is time to stop staying in abusive jobs or abusive relationships because of fear of abandonment. And your body lets you know that staying in an abusive situation isn't such a hot idea.

I believe that the patients we attract are a direct reflection of where we are personally in our lives. I am convinced that the patients we see are teachers for us. After we announced that we wanted women who would be partners in their healthcare, the type of person who came here changed. They are different and more fun than those we saw in 1986.

The Practice

In Maine, you can't have a professional corporation in which people with different licenses are partners. Accountants cannot be partners with lawyers in a professional corporation. In the beginning, we created an elaborate business structure so the nurse practitioners and MDs could be equal entities in the business. But as I said, we're in a transition phase. Now Women to Women, the business corporation, is a central pod, and each of us will have an individuated practice off of it. So we are moving toward more individuality.

But the group is still important. At first we were going to let the whole thing break up, but then we realized what tremendous support we got from each other. This individualized model feels right. We've divided the space into what it costs for the reception area and what it costs to have individual offices and what part of the staff each practitioner is using. Of course everybody will have a slightly different way that they use the staff and space, but we no longer have to be an undifferentiated mass of individual practitioners, which is what women have been trained to do. Women have been trained that anyone with lively energy has to be subservient to the group or else everyone will hate her. But it's okay to have your individuality.

We will continue to have monthly meetings for visioning the central vision for Women to Women. I think what we're about is becoming vessels for the spiritual parts of us to cocreate on earth. We're moving beyond the duality of the idea that to serve, one must be overworked, harried, tired, and poor. We don't need to do that anymore. If we keep participating in that model, then we can't create a morphogenic field, a resonating field, of what abundance and a fulfilled life would look like for a woman. Until now, we've had an either/or model: you can be a great businesswoman or artist, but your family life is a shambles. Or you can have a family, but you lose in business. We're interested in both.

We were just at a legal meeting, and the way lawyers were posturing made me laugh. I had to look at the floor. I thought, "These people go through life thinking that this is the way you do it." The way we go through life here is, we'll begin a meeting by calling in our higher selves or calling in the spiritual guidance that's available to us for the task at hand. For instance, we are having a lot of dialogue on insurance companies at this point. We are clear, as medical insurance consumers, that none of us receives anything close to what I call value for what we're paying for.

Another one of the big issues you hear about is how do you get reimbursed for alternative practice? But I think we shouldn't even bother trying. I would like the public to know that what they are participating in with insurance companies is a gigantic lottery. It's like going to Las Vegas, where the odds on the house games aren't in your favor. The casino will always win. That's how insurance companies are set up.

You don't have to be a healthcare practitioner for very long to see the games that are played. It's part of the victim mentality to think that a company whose job is to make money is actually going to be there for you. Health insurance, to me, is for preventing you from being completely wiped out financially, should you get a major illness. That's what it's for.

Day-to-day care should be our own personal responsibility. If each of us, in our businesses, took the money we were paying in to a premium every month and used it for acupuncture, massage, health foods, and vitamin supplements, then we'd get a return on our dollar. We now have a population that thinks every cold should be covered when they go in to their doctor. What it sets up is a belief that "I don't own my body. They own my body." I tell people what they need to do to get well, and they say to me, "It's not covered." I say, "Well, then I guess you've given your power to the insurance company, haven't you?"

In this particular office, we are now looking at every contract we have with every insurance company and every HMO, and we are deciding which ones are worth our time and which aren't. And we are gradually beginning the process of dropping the ones that are far too much of a hassle to keep.

This disease-care system is the tail wagging the dog. We need to wake up and create health-care systems within businesses to keep people healthy. The way it's set up now is that illness is the only acceptable form of Western meditation. You hate your job, and you have no way to go to bat for yourself, so you get sick. It's what Anne Schaef calls "dying for your benefits."

What Is Health?

Health is a state of balance in which your life is defined by purpose, freedom, growth, and joy. Illness is a sign of imbalance that says, "You're off track a little, make a correction." And sometimes, health requires some major illnesses to occur so that health can happen. In a way, health and disease are a duality, like life and death.

The people who are the healthiest, in my experience, are the ones who, if they died tomorrow, could say, "I lived a full life. I accomplished what I wanted to accomplish." Niro Assistent is a woman who had AIDS, but she wasn't afraid of death. She said there was a woman inside her, and she wanted to be sure that that woman lived before she died. So she brought her out. That's what health is. It is about living your life in such a way that it is an expression of your individuality and who you really are. Then you've got health.

I'm certain that there are seventh-chakra contracts that people have made about illness, where the illness is absolutely necessary for them to complete their life purpose. Think about Stephen Hawking with amyotrophic lateral sclerosis (ALS). As Elisabeth Kübler-Ross used to say, "When the physical quadrant closes down early, then the spiritual quadrant, the emotional quadrant, the mental quadrant, often take over and expand in ways that they never would have if the physical quadrant were functioning fully."

So we never want to make a judgment about what the disease is. But I do believe that our lives are enriched enormously if we can say, "What is the purpose that my cold, or my headache, serves?" I don't think we were meant by any universal intelligence that created this earth to have 50% of the people who are over age 80 have Alzheimer's disease. Or for 60% of women to suffer from menstrual cramps. That doesn't make any sense at all. So when that's happening, we have to look at the whole culture and ask why that is.

Our culture, our society, actually creates certain diseases. I think it's absolutely that simple. They're holographic diseases. In a hologram, any little, tiny part looks like the whole. So I think about breast cancer, and I think of all the potential causes of breast cancer. We have excess fat in the diet, too much estrogen, not enough progesterone, possibly DDT, PCBs, environmental toxins, artificial light. And then the emotional/psychological aspect of breast cancer, which is the mother archetype gone sour, which is "give, give, give, give, give," without any receiving. The breast cancer archetype is keeping a brave face in front of the world, while inside, you're furious or sad. Now, all those things are related to nurturing. There isn't any way that a culture has a right relationship with nurturing and giving and receiving when we're putting toxins into the environment. Our relationship with Mother Earth is out of whack, and it's reflected in individual women's bodies.

Each of us has to take complete responsibility for how we live our lives. We also have to get out of our self-centeredness, that we've created it all with our egos. I believe we've created it all with this higher part of our selves. But the ego, the part of us that's feeling the pain of an illness, is not the part that created it. The part that created it is our eternal soul, and it knows we're okay—that even if we die, we're always okay.

New Assumptions about the Nature of Reality

The number-one assumption we hold that is completely different is that we don't heal the patient. The patient heals herself. And I'm telling you, that's a new assumption.

Number two, we're not responsible for the patient. We are sharing responsibility. We bring our knowledge to the situation, and she brings her knowledge to the situation, and both of these are crucial to the outcome of the healing. The old paradigm is—and I've had this happen—I ask a woman to tell me what's going on, and she says, "You tell me. You're the doctor." As though she has nothing to offer.

Women in the old paradigm are led to believe that the fibroid popped out of the closet and landed on their uterus, that the abnormal Pap smear happened because their luck was bad, and that they didn't bring anything to the equation, that it just happened. It's the most disempowering paradigm you can imagine.

We stay out of the new one because we've been shamed and blamed since childhood, and we don't feel like we're a living, breathing part of the universe. So when you bring up cocreation, people have to move through their own shame and self-centeredness.

The third assumption is that people can heal. It's always possible to heal. There's always hope. So those are our working assumptions.

Let me give you a concrete example of how to empower patients. This has to do with sending out cards every year that say, "It's time for your annual Pap smear." We decided that it is not in our vision to be the Pap smear monitors of our patients. We don't own their cervixes, they own their cervixes. But the medical profession is set up very parent-child.

Now, when someone comes in for an annual, we say, "In keeping with our vision of empowering women on every level, we will assume that you can take responsibility for making your annual visit at the time when you're due for your annual visit, and we will not be sending out a reminder card."

The truth is we have patients who are furious with us if we don't call and remind them about their appointments. But isn't that parent-child? So we say, "In concert with our vision, we believe that you are able to take responsibility for your cervix, for your breasts, for your body, and we know you will call when it's time." So, that's an example of where we're headed, although we are not completely there yet.

I am currently working on an article about tamoxifen. It's the antiestrogen drug for women who have estrogen-receptor-positive breast cancer. There are side effects from the drug, depression and that kind of thing. The conventional medical opinion, after 20 years, is that tamoxifen decreases recurrence rates in breast tumors that are positive for estrogen receptors. So that's what "Dad" says to do. Often a woman will say that she wants to get off the drug, and she wants my permission. If I say, "My opinion is that you should get off it," and Dad says, "Don't get off it," then what is she doing? She's going to play Mom against Dad. And then if she gets a recurrence, she gets to blame somebody. That's the way the game works.

So if I have a patient who wants to go off tamoxifen, she has to absolutely say, "I don't want to be on this drug. I don't like the way I feel, and I believe that my body is healed enough that I don't need it, but I know there are no guarantees, and I am making this decision." This is what Carolyn Myss calls "the initiation of the fourth chakra." There are no guarantees.

We used to think there were guarantees. If you clean your plate, you'll grow up to be big and healthy. If you get straight As, you will get into Harvard. Except now, in our culture, all bets are off. There aren't any guarantees. In my experience, when you're in the old mode of guarantees, there is not a lot of hope for true help. You're like a piece of seaweed in the ocean. You just flow, depending on what the tides and the wind are doing. And the wind is whatever the collective culture is telling you to do or think.

Carolyn Myss says that a lawyer's job is to serve the illusion of their clients' egos that it is possible to control every variable. Now think about this. A lawyer's job is to buy into the illusion that it is possible to make outcomes certain for their clients. That is how they work. And in that legal belief system, your spirit won't come in and participate, because it's totally an ego game. It's serving the illusion that the ego is in control.

See, it's, "I'll get even." It's the vendetta. It's an eye for an eye, a tooth for a tooth. When you move into forgiveness, and when you understand it, it doesn't mean that what happened to you in the past was okay. It just means that you're not going to let it bog you down in the present. When you call your soul back to the present, you're operating in a different system. But there's no healing in the legal system.

Now, I am not a neophyte to lawsuits. I have been in the legal arena over and over. And what always heals it for me is when I make a shift inside, where I say that I could leave my practice. I could leave medicine. If my higher power is asking me to leave medicine through this lawsuit, I'm going. It's okay. And when I get to that place where I don't care and can let it go and I'm free, the lawsuits have all gone away. I've never had to go to court.

You can tell the doctors reading this that 80% of ob/gyns have had two lawsuits. I have had more than that. So I'm not a Pollyanna who's saying, "Let's live in the light." Because when you only think you're supposed to live in the light, it means you're terrified of the dark. I am not terrified of the dark. I have been there.

Consciousness Creates the Body

What I was saying when I wrote in my book that "consciousness creates the body" is that quantum mechanics and everything we know about physics says that matter and energy are interconvertible. So I believe that this earth and our bodies are a manifestation of divine mind and that each of us has our own little piece of divine mind that operates within us. I did not talk about this in the book because I consciously wanted a text that would be useful to people in any number of belief systems. But what I really believe is we didn't start as babies. We're infinite souls. Then, once you are in the body, your connection with your divine guidance recreates the cells.

Look at Deepak Chopra's work and how eloquently he speaks about the fact that our liver is regenerated every 30 days. He's seeding the world with these pushing-the-envelope ideas. It's wonderful. So we get this body initially, and the body is created by our own DNA and our mother's environmental interaction, and all of that. But then, as Deepak says, our biologic systems—all biologic systems—have a central nervous system that, despite the fact that it is bombarded with billions of stimuli daily about what is the truth or what is real, only processes those pieces of data that reinforce what we already believe. The belief system we have literally pulls to us the events, foods, and atoms that then become our bodies. And our bodies are constantly being replaced, so we could heal anything if we could pop out of that collective jar that we're all in that says, "This is possible, but this isn't."

On a practical level, I have occasional patients who will not go to a support group for breast cancer. They will say—and they're on to something—"I do not want to participate in the morphogenic field of this disease." Now, if they're doing it from denial, it's a bad thing. But if they're doing it because they are moving on with their lives and are not going to let this diagnosis interfere with their lives, it's a very good thing. But only the person herself can decide that.

I have a friend in Denver who had to go through chemotherapy for a cancer, and the doctor said, "You'll lose your hair." He said, "Not a chance. I'm not losing my hair." And he never lost his hair.

I think these types of miracles are an everyday occurrence. But our culture doesn't believe. In the old days, you went to the priest and paid money for salvation. Now you go to the doctor and pay money for salvation. But what if people understood that they had their own connection to the divine and they didn't need an intermediary that they paid, be it an insurance company, a doctor, or a priest? What if they realized that you gathered together in community because we're community creatures, not because you can buy salvation. Look at the way the church used to operate in the Middle Ages. It seems to me that medicine is operating the same way now. You pay this healthcare premium, and you'll be saved. But it's not working.

You asked me what I believe about shamans and faith healers, these people who can perform miracles on others, and how that fits with people taking responsibility for their own heath. Well, I did a lot of research on Philippine psychic surgeons. I watched this healer, and his hands went right into the body. It's true. They operate in the realm where energy and matter are interconvertible, so of course you can put your hands in a body. Two of my colleagues went to a psychic surgeon. One got rid of her menstrual cramps. They have never come back, and she has documented endometriosis. Both said it was much easier to believe before they went than after. They said they could feel the guy's hands inside their bellies and that that was very hard on their belief systems.

But what I have since found out about the Philippine psychic surgeons is they may, in the moment, be severing the energetic ties of that disease with your body. So they'll say to you, "The tumor is gone." And in the moment, I believe that is true. But if the emotional/psychological patterns that created it are not interrupted, it will just come back.

Of course, some things are in the realm of the miraculous. Some people don't change their belief system or do anything, and they're healed. And now we're back in mystery. In Newtonian physics, which is our culture, we believe in cause and effect, that something always has to have a cause and it always has to have an effect. Sometimes, I don't think it does. It's just a mystery. There are reasons, and we don't know what they are.

One type of healing I'm very interested in at this point is shamanic soul-retrieval work. That makes a lot of sense to me. Past life therapy also makes sense.

I had classical migraines from when I was 12 until my sophomore year in college. The migraines went away on the night that I decided to throw myself in front of a car rather than do a critique of a poem by Keats for my English professor. I hated the library. I hated critiquing poetry, and I didn't know what "Ode to a Grecian Urn" was supposed to represent. It was a snowy night in Cleveland, and for a fleeting second, I thought, "I'm going to throw myself in front of a car." Then I thought, "Except I'll break my leg and I'll be wandering around with a cast, and I'll just have to do the poem and haul around the cast." So I called my parents and said, "I hate it here. I want to come home." My father said, "Good. Come home." Then I got it. I had the choice.

Something fundamental happened in my soma-psyche. I didn't get migraine headaches after that. Now, I've had one or two since. Each time they have been associated with an intellectual overdrive, where I'm pushing myself mercilessly and ignoring my body completely. But I stopped that pattern, in general, in my sophomore year of college. The reason the migraines left is that I began to perceive the world in a different, lighter way.

When I got to medical school, I met people who were so bright that they could look at a page and they had it. They didn't have to study. For the first time in my life, I was in the middle of the group, and no amount of overdrive would put me at the top of the class. The innate gifts and talents for intellectual material of these people were so far above anything I was born with that I said, "Relax." So I was in the middle of my class in medical school, and I learned that this could work. I see med students coming up to me sometimes who look battered, and I realize that their job is to just get through the training and lighten up. Don't take it so seriously.

Dartmouth, my alma mater, is making an effort to humanize things, but most mentors—certainly surgical mentors—have a battlefield mentality. And if you're ever in an intensive care unit or in general surgery, believe me, a battlefield mentality helps you get through your day. But I had to get out of that because I was tired of the incoming wounded. I began to wonder, "why do we have all these incoming wounded? Could we be doing something different so that people aren't caught in the crossfire?" And that was my soul's purpose.

I could do incoming wounded really well. I was a good guy. I could participate, and I liked my colleagues. But this is my next step. I have a quote I use in lectures: "Masculinity expresses the idea that there are things worth dying for. Femininity expresses the idea that there are things worth living for." Now, I think all of us—men and women both—need to figure out what in our lives is worth living for. Usually, we don't even ask that question until someone is sick.

My Own Healthcare

I don't consume much conventional healthcare. I think that a lot of doctors would tell you that they don't think they're getting real value from it. You know, if someone were to say to me, "We're going to get some routine blood work on you," I'd ask why.

Most of the people I see have family doctors or gynecologists whom they see for routine care, and they see me in consultation. I'm bridging for them. What I want people to get is that they don't need a lot of conventional care. My mother comes up here once every 4 years. She's 69. She doesn't want any more than that. We're led to believe that you need all these tests and all this disease screening to stay healthy. But any time you order routine blood work, there will be one or two things that are abnormal. Always! It's part of the law of averages. Then people fixate around that. Sometimes I wonder if I should get cholesterol levels on people because then they begin to focus only on what's wrong. And by the law of manifestation, that expands.

Andrew Weil said it best: "It is one of the most destructive powers of modern medicine to undermine people's belief about how they are." And it's true. They go in feeling great and they come out with a disease.

By the way, to get anything covered by your insurance, you do need a disease. But once you get a disease on your record in the giant computer in the sky, try getting it off! Then you can't get insurance. Preexisting condition. They have you coming and going!

So to all the practitioners out there, I would say, "There are other models." If you regard your work with patients and your work on yourself as the same, then to have their souls touched, people will come from a long way away. We have patients from all over the United States. They don't need to come very often, and they say, "If I'm going to have my body touched and examined, then it's going to be a sacred experience."

A woman named Peggy Huddleston just finished a book called *How to Prepare for Surgery: Mind/Body Techniques to Enhance the Healing Process*. It's a fabulous book about how to access your inner wisdom and ask that your surgeon and your anesthesiologist do the same during your surgery. That's what I want to see—where enough of us have the courage to live our light in the middle of grand rounds, in the operating room, in the radiology department, or in the offices that we create.

The answers will always come from your own inner process. You will draw the circumstances to you that you need.

CHAPTER 44

ROGER WALSH, MD, PHD

The Heart of Healing: Essential Spirituality for Healing Professionals

Roger Walsh, MD, PhD, was born in Brisbane, Australia and graduated from the University of Queensland with degrees in psychology, physiology, neuroscience, and medicine. He then went to Stanford University, Palo Alto, California, on a Fulbright scholarship; trained in psychiatry; and passed licensing exams in medicine, psychology, and psychiatry. His research has focused on topics such as meditation, Asian psychologies and philosophies, the nature of psychological health and well-being, transpersonal psychology, spirituality, contemplative disciplines, and the psychological roots of our contemporary global crises.

Dr. Walsh is currently professor of psychiatry, philosophy, and anthropology at the University of California-Irvine. His recent publications include *Paths Beyond Ego: The Transpersonal Vision*, *The Spirit of Shamanism*, and *Essential Spirituality: The Seven Central Practices*, with a foreword by His Holiness the Dalai Lama.

I interviewed Dr. Walsh in 2001 in his offices at the University of California-Irvine, in Irvine, California.

It's curious, but I'm the last person I would have ever expected to be doing this kind of work. From early adolescence, science was my god, and the only question was "What kind of scientist am I going to be?" My first love was astronomy, but in medical school I became a hardcore neuroscientist and assumed I would do that kind of work for the rest of my life. But California has a way of changing things; psychiatry has a way of changing things; and being in therapy has a way of changing things—or at least they all did for me. I went to medical school in Australia, then came to the United States for a psychiatry residency at Stanford. And promptly I found myself in a completely different world. People were talking about accessing the unconscious, getting in touch with emotions, and so forth. It was just nuts to me. Yet I began to appreciate that some of these people seemed to have a sensitivity and wisdom that I was missing.

Since I was doing therapy on people, I felt I had a moral obligation to try it for myself. I started working with a humanistic-existential therapist named Jim Bugental. It was the most transformative experience of my life. Perhaps the most crucial change was that I became aware of my internal subjective experiences. Eventually, this unveiled the inner world of emotions, images, intuitions, and thoughts that I had been oblivious to. I'd been absolutely out of contact with myself. I felt that I had spent my entire life living on just the top 6 inches of a wave on top of an ocean that I hadn't known existed. It blew me away that there was an inner universe as vast and mysterious as the outer universe and that I could have spent my entire life unaware of it.

I started exploring everything the human potential movement had to offer. You name it— I went through it. There was a lot of nonsense, but there were also things of value. Gradually I found myself gravitating toward religious practices like meditation and yoga, even though at the time I thought religion was the opiate of the masses.

436

I was puzzled—why did these practices seem to be helpful if religion was just a relic of primitive culture? Then there was a moment that changed my life. I was walking toward the bathroom to wash up for dinner, and as I opened the door it suddenly hit me. At the contemplative core of the great religions lie techniques for developing and road maps for describing the same kind of understandings and states of mind realized by the founders, saints, and sages. The great religions contain state-specific psychologies, philosophies, and technologies. At their best, they can offer disciplines for producing and understanding higher states of mind and stages of development. That recognition was a life-changing moment.

I then dove into various meditative and contemplative practices, and it became clear that these are powerful and profound techniques. Associated with them are sophisticated maps of multiple states of consciousness and stages of psychological development beyond those Western psychology has recognized, at least until transpersonal psychology began to include them.

I have spent much of the last 25 years trying to do these practices on the one hand, and on the other trying to make intellectual sense of them. I have been trying to create bridges between contemplative wisdom and contemporary knowledge. I guess I've been called to become what Carl Jung called a *gnostic intermediary*. He initially used that term about Wilhelm, the translator of the *I-Ching*. Jung said a gnostic intermediary is someone who imbibes a wisdom tradition and then transmits it into the language and concepts of another culture.

What is required of a gnostic intermediary is a threefold process. First, you have to begin to imbibe the wisdom. Second, you have to learn the language and conceptual system of the people to whom you are trying to communicate. Third, you have to translate in a way that creates an "Aha!" experience, so that it makes sense to people. I think that's what a lot of us who have explored contemplative traditions have been trying to do.

Contemplative Wisdom

Integrating contemplative wisdom into our culture is, of course, an ongoing perennial challenge. Of course there are strong forces within us and around us—the media being a relatively recent one—that hinder this. In the intellectual arena, transpersonal psychology was the first contemporary discipline to incorporate a multistage worldview and the understanding that there are stages of development beyond the conventional. It also recognized that the conventional level of psychological development—what we have called *normality* and taken to be the ceiling of human possibilities—is really a stage of collective developmental arrest. The implications of this recognition are extraordinary: we are half-grown and half-awake, and a remarkable array of psychological potentials and capacities await us as our human birthright. But to experience them we have to take up practices that develop them and us. And that's what authentic spiritual practices—properly applied—can do.

With these novel perspectives, we can now recognize that disciplines such as, for example, Buddhist Abhidhamma psychology, Vedantic philosophy, and Christian mysticism are multistate disciplines that aim for and describe transpersonal stages. But they use outdated languages and conceptual systems wedded to ancient mythologies that no longer work for many of us today. It's not the first time that these concepts have migrated to new cultures, and there's always been the challenge of translating across cultures. But translating across centuries from a mythic agrarian to a postmodern worldview is an entirely novel challenge.

So in writing *Essential Spirituality* I was trying to do several things: one was to make sense of and legitimize spiritual practice. A second was to show that practice is what's really crucial. Many books offer nice stories about spirituality and help you feel good but don't offer truly transformative practices. In Ken Wilber's language, these books are more about translation than transformation—that is, they satisfy people at their current developmental stage rather than offer them tools that will help move them beyond that stage.

States of Development

It's becoming increasingly clear that there are developmental stages available to all of us beyond the conventional level. What we think of as the ceiling of development—whether it's moral or cognitive development or motivation or any number of dimensions of capacities—is not the ceiling. In fact, current mainstream research shows that there are postconventional transpersonal stages. Contemplative traditions, in my understanding, are designed to take people from conventional to postconventional stages.

For example, contemplative practices aim at fostering emotional development to transpersonal levels in two general ways. First, they offer ways of transforming and reducing difficult and damaging emotions such as anger, jealousy, and fear. Second, they offer techniques for cultivating beneficial emotions such as love, compassion, and joy. Moreover, contemplative techniques aim to expand the scope of our positive emotions so they are not just limited to one person, but encompass many people and eventually all life.

A second dimension of growth and development centers on motivation. In traditional language this was referred to as *purifying motivation*. We can now think of it as, in part, moving up Maslow's hierarchy of needs. Authentic spiritual traditions have practices to reduce compulsive egocentric motives such as greed and aversion and to foster beneficent motives such as generosity and service. Recently, psychologist C. Daniel Batson, among others, has built a strong case that there really is an independent motive for altruism. This is vitally important in painting a more optimistic picture of human nature and potential. Yet Western psychologists lament that we don't have any way of cultivating and increasing altruism. But if you turn to, say, Christian contemplation or Tibetan Buddhism, you find literally dozens of practices for the generation of altruism and compassion. So there are two worlds—Western psychology and contemplative practices—ripe for integration.

Of course, such practices are crucial for healers. People enter medical school or other healing professions with altruistic motives, yet studies show that empathy can be reduced by doctoral training programs. This is tragic. But meditation has been found to increase empathy. And empathy, as Carl Rogers discovered, is one of the characteristics of good therapists and healers. So within the ancient traditions, we have techniques for fostering the altruism and compassion that are so crucial to healing professionals.

So far, I've been talking very generally about the full range of meditations, which are practices that train awareness and attention to foster psychological and spiritual well-being and development. It's useful to recognize that there are spiritual practices for general development and also specific practices for the cultivation of particular mental qualities and capacities. So one might think of practices like yogic breath or mantra meditation, Taoist yoga, or Buddhist awareness as general enhancers of well-being and maturation. But there are also a host of very specific practices for the cultivation of, say, love and compassion. These include specific Jewish, Christian, and Sufi contemplations, as well as Buddhist loving kindness meditation and Bhakti Yoga. Another specific capacity, with corresponding practices to elicit it, are the Sufi, yogic, and Tibetan Buddhist practices for lucid dreaming.

Lucid Dreaming

Let me repeat a story the Dalai Lama told a group of transpersonal psychologists about Tibetan dream yoga. The Dalai Lama said that first, they teach yogis to be aware while they're dreaming.

That's done by practicing mindfulness throughout the day, by creating a very strong intention before falling asleep, by holding a visualization in the mind as you fall asleep, and by sleeping in particular postures. Once practitioners recognize they're dreaming—i.e., become lucid—they undertake specific exercises within the dream. For example, they practice changing their dream bodies, perhaps seeing themselves as enlightened teachers, and thereby gain a sense of the power and potentials of consciousness. Another traditional practice is to meet the Buddha in your dream and listen to him teach. Actually, there is a whole tradition in Tibetan Buddhism of receiving wisdom through dreams.

According to the Dalai Lama, once yogis have mastered awareness in dreams, they next learn to be aware in nondream sleep between dreams. So now they maintain continuous awareness throughout the night. They watch themselves fall asleep; they watch themselves beginning to dream; they watch the dream end; and they watch themselves wake up. Basically they are continuously aware 24 hours a day. Then the Dalai Lama said—and by this stage I realized I was totally out of my league—that once yogis are able to maintain this continuity of awareness, they are taught to recognize that the waking state is also a dream. So now they're continuously aware 24 hours a day, without breaking consciousness, and they're aware that it's all a reflection of mind.

This still is not unique to Tibetan Buddhists. Some advanced Sufis, Christian contemplatives, Hindu yogis, and Transcendental Meditation (TM) practitioners also claim to be able to develop lucid dreaming and continuous awareness. TM calls this continuous awareness *cosmic consciousness*, while Hindu Vedanta calls it *Turya*, meaning "the fourth"—a fourth state of consciousness distinct from and transcendent to the usual three states of waking, dreaming, and nondream sleep.

A recent electroencephalographic (EEG) study of a group of TM practitioners who claimed to have this continuous awareness was absolutely fascinating. It showed a unique EEG pattern in which the fast rhythm of waking activity was superimposed on the slow waves of deep sleep. So we now have laboratory confirmation of this millennia-old claim for a capacity that psychologists had totally dismissed.

The Practice of Cultivating Love

In all the great contemplative disciplines, the cultivation of love is a crucial part of spiritual practice. As such, it both depends on and contributes to a full spiritual practice. The deepest love will therefore only flower to the extent one has developed other spiritual qualities.

There are a variety of techniques for this. In Buddhism, a classic one is the practice of the cultivation of loving kindness. One begins by the recitation of a phrase such as: "May you be happy, joyous, loving, and peaceful," or something similar. If you are doing this loving-kindness meditation as part of your daily meditation, you might spend 20 minutes focusing on a particular person. If you are doing it full time in retreat, then you repeat the phrase from the moment you wake up until the moment you fall asleep, whether you're walking or sitting, eating, or showering.

Not surprisingly, sooner or later a couple of things start to happen. One is that you may start to feel happy, joyous, loving, and peaceful. Second, the bestiary of barriers in the way of feeling happy, joyous, loving, and peaceful begin to arise from the unconscious. For example, anger and fear, jealousy, and greed start to surface. What do you do then? You simply continue the practice and allow these conflicting emotions to boil off. When the feelings of happiness and love are relatively strong and continuous, then you move from focusing on your self to focusing on a benefactor and generate these same feelings toward that person. Then in turn you do the same toward a friend, a neutral person, and an enemy. When you start on an enemy, usually a lot of anger comes up. You don't fight or resist the anger in any way; you just keep the practice going, the anger dissipates by itself, and gradually warm feelings toward your enemy begin. Then you move to larger and larger groups of people until eventually you include all conscious life and are saying, "May all beings be happy, joyous, loving, and peaceful." When these practices are done in retreat continuously for days at a time, the effects can be remarkably powerful.

What you're doing is essentially the opposite of what Western psychologists do with systematic desensitization. There you take a trauma, fear, or phobia, then use an emotion or physiological state that is incompatible with it, such as relaxation, to counteract it. The Buddhists get people to visualize and repeat phrases consistent with love, calmness, and happiness while in situations that once would have evoked anger, jealousy, and fear. So it's the same counter-conditioning process, but instead of trying to reduce difficult emotions, you're cultivating positive emotions. This is the practice for cultivating love.

There are also similar practices for cultivating other helpful emotions, such as compassion and sympathetic joy, which is feeling joy at other people's joy. The Buddhists offer detailed technology, a very precise and carefully laid out program for fostering positive emotions, and clearly it's possible to develop these emotions beyond what we think of as "normal."

Compassion and the Healthcare Practitioner

How do these practices help those of us who are healthcare practitioners? In a variety of ways, first perhaps by shifting motivation. For example, since these practices have become important to me, I now take time before doing a therapy session to cultivate some of these feelings and motives. So instead of just jumping into my chair and saying, "What do you want to talk about today?" I try for just a few minutes beforehand to cultivate feelings of care and compassion and of really wanting to be of service. So the motivational stance is different.

Another benefit I've noticed is that, although I'm clearly a student of these things, not a master, I seem to be calmer and more sensitive than I used to be, so my capacity for noticing and empathizing with someone else's feelings is improved. Then there's a deeper understanding of the mind that comes from meditation. These days I find myself feeling that an awful lot of the problems that people come up with I've run into myself, not only in life, but also in meditation practice.

So if someone comes in feeling depressed and angry, I've certainly also spent time in life being depressed and angry. But more valuable, I've also spent time in retreat exploring those emotions and learning some way to work with them. I find that my own experience in working with mental states is enormously valuable in helping other people work with theirs.

It's also rewarding to be able to do one's work as spiritual practice. I try to do my work as karma yoga, as awakening service. My hope, imperfect as I may be at it, is that my work will be of benefit to people. And this is the first part of karma yoga: to dedicate one's work and service in the world to a higher good. The second element is to work as impeccably as one can toward that goal.

The third element is to let go of attachment to how the work turns out. There's the paradox: you work as fully and impeccably and helpfully as you can while simultaneously trying—I emphasize trying—to let go of your attachment to the results. As the *Bhagavad Gita*, the classic karma yoga text says, "To the work you are entitled, but not to the fruits thereof." So this means attempting to let go of obsessing about egocentric goals such as looking good, and what people think of you, and all of that. And here's where it gets really hard for healers: it even means working to relinquish the attachment to your clients getting better. This sounds paradoxical. Yet we can only help people to the extent we don't need anything from them.

Karma yoga—awakening service—is a wonderful practice for those of us who are busy with work and responsibilities in the world, because it doesn't require renouncing those activities; rather, it reframes and refines them and us.

The Path to Here

I was raised in Christianity, then went through my scientismic agnostic phase in late adolescence and early adulthood. After discovering meditation, I did my journey to the East and studied Buddhism and yoga. When I came back, I delved into some of the Sufi and Jewish practices and also studied shamanism and Christian contemplation.

One thing that drove my study of shamanism was that I just couldn't understand it. Even after I'd seen some common threads in the different great traditions, shamanism remained an enigma. Then I was reading Mircea Eliade's classic book *Shamanism*, and I suddenly realized that a central practice of shamanism was the "journey," or the out-of-body experience.

I came to think of shamanism as the earliest tradition of systematic spiritual practitioners. They were the first people to create a systematic technology of altered states. In *The Spirit of Shamanism*, I define shamanism as a tradition marked by six key characteristics: (1) shamans systematically alter their consciousness to (2) undertake a journey (3) during which they experience themselves or their spirit going to other realms (4) in which they are able to meet beings (5) from whom they gain knowledge or power (6) to bring back for the benefit of the tribe.

That finally helped make sense of shamanism for me. Of course, as part of my learning process I wanted to taste these experiences for myself. One of the great benefits of shamanism is that most people can fairly easily and quickly learn a number of shamanic techniques. This contrasts with some other traditions where it may take quite some time for people to gain a sense of mastery. So there's an ease that makes shamanism relatively accessible. Of course, there is major debate over the use of shamanic techniques as weekend workshop experiences as opposed to part of a lifelong tribal role.

One question that is frequently raised is: Does the practice of shamanism elicit the same transpersonal states that meditative practices do? But what is really being asked by this question is: Do all roads lead up to the same mountain and to the same heights? And I think the answer is no, not necessarily. Different roads can lead "upward" in the sense of fostering transpersonal development, but they may do so in different ways and with different degrees of effectiveness. Some may move people through further stages than others or with greater speed and effectiveness. And different practices may also induce quite different experiences along the way.

The Power of Images

For example, even though shamans, yogis, Christian contemplatives, Jewish cabbalists, and Tibetan Buddhists may all experience and explore archetypal imagery, it's going to be very different imagery for the different practitioners. For shamans, it's likely to be power animals; for the yogi, it may be an image of Shiva; and for the Christian contemplative, it may be angelic forms or a vision of Christ. So those are very different experiences even though the underlying deep structure in all of the experiences is an archetypal image.

Of course, images are "polyvalent" meaning that they can carry many meanings. Speaking psychologically, images can express different beliefs and experiences and come from different levels of the psyche. Speaking religiously or spiritually, images can express different experiences and levels of spiritual realization. But what's crucial spiritually is, as Joseph Campbell put it so exquisitely, that images should be "transparent to the transcendent."

For example, consider an image of the Hindu deity Shiva. At one function and level of the psyche, the image might either spontaneously or intentionally evoke feelings of gratitude and devotion or, recalling Shiva's mythic role as a warrior, feelings of strength and courage. At another level—on the borderline between the mythic and cosmological—the Shiva image might recall the "dance of Shiva": the continuous change and destruction of all forms. Beyond that, Shiva might recall the infinite *sat-chit-ananda* (boundless Being, consciousness, and bliss) from which all forms arise. Finally, there might be the recognition that the inner image of Shiva—and all he symbolizes—is none other than your own true nature, which awaits only your recognition and remembrance. *Shiva soham,* "I am Shiva," has been the mantra of countless yogis across the centuries and *Tat tvam asi,* "I am that too," is what the Upanishads so famously proclaimed.

Of course, not all images are archetypal. Most are idiosyncratic and unique to the person having them. But even these can convey valuable information. For example, images can arise that exquisitely symbolize one's subconscious or unconscious states of mind, beliefs, and feelings. These are called autosymbolic images.

In a classic example, a person in therapy who's out of touch with his or her feelings—a so-called dyslexithymic—says to the therapist, "No, I'm not angry with you, but I am having this image of cutting you up with a knife." It doesn't take 5 years of psychiatric training to figure that one out. So images can be very informative about one's own mental state. For psychologists, and for Jungians especially, the unconscious can communicate with the conscious mind through deeply symbolic and potentially healing imagery.

For contemplatives—and for Sufis and Tibetan Buddhists especially—the depths of the unconscious and its images can be informed by the spiritual and the sacred. "If there is a prophet among you, I the Lord, make Myself known to him. I speak with him in a dream," claims the Jewish Torah.

The Seven Central Practices to Awaken Heart and Mind

One of the unique features of our era is that this is the first time in human history that we have had access to all the world's religious and spiritual traditions. Like a growing number of people, I've been exploring these traditions and have been struck by the fact that, at their contemplative core, they contain a number of common understandings—the so-called perennial philosophy— and a number of common practices—what we might call the perennial practices. There seem to be seven practices that are widely regarded as central and essential. I outlined these in *Essential Spirituality: The Seven Central Practices to Awaken Heart and Mind.* The first three were given to me by Ram Dass, who said in one of his talks that all traditions emphasize three practices: ethics, concentration, and wisdom. That had a powerful impact on me. I can still remember the exact moment I heard him say that, and it hit me that there are common denominators across traditions. Gradually, I became aware that there are other practices within authentic traditions that seem to be universal as well. Here, I'm using authentic in Ken Wilber's sense, meaning that a tradition is authentic to the extent to which it aims to move people up through various transpersonal stages. These other four practices are redirecting motivation, transforming emotions, refining perception, and cultivating service to others.

First, it became apparent that shifting motivation is crucial. In fact, all the great traditions emphasize the importance of redirecting our motives. At the most general level they aim for what traditionally was called *purification,* which in our contemporary psychological language overlaps with movement up Maslow's hierarchy of needs. More specifically, they aim to reduce egocentric compulsivity and to strengthen self-transcendence and altruism.

Next, I began to appreciate that all authentic traditions emphasize—and often have sophisticated disciplines for—transforming emotions. The transformations they aim for are of three general kinds. They are first, reducing painful, destructive emotions such as anger, fear, and jealousy; second, enhancing positive emotions such as love, compassion, and joy. Some traditions also emphasize the importance of developing equanimity, which the stoics called *apathiea* and which has been tragically mistranslated as apathy. By contrast, Western therapy has some excellent techniques for reducing negative emotions but virtually nothing for directly cultivating positive emotions or equanimity. There is an obvious integration of contemplative and therapeutic perspectives crying out to be done here, and hopefully transpersonal psychologists and others will work on this.

Developing concentration is also a crucial practice. Our minds are unbelievably out of control. William James said that the longest any of us can attend to an unchanging stimulus is 3 seconds, and Western psychologists accepted that for a century. We said that attention cannot be sustained.

On the other hand, the contemplative traditions say that not only can attention be sustained but that it has to be sustained if you want to live a full spiritual life. So whereas Western psychology threw up its hands at the problem, the contemplative traditions solved it. They solved it with a variety of meditative practices for training, taming, and sustaining attention, thereby creating a laserlike awareness with the enormous focus, penetrating power, and clarity that a concentrated mind gives. This enables one to penetrate into the depths of the mind and to recognize and transform deeper structures, presuppositions, and problems.

Developing concentration facilitates the next practice, which is the training of awareness, which has two aspects. The first is refining awareness so that we see more accurately, clearly, and sensitively. Interestingly, there are now several studies showing that meditators have greater perceptual sensitivity and processing speed.

The second component of awareness training is recognizing the sacred. It's a shift in the kind of lens through which we see the world—for example, seeing the world less through eyes darkened by fear and anger and more through eyes lit by love and compassion. Of course, the more we see others with love, the more we're likely to see the sacred in them. Also, the deeper we go into ourselves, the more we are able to recognize the sacred in ourselves and others.

The result is a transformation of perception. The general direction of the transformation is a movement from paranoia to pronoia to transnoia. In paranoia we look out at the world through lenses of fear and anger, and—not surprisingly—we see an angry, threatening world. With pronoia we look out through the lens of love and kindness and see people wanting and willing to help us. With transnoia, our perception is tinged by the transcendent. Transnoia is spiritual vision in which the world seems like a sacred setting and a schoolhouse that is all part of the divine plan for our awakening.

Yet if I could choose only one of the seven central practices to get out into the culture, I think it would be ethics. But it would be a different understanding of ethics from the current under-standing. The conventional religious understanding is—to parody it somewhat—"be good or God will get you." The contemplative traditions, on the other hand, have a much more profound understanding of ethics, based on a sophisticated understanding of the way the mind works.

We can think of unethical intentions as those in which we act in ways designed to harm anyone, including ourselves. If we look inward at those times, we find that our harmful acts are powered by painful, destructive mental states: motives and emotions such as fear, anger, greed, and jealousy.

Now here's where it gets really interesting and we discover just how crucial our ethical choices are. If we act on these painful motives and emotions, we strengthen them and drive them deeper into our psyches. In psychological terms, we reinforce and condition them; in neurological terms, we create greased pathways; and in Eastern terms, we strengthen our karma. But whatever framework you want to use, we're strengthening destructive qualities.

On the other hand, when we look inward when we are acting ethically—when we are being helpful—we find pleasant, healthy motives and emotions such as love, joy, and generosity. And, most crucially, we strengthen these. So an ethical lifestyle turns out to be not only good for others but good for us as well. It's a win-win lifestyle.

I think we need to define ethics in terms of intentions. I define an intention as ethical to the extent to which it aims to enhance well-being and minimize harm for all beings, including oneself. It's not a moralistic definition. It's not looking at intentions or behavior in terms of conventional right or wrong. It's looking pragmatically in terms of what works to enhance well-being. Of course, the capacity to see clearly what enhances well-being is a function of wisdom, which is a nice example of the way spiritual practices and capacities support and foster one another. Let me give an example of ethical and unethical behavior from my own life. I've been audited by the Internal Revenue Service (IRS) several times and had some of my deductions dismissed because of sloppy bookkeeping. The first couple of times it happened I blamed the IRS and was very irate. Of course, all this did was make me an angrier person. It didn't change my finances, my bookkeeping, or the IRS one iota.

Finally, I had a blinding insight into the obvious. I got the idea that the people in the IRS were my teachers and were showing me where I wasn't being careful, conscientious, or ethical. So I decided to do my taxes as a part of ethical training. It was an interesting challenge because each time I wanted to fudge, if I looked inside, I found that I was attached to something, either money or something it could get me. So it became a training in nonattachment. It also became a training in awareness, because every time I started to feel tense or uptight or greedy, that was feedback about what was going on. So I learned a great deal in the process, and an additional award was that in the next couple of audits, all my claims were accepted.

This brings us to the sixth central and essential practice outlined in *Essential Spirituality*—the cultivation of wisdom. Wisdom is deep understanding of, and practical skill in dealing with, the central existential issues of life. These are issues that all of us face simply because we are human—issues such as pain and suffering, loneliness and loss, sickness, and ultimately death.

It's crucial to recognize that there is an enormous difference between knowledge and wisdom. Knowledge comes from acquiring facts, but wisdom comes from reflection on experience. Knowledge informs, but wisdom transforms. Knowledge is something you have; wisdom is something you must become. They're very, very different.

Our culture and universities worship knowledge. Yet you can know a hell of a lot and not be very wise, and for me it was painful to recognize that universities have very little to do with wisdom. These days, universities are more and more about the discovery of knowledge and less and less about the uncovering of wisdom.

The last practice—and in many ways the culmination of all the previous ones—is service. We practice not for ourselves alone but also to be of optimal service. We usually think of service as trying to feed the hungry or relieve pain or perhaps trying to do one's bit for peace, all of which are crucial.

But there's also another level of service that comes from appreciating that so much of human suffering and so many of our global problems reflect our individual and collective states of mind. An enormous amount of suffering is created out of ignorance, fear, greed, jealousy, and so forth. And to help heal these underlying causes of suffering in the world requires that you have, to some degree, healed and understood them in yourself. So the depth of your own inner work is a major factor determining how effective you can be in helping to relieve the inner causes of suffering of others and of the world.

This is obviously not a new idea. Jesus exclaimed, "Why do you complain about the speck in someone else's eye when you've got a beam in your own?" Five hundred years earlier, Buddha pointed out that "To help others you must first do a harder thing, help yourself." So there's a common message.

Global Problems as Global Symptoms

It's remarkable that, for the first time in history, each and every one of the global crises we're facing is human-caused. Whether you think of overpopulation, pollution, nuclear weapons, or terrorism—they are all human-caused. Our global problems are really global symptoms; they're symptoms of our individual and collective minds. The world is our own psyche writ large, and so far the major responses have been military, political, and economic.

Yes, it's absolutely crucial for us to work to feed the hungry, reduce the population explosion, and disarm nuclear stockpiles, but we also have to address the underlying causes. Things change once you begin to appreciate that all these problems stem from our individual and collective psyches and from the disruptive forces within us and between us. Then you begin to appreciate that military, political, and economic "solutions" are merely symptomatic treatments, like giving aspirin to someone with an infectious fever. Of course, giving aspirin to reduce the fever can be crucial, but you can't expect it to cure the underlying infection.

It's the same with our current social and global problems. It's crucial that we address not only the symptoms—the crises—but also the underlying causes as well. And what determines our effectiveness in treating the underlying psychological and spiritual causes is our own understanding of them and how effectively we have worked with them in ourselves. So spiritual practices may be crucial, not only to our individual well-being but to the well-being and even survival of our society, our civilization, and our planet.

Of course, ideally we will want to tackle our social and global problems in as many ways as we can—psychological, spiritual, organizational, political, educational, and more. As Aldous Huxley wrote in *Island*, "Where do we start? We start everywhere at once." And the optimal way of contributing, in any arena, may be to perform our contributions as karma yoga or awakening service.

When you do karma yoga, then each and every experience is a chance for learning. For example, things get very interesting once you begin to see that painful emotions are giving you feedback, telling you that you're in the grip of an attachment.

In fact, if you look very carefully at negative or difficult emotions, you see that they're intimately related to attachments. For example, fear comes from thinking that we're going to lose something we're attached to, or (its mirror image) get something we're averse to. Worry overwhelms us when we obsess over getting or losing something we're attached to. Jealousy overwhelms us when someone else has what we crave. Anger arises when someone comes in the way of our getting what we're attached to. We become depressed when we lose hope of getting what we crave.

Once you understand this, you realize there are two kinds of experiences: there's pleasant experience, and there's feedback that there's an attachment operating. Then the challenge is to let it go.

But, of course, that's easier said than done, as we all know. For example, it's hard not to get attached to the outcome of your work, particularly if you're working for an idealistic cause. But if you are trying to be helpful and things don't work out, and if you're attached to the outcome, you are going to get angry and upset. We probably all know a number of angry social activists.

If you're doing healing work, perhaps the most universal and tricky attachment of all is to having your clients get better. This is perfectly understandable, but it leads to several problems and lots of suffering. First, you have just made your happiness dependent on your clients' healing. Yet the reality is that some clients heal and others don't. Second, if there is any conflict or competition between you and your clients—and there often is at some stage of therapy—then all they have to do to win is not get better.

The third problem is that, paradoxically, the attachment to having clients heal can actually reduce their healing. You can only be of as much help to someone as you don't need anything from them. Of course, it's easier for all of us to talk about these attachments than it is to reduce them, but recognizing and talking about them is a first step.

Human Possibilities

There's long been a tradition suggesting that there is much more to our human condition than meets the eye. There are potentials of body, mind, and spirit available to us that far exceed conventional limits, and there's a growing body of research to support this. In the psychological domain, it's possible to cultivate qualities such as love and compassion, concentration and calm, awareness and wisdom, to remarkable degrees, and there are techniques to do this. But they take practice, and while some of them can be quite simple, they aren't necessarily fast.

Most contemplative practices are slow and cumulative. They have to be done over a period of time and on a regular basis. Yet doing these practices is enormously valuable and can enhance our own well-being and the well-being of everyone whose lives we touch.

Index

Page numbers followed by the letter *b* indicate boxes.

Page numbers followed by the letter *b* indicate boxes.

Page numbers followed by the letter *b* indicate
boxes.

Page numbers followed by the letter *b* indicate boxes.